Evidence Based Treatments for
Trauma-Related Psychological Disorders

Ulrich Schnyder • Marylène Cloitre
Editors

Evidence Based Treatments for Trauma-Related Psychological Disorders

A Practical Guide for Clinicians

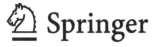
Springer

Editors
Ulrich Schnyder
Department of Psychiatry
and Psychotherapy
University Hospital Zurich
Zurich
Switzerland

Marylène Cloitre
Dissemination and Training Division
National Center for PTSD
San Franciso, California
USA

ISBN 978-3-319-07108-4   ISBN 978-3-319-07109-1   (eBook)
DOI 10.1007/978-3-319-07109-1
Springer Cham Heidelberg New York Dordrecht London

Library of Congress Control Number: 2015931248

Printed on acid-free paper

Springer is part of Springer Science+Business Media (www.springer.com)

Contents

Introduction

1

Ulrich Schnyder and Marylène Cloitre

1.1 Why This Book?

Over the last three decades, the field of traumatic stress-related research and clinical practice has developed tremendously. In the aftermath of the war in Vietnam, similar to other periods in recent history such as following World War I and World War II, mental health professionals, policy makers, and the general public became aware of the bio-psycho-social impact that overwhelming traumatic experiences can have on both soldiers and the civilian population (Weisæth 2014). However, unlike earlier periods, this time the interest among professionals and the public did not abate and has led to profound changes in government policies, mental health services, and social perceptions. Never before has the trauma field encountered such a long period of ever-increasing interest among scientists as well as clinicians. The introduction of the new diagnostic category of posttraumatic stress disorder (PTSD) in the DSM-III in 1980 (APA 1980) sparked an unprecedented and, at least to some degree, unexpected development. Few areas in mental health have enjoyed such a dynamic and steady growth over the last 35 years. The number of trauma-related publications in basic and clinical research, and thus the body of knowledge in the trauma field, has increased exponentially and continues to grow.

In parallel with the steady accumulation of basic knowledge, therapeutic approaches have been developed to treat people suffering from PTSD and other trauma-related

U. Schnyder (✉)
Department of Psychiatry and Psychotherapy, University Hospital Zurich,
Zurich, Switzerland
e-mail: ulrich.schnyder@access.uzh.ch

M. Cloitre
Dissemination & Training Division, National Center for PTSD,
San Francisco, CA, USA
e-mail: marylene.cloitre@nyumc.org

© Springer International Publishing Switzerland 2015
U. Schnyder, M. Cloitre (eds.), *Evidence Based Treatments for Trauma-Related Psychological Disorders: A Practical Guide for Clinicians*,
DOI 10.1007/978-3-319-07109-1_1

psychological problems. Today, a number of evidence-based psychological and pharmacological treatments are available (Bisson et al. 2013; Bradley et al. 2005; Watts et al. 2013). Overall, effect sizes appear to be larger for psychotherapy as compared to medication. Many well-controlled trials studying outcomes for a variety of trauma survivors have demonstrated that trauma-focused psychotherapies are effective in treating PTSD. Still, dropout rates are relatively high, and the majority of patients who complete psychotherapy and/or pharmacotherapy still retain their PTSD diagnosis and do not achieve good end-state functioning at posttreatment assessment. Therefore, new developments are needed (Schnyder 2005). One way forward is to further refine well-established, empirically supported psychotherapies. By means of dismantling studies, mechanisms of change can be established, the most effective treatment components can be identified, and less effective elements can be eliminated. In addition, new and alternative therapies (psychopharmacological interventions, alternative or complementary therapies) must be considered and systematically tested as should strategies to increase access to mental health resources globally (e.g., the use of technology and telemental health approaches, Chap. 25).

So, why this book? There are so many excellent and up-to-date books already on the market on various aspects of traumatic stress. However, most of these books are either written by scientists for scientists or written by clinical practitioners for clinical practitioners. The motivation for publishing yet another book lay in our desire to edit a book written by clinically experienced researchers and scientifically trained clinicians, a book firmly rooted in sound science but written in a language that appeals to clinicians. The contributors to this book are writing for therapists in clinical settings who may be academically trained but are primarily interested in how they can best treat their traumatized patients.

This book offers an evidence-based guide for clinical psychologists, psychiatrists, psychotherapists, and other clinicians working with trauma survivors in various settings. It provides easily digestible, up-to-date information on the basic principles of traumatic stress research and practice, including psychological and sociological theories as well as epidemiological, psychopathological, and neurobiological findings. However, given the therapists' aforementioned primary interest, the core focus of the book is on evidence-based psychological treatments for trauma-related mental disorders. Importantly, the full range of trauma and stress-related disorders is covered, including acute stress reaction, complex PTSD, and prolonged grief disorder, reflecting important anticipated developments in the ICD-11 diagnostic classification. Additional chapters are devoted to the treatment of comorbidities, special populations and special treatment modalities, and pharmacological treatments for trauma-related disorders. The book concludes by addressing the fundamental question of how to treat whom and when.

1.2   The Content of the Book

Part I of the book lays the foundation for understanding the effects of trauma and implications for treatment by providing a short and concise overview of the basic principles of what we know today about traumatic stress. Starting with the epidemiology of potentially traumatic events and trauma-related disorders, it becomes clear from the very beginning of this book that trauma is a major public health issue. The most important psychological and sociological theories of PTSD are described, such as fear conditioning, dual representation theory, cognitive theory and "hotspots," psychodynamic theories, and PTSD from a social and societal perspective. This is followed by an update on neurobiological findings in PTSD and a chapter on the relationship between traumatic exposure, PTSD, and physical health.

Part II describes the current diagnostic spectrum of trauma-related disorders. It covers PTSD, acute stress disorder and acute stress reactions, complex PTSD, and prolonged grief disorder. Similarities and differences between the two major diagnostic classification systems, the DSM and the ICD, are discussed. While the DSM-5 was published in May 2013, the release of the ICD-11 is not expected until 2017. It currently looks like there will be greater differences between DSM-5 and ICD-11 than there were between DSM-IV and ICD-10. This will create interesting challenges but also opportunities for the trauma field to further grow, diversify, and differentiate.

Part III is the core part of the book, and, accordingly, the largest one. In nine chapters, empirically supported psychological interventions in the trauma field are presented. Part III starts with early interventions in both unselected populations of recent trauma survivors and preselected groups of trauma survivors who have been screened and identified as being at high risk of developing chronic trauma-related disorders. Empirically supported psychotherapies for PTSD are next: prolonged exposure (PE) therapy, cognitive therapy, cognitive processing therapy (CPT), eye movement desensitization and reprocessing (EMDR) therapy, narrative exposure therapy (NET), and brief eclectic psychotherapy (BEPP) each are thoroughly described in separate chapters. Skills training in affective and interpersonal regulation (STAIR) narrative therapy for more complex conditions such as complex PTSD is addressed in a separate chapter, as is complicated grief treatment (CGT) for prolonged grief disorder.

To provide some consistency across treatment approaches, we asked the authors of this part of the book to organize their chapters in a similar way, beginning with a short summary of the theoretical underpinnings of their approach, using language that can be understood and digested by clinicians who do not necessarily read the research literature. The main part of the chapter then demonstrates how the treatment is applied in clinical practice. Invariably, the treatment protocol is illustrated by one or several case presentations. Having read this part of any given chapter, we hope that readers will get a clear picture of how the treatment works in real-world clinical practice. This is followed by a section on the challenges that are typically met by clinicians when applying this treatment with a wide range of trauma survivors and how to deal with them. Each chapter ends with a summary of empirically established treatment outcomes and other research findings related to this treatment approach.

Part IV concerns the treatment of those comorbidities that can be found most frequently in people with trauma-related disorders: substance use disorders, borderline personality disorder, and chronic pain conditions such as somatoform pain disorder.

Part V addresses clinical challenges related to the treatment of special populations: children and adolescents, elderly people, refugees, and war veterans. When planning this part of the book, we recognized that the field of child and adolescent psychotraumatology has developed and expanded dramatically over the past years. In some aspects, the field is now more advanced than the "mainstream" of trauma work with adults. Therefore, we decided to ask the contributing authors to write a chapter that differs a bit from the other chapters and to provide a general overview of evidence-based treatments for traumatized children and adolescents, rather than an in-depth description of one particular approach. We also decided to edit another volume on empirically supported treatments for traumatized children and adolescents, once this book is published.

Part VI is on special treatment modalities such as group treatment and couple treatment for PTSD and on the dynamically emerging field of telemental health and technology-based approaches to assess and treat trauma survivors.

Part VII covers pharmacological treatments for PTSD.

The concluding Part VIII of the book is devoted to discussing what treatments work best for which patients. It describes research and clinical advances in other fields regarding patient-treatment matching that are applicable to trauma work. This includes collaborative decision-making between patient and therapist to determine focus of treatment, strategies for building streamlined multicomponent interventions, and the use of "measurement-based care" to guide decisions about duration of interventions and of treatment.

In line with its title, the main focus of this book is on evidence-based treatments. Chambless and Hollon (1998) postulated that the following criteria would have to be met for a therapeutic approach to be "evidence-based" or "empirically supported." First, the efficacy of the approach must have been demonstrated by a series of randomized controlled trials (RCTs), using appropriate samples and control groups. In these trials, the samples must have been adequately described and valid and reliable outcome assessments must have been used. Finally, the results must have been replicated by at least one independent group of researchers. Foa and colleagues make the point that the use of more rigorous scientific methods in psychotherapy outcome research in the trauma field has increased substantially in the course of the past 25 years (Foa et al. 2009). However, evidence-based medicine is by definition oriented towards the past, as it only informs us about the well-established, empirically supported treatments that have already proven their efficacy. If we rely only on the currently available scientific evidence, new developments will be substantially impeded. Since many patients decline treatment or do not seek professional help at all, there is a need for improvements regarding acceptance of established therapies. Also, there ought to be scope for new, creative approaches, for which scientific evidence is not yet available.

It appears that the state of the science varies greatly across fields covered in this book. On the one hand, there is quite an array of empirically supported treatments for PTSD from which both clinicians and patients can choose. On the other hand, when it comes to, for example, treating trauma-related disorders and comorbid chronic pain in tortured refugees, the level of scientific evidence is still very poor.

As mentioned before, there is room for improvement and a need for further development. Promising developments may include, e.g., mindfulness-based approaches, "mini-interventions" for specific problems trans-diagnostically, or web-based therapies and other telemental health and technology-based approaches.

1.3 Commonalities Across Psychological Treatments

When reading through the various chapters, and particularly those of Part III, what emerges very clearly is that the empirically supported psychotherapies for trauma survivors have a lot in common. We think that while there are some important differences across approaches, the commonalities outweigh the differences by far. Interventions and characteristics of treatments that are frequently shared are as follows:

- *Psychoeducation* offers information on the nature and course of posttraumatic stress reactions, affirms that they are understandable and expectable, identifies and helps with ways to cope with trauma reminders, and discusses ways to manage distress (Schnyder et al. 2012). In short, as defined by Wessely and colleagues, psychoeducation provides "information about the nature of stress, posttraumatic and other symptoms, and what to do about them" (Wessely et al. 2008). Psychoeducation is provided in the immediate aftermath of individual or large-scale, collective trauma, such as in the context of psychological first aid (PFA), with the aim of preventing acute and chronic trauma-related psychiatric disorders, as well as fostering resilience. Psychoeducation also is an important component of trauma-focused psychotherapies for PTSD; here, psychoeducation aims at facilitating therapeutic interventions, optimizing patient cooperation, and preventing relapse. Although most mental health professionals consider trauma education or psychoeducation to be an important tool, there is no generally accepted definition of its aims and core components. Accordingly, there are no standardized procedures for its delivery, and not surprisingly, barely any research has been published regarding its effectiveness (Schnyder et al. 2012).
- *Emotion regulation and coping skills* are frequently taught and trained across many therapeutic approaches. In some instances, this is done more implicitly, in others very explicitly to the degree that, e.g., in Cloitre's skills training in affective and interpersonal regulation (STAIR) narrative therapy, the training in emotion regulation skills takes center stage in the first part of the treatment protocol. In most therapies, emotion regulation skills are introduced in the beginning or first stages of treatment. Viewed from a different angle, teaching emotion regulation skills may also be seen as a treatment element that aims at promoting trauma survivors' resilience.
- *Imaginal exposure* is emphasized most strongly in prolonged exposure (PE) therapy: Imaginal exposure to trauma memories is combined with in vivo exposure to reminders of the trauma. However, some form of exposure to the patients' memory of their traumatic experiences can be found in virtually all evidence-based

psychological treatments for trauma-related disorders. In EMDR therapy, patients focus their attention on the trauma while remaining silent and performing saccadic, horizontal eye movements; in cognitive processing therapy (CPT), they produce a written account at home and read from it to the therapist during therapy sessions; in brief eclectic psychotherapy for PTSD (BEPP), imaginal exposure is done to promote catharsis; etc.

- *Cognitive processing and restructuring* is another element that can be found in almost all of the empirically supported psychological treatments for PTSD (and other trauma-related disorders). While in cognitive therapy for PTSD as well as in CPT, Socratic dialogue and cognitive restructuring are the most important treatment ingredients, in other approaches such as PE or EMDR, cognitive restructuring is seen as part of the integration that takes place after exposure or following a set of eye movements.

- *Emotions* are targeted more or less in all psychotherapies. Some (NET, PE) predominantly tackle the patients' trauma or fear network, others focus more on guilt and shame (CPT), anger (STAIR), or grief and sadness (BEPP). Moral injury can occur in particularly complex traumatic experiences and involves a mixture of partially conflicting emotions that arise from being exposed to ethical dilemmas. Although not (yet) explicitly described in most treatment manuals, moral injury is increasingly recognized as a relevant issue that needs to be addressed in psychotherapy with traumatized veterans, tortured refugees, and other populations that survived complex traumatic exposure.

- *Memory processes* also play an important role in treating trauma-related disorders. PTSD can be understood as a memory disorder. According to Brewin's dual representation theory, sensation-near representations are distinguished from contextualized representations, previously referred to as the situationally accessible memory (SAM) and the verbally accessible memory (VAM) systems (Brewin et al. 2010) (Chap. 3). NET therapists work on transforming hot memories into cold memories. No matter which technical terms are used, the restoration of memory functions and the creation of a *coherent trauma narrative* appear to be central goals of all trauma-focused treatments.

1.4   The Cultural Dimension

Wen-Shing Tseng, the founding president of the World Association of Cultural Psychiatry, defined culture as a dynamic concept referring to a set of beliefs, attitudes, and value systems, which derive from early stages of life through enculturation, and become an internal mode of regulating behavior, action, and emotion (Tseng and Streltzer 2001). Thus, culture is not static, but changing continuously across generations, responding to ever-changing environmental demands. Furthermore, culture in Tseng's sense is specific for each individual and therefore much more important than ethnicity or race. Experienced therapists usually tailor psychotherapy to each patient's particular situation, to the nature of psychopathology, to the stage of therapy, and so on. Treatment could be even more effective, however, if the cultural dimension were to be incorporated. Culturally relevant, culture-sensitive, or culture-competent psychotherapy involves trying to understand how culture enhances the meaning of the patient's life history, the cultural components of a patient's illness and help-seeking behaviors, as well as the patient's expectations with regard to treatment.

Trauma is a global issue (Schnyder 2013). Our traumatized patients come from all over the world. We can no longer take for granted that they all speak our language or share our cultural values. Therefore, we need to increase our cultural competencies. Being sensitive to cultural issues has become a sine qua non for being a good therapist. Only few of us will conduct psychotherapies with the help of professional interpreters on a regular basis (Chap. 21). On the one hand, taking into account the cultural dimension adds yet one more challenge to our already demanding profession. On the other hand, it also enriches our work, providing us with opportunities to learn how diverse human beings are and how different a phenomenon such as a flashback or a certain aspect of a traumatic experience can be understood and interpreted depending on the patient's and their therapist's cultural backgrounds.

Acknowledgments Editing this book has been a greatly rewarding pleasure throughout the process. We feel privileged to have been able to work with a truly outstanding panel of contributing authors, many of whom are world leaders and scholars in the trauma field. Not only did the authors submit their manuscripts in a timely fashion, they were extremely responsive to our editorial feedback and suggestions. We also learned a lot from them. Working with such a group of colleagues is simply wonderful: Thank you to all our authors!

Thank you to Corinna Schaefer and Wilma McHugh of Springer International Publishing. From the very first, tentative ideas of a book outline, and during the whole publishing process, Corinna and Wilma provided us with the professional support that is necessary for a successful outcome. Thank you for your patience and continuous encouragement!

Lastly, this book contains many, many clinical case examples. Thank you to all the patients who, through the chapter authors, shared their stories with us so that we can learn from them to become better therapists.

References

APA. (1980). *Diagnostic and statistical manual of mental disorders* (3rd ed.). Washington, DC: American Psychiatric Association.

Bisson, J. I., Roberts, N. P., Andrew, M., Cooper, R., & Lewis, C. (2013). Psychological therapies for chronic post-traumatic stress disorder (PTSD) in adults. *Cochrane Database Systematic Review*. doi:10.1002/14651858.CD003388.pub4.

Bradley, R., Greene, J., Russ, E., Dutra, L., & Westen, D. (2005). A multidimensional meta-analysis of psychotherapy for PTSD. *American Journal of Psychiatry, 162*(2), 214–227.

Brewin, C. R., Gregory, J. D., Lipton, M., & Burgess, N. (2010). Intrusive images in psychological disorders: Characteristics, neural mechanisms, and treatment implications. *Psychological Review, 117*, 210–232.

Chambless, D. L., & Hollon, S. D. (1998). Defining empirically supported therapies. *Journal of Consulting and Clinical Psychology, 66*(1), 7–18.

Foa, E. B., Keane, T. M., Friedman, M. J., & Cohen, J. A. (2009). *Effective treatments for PTSD. Practice guidelines from the International Society for Traumatic Stress Studies* (2nd ed.). New York: Guilford.

Schnyder, U. (2005). Why new psychotherapies for posttraumatic stress disorder? Editorial. *Psychotherapy and Psychosomatics, 74,* 199–201.

Schnyder, U. (2013). Trauma is a global issue. *European Journal of Psychotraumatology, 4,* 20419. doi:http://dx.doi.org/10.3402/ejpt.v4i0.20419.

Schnyder, U., Pedretti, S., & Müller, J. (2012). Trauma education. In C. R. Figley (Ed.), *Encyclopedia of trauma: An interdisciplinary guide* (pp. 709–714). Thousand Oaks: SAGE.

Tseng, W.-S., & Streltzer, J. (Eds.). (2001). *Culture and psychotherapy. A guide to clinical practice.* Washington, DC: American Psychiatric Press.

Watts, B. V., Schnurr, P. P., Mayo, L., Young-Xu, Y., Weeks, W. B., & Friedman, M. J. (2013). Meta-analysis of the efficacy of treatments for posttraumatic stress disorder. *Journal of Clinical Psychiatry, 74*(6), e541–e550. doi:10.4088/JCP.12r08225.

Weisæth, L. (2014). The history of psychic trauma. In M. J. Friedman, T. M. Keane, & P. A. Resick (Eds.), *Handbook of PTSD – Science and practice* (2nd ed., pp. 38–59). New York: Guilford.

Wessely, S., Bryant, R. A., Greenberg, N., Earnshaw, M., Sharpley, J., & Hughes, J. H. (2008). Does psychoeducation help prevent post traumatic psychological distress? *Psychiatry, 71*(4), 287–302.

Part I

Traumatic Stress: The Basic Principles

Trauma as a Public Health Issue: Epidemiology of Trauma and Trauma-Related Disorders

2

Sarah R. Lowe, Jaclyn Blachman-Forshay, and Karestan C. Koenen

Reports in the mainstream media suggest that traumatic events, such as natural disasters, sexual assault, and child abuse, are frequent occurrences throughout the world and take a tremendous psychological toll on individuals and communities. In this chapter, we aim to present the global public health burden posed by trauma exposure. To accomplish this goal, we review the prevalence and distribution of traumatic events and trauma-related disorders from epidemiologic studies. Epidemiology is the cornerstone of public health and focuses on the distribution and causes of disease in human populations and on developing and testing ways to prevent and control disease. Epidemiological studies have provided empirical evidence on the high prevalence of trauma and the devastating effects of trauma-related disorders and have shown that trauma is not equally distributed across populations. When presenting the results, we note methodological considerations that make cross-study comparisons difficult. Finally, we use the epidemiologic data presented to discuss public health approaches to addressing trauma and trauma-related disorders. We conclude that trauma exposure is a major public health problem whose health burden has only begun to be appreciated.

2.1 Epidemiology of Trauma Exposure

Table 2.1 summarizes the results of epidemiological studies documenting the prevalence of various traumatic events. To be included in this review, studies had to meet at least one of the following criteria: (1) a nationally representative sample of any

S.R. Lowe (✉) • J. Blachman-Forshay • K.C. Koenen
Department of Epidemiology, Mailman School of Public Health, Columbia University, New York, NY, USA
e-mail: srlowe@gmail.com

© Springer International Publishing Switzerland 2015
U. Schnyder, M. Cloitre (eds.), *Evidence Based Treatments for Trauma-Related Psychological Disorders: A Practical Guide for Clinicians*,
DOI 10.1007/978-3-319-07109-1_2

Table 2.1 Epidemiological studies on the prevalence of potentially traumatic events (PTEs) and posttraumatic stress disorder (PTSD)

Study	Country	Design	N	PTE prevalence	PTSD assessment (instrument; criteria; index event)	PTSD prevalence
de Jong et al. (2001)**	Algeria	Randomly selected residents from Gouvernorat d'Algiers	653	War related (1*): 91.9 %	CIDI; DSM-IV; all PTEs	Lifetime: 37.4 %
Chapman et al. (2010); Mills et al. (2011)	Australia	Australian National Survey of Mental Health and Wellbeing (2007). Nationally representative sample (18–65)	8,841	Any PTE (29), 74.9 %; childhood (1*), 10.1 %; sexual (1*), 9.6 %	CIDI, modified; DSM-IV; worst	Lifetime, 7.2 %; past year, 4.4 %
				War related (1*), 4.1 %; disaster (1*), 8.4 %; bereavement (1), 34.4 %		
Ikin et al. (2004)**	Australia	Entire cohort of Gulf War veterans	1,381	–	CIDI; DSM-IV; unspecified	Lifetime, 1.3 % (prewar onset), 5.3 % (postwar onset); past year, 5.1 %
Rosenman (2002)	Australia	National Survey of Mental Health and Wellbeing (1997). Nationally representative sample (18+)	10,641	Any PTE (10), 57.4 %; sexual (1*), 10.6 %; war related (1), 3.2 %; disaster (1), 16.8 %	CIDI, modified; DSM-IV, ICD-10; worst	Past year: 1.5 % (DSM-IV), 3.6 % (ICD-10)
O'Toole et al. (1996)**	Australia	Australian Vietnam Veterans Health Study. National random sample of veterans who served from 1962 to 1972	641	–	DIS, AUSCID, Mississippi Scale; DSM-III; various	Lifetime, 17.1 % (DIS, all events), 11.7 % (DIS, combat related, 20.9 % (AUSCID); current, 11.6 % (AUSCID), 8.1 % (Mississippi)

Darves-Bornoz et al. (2008)	Belgium	ESEMeD. Nationally representative sample (18+)	1,043	–	CIDI; DSM-IV; worst	Past year: 0.8 %
Karam et al. (2013)	Brazil	São Paulo Megacity Study. Representative sample of the São Paulo metropolitan area (18+)	2,942	–	CIDI; DSM-IV; worst and random	Past year: 1.0 %
Karam et al. (2013)	Bulgaria	Bulgaria National Survey of Health and Stress. Nationally representative sample (18+)	2,233	–	CIDI; DSM-IV; worst and random	Past year: 0.9 %
de Jong et al. (2001)**	Cambodia	Randomly selected residents from three areas: (1) Odamgang I Commune in Sangke District in the Battambang province; (2) Veal Pong Commune in the Udong District in the Kampong Speu province; (3) Sang Kat Psar Doeum Kor in the capital, Phnom Penh	610	War related (1*): 74.4 %	CIDI; DSM-IV; all PTEs	Lifetime: 28.4 %
Nelson et al. (2011); Fikretoglu and Liu (2012)**	Canada	Canadian Community Health Survey – Canadian Forces Supplement. Representative sample of active Canadian Forces members (16–64)	8,441	–	CIDI; DSM-IV: worst	Lifetime, 6.5 %; past year, 2.3 %
Van Ameringen et al. (2008)	Canada	Nationally representative sample (18+)	2,991	Any PTE (18), 75.9 %; childhood (1), 9.3 %; sexual (1*), 21.9 %; war related (1*), 4.3 %; disaster (1), 15.6 %; bereavement (1), 41.1 %	Canadian Community Health Survey (based on CIDI); DSM-IV; worst	Lifetime, 9.2 %; current, 2.4 %

(continued)

Table 2.1 (continued)

Study	Country	Design	N	PTE prevalence	PTSD assessment (instrument; criteria; index event)	PTSD prevalence
Benitez et al. (2009)	Chile	Chilean Study of Psychiatric Prevalence. Representative household sample in Santiago, Concepción, Cautín, and Iquique (15+)	2,978	Any PTE (11), 46.7 % (males), 33.2 % (females); sexual (1), 3.8 % (females), 1.0 % (males); war related (1), 0.1 % (females), 0.7 % (males); disaster (1), 5.6 % (females), 8.0 % (males); bereavement (1), 3.4 % (females), 1.8 % (males)	CIDI; DSM-III-R; unspecified	Lifetime: 4.4 %
Karam et al. (2013)	Colombia	Colombian National Study of Mental Health. Representative sample of urban areas (18–65)	2,381	–	CIDI; DSM-IV; worst and random	Past year: 0.3 %
Elkit (2002)	Denmark	Nationally representative sample of 8th graders (13–15)	390	Any PTE (20), 88.0 %; childhood (1*), 7.4 %; sexual (1*), 1.8 %; bereavement (1), 51.8 %	HTQ; DSM-III-R; worst	Lifetime: 9.0 %
Soosay et al. (2012)	East Timor	Whole population survey of two villages, one urban and one rural, broadly representative of the national population (18+)	1,245	Any PTE (16), 100 %; war related (1), 34.3 %; disaster (1*), 76.3 %; bereavement (1*), 18.3 %	HTQ; DSM-IV; unspecified	Current: 5.0 %

Study	Country	Sample	N	PTE	Instrument	Prevalence
de Jong et al. (2001)**	Ethiopia	Randomly selected Eritrean refugees from temporary shelters in Addis Ababa	1,200	War related (1*), 78.0%	CIDI; DSM-IV; all PTEs	Lifetime: 15.8%
Darves-Bornoz et al. (2008)	France	ESEMeD. Nationally representative sample (18+)	1,436	–	CIDI; DSM-IV; worst	Past year: 2.3%
de Jong et al. (2001)**	Gaza	Randomly selected residents of 3 refugee camps, 3 cities, and 2 resettlement areas	653	War related (1*): 59.3%	CIDI; DSM-IV; all PTEs	Lifetime: 17.8%
Hauffa et al. (2011)	Germany	Nationally representative household sample (14+)	2,510	Any PTE (12), 23.8%; childhood (1). 1.5%; sexual (1), 1.2%; war related (1*), 5.5%; disaster (1), 0.6%	PSS; DSM-IV; unspecified	Lifetime: 2.9%
Darves-Bornoz et al. (2008)	Germany	ESEMeD. Nationally representative sample (18+)	1,323	–	CIDI; DSM-IV; worst	Past year: 0.7%
Maercker et al. (2008)	Germany	Nationally representative sample (14–93)	2,426	Any PTE (12), 28.0% (females), 20.9% (males); childhood (1), 1.2%; sexual (1), 0.8%; war related (1*), 8.2%; disaster (1), 0.8%	PSS, modified; DSM-IV; unspecified	Past month: 2.3%
Bödvarsdottír and Elklit (2007)	Iceland	Nationally representative sample of 9th graders (13–15)	206	Any PTE (20), 77%; sexual (1*), 3.9%; childhood (1*), 5.8%; bereavement (1), 42.7%	HTQ; DSM-IV; worst	PTSD-like state at time of the event: 6.0%

(continued)

Table 2.1 (continued)

Study	Country	Design	N	PTE prevalence	PTSD assessment (instrument; criteria; index event)	PTSD prevalence
Alhasnawi et al. (2009)	Iraq	Iraq Mental Health Survey. Nationally representative household sample (18+)	4,332	–	CIDI; DSM-IV; unspecified	Lifetime, 2.5 %; past year, 1.1 %
Karam et al. (2013)	Israel	Israel National Health Survey. Nationally representative sample (21+)	4,849	–	CIDI; DSM-IV; worst	Past year: 0.4 %
Darves-Bornoz et al. (2008)	Italy	ESEMeD. Nationally representative sample (18+)	1,779	–	CIDI; DSM-IV; worst	Past year: 0.7 %
Kawakami et al. (2014)	Japan	WMH Japan Survey. Random sample from 1 metropolitan city, 2 urban cities, 8 rural municipalities (20+)	1,682	Any PTE (29), 60.7 %; childhood (1), 6.9 %; sexual (3), 4.3 %; war related (7), 8.7 %; bereavement (1), 23.7 %	CIDI; DSM-IV; worst and random	Lifetime, 1.3 %; past year, 0.7 %; past month, 0.2 %
Karam et al. (2013); Karam et al. (2008)	Lebanon	Lebanese Evaluation of the Burden of Ailments and Needs of the Nation study. Nationally representative (18+)	2,857	War related (10): 68.8 %	CIDI; DSM-IV; unspecified	Lifetime, 3.4 %; past year, 1.6 %
Johnson et al. (2008)	Liberia	Nationally representative household sample (18+)	1,666	Sexual (1), 42.3 % (female former combatants), 9.2 % (female noncombatants), 32.6 % (male former combatants), 7.4 % (male former combatants); war related (1), 33.0 %	PSS, modified; DSM-IV; unspecified	Past month: 44 %

Study	Country	Sample	N	PTE	Instrument	Prevalence
Domanskaité-Gota et al. (2009)	Lithuania	National representative sample of 9th graders (13–17)	183	Any PTE (2): 80.2 %. Childhood (1*), 4.4 %; sexual (1*), 4.4 %; bereavement (1), 24.2 %	HTQ: DSM-IV; worst	Lifetime: 6.1 %
Medina-Mora et al. (2003); Medina-Mora et al. (2005); Karam et al. (2013)	Mexico	National Study of Psychiatric Epidemiology. Nationally representative sample (18–65)	5,286	Any PTE (28), 68 %; childhood (1), 18.3 %; sexual (1*), 5.4 %; war related (1), 1.0 %; disaster (1), 13.7 %; bereavement (1), 26.9 %	CIDI; DSM-IV, ICD-10; worst	Lifetime, 1.5 % (DSM-IV), 2.6 % (ICD-10); past year, 0.3 % (DSM-IV), 0.6 % (ICD-10); past month, 0.2 % (ICD-10)
Kadri et al. (2007)	Morocco	Representative household sample of Casablanca City residents (15+)	800	Any PTE (unspecified): 12.1 %	MINI; DSM-IV; unspecified	Current: 3.4 %
Bronner et al. (2009)	Netherlands	National representative sample (18+)	2,238	Any PTE (12), 52.2 %; sexual (1*), 7.6 %; war related (1), 1.9 %; disaster (1), 11.1 %; bereavement (1), 9.3 %	–	–
de Vries and Olff (2009)	Netherlands	Nationally representative sample (18–80)	1,087	Any PTE (36): 80.7 %. Childhood (1), 3.9 %; sexual (1*), 3.7 %; war related (1*), 16.3 %; disaster (1*), 7.5 %; bereavement (5), 51.4 %	CIDI; DSM-IV; worst	Lifetime: 7.4 %
Darves-Bornoz et al. (2008)	Netherlands	ESEMeD. Nationally representative sample (18+)	1,094	–	CIDI; DSM-IV; worst	Past year: 2.6 %

(continued)

Table 2.1 (continued)

Study	Country	Design	N	PTE prevalence	PTSD assessment (instrument; criteria; index event)	PTSD prevalence
Karam et al. (2013)	New Zealand	New Zealand Mental Health Survey. Nationally representative sample (18+)	7,312	–	CIDI; DSM-IV; worst and random	Past year: 2.1 %
Bunting et al. (2013)	Northern Ireland	Northern Ireland Study of Health and Stress. Nationally representative household sample (18+)	1,986	Any PTE (28): 60.6 %. War related (12): 39.0 %	CIDI; DSM-IV; worst	Lifetime: 8.8 %; past year: 5.1 %
Karam et al. (2013)	People's Republic of China	Beijing and Shanghai WMH Surveys. Representative sample of Beijing and Shanghai metropolitan areas (18–70)	1,628	–	CIDI; DSM-IV; worst and random	Past year: 0.2 %
de Albuquerque et al. (2003)	Portugal	Nationally representative sample of adults (18+)	2,606	Any PTE (10), "around 75 %"; sexual (1*), 0.9 %; war related (1), 7.4 %; disaster (1), 16.7 %; bereavement (1), 29.3 %	Short screening scale; DSM-IV; worst	Current: 7.9 %
Florescu et al. (2009)	Romania	Mental Health Study in Romania. Nationally representative household sample (18+)	2,357	–	CIDI; DSM-IV; unspecified	Past year: 0.7 %
Atwoli et al. (2013)	South Africa	South African Stress and Health Study. Nationally representative sample of household and hotel residents (18+)	4,315	Any PTE (27), 73.8 %; childhood (1), 12.9 %; sexual (3), 7.6 %; war related (6), 12.2 %; disaster (1*), 4.1 %; bereavement (1), 39.2 %	CIDI; DSM-IV; random	Lifetime, 2.3 %; past year, 0.7 %

Study	Country	Sample	N	PTE prevalence	Measure	PTSD prevalence
Jeon et al. (2007)	South Korea	Korean Epidemiologic Catchment Area study. Nationally representative household sample (18–64)	6,258	Any PTE (1): 33.3 %. Sexual (1): 2.3 %. War related (1): 1.6 %. Disaster (1): 5.4 %	CIDI, Korean version; DSM-IV; worst	Lifetime: 1.7 %
Karam et al. (2013)	Spain	ESEMeD. Nationally representative sample (18+)	2,121	–	CIDI; DSM-IV; worst	Past year: 0.6 %
Landolt et al. (2013)	Switzerland	Nationally representative sample of 9th grade public school students (ages 12–20+, mean: 15.5)	6,787	Any PTE (13), 56.4 %; childhood (1), 6.9 %; sexual (1), 3.1 %; war related (1), 5.6 %; disaster (1*), 14.4 %; bereavement (1). 22.4 %	Adolescent version of the UCLA PTSD Reaction Index; DSM-IV; unspecified	Lifetime (for participants who experienced PTEs): 7.4 %
Karam et al. (2013)	Ukraine	Comorbid Mental Disorders during Periods of Social Disruption. Nationally representative sample (18+)	1,719	–	CIDI; DSM-IV; worst and random	Past year: 2.0 %
Weich et al. (2011); Bentall et al. (2012)	United Kingdom	2007 Adult Psychiatric Morbidity Survey. Nationally representative household sample (16+)	7,353	Childhood (1), 2.9 %; sexual (1*), 8.7 %	Trauma Screening Questionnaire; DSM-IV; unspecified	Past week (for n=7,325): 2.9 %
Fear et al. (2010)**	United Kingdom	Three random military samples: (1) members deployed to Iraq from 1/2003 to 4/2003; (2) members deployed to Afghanistan from 4/2006 to 4/2007; and (3) replenishment sample of enlistees since 4/2003	9,990	–	PCL; DSM-IV; unspecified	Current: 4.2 % (regulars, deployed), 4.0 % (regulars, not deployed), 5.0 % (reservists, deployed), 1.8 % (reservists, not deployed)

(continued)

Table 2.1 (continued)

Study	Country	Design	N	PTE prevalence	PTSD assessment (instrument; criteria; index event)	PTSD prevalence
McLaughlin et al. (2013)	United States	National Comorbidity Survey-Replication, Adolescent Supplement. Nationally representative household and school sample (13–17)	10,123	Any PTE (19), 61.8 %; childhood (1), 2.0 %; sexual (1*), 3.8 %; disaster (1), 14.8 %; bereavement (1), 28.2 %	CIDI; DSM-IV; worst	Lifetime: 4.7 %
Pietrzak et al. (2011); Breslau et al. (2013)	United States	National Epidemiological Survey of Alcohol and Related Conditions. Nationally representative sample of noninstitutionalized adults (18+) living in households or group quarters; oversampling of Blacks, Hispanics, and persons 18–24 years old	34,653	Sexual (1), 8.7 %; disaster (1), 15.7 %; bereavement (1), 41.6 %	Module from the Alcohol Use Disorders and Associated Disabilities Interview Schedule; DSM-IV; worst	Lifetime: 6.4 %
McCauley et al. (2010); Cisler et al. (2011)	United States	National Survey of Adolescents-Replication. Nationally representative household sample of English-speaking adolescents (12–17)	3,614	Sexual (1): 7.5 %	PTSD module of the National Survey of Adolescents and National Women's Study; DSM-IV; unspecified	Past 6 months: 3.9 %

Study	Country	Sample	N	PTE	Measure	Prevalence
Smith et al. (2008)**	United States	Millennium Cohort Study. National population-based study of active duty and Reserve/National Guard personnel, pre- and post-deployment	50,128	–	PCL-C; DSM-IV; unspecified	Current, new onset, 7.6 % (deployed, exposed), 1.4 % (deployed, not exposed), 2.3 % (not deployed); current, persistent, 43.5 % (deployed, exposed), 26.2 % (deployed, not exposed), 47.6 % (not deployed)
Kessler et al. (2005); Nickerson et al. (2012)	United States	National Comorbidity Survey-Replication. Nationally representative sample of English-speaking adults (18+)	5,692	Any PTE (26), 86.9 %; childhood (1*), 19.0 %; sexual (1*), 19.1 %; war related (5), 10.4 %	CIDI; DSM-IV; worst and random	Past year: 3.5 %
Kang et al. (2003)**	United States	National Health Survey of Gulf War Era Veterans and Their Families. Random samples of Gulf and non-Gulf veterans	20,917	–	PCL; DSM-III; unspecified	Current: 12.1 % (Gulf veterans), 4.2 % (non-Gulf veterans)
Acierno et al. (2000); Rheingold et al. (2004); Ford et al. (2010)	United States	National Survey of Adolescents. Nationally representative sample (12–17)	4,023	Any PTE (24), 83.3 %; sexual (1), 13.0 % (females), 3.4 % (males)	Modified PTSD module from the National Women's Study; DSM-IV; unspecified	Past 6 months: 5.0 %

(continued)

Table 2.1 (continued)

Study	Country	Design	N	PTE prevalence	PTSD assessment (instrument; criteria; index event)	PTSD prevalence
Kessler et al. (1995)	United States	National Comorbidity Survey, Phase II. Representative sample of the noninstitutionalized civilian population (15–54) in the 48 contiguous states	5,877	Any PTE (10), 51.2 % (females), 60.7 % (males); childhood (1*), 4.8 % (females), 3.2 % (males); sexual (1*), 12.3 % (females), 2.8 % (males); war (1), 0.0 % (females), 6.4 % (males); disaster (1), 15.2 % (females), 18.9 % (females)	Revised DIS, CIDI; DSM-III-R; worst	Lifetime: 7.8 %
Finkelhor and Dziuba-Leatherman (1994)	United States	Nationally representative sample of adolescents (10–16) and their caretakers	2,000	Any PTE (6), 35.1 %; childhood (1*), 22.2 %; sexual (1*, 7.5 %	–	–
Resnick et al. (1993)	United States	National Women's Study. Nationally representative sample; oversample of women aged 18–34	4,008	Any PTE (11), 68.9 %; sexual (1*), 14.3 %; bereavement (1), 13.4 %	Modified DIS from the National Vietnam Veterans Readjustment Study; DSM-III-R; unspecified	Lifetime, 12.3 %; current, 4.6 %
CDC (1988)**	United States	Vietnam Experience Study. Random sample of Vietnam veterans	2,490	–	DIS; DSM-III; combat related	Lifetime, 14.7 %; past month, 2.2 %

Kulka et al. (1988)**	United States	National Vietnam Veterans Readjustment Study. Representative sample of Vietnam veterans	1,632	–	SCID, Mississippi Scale for Combat-Related PTSD, Minnesota Multiphasic Personality Inventory; DSM-III; various	Lifetime, 30.9 % (males), 26.9 % (females); current, 15.2 % (males), 8.5 % (females)
Darves-Bornoz et al. (2008)	Western Europe (Spain, Italy, Germany, the Netherlands, Belgium, France)	ESEMeD. Representative samples (18+)	8,797	Any PTE (28), 63.6 %; childhood (1), 3.6 %; sexual (1*), 3.4 %; war related (1*), 3.4 %; disaster, 5.9 %; bereavement, 24.6 %	–	–

Notes: Selected studies included nationally representative samples or, when unavailable, regionally representative samples, as well as studies of special populations (e.g., refugees, nationally representative military samples; denoted with **). Age range listed in parentheses. Trauma types included: *Childhood*, non-sexual events, e.g., abuse, neglect; *sexual*, e.g., child sexual abuse, rape; *war related*, e.g., combat, civilian in war zone; *disaster*, e.g., natural, man-made; *bereavement*, e.g., loss of family member due to homicide, sudden death of a close friend. Number of events included listed in parentheses; * denotes that more events in category were included, but total prevalence not reported; value represents the event with highest prevalence.

Abbreviations: *CIDI* World Health Organization Composite International Diagnostic Interview, *DIS* Diagnostic Interview Schedule, *HTQ* Harvard Trauma Questionnaire, *PSS* PTSD Symptom Scale, *MINI* Mini International Neuropsychiatric Interview, *ESEMeD* European Study of the Epidemiology of Mental Disorders, *WMH* World Mental Health age group; (2) if no nationally representative sample was available for the given country, a regionally representative sample; or (3) an epidemiological study of a special population (e.g., refugees, nationally representative military samples). As shown, nationally representative studies in the USA, including the National Comorbidity Study (NCS; Kessler et al. 1995), the National Comorbidity Study-Replication (NCS-R; Nickerson et al. 2012), and the National Women's Study (Resnick et al. 1993), have found that the majority of US adults have experienced at least one potentially traumatic event (PTE). The most commonly experienced PTEs in US studies include the sudden, unexpected death of a close friend or family member, witnessing someone being badly hurt or injured, and exposure to a man-made or natural disaster (c.f., McLaughlin et al. 2013; Nickerson et al. 2012). Nationally representative studies of adult household residents in other high-income countries, including Australia (Mills et al. 2011), Canada (Van Ameringen et al. 2008), Northern Ireland (Bunting et al. 2013), and the Netherlands (Bronner et al. 2009), have similarly found that the majority of adults have experienced at least one PTE. Lower national prevalences have been reported in Germany and South Korea, wherein a third or fewer respondents reported lifetime trauma exposure (Hauffa et al. 2011; Jeon et al. 2007). Extant studies suggest that trauma exposure is also quite common in middle- and lower-income countries (e.g., Cambodia [de Jong et al. 2001], East Timor [Soosay et al. 2012], Mexico [Medina-Mora et al. 2005], South Africa [Atwoli et al. 2013]). However, characteristics of many of these studies, including their focus on specific regions (e.g., metropolitan areas) or groups (e.g., adolescents), limit the ability to make generalizations to the entire population.

Although trauma exposure is common across the globe, there is marked variation among different countries in the incidence of specific events. At least four factors may influence cross-national differences. First, this divergence could reflect real differences in rates. For example, rape may be more common in high conflict zones and therefore result in higher prevalences (cf., higher rates among Liberian former combatants vs. noncombatants; Johnson et al. 2008). Second, there is cultural variation in the acceptability of reporting traumatic events, particularly sexual assault. Respondents' embarrassment or fear of retaliation, which could be culturally mediated, likely influences reporting (e.g., Chan et al. 2013). Third, respondents might be less likely to report events that are considered normative. In this vein, regions in which one might expect more trauma exposure do not necessarily show a higher prevalence of traumatic events (e.g., marked variation in the prevalence of PTEs in postconflict settings; de Jong et al. 2001). Fourth, measurement issues, including inadequately worded questions, might also influence the accuracy of reports.

An additional consideration in making cross-study comparisons concerns variation in which traumatic events were assessed. Trauma inventories differ in both the number and types of events listed and each only provides information about the events that were included. More extensive inventories have been found to yield a higher prevalence of trauma exposure solely due to inclusion of additional events (Mills et al. 2011). Variation in which events are included is due in part to changing definitions of trauma in the *Diagnostic and Statistic Manual of Mental Disorders*

(DSM*)*. In the DSM-III and DSM-III-R, traumatic events were described as those that "occur outside the range of usual human experience." In contrast, the DSM-IV and DSM-IV-R classified traumatic events as involving "actual or threatened death or serious injury, or threat to the physical integrity of self or others" (criterion A1), as well as an emotional response of "fear, helplessness, or horror" (criterion A2). This change increased prevalence of trauma exposure, although did not substantially alter the prevalence of posttraumatic stress disorder (PTSD) (Breslau and Kessler 2001). The recently released DSM-5 does not require an emotional response for an event to be considered traumatic, which is likely to further increase the prevalence of traumatic events.

2.2 Predictors and Correlates of Trauma Exposure

Within countries, trauma exposure varies by individual and group level characteristics. Three categories of predictors of traumatic events have been documented in epidemiological studies: demographic characteristics, within-individual factors, and social contextual factors.

2.2.1 Demographic Characteristics

Demographic variation in trauma exposure depends in part on the nature of the traumatic event. Some traumatic events are, by definition, confined to specific phases of the life span. For example, various traumatic events specify that the victim is a minor, such as child physical, sexual, and emotional abuse, and therefore occur only in childhood and adolescence. On the other end of the spectrum, elder abuse – including physical abuse, neglect, and exploitation by caregivers – is by definition specific to persons 65 years and older (e.g., Lowenstein et al. 2009). For traumatic events that can occur at any point during the life span, exposure generally decreases with age (e.g., Norris 1992), although there is variation among different classes of events. In the 1996 Detroit Area Survey of Trauma, for example, which surveyed adults up to 45 years old, exposure to assaultive violence, injuries, and trauma to a close friend or family member peaked between the ages of 16 and 20, and assaultive violence in particular declined sharply thereafter (Breslau et al. 1998). In contrast, the same study found the unexpected death of a loved one to be most frequent between the ages of 40 and 45.

Men are at increased risk of trauma exposure, both single and cumulative events, compared to women (e.g., Hatch and Dohrenwend 2007). However, gender differences depend on the specific characteristics of traumatic events. An epidemiological study in Mexico, for example, found gender differences by *type* of trauma (women reported more sexual assault; men reported more physical assault), *timing* of trauma (women reported more trauma in childhood; men reported more trauma in adolescence and adulthood), and *relationship context* (women reported more intimate partner and family violence; men reported more violence perpetrated by friends, acquaintances, and strangers) (Baker et al. 2005).

Only recently have researchers begun to study risk of traumatic events among sexual minorities. One epidemiological study found that lesbians, gay men, bisexuals, and heterosexuals with a history of same sex activity had a greater risk of childhood maltreatment, interpersonal violence, trauma to a loved one, or unexpected death of someone close than heterosexuals with no same sex attractions or partners (Roberts et al. 2010).

Lastly, findings on variation in trauma exposure by race and ethnicity have been mixed (Hatch and Dohrenwend 2007). Again, differences likely depend in part on the type of event. For example, studies have found that African Americans are at increased risk for physical assault and unexpected death of a friend or family member relative to Whites (e.g., Rheingold et al. 2004), whereas others have found them to be at lower risk of lifetime exposure and sexual assault (e.g., Norris 1992).

2.2.2   Within-Individual Factors

Prospective studies of children into early adulthood have identified several early risk factors – including aggressive, disruptive, and antisocial behaviors, hyperactivity, difficult temperament, and lower intelligence – for later trauma, particularly assaultive events (e.g., Breslau et al. 2006; Koenen et al. 2007; Storr et al. 2007). Other studies have shown that adolescents with a history of child physical and sexual abuse are at increased risk of exposure (e.g., Amstadter et al. 2011; Elwood et al. 2011). In contrast, a longitudinal birth cohort study in New Zealand found the presence of any juvenile psychiatric disorder (including anxiety, depressive, conduct, and attentional disorders), but not childhood maltreatment, to be a significant predictor of trauma exposure in early adulthood (Breslau et al. 2013).

Additional prospective studies have examined the role of adults' psychological symptoms in predicting subsequent trauma exposure and suggest that classes of symptoms might be differentially related to different forms of exposure. For example, in the National Study of Women, PTSD symptoms were predictive of rape, whereas depression and drug use were predictive of physical assault (Acierno et al. 1999). In contrast, in a cohort of German adolescents and young adults, anxiety disorders and drug use were significantly associated with both assaultive and sexual trauma, whereas depression and alcohol and nicotine use were not (Stein et al. 2002).

2.2.3   Social Contextual Factors

Several studies have found income and education to be negatively associated with exposure, although others have shown either positive or no associations (Hatch and Dohrenwend 2007). Variation in findings is likely a function of both context and the type of trauma assessed. For example, a Mexican epidemiological study found that lower education and income increased risk for some events (e.g., sexual and physical assault, combat) and decreased risk for others (e.g., accidents, threats with weapons) (Norris et al. 2003).

In the same study, there was significant variation in the frequency of traumatic events among the four Mexican cities from which participants were recruited, indicating that geographic location or community characteristics influence exposure. Along these lines, studies in the USA have suggested that rates of assaultive violence are higher in urban, versus suburban, areas (e.g., Breslau et al. 1996).

Within communities, the family environment is an important factor in determining risk. Adolescents whose parents have lower education or who live with only one biological parent have higher rates of exposure than their counterparts (e.g., Landolt et al. 2013; McLaughlin et al. 2013). Parents' psychological symptoms, including posttraumatic stress and drug abuse, also increase risk (e.g., Amstadter et al. 2011; Roberts et al. 2012).

2.3 Consequences of Trauma Exposure

The consequences of trauma exposure on psychological health can be profound and include PTSD, acute stress disorder (ASD), bereavement-related disorder (BRD), and other conditions.

2.3.1 PTSD

Table 2.1 summarizes the results of epidemiological studies documenting the prevalence of PTSD. A consideration in comparing these figures is that some studies have reported on past-month, past-6-month, or past-year prevalence, whereas others have reported lifetime prevalence. An additional source of variation is the traumatic event or events to which PTSD symptoms are linked, for example, whether participants report on symptoms linked to the event identified as the "worst," to a randomly selected traumatic event, or to all traumatic events endured. Studies have also varied in the measures used to assess PTSD (e.g., World Mental Health Organization Composite International Diagnostic Interview [CIDI], PTSD Symptom Scale, Harvard Trauma Questionnaire) and in the criteria used to define cases (e.g., DSM-IV, ICD-10). Among nationally representative studies of adult household residents that used the CIDI, the "worst event" method, and DSM-IV criteria, lifetime prevalence ranges from 1.7 % in South Korea (Jeon et al. 2007) to 8.8 % in Northern Ireland (Breslau et al. 2013), and past-year prevalence ranges from 0.6 % in Spain (Karam et al. 2013) to 5.1 % in Northern Ireland (Breslau et al. 2013).

Risk for PTSD varies by type of traumatic event experienced, such that assaultive events, particularly rape and sexual assault, are most likely to yield PTSD, and learning of a traumatic event that happened to someone else or witnessing an injury is least likely (e.g., Breslau et al. 1996; Bronner et al. 2009). However, cases of PTSD are most often attributed to the unexpected death of a loved one due to the high frequency of this trauma (e.g., Breslau et al. 1996). Studies also suggest that the number of exposures contributes to PTSD risk, such that exposure to more events is associated with a higher prevalence of PTSD (e.g., Finkelhor et al. 2007; Neuner et al. 2004).

A methodological limitation of this research is that the majority of studies to date have been cross-sectional. A handful of studies have explored longitudinal trajectories of posttraumatic stress among survivors of single incident events – that is, studies in which participants experienced the same traumatic event or type of event, including disaster (Norris et al. 2009), traumatic injury (deRoon-Cassini et al. 2010), sexual assault (Steenkamp et al. 2012), and military deployment (Dickstein et al. 2010). These studies have found that, although the majority of participants exhibit a trajectory of consistently low symptoms, some experience other patterns. Most notably, trajectories of chronically high symptoms were evident in each study, with prevalences ranging from 3 % to 22 %. Variation in prevalences is likely due to a variety of factors, including the measure used to assess posttraumatic stress, the nature of the traumatic event, and the duration of follow-up. Only one published study to date has explored posttraumatic stress trajectories among adults with a broader range of traumatic experiences (e.g., Lowe et al. 2014). In this study of urban residents, the majority of participants reported consistently low posttraumatic stress, whereas nearly a quarter were in a trajectory of consistent subthreshold PTSD, and approximately 10 % were in chronic PTSD trajectories. Posttraumatic stress trajectory studies have identified several correlates of trajectories of higher, versus lower, PTSD, among them demographic characteristics associated with socioeconomic disadvantage (e.g., younger age, lower income), more extensive trauma exposure (e.g., exposure to a greater number of events, more severe exposure), fewer social resources (e.g., lower social support), and more severe comorbid symptoms (e.g., higher levels of depression and alcohol use) (Dickstein et al. 2010; Lowe et al. 2014).

Epidemiological studies have not yet provided much insight into the prevalence of the dissociative subtype of PTSD, which was introduced in the DSM-5. An exception is the World Mental Health Surveys, which found that, among over 25,000 participants from 16 countries, 14.4 % reported dissociative experiences (Stein et al. 2013). Dissociative symptoms in this sample were significantly associated with higher levels of reexperiencing, male sex, childhood-onset PTSD, exposure to a greater number of traumatic events and childhood adversities (e.g., family violence, parent mental illness) prior to PTSD onset, history of separation anxiety disorder and specific phobia, severe role impairment, and suicidality. Future studies using measures based on the DSM-5 criteria will shed additional light on the prevalence of the dissociative subtype. Similarly, future epidemiological studies are needed to document the prevalence of complex PTSD, characterized by affect dysregulation, negative self-concept, and interpersonal disturbances in addition to classic PTSD symptoms, in the WHO International Classification of Diseases, 11th version (ICD-11) (Cloitre et al. 2013).

2.3.2 ASD

The epidemiological literature has provided relatively less insight into the prevalence of ASD. This is likely due to the very nature of the disorder, that is, it can occur only within the first month of the traumatic event. In a normative population-based survey, it is likely that few participants who had experienced a lifetime traumatic event had done so within the prior month, and therefore the point prevalence of ASD would be inherently very small. An alternative approach would be to assess lifetime prevalence of ASD by asking participants if they ever experienced symptoms and, if so, whether symptoms were confined to the first month after the event. This would rely on participants' accuracy regarding the timing of symptoms and could be affected by retrospective bias. A third approach would be an epidemiological study of ASD in the aftermath of a mass traumatic event, such as a natural disaster. This too might be difficult given the time it would take for researchers to secure necessary funding and resources to launch an investigation. Despite these challenges, Cohen and Yahav (2008) conducted a population-based survey in northern and central Israel during the second Lebanon war in 2006 and found that 6.8 % of the northern sample and 3.9 % of the central sample met DSM-IV criteria for ASD. A further analysis found that, among the northern sample, 20.3 % of Arab participants met criteria for ASD, compared to 5.5 % of Jewish participants (Yahav and Cohen 2007).

As an alternative to population-based surveys, researchers have drawn upon hospital samples to assess the prevalence of ASD in relation to traumatic illness, such as myocardial infarction (Roberge et al. 2008) and cancer (e.g., Pedersen and Zachariae 2010), and traumatic injury from such causes as motor vehicle accidents (e.g., Kassam-Adams and Winston 2004) and burns (Saxe et al. 2005). The prevalence of ASD across these studies ranges from 1.0 % among admissions to a Level 1 trauma center (Creamer et al. 2004) to 54.3 % among injured child and adolescent earthquake survivors (Liu et al. 2010). More recently, a longitudinal study of 1054 consecutive admissions to five major trauma hospitals in Australia found that 10 % of participants met DSM-IV criteria for ASD (Bryant et al. 2012). Notably, several changes in the diagnostic criteria for ASD were made in DSM-5, and no published study to our knowledge has documented the prevalence of DSM-5 ASD.

2.3.3 BRD

BRD was introduced to the DSM-5, informed by literature on how normal grief after the death of a loved one becomes pathological, including research on complicated grief (CG). Although no published epidemiological studies have explored the prevalence of BRD, at least four studies have investigated CG in epidemiological samples and shed some light onto this issue. First, a study of the general German population reported a 3.7 % prevalence of CG, assessed via the Inventory of Complicated Grief-Revised (ICG-R) (Kersting et al. 2011; Prigerson et al. 1995). Second, a 4.8 % prevalence of CG was found among Dutch older adults using the ICG-R (Newson et al. 2011). Third, a study of Swiss older adults found the prevalence of CG to be 4.2 % using the Complicated Grief Module (Horowitz et al. 1997), and 0.9 % using the Inventory of Traumatic Grief-Revised (Forstmeier and Maercker 2006). Lastly, using the Brief Grief Questionnaire, a study of bereaved Japanese adults found 2.4 % to have CG (Fujisawa et al. 2010; Shear et al. 2006). Taken together, the findings suggest that BRD may be quite common and, like PTSD, related to demographic, trauma-related, and psychological characteristics. The studies also underscore that variability in prevalence estimates depend on the measure employed.

2.3.4 Other Psychological Disorders

Although other disorders are not necessarily precipitated by a traumatic event, epidemiological studies have found trauma exposure to be associated with mood disorders (major depression, dysthymia), anxiety disorders (panic disorder, agoraphobia, social phobia, specific phobia), substance use disorders (alcohol and drug abuse, nicotine dependence), and antisocial personality disorder (e.g., Bunting et al. 2013; Zlotnick et al. 2008).

2.3.5 Physical Health Consequences

Emerging evidence suggests that trauma exposure may also increase risk of adverse physical health conditions, beyond the influence of PTSD and other psychological symptoms. First, childhood trauma has been associated with increased risk of a range of health outcomes. For example, among adults in the NCS, childhood physical abuse was associated with increased risk of lung disease, peptic ulcer, and arthritic disease; childhood sexual abuse was associated with increased risk of cardiovascular disease; and childhood neglect was associated with increased risk of diabetes and autoimmune disorder (Goodwin and Stein 2004). Analyses of the Nurses Health Study 2 (NHS2) have provided further evidence that experiences of physical and sexual abuse and childhood and adolescence increase risk of a variety of adult health conditions, including myocardial infarction, stroke, hypertension, and type 2 diabetes (Rich-Edwards et al. 2010, 2012; Riley et al. 2010).

Second, there is evidence of a dose-response relationship between trauma exposure and physical health conditions. In the NCS-R, the number of traumatic events experienced was significantly associated with greater odds of 13 health conditions, including arthritis, chronic pain, cardiovascular disease, asthma, diabetes, and cancer (Sledjeski et al. 2008). Similarly, in an epidemiological sample of urban adults, Keyes and colleagues (2013) found that the number of lifetime traumatic events significantly increased risk for arthritis and, moreover, that participants who had experienced more events tended to have earlier onset of any of six physical health conditions than those who had experienced fewer or no lifetime trauma. A larger study of adults from 14 countries in the World Mental Health surveys also detected a dose-response effect between traumatic events and the onset of any physical health condition (Scott et al. 2013). The pattern of results was consistent among the 14 countries, 11 different health conditions, and 14 different forms of trauma, with a few notable exceptions: lifetime traumatic events were not associated with increased risk for cancer and stroke, and combat and other war-related events reduced the odds of physical health problems. An analysis of Wave 2 of the NESARC further suggested that associations might depend on both the nature of the traumatic event and physical health condition (Husarewycz et al. 2014). The authors assessed relationships between six different forms of trauma and six health outcomes (cardiovascular disease, arteriosclerosis or hypertension, gastrointestinal disease, diabetes, arthritis, and obesity) and found variation in the patterns of statistical significance in multivariate models: traumatic injuries and witnessing trauma increased risk of all six health conditions; psychological trauma increased risk of cardiovascular and gastrointestinal disease; disasters increased risk of cardiovascular disease, gastrointestinal disease, and arthritis; and war related and other trauma were not associated with increased risk of any physical health outcome. For more details on the physical health consequences of trauma exposure, see Chap. 5.

2.3.6 Intergenerational Effects

A novel area of epidemiological research focuses on the intergenerational effects of maternal exposure to trauma on offspring mental and physical health. Two published studies have emerged from linked longitudinal data from large cohorts of mothers in the NHS2 and their children in the Growing Up Today Study (GUTS). First, NHS2 mothers' PTSD symptoms were significantly and positively associated with GUTS participants' number of lifetime traumatic events and PTSD symptoms (Roberts et al. 2013). Second, NHS2 mothers' exposure to childhood physical, sexual, and emotional abuse was associated with an increased likelihood of GUTS participants reporting a high-risk smoking trajectory characterized by early initiation and increasing use, as well as being overweight or obese (Roberts et al. 2014). In a third study of NHS2 participants, exposure to childhood trauma increased risk of a host of adverse perinatal experiences (e.g., toxemia, gestational diabetes, low birth weight, premature birth) and, beyond these experiences, increased risk of autism in their children (Roberts et al. 2013).

2.4 Public Health Perspectives on Treatment

Thus far, we have shown that traumatic events are common occurrences across the life span, are not distributed equally across populations, and can have major consequences for mental and physical health that extend across generations. A remaining consideration is how to address trauma and its consequences from a public health perspective. There are three general approaches in this regard, each defined by its timing relative to the traumatic event: primary, secondary, and tertiary prevention.

2.4.1 Primary Prevention

Primary prevention strategies aim to either prevent traumatic events from occurring or trauma-related disorders from developing. General approaches include interventions that shift attitudes and norms surrounding potentially traumatic events to decrease their acceptability and incidence. An example of such an approach is the Northeastern Center for Sport and Society Mentors in Violence Prevention (MVP) program (www.northeastern.edu/sportandsociety). Through the MVP program, former college-level and professional athletes lead workshops that encourage youth participants to evaluate societal norms that encourage or condone gender-based violence and to brainstorm strategies for bystanders to intervene. Public policies and legislation also have the potential to reduce the incidence of traumatic events. In the case of natural disasters, such as floods and hurricanes, for example, sound plans for evacuation of residents in low-lying areas and transfer of medical care can prevent exposure to potentially life-threatening events. Legislation that assigns responsibility to perpetrators and other entities that have caused harm could also influence the likelihood that such events reoccur (Sorenson 2002). Additionally, legislation, such as the International Violence Against Women Act, has proposed to integrate measures to address violence against women into governments' foreign policy and would potentially have a global impact on various forms of gender-based traumatic events, including rape, domestic violence, and human trafficking (Amnesty International 2013/2014).

Of course, trauma exposure cannot be eliminated completely, and, as such, other primary prevention strategies focus on preventing trauma-related disorders after an event has occurred through early intervention. Early pharmacologic interventions, such as administration of the β-adrenergic blocker propranolol, have been found to reduce PTSD among trauma-exposed medical patients, although the results have been inconsistent (Chap. 7). Recent studies of trauma-exposed emergency room patients have also provided evidence for the promise of early cognitive behavioral interventions to prevent symptom development (Chap. 7).

2.4.2 Secondary Prevention

Unlike primary prevention efforts to prevent trauma and the development of trauma-related disorders, secondary prevention efforts target early cases of disorders before significant and/or chronic morbidity has occurred. A major aspect of secondary prevention consists of accurate identification of cases. Clinicians' assessment of patients' trauma histories in initial evaluations to determine whether presenting problems are indicative of a trauma-related condition is essential to case identification. Of course, not all persons suffering from PTSD and other trauma-related conditions will present to mental health treatment. As such, other practitioners who could potentially come in contact with persons suffering from PTSD, such as primary care and specialty physicians and personnel at social service agencies, should be educated about the psychological effects of trauma and how to screen for trauma-related psychopathology. Collaborative medical teams including physicians, social workers, and psychologists would also facilitate referrals for identified cases.

Once cases are identified, empirically supported treatments could be employed to reduce trauma-related psychopathology. To date, several treatments have received empirical support for reducing PTSD symptoms, including selective serotonin reuptake inhibitors, cognitive behavioral therapies (e.g., cognitive restructuring), prolonged exposure, and eye movement desensitization and reprocessing (Chaps. 8, 9, 10, 11, 12, and 13). The more limited research on the treatment of traumatic grief, including bereavement-related disorder (BRD) and prolonged grief disorder (PGD, as defined in ICD-11), has provided some evidence for the efficacy of cognitive behavioral and interpersonal psychotherapies (Chap. 15).

2.4.3 Tertiary Prevention

Finally, tertiary prevention involves methods to reduce the negative impact of existent disease by restoring functioning and reducing disease-related complications. As with secondary prevention, a major facet of tertiary prevention is the identification of PTSD and other trauma-related disorders. The difference is that such efforts pertain to identifying chronic cases and cases in which trauma-related symptoms may have already contributed to comorbid mental health conditions (e.g., substance abuse), physical health problems (e.g., obesity, migraine headaches, Chap. 5), and psychosocial impairment (e.g., unemployment, relationship problems).

Once cases are identified, tertiary prevention strategies also include empirically supported treatments to decrease trauma-related symptom severity. However, in some cases, treatment of comorbid conditions should be prioritized over trauma-related pathology to restore a level of functioning conducive to trauma-focused therapies (Part IV, Chaps. 16, 17, and 18). Similarly, interventions that target functional impairment – including parenting strategies, couples therapy, and job training – could address pressing concerns that prevent patients from facing their traumatic histories (Chaps. 14 and 24). Again, collaboration between mental health practitioners and other professionals, including caseworkers and physicians, as well as engagement of loved ones in treatment, is essential to tertiary prevention.

2.5 Conclusion: The Public Health Burden of Trauma Exposure

The global burden of trauma exposure for mental and physical health over the life course has not, to our knowledge, been quantified at this writing. However, based on our review of the literature, we conclude that it is likely to be profound.

The reviewed literature indicates that exposure to traumatic events is widespread. The majority of adults in higher-income countries have experienced at least one lifetime trauma, and emerging evidence suggests that this is the case in middle- and lower-income countries as well. Traumatic events, in turn, increase the risk of a wide range of negative outcomes.

First, trauma exposure is a necessary condition for three psychiatric conditions: PTSD, ASD, and BRD. Although the majority of trauma survivors do not go on to develop these disorders, the review above indicates that a substantial number of survivors do. The lifetime prevalence of PTSD in population-based samples is as high as 8.8 %, and trajectory studies suggest that a sizeable minority of trauma-exposed persons will exhibit chronic severe PTSD. Although less research has been conducted on ASD and BRD, the extant literature suggests that approximately 10 % of trauma survivors develop ASD and that the lifetime prevalence of BRD in the general population is as high as 4.8 %.

Second, trauma exposure has been found to increase the risk of a host of other mental health conditions, including anxiety disorders, substance use disorders, and, most notably, major depression. As of 2011, major depression is the third leading cause of disease burden, accounting for 4.3 % of the global disease burden, and is estimated to become the leading cause of global disease burden by 2030 (World Health Organization 2011). The burden of trauma is likely to exceed these estimates, as exposure also increases risk for a range of chronic physical health conditions, including cardiovascular disease, diabetes, and cancer, and its effects appear to extend across generations.

Taken together, the evidence provides strong support for our contention that trauma is a critical public health issue. Effective prevention of trauma exposure may have profound and wide-ranging health effects both within and across generations.

References

Acierno, R., Resnick, H., Kilpatrick, D. G., Saunder, B., & Best, C. L. (1999). Risk factors for rape, physical assault, and posttraumatic stress disorder in women: Examination of differential multivariate relationships. *Journal of Anxiety Disorders, 13*, 541–563. doi:10.1016/S0887-6185(99)00030-4.

Acierno, R., Kilpatrick, D. G., Resnick, H., Saunders, B., de Arellano, M., & Best, C. (2000). Assault, PTSD, family substance use, and depression as risk factors for cigarette use in youth: Findings from the National Survey of Adolescents. *Journal of Traumatic Stress, 13*, 381–396. doi:10.1023/A:1007772905696.

Alhasnawi, S., Sadik, S., Rasheed, M., Baban, A., Al-Alak, M. M., Othman, A. Y., Ismet, N., Shawani, O., Murthy, S., Aljadiry, M., Chatterji, S., Al-Gasseer, N., Streel, E., Naidoo, N., Mahomoud Ali, M., Gruber, M. J., Petukhova, M., Sampson, N. A., Kessler, R. C., & the Iraq Mental Health Survey Study Group. (2009). The prevalence and correlates of DSM-IV in the Iraq Mental Health Survey (IMHS). *World Psychiatry, 8*, 97–109.

Amnesty International. (2013/2014). *The International Violence Against Women Act (I-VAWA).* Issue Brief, No. 3. Retrieved from www.amnestyusa.org

Amstadter, A. B., Elwood, L. S., Begle, A. M., Gudmundsdottir, B., Smith, D. W., Resnick, H., Hanson, R. F., Saunders, B. E., & Kilpatrick, D. G. (2011). Predictors of physical assault victimization: Findings from the National Survey of Adolescents. *Addictive Behaviors, 36*, 814–820. doi:10.1016/j.addbeh.2011.03.008.

Atwoli, L., Stein, D. J., Williams, D. R., Mclaughlin, K. A., Petukhova, M., Kessler, R. C., & Koenen, K. C. (2013). Trauma and posttraumatic stress disorder in South Africa: Analysis from the South African stress and health study. *BMC Psychiatry, 13*, 182. doi:10.1186/1471-244X-13-182.

Baker, C. K., Norris, F. H., Diaz, D. M. V., Perilla, J. L., Murphy, A. D., & Hill, E. G. (2005). Violence and PTSD in Mexico: Gender and regional differences. *Social Psychiatry and Psychiatric Epidemiology, 40*, 519–528. doi:10.1007/s00127-005-0921-2.

Benitez, C. P., Vicente, B., Zlotnick, C., Kohn, R., Johnson, J., Valdivia, S., & Rioseco, P. (2009). Estudio epidemiológico de sucesos traumáticos, trastorno de estrés post-traumático y otros trastornos psiquiátricos en una muestra representativa de Chile. *Salud Mental, 31*, 145–153.

Bentall, R. P., Wickham, S., Shevlin, M., & Varese, F. (2012). Do specific early-life adversities lead to specific symptoms of psychosis? A study from the 2007 Adult Psychiatric Morbidity Survey. *Schizophrenia Bulletin, 38,* 734–740. doi:10.1093/schbul/sbs049.

Bödvarsdottír, I., & Elklit, A. (2007). Victimization and PTSD-like states in an Icelandic youth sample. *BMC Psychiatry, 7,* 1–7. doi:10.1186/1471-244X-7-51.

Breslau, N., & Kessler, R. C. (2001). The stressor criterion in DSM-IV Posttraumatic Stress Disorder: An empirical investigation. *Biological Psychiatry, 50,* 699–704. doi:10.1016/S0006-3223(01)01167-2.

Breslau, N., Kessler, R. C., Chilcoat, H. D., Schultz, L. R., Davis, G. C., & Andreski, P. (1998). Trauma and posttraumatic stress disorder in the community. *Archives of General Psychiatry, 55,* 626–632. doi:10.1001/archpsyc.55.7.626.

Breslau, N., Lucia, V. C., & Alvarado, G. F. (2006). Intelligence and other predisposing factors in exposure to trauma and posttraumatic stress disorder. *Archives of General Psychiatry, 63,* 1238–1245. doi:10.1001/archpsyc.63.11.1238.

Breslau, N., Troost, J. P., Bohnert, K., & Luo, Z. (2013). Influence of predispositions on posttraumatic stress disorder: Does it vary by trauma severity? *Psychological Medicine, 43,* 381–390. doi:10.1017/S0033291712001195.

Bronner, M. B., Peek, N., de Vries, M., Bronner, A. E., Last, B. F., & Grootenhuis, M. A. (2009). A community-based survey of Posttraumatic Stress Disorder in the community. *Journal of Traumatic Stress, 22,* 74–78. doi:10.1002/jts.20379.

Bryant, R. A., Creamer, M., O'Donnell, M., Silove, D., & McFarlane, A. C. (2012). The capacity of acute stress disorder to predict posttraumatic psychiatric disorders. *Journal of Psychiatric Research, 46,* 168–173. doi:10.1016/j.jpsychires.2011.10.007.

Bunting, B. P., Ferry, F. R., Murphy, S. D., O'Neill, S. M., & Bolton, D. (2013). Trauma associated with civil conflict and Posttraumatic Stress Disorder: Evidence from the Northern Ireland Study of Health and Stress. *Journal of Traumatic Stress, 26,* 134–141. doi:10.1002/jts.21766.

Centers for Disease Control. (1988). Health status of Vietnam veterans. I. Psychosocial characteristics. *JAMA, 259,* 2701–2707.

Chan, K. L., Yan, E., Brownridge, D. A., & Ip, P. (2013). Associating childhood sexual abuse with child victimization in China. *Journal of Pediatrics, 162,* 1028–1034. doi:10.1016/j.jpeds.2012.10.054.

Chapman, C., Mills, K., Slade, T., McFarlane, A. C., Bryant, R. A., Creamer, M., Silove, T., & Teesson, M. (2010). Remission from post-traumatic stress disorder in the general population. *Psychological Medicine, 42*(8), 1695–1703. doi:10.1017/S0033291711002856.

Cisler, J. M., Amstadter, A. B., Begle, A. M., Resnick, H. S., Danielson, C. K., Saunders, B. E., & Kilpatrick, D. G. (2011). A prospective examination of the relationship between PTSD, exposure to assaultive violence, and cigarette smoking among a national sample of adolescents. *Addictive Behaviors, 36,* 994–1000. doi:10.1016/j.addbeh.2011.05.014.

Cloitre, M., Garvert, D. W., Brewin, C. R., Bryant, R. A., & Maercker, A. (2013). Evidence for proposed ICD-11 PTSD and complex PTSD: A latent profile analysis. *European Journal of Psychotraumatology, 4,* 1–12. doi:10.3402/ejpt.v4i0.20706.

Cohen, M., & Yahav, R. (2008). Acute stress symptoms during the Second Lebanon War in a random sample of Israeli citizens. *Journal of Traumatic Stress, 21,* 118–121. doi:10.1002/jts.20312.

Creamer, M., O'Donnell, M. L., & Pattison, P. (2004). The relationship between acute stress disorder and posttraumatic stress disorder in severely injured trauma survivors. *Behaviour Research and Therapy, 42,* 315–328. doi:10.1016/S0005-7967(03)00141-4.

Darves-Bornoz, J. M., Alonso, J., de Girolamo, G., de Graar, R., Haro, J. M., Kovess-Masfety, V., Lepine, J. P., Nachbaur, G., Negre-Pages, L., Vilagut, G., & Gasquet, I. (2008). Main traumatic events in Europe: PTSD in the European study of the epidemiology of mental disorders survey. *Journal of Traumatic Stress, 21,* 455–462. doi:10.1002/jts.20357.

de Albuquerque, A., Soares, C., de Jesus, P. M., & Alves, C. (2003). Perturbação pós-traumática do stress (PTSD): Avaliação da taxa de ocorrência na população adulta portuguesa. *Acta Médica Portuguesa, 16,* 309–320.

de Jong, J. T., Komproe, I. H., Ommeren, M. V., Masri, M. E., Araya, M., Khaled, N., van De Put, W., & Somasundaram, D. (2001). Lifetime events and posttraumatic stress disorder in 4 post-conflict settings. *Journal of the American Medical Association, 286*, 555–562. doi:10.1001/jama.286.5.555.

de Vries, G., & Olff, M. (2009). The prevalence of traumatic events and posttraumatic stress disorder in the Netherlands. *Journal of Traumatic Stress, 22*, 259–267. doi:10.1002/jts.20429.

deRoon-Cassini, T. A., Mancini, A. D., Rusch, M. D., & Bonanno, G. A. (2010). Psychopathology and resilience following traumatic injury: A latent growth mixture model analysis. *Rehabilitation Psychology, 55*, 1–11. doi:10.1037/a0018601.

Dickstein, B. D., Suvak, M., Litz, B. T., & Adler, A. B. (2010). Heterogeneity in the course of posttraumatic stress disorder: Trajectories of symptomatology. *Journal of Traumatic Stress, 23*, 331–339. doi:10.1002/jts.20523.

Domanskaité-Gota, V., Elklit, A., & Christiansen, D. M. (2009). Victimization and PTSD in a Lithuanian national youth probability sample. *Nordic Psychology, 61*, 66–81. doi:10.1027/1901-2276.61.3.66.

Elklit, A. (2002). Victimization and PTSD in a Danish national youth probability sample. *Journal of the American Academy of Child and Adolescent Psychiatry, 41*, 174–181. doi:10.1097/00004583-200202000-00011.

Elwood, L. S., Smith, D. W., Resnick, H. S., Gudmundsdottir, B., Amstadter, A. B., Hanson, R. F., Saunders, B. E., & Kilpatrick, D. G. (2011). Predictors of rape: Findings from the National Survey of Adolescents. *Journal of Traumatic Stress, 24*, 166–173. doi:10.1002/jts.20624.

Fear, N. T., Jones, M., Murphy, D., Hull, L., Iverson, A. C., Coker, B., Machell, L., Sundin, J., Woodhead, C., Jones, N., Greenberg, N., Landau, S., Dandeker, C., Rona, R. J., Hotopf, M., & Wessely, S. (2010). What are the consequences of deployment to Iraq and Afghanistan on the mental health of the UK armed forces? *Lancet, 375*, 1783–1797. doi:10.1016/S0140-6736(10)60672-1.

Fikretoglu, D., & Liu, A. (2012). Prevalence, correlates, and clinical features of delayed posttraumatic stress disorder in a nationally representative military sample. *Social Psychiatry and Psychiatric Epidemiology, 47*, 1359–1366. doi:10.1007/s00127-011-0444.

Finkelhor, D., & Dziuba-Leatherman, J. (1994). Children as victims of violence: A national survey. *Pediatrics, 94*, 413–420.

Finkelhor, D., Ormrod, R. K., & Turner, H. A. (2007). Poly-victimization: A neglected component in childhood victimization. *Child Abuse and Neglect, 31*, 7–26. doi:10.1016/j.chiabu.2006.06.008.

Florescu, S., Moldovan, M., Mihaescu-Pintia, C., Ciutan, M., & Sorel, G. E. (2009). The Mental Health Study Romania 2007: Prevalence, severity, and treatment of 12-month DSM-IV disorders. *Management in Health, 4*, 23–31. doi:10.5233/mih.2009.0028.

Ford, J. D., Elhai, J. D., Connor, D. F., & Frueh, B. C. (2010). Poly-victimization and risk of posttraumatic, depressive, and substance use disorders and involvement in delinquency in a national sample of adolescents. *Journal of Adolescent Health, 46*, 545–552. doi:10.1016/j.jadohealth.2009.11.212.

Forstmeier, S., & Maercker, A. (2006). Comparison of two diagnostic systems for Complicated Grief. *Journal of Affective Disorders, 99*, 203–211. doi:10.1016/j.jad.2006.09.013.

Fujisawa, D., Miyashita, M., Nakajima, S., Ito, M., Kato, M., & Kim, Y. (2010). Prevalence and determinants of complicated grief in a general population. *Journal of Affective Disorders, 127*, 352–358. doi:10.1016/j.jad.2010.06.008.

Goodwin, R. D., & Stein, M. B. (2004). Association between childhood trauma and physical disorders among adults in the United States. *Psychological Medicine, 34*, 509–520. doi:10.1017/S003329170300134X.

Hatch, S. L., & Dohrenwend, B. P. (2007). Distribution of traumatic events and other stressful life events by race/ethnicity, gender, SES and age: A review of the research. *American Journal of Community Psychology, 40*, 313–332. doi:10.1007/s10464-007-9134-z.

Hauffa, R., Rief, W., Brahler, E., Martin, A., Mewes, R., & Glaesmer, H. (2011). Lifetime traumatic experiences and posttraumatic disorder in the German population. *Journal of Nervous and Mental Disease, 199*(12), 934–939. doi:10.1097/NMD.0b013e3182392c0d.

Horowitz, M. J., Siegel, B., Holen, A., Bonanno, G. A., Milbrath, C., & Stinson, C. H. (1997). Diagnostic criteria for complicated grief disorder. *American Journal of Psychiatry, 154,* 904–910.

Husarewycz, M. N., El-Gabalawy, R., Logsetty, S., & Sareen, J. (2014). The association between number and type of traumatic life experiences and physical conditions in a nationally representative sample. *General Hospital Psychiatry, 36,* 26–32. doi:10.1016/j.genhosppsych.2013.06.003.

Ikin, J. F., Sim, M. R., Creamer, M. C., Forbes, A. B., McKenzie, D. P., Kelsall, H. L., Glass, D. C., McFarlane, A. C., Abramson, M. J., Ittak, P., Dwyer, T., Blizzard, L., Delaney, K. R., Horsley, K. W., Harrex, W. K., & Schwarz, H. (2004). War-related psychological stressors and risk of psychological disorders in Australian veterans of the 1991 Gulf War. *British Journal of Psychiatry, 185,* 116–126. doi:10.1192/bjp.185.2.116.

Jeon, H. J., Suh, T., Lee, H. J., Hahm, B. J., Lee, J. Y., Cho, S. J., Lee, Y. R., Chang, S. M., & Cho, M. J. (2007). Partial versus full PTSD in the Korean community: Prevalence, duration, correlates, comorbidity, and dysfunctions. *Depression and Anxiety, 24,* 577–585. doi:10.1002/da.20270.

Johnson, K., Asher, J., Rosborough, S., Raja, A., Panjami, R., Beadling, C., & Lawry, L. (2008). Association of combatant status and sexual violence with health and mental health outcomes in postconflict Liberia. *Journal of the American Medical Association, 300,* 676–690. doi:10.1001/jama.300.6.676.

Kadri, N., Agoub, M., El Gnaoui, S., Berrada, S., & Moussaoui, D. (2007). Prevalence of anxiety disorders: A population-based epidemiological study in metropolitan area of Casablanca, Morocco. *Annals of General Psychiatry, 6.* doi:10.1186/1744-859X-6-6.

Kang, H. K., Natelson, B. H., Mahan, C. M., Lee, K. Y., & Murphy, F. M. (2003). Post-traumatic stress disorder and chronic fatigue syndrome-like illnesses among Gulf War veterans: A population-based survey of 30,000 veterans. *American Journal of Epidemiology, 157,* 141–148. doi:10.1093/aje/kwf187.

Karam, E. G., Mneimneh, Z. N., Dimassi, H., Fayyad, J. A., Karam, A. N., Nasser, S. C., Chatterji, S., & Kessler, R. C. (2008). Lifetime prevalence of mental disorders in Lebanon: First onset, treatment, exposure to war. *PLoS Medicine, 5,* e61. doi:10.1371/journal.pmed.0050061.

Karam, E. G., Friedman, M. J., Hill, E. D., Kessler, R. C., McLaughlin, K. A., Petukhova, M., Sampson, L., Shahly, V., Angermeyer, M. C., Bromet, E. J., de Girolamo, G., de Graaf, R., Demyttenaere, K., Ferry, F., Florescu, S. E., Haro, J. M., He, Y., Karam, A. N., Kawakami, N., Kovess-Masfety, V., Medina-Mora, M. E., Browne, M. A., Posada-Villa, J. A., Shalev, A. Y., Stein, D. J., Viana, M. C., Zarkov, Z., & Koenen, K. C. (2013). Cumulative traumas and risk thresholds: 12-month PTSD in the World Mental Health (WMH) surveys. *Depression and Anxiety, 31,* 130–142. doi:10.1002/da.22169.

Kassam-Adams, N., & Winston, F. K. (2004). Predicting child PTSD: The relationship between acute stress disorder and PTSD in injured children. *Journal of the American Academy of Child and Adolescent Psychiatry, 43,* 403–411. doi:10.1097/01.chi.0000112486.08386.c2.

Kawakami, N., Tsuchiya, M., Umeda, M., Koenen, K. C., & Kessler, R. C. (2014). Trauma and posttraumatic stress disorder in Japan: Results from the World Mental Health Japan Survey. *Journal of Psychiatric Research, 53,* 157–165. doi:10.1016/j.jpsychires.2014.01.015.

Kersting, A., Brahler, E., Glaesmer, H., & Wagner, B. (2011). Prevalence of complicated grief in a representative population-based sample. *Journal of Affective Disorders, 131,* 339–343. doi:10.1016/j.jad.2010.11.032.

Kessler, R. C., Sonnega, A., Bromet, E., Hughes, M., & Nelson, C. B. (1995). Posttraumatic stress disorder in the National Comorbidity Survey. *Archives of General Psychiatry, 52,* 1048–1060. doi:10.1001/archpsyc.1995.03950240066012.

Kessler, R. C., Chiu, W. T., Demler, O., & Walters, E. E. (2005). Prevalence, severity, and comorbidity of 12-month DSM-IV disorders in the National Comorbidity Survey Replication. *Archives of General Psychiatry, 62,* 617–627. doi:10.1001/archpsyc.62.6.617.

Keyes, K. M., McLaughlin, K. A., Demmer, R. T., Cerdá, M., Koenen, K. C., Uddin, M., & Galea, S. (2013). Potentially traumatic events and the risk of six physical health conditions in a population-based sample. *Depression & Anxiety, 30,* 451–460. doi:10.1002/da.22090.

Koenen, K. C., Moffitt, T. E., Poulton, R., Martin, J., & Caspi, A. (2007). Early childhood factors associated with the development of post-traumatic stress disorder: Results from a longitudinal birth cohort. *Psychological Medicine, 37*, 181–192. doi:10.1017/S0033291706009019.

Kulka, R. A., Schlenger, W. E., Fairbank, J. A., Hough, R. L., Jordan, B. K., Marmar, C. R., & Weiss, D. S. (1988). *Contractual report of findings from the National Vietnam Veterans Readjustment Study*. Research Triangle Park: Research Triangle Institute.

Landolt, M. A., Schnyder, U., Maier, T., Schoenbucher, V., & Mohler-Kuo, M. (2013). Traumatic exposure and posttraumatic stress disorder in adolescents: A national study in Switzerland. *Journal of Traumatic Stress, 26*, 209–216. doi:10.1002/jts.21794.

Liu, K., Liang, X., Guo, L., Li, Y., Li, X., Xin, B., Huang, M., & Li, Y. (2010). Acute stress disorder in the paediatric surgical children and adolescents injured during the Wenchuan earthquake in China. *Stress and Health, 26*, 262–268. doi:10.1002/smi.1288.

Lowe, S. R., Galea, S., Uddin, M., & Koenen, K. C. (2014). Trajectories of posttraumatic stress among urban residents. *American Journal of Community Psychology, 53*, 159–172. doi:10.1007/s10464-014-9634-6.

Lowenstein, A., Eisikovits, Z., Band-Winterstein, T., & Enosh, G. (2009). Is elder abuse and neglect a social phenomenon? Data from the first national prevalence survey in Israel. *Journal of Elder Abuse & Neglect, 21*, 253–277. doi:10.1080/08946560902997629.

Maercker, A., Forstmeier, S., Wagner, B., Glaesmer, H., & Brahler, E. (2008). Posttraumatische Belastungsstörungen in Deutschland: Ergebnisse einer gesamtdeutschen epidemiologischen Untersuchung. *Nervenarzt, 79*, 577–586. doi:10.1007/s00115-008-2467-5.

McCauley, J. L., Danielson, C. K., Amstadter, A. B., Ruggiero, K. J., Resnick, H. S., Hanson, R. F., & Kilpatrick, D. G. (2010). The role of traumatic event history in non-medical use of prescription drugs among a nationally representative sample of US adolescents. *Journal of Child Psychology and Psychiatry, 51*, 84–93. doi:10.1111/j.1469-7610.2009.02134.x.

McLaughlin, K. A., Koenen, K. C., Hill, E. D., Petukhova, M., Sampson, N. A., Zaslavsky, A. M., & Kessler, R. C. (2013). Trauma exposure and posttraumatic stress disorder in a nationally representative sample of adolescents. *Journal of the American Academy of Child & Adolescent Psychiatry, 52*, 815–830. doi:10.1016/j.jpsychires.2011.08.005.

Medina-Mora, M. E., Borges, G., Muñoz, C. L., Benjet, C., Jaimes, J. B., Bautista, C. F., & Aguilar-Gaxiola, S. (2003). Prevalencia de trastornos mentales y uso de servicios: Resultados de la Encuesta Nacional de Epidemiología Psiquiátrica en México. Salud Mental, 26, 1–16

Medina-Mora, M. E., Borges-Guimaraes, G., Lara, C., Ramos-Lira, L., Zambrano, J., & Fleiz-Bautista, C. (2005). Prevalencia de sucesos violentos y de trastorno por estrés postraumático en la población mexicana. *Salud Pública de México, 47*, 8–22. doi:10.1590/S0036-36342005000100004.

Mills, K. L., McFarlane, A. C., Slade, T., Creamer, M., Silove, D., Teeson, M., & Bryant, R. (2011). Assessing the prevalence of trauma exposure in epidemiological surveys. *Australian and New Zealand Journal of Psychiatry, 45*, 407–415. doi:10.3109/00048674.2010.543654.

Nelson, C., Cyr, K. S., Corbett, B., Hurley, E., Gifford, S., Elhai, J. D., & Richardson, J. D. (2011). Predictors of posttraumatic stress disorder, depression, and suicidal ideation among Canadian Forces personnel in a National Canadian Military Health Survey. *Journal of Psychiatric Research, 45*, 1483–1488. doi:10.1016/j.jpsychires.2011.06.014.

Neuner, F., Schauer, M., Karunakara, U., Klaschik, C., Robert, C., & Elbert, T. (2004). Psychological trauma and evidence for enhanced vulnerability for posttraumatic stress disorder through previous trauma among West Nile refugees. *BMC Psychiatry, 4*, 34. doi:10.1186/1471-244X-4-34.

Newson, R. S., Boelen, P. A., Hek, K., Hofman, A., & Tiemeier, H. (2011). The prevalence and characteristics of complicated grief in older adults. *Journal of Affective Disorders, 132*, 231–238. doi:10.1016/j.jad.2011.02.021.

Nickerson, A., Aderka, I. M., Bryant, R. A., & Hoffman, S. G. (2012). The relationship between childhood exposure to trauma and intermittent explosive disorder. *Psychiatry Research, 197*, 128–134. doi:10.1016/j.psychres.2012.01.012.

Norris, F. H. (1992). Epidemiology of trauma: Frequency and impact of different potentially traumatic events on different demographic groups. *Journal of Consulting and Clinical Psychology, 60*, 409–418. doi:10.1037/0022-006X.60.3.409.

Norris, F. H., Murphy, A. D., Baker, C. K., Perilla, J. L., Rodriguez, F. G., & Rodriguez, J. J. G. (2003). Epidemiology of trauma and posttraumatic stress disorder in Mexico. *Journal of Abnormal Psychology, 112*, 646–656. doi:10.1037/0021-843X.112.4.646.

Norris, F. H., Tracy, M., & Galea, S. (2009). Looking for resilience: Understanding the longitudinal trajectories of responses to stress. *Social Science & Medicine, 68*, 2190–2198. doi:10.1016/j.socscimed.2009.03.043.

O'Toole, B. I., Marshall, R. P., Grayson, D. A., Schureck, R. J., Dobson, M., Ffrench, M., Pulvertaft, B., Meldrum, L., Bolton, J., & Vennard, J. (1996). The Australian Vietnam Veterans Study: III. Psychological health of Australian Vietnam veterans and its relationship to combat. *International Journal of Epidemiology, 25*, 331–340. doi:10.1093/ije/25.2.331.

Pedersen, A. F., & Zachariae, R. (2010). Cancer, acute stress disorder, and repressive coping. *Scandinavian Journal of Psychology, 51*, 84–91. doi:10.1111/j.1467-9450.2009.00727.x.

Pietrzak, R. H., Goldstein, R. B., Southwick, S. M., & Grant, B. F. (2011). Prevalence and Axis I comorbidity of full and partial posttraumatic stress disorder in the United States: Results from Wave 2 of the National Epidemiological Survey on Alcohol and Related Conditions. *Journal of Anxiety Disorders, 25*, 456–465. doi:10.1016/j.janxdis.2010.11.010.

Prigerson, H. G., Maciejewski, P. K., Reynolds, C. F., Bierhals, A. J., Newsom, J. T., Fasiczka, A., Frank, E., Doman, J., & Miller, M. (1995). Inventory of complicated grief: A scale to measure maladaptive symptoms of loss. *Psychiatry Research, 59*, 65–79.

Resnick, H. S., Kilpatrick, D. G., Dansky, B. S., Saunders, B. E., & Best, C. L. (1993). Prevalence of civilian trauma and posttraumatic stress disorder in a representative sample of women. *Journal of Consulting and Clinical Psychology, 61*, 984–991. doi:10.1037/0022-006X.61.6.984.

Rheingold, A. A., Smith, D. W., Ruggiero, K. J., Saunders, B. J., Kilpatrick, D. G., & Resnick, H. S. (2004). Loss, trauma exposure, and mental health in a representative sample of 12-17-year-old youth: Data from the National Survey of Adolescents. *Journal of Loss and Trauma, 9*, 1–19. doi:10.1080/15325020490255250.

Rich-Edwards, J. W., Spiegelman, D., Hibert, E. N. L., Jun, H., Todd, T. J., Kawachi, I., & Wright, R. J. (2010). Abuse in childhood and adolescence as a predictor of type 2 diabetes in adult women. *American Journal of Preventive Medicine, 39*, 529–536. doi:10.1016/j.amepre.2010.09.007.

Rich-Edwards, J. W., Mason, S., Rexrode, K., Spiegelman, D., Hibert, E., Kawachi, I., Jun, H. J., & Wright, R. J. (2012). Physical and sexual abuse in childhood as predictors of early-onset cardiovascular events in women. *Circulation, 126*, 920–927. doi:10.1161/CIRCULATIONAHA.111.076877.

Riley, E. H., Wright, R. J., Jun, H. J., Hibert, E. N., & Rich-Edwards, J. W. (2010). Hypertension in adult survivors of child abuse: Observations from the Nurses' Health Study II. *Journal of Epidemiology and Community Health, 64*, 413–418. doi:10.1136/jech.2009.095109.

Roberge, M., Dupuis, G., & Marchand, A. (2008). Acute stress disorder after myocardial infarction: Prevalence and associated factors. *Psychosomatic Medicine, 70*, 1028–1034. doi:10.1097/PSY.0b013e318189a920.

Roberts, A. L., Austin, S. B., Corliss, H. L., Vandermorris, A. K., & Koenen, K. C. (2010). Pervasive trauma exposure among sexual orientation minority adults and risk of posttraumatic stress disorder. *American Journal of Public Health, 100*, 2433–2441. doi:10.2105/AJPH.2009.168971.

Roberts, A. L., Galea, S., Austin, S. B., Cerdá, M., Wright, R. J., Rich-Edwards, J. W., & Koenen, K. C. (2012). Posttraumatic stress disorder across generations: Concordance and mechanisms in a population-based sample. *Biological Psychiatry, 72*, 505–511. doi:10.1016/j.biopsych.2012.03.020.

Roberts, A. L., Lyall, K., Rich-Edwards, J. W., Ascherio, A., & Weisskopf, M. G. (2013). Association of maternal exposure to child abuse with elevated risk for autism in offspring. *JAMA Psychiatry, 70*, 508–515. doi:10.1001/jamapsychiatry.2013.447.

Roberts, A. L., Galea, S., Austin, S. B., Corliss, H. L., Williams, M. A., & Koenen, K. C. (2014). Women's experiences of abuse in childhood and their children's smoking and overweight. *American Journal of Preventive Medicine, 46*, 249–258. doi:10.1016/j.amepre.2013.11.012.

Rosenman, S. (2002). Trauma and posttraumatic stress disorder in Australia: Findings in the population sample of the Australian National Survey on Health and Wellbeing. *Australian and New Zealand Journal of Psychiatry, 36*, 515–520. doi:10.1046/j.1440-1614.2002.01039.x.

Saxe, G., Stoddard, F., Chawla, N., Lopez, C. G., Hall, E., Sheridan, R., King, D., & King, L. (2005). Risk factors for acute stress disorder in children with burns. *Journal of Trauma and Dissociation, 6*, 37–49. doi:10.1300/J229v06n02_05.

Scott, K. M., Koenen, K. C., Aguilar-Gaxiola, S., Alonso, J., Angermeyer, M. C., Benjet, C., Bruffaerts, R., Caldas-de-Almeida, J. M., de Girolamo, G., Florescu, S., Iwata, N., Levinson, D., Lim, C. C. W., Murphy, S., Ormel, J., Posada-Villa, J., & Kessler, R. C. (2013). Associations between lifetime traumatic events and subsequent chronic physical conditions: A cross-national, cross-sectional study. *PLoS ONE, 8*, e80573. doi:10.1371/journal.pone.0080573.

Shear, K. M., Jackson, C. T., Essock, S. M., Donahue, S. A., & Felton, C. J. (2006). Screening for complicated grief among Project Liberty service recipients 18 months after September 11, 2001. *Psychiatric Services, 57*, 1291–1297. doi:10.1176/appi.ps.57.9.1291.

Sledjeski, E. M., Speisman, B., & Dierker, L. C. (2008). Does number of lifetime traumas explain the relationship between PTSD and chronic medical conditions? Answers from the National Comorbidity Study-Replication (NCS-R). *Journal of Behavioral Medicine, 31*, 341–349. doi:10.1007/s10865-008-9158-3.

Smith, T. C., Ryan, M. A. K., Wingard, D. L., Slymen, D. J., Sallis, J. F., & Kritz-Silverstein, D. (2008). New onset and persistent symptoms of post-traumatic stress disorder self reported after deployment and combat exposures: Prospective population based US military cohort study. *British Medical Journal, 336*, 366–371. doi:10.1136/bmj.39430.638241.AE.

Soosay, I., Silove, D., Bateman-Steel, C., Steel, Z., Bebbington, P., Jones, P. B., Chey, T., Ivancic, L., & Marnane, C. (2012). Trauma exposure, PTSD and psychotic-like symptoms in post-conflict Timor Leste: An epidemiological survey. *BMC Psychiatry, 12*, 229. doi:10.1186/1471-244X-12-229.

Sorenson, S. B. (2002). Preventing traumatic stress: Public health approaches. *Journal of Traumatic Stress, 15*, 3–7. doi:10.1023/A:1014381925423.

Steenkamp, M. M., Dickstein, B. D., Salters-Pedneault, K., Hofmann, S. G., & Litz, B. T. (2012). Trajectories of PTSD symptoms following sexual assault: Is resilience the modal outcome? *Journal of Traumatic Stress, 25*, 469–474. doi:10.1002/jts.21718.

Stein, M. B., Höfler, M., Perkonigg, A., Lieb, R., Pfister, H., Maercker, A., & Wittchen, H.-U. (2002). Patterns of incidence and psychiatric risk factors for traumatic events. *International Journal of Methods in Psychiatric Research, 11*, 143–153. doi:10.1002/mpr.132.

Stein, D. J., Koenen, K. C., Friedman, M. J., Hill, E., McLaughlin, K., Petukhova, M., Ruscio, A. M., Shahly, V., Spiegel, D., Borges, G., Bunting, B., Caldas-de-Almeida, J. M., de Girolamo, G., Demyttenaere, K., Florescu, S., Haro, J. M., Karam, E. G., Kovess-Masfety, V., Lee, S., Matschinger, H., Mladenova, M., Posada-Villa, J., Tachimori, H., Viana, M. C., & Kessler, R. C. (2013). Dissociation in posttraumatic stress disorder: Evidence from the World Mental Health Surveys. *Biological Psychiatry, 73*, 302–312. doi:10.1016/j.biopsych.2012.08.022.

Storr, C. L., Ialongo, N. S., Anthony, J. C., & Breslau, N. (2007). Childhood antecedents of exposure to traumatic events and posttraumatic stress disorder. *American Journal of Psychiatry, 164*, 119–125. doi:10.1176/appi.ajp.164.1.119.

Van Ameringen, M., Mancini, C., Patterson, B., & Boyle, M. H. (2008). Post-traumatic stress disorder in Canada. *CNS Neuroscience & Therapeutics, 14*, 171–181. doi:10.1111/j.1755-5949.2008.00049.x.

Weich, S., McBride, O., Hussey, D., Exeter, D., Brugha, T., & McManus, S. (2011). Latent class analysis of co-morbidity in the Adult Psychiatric Morbidity Survey in England 2007: Implications for DSM-V and ICD-11. *Psychological Medicine, 41*, 2201–2212. doi:10.1017/S0033291711000249.

World Health Organization. (2011). *Global burden of mental disorders and the need for a comprehensive, coordinated response from health and social sectors at the country level.* Retrieved from http://apps.who.int/gb/ebwha/pdf_files/EB130/B130_9-en.pdf

Yahav, R., & Cohen, M. (2007). Symptoms of acute stress in Jewish and Arab Israeli citizens during the Second Lebanon War. *Social Psychiatry and Psychiatric Epidemiology, 42*, 830–836. doi:10.1007/s00127-007-0237-5.

Zlotnick, C., Johnson, J., Kohn, R., Vicente, B., Rioseco, P., & Saldivia, S. (2008). Childhood trauma, trauma in adulthood, and psychiatric diagnoses: Results from a community sample. *Comprehensive Psychiatry, 49*, 163–169. doi:10.1016/j.comppsych.2007.08.007.

Psychological and Social Theories of PTSD

3

Mirjam J. Nijdam and Lutz Wittmann

3.1 Introduction

Psychological theories have been developed to explain why certain trauma survivors go on to develop PTSD and others do not. These theories try to capture what happens at the level of the trauma survivor's personal experiences, in terms of thoughts, memory, emotions, behaviours, and underlying processes of which the person is unaware. Symptoms of PTSD in DSM-5 include recurrent involuntary and intrusive memories of the trauma, flashbacks that make the person feel like he or she is experiencing the trauma again, inability to recall key features of the trauma, and impaired concentration (American Psychiatric Association 2013). Because these symptoms are linked to memory functioning and the way the trauma is processed, PTSD has been termed a disorder of memory by various theorists (Brewin 2003; McNally 2003; van der Kolk 2007). Trauma-focused psychotherapies could also be called memory-focused psychotherapy for PTSD, because patient and therapist work with the memory of the trauma (Grey and Holmes 2008).

Psychological theories are also essential to understanding the working mechanisms of psychological treatments for PTSD. It can sound quite counterintuitive that imaginal exposure to the traumatic memory works, as some memory theories predict that repeated exposure to a memory would only strengthen it (f.i. Crowder 1976). In the first part of this chapter, we will successively focus on theories of fear

M.J. Nijdam (✉)
Department of Psychiatry, Center for Psychological Trauma, Academic Medical Center at the University of Amsterdam, Meibergdreef 5, 1105 AZ Amsterdam, The Netherlands
e-mail: m.j.nijdam@amc.uva.nl

L. Wittmann
International Psychoanalytic University Berlin, Stromstraße 3, 10555 Berlin, Germany
e-mail: lutz.wittmann@ipu-berlin.de

© Springer International Publishing Switzerland 2015
U. Schnyder, M. Cloitre (eds.), *Evidence Based Treatments for Trauma-Related Psychological Disorders: A Practical Guide for Clinicians*,
DOI 10.1007/978-3-319-07109-1_3

conditioning, dual representation theory, cognitive theory and 'hotspots', and psychodynamic theories. We will first discuss the most important concepts used by these theories and then focus on their accounts of natural recovery from PTSD and their proposed working mechanisms for psychological treatments. In the second part of this chapter, we will outline PTSD from a societal perspective and discuss the most important ideas in this realm. Case examples will provide illustrations of important concepts of these theories.

3.2 Fear Conditioning Theories

The overarching idea of these theories is that a traumatic event is stored in a way that hinders the person's recovery from the trauma and from PTSD. This can, for instance, be apparent in recollections of the trauma that keep the person from maintaining his or her daily routines and vivid nightmares from which the person awakens, reducing the individually necessary amount of sleep the person needs. In the elementary version of these theories, two processes were hypothesized in the process that led to PTSD symptoms after having experienced a traumatic event. Mowrer's two-factor theory (1960) assumes that these processes play a role in all anxiety disorders, and this theory has been further elaborated for PTSD by Keane and colleagues (1985). A classical conditioning process is hypothesized to be crucial in the *development* of PTSD. This classical conditioning process holds that previously neutral stimuli present at the time of the traumatic event (conditioned stimuli, such as the tunnel where an accident happened) become fear-laden through their coupling with the trauma, for instance, the accident itself (termed the unconditioned stimulus). When a person encounters a conditioned stimulus such as the tunnel again, it would evoke the memory of, for instance, the car that was shred to pieces and the people who were severely wounded in the accident. An operant conditioning process is proposed to be responsible for the *maintenance* of the PTSD symptoms in the longer run. This operant conditioning process would involve people avoiding thinking about or being reminded of the traumatic event, because this memory is painful and evokes anxiety and tension. Avoiding the fear-conditioned stimuli or thinking of the incident itself in one's mind would be reinforced by a short-term decrease of fear or even the absence of fear and tension. One can imagine how this may be for an accident survivor who may want to avoid the tunnel in which the accident took place altogether or try to block the thoughts of the traumatic incident when it is necessary to drive through the tunnel because he has no other option. However, such avoidance would make the person even more anxious and tense to think of the traumatic event in the future and thus reinforce the fear responses in the long run.

Lang's theory (1979, 1985) assumes that frightening events are stored in a broader cognitive framework and that they are represented within memory as interconnections between nodes in an associative network. These networks function as a kind of prototypes for recognizing and coping with meaningful situations. Three types of information were proposed: stimulus information about the trauma, such as sights and sounds, information about the emotional and physiological response to the event, and meaning information (most importantly about the degree of threat). These nodes are interconnected, so if the person encounters one sort of information belonging to the traumatic event, the other modes of information would be activated automatically. As soon as sufficient elements of the network are activated, the whole network of fear is activated together with the subjective experience and the corresponding behaviours. Lang proposes that fearful memories are easily activated by ambiguous stimuli, which are in some respect similar to the content of the original anxiety-provoking memory. PTSD may then be explained as a permanent activation of the fear network because of the very tight connections in this kind of fear network and the very strong emotional and physiological responses. Knowledge about the traumatic experience can change by strengthening associations between a certain emotional network and other incompatible networks. If the above-mentioned accident survivor approaches many tunnels and experiences that physiological responses such as panic do not occur, this response is incompatible with anxiety and avoidance.

Foa's emotional processing theory (1989, 1998) draws on these principles but emphasizes that the representation of traumatic events in memory is different from that of 'normal' events. An assumption made by this theory is that traumatic events violate the basic concepts of safety that people hold. A central concept in this theory is the *fear network*, the cognitive representation of fear that includes both emotional reactions and ongoing beliefs about threats in the environment. Foa and colleagues hypothesize that activation of one node (the place of the accident) would automatically and selectively evoke the fear node and behavioural and physiological responses (such as sweating and heart palpitations) that coincide with very frightening events. Activation of the fear network could be caused by a large number of environmental cues and would have a low threshold to be activated. A person with PTSD would notice this activation in terms of hypervigilance to trauma cues, information of the traumatic experience entering consciousness and re-experiencing parts of it, having very strong physiological responses when being reminded of the trauma, and attempting to avoid and suppress intrusions. Updates to this theory have focused on the role of pre-trauma views and vulnerability for PTSD as well as negative appraisals of responses and behaviours which could exacerbate the perception of incompetence (Foa and Rothbaum 1998; Brewin and Holmes 2003; Foa et al. 2007). Pre-trauma views that are more rigid (either rigid positive views or rigid negative views) would lead to increased vulnerability for PTSD. Rigid positive views about the self as extremely competent and the world as extremely safe would be contradicted by the trauma. Rigid negative views about the self as extremely incompetent and the world as extremely dangerous would be confirmed by the traumatic event. These rigid negative beliefs (or the shattering of the positive ones) make a person likely to interpret many situations or people as harmful and overgeneralize danger. Emphasis is also placed on beliefs present before, during, and after the trauma, which may lead to negative appraisal of one's reactions to the trauma and exacerbation of feeling incompetent or feeling very much in danger.

Foa and Rothbaum (1998) further suggest that trauma memories can be reactivated and changed by incorporating new information. Natural recovery would mean that this fearful memory would be integrated with the rest of a person's memories, and the overly strong reactions need to be weakened for this. This could be achieved by repeated exposure to the fearful places and memories and by integrating information that is inconsistent with the fearful character of the acquired traumatic memory (for instance, driving through the same tunnel and not being in an accident). Foa et al. (1989) assume that PTSD will persist if this exposure to all the fearful elements of the memory does not take place sufficiently or long enough for anxiety to habituate. In that case, only some associations are weakened and others stay intact. Excessive arousal or thinking errors and simply the strong tendency to avoid re-exposure are examples of ways in which this process does not take place in an optimal fashion. Trauma survivors may then continue to believe that the world is threatening.

The treatment method that is rooted in this theory, prolonged exposure therapy (Foa and Rothbaum 1998; Foa et al. 2007), has proven to be very effective and is recommended in various treatment guidelines as treatment of choice for PTSD (NICE 2005; Foa et al. 2008). Repeated exposure to the trauma memory is applied in this treatment with the aim of achieving fear extinction. For emotional processing to occur, Foa and colleagues think that it is essential that survivors are emotionally engaged with their traumatic memories, that they articulate and organize their chaotic experience, and that they learn to develop a balanced view of the world – to come to believe that the world is not a terrible place, despite the trauma (Foa and Riggs 1995; Foa and Street 2001). Effective processing changes the unrealistic associations and erroneous cognitions are corrected (Foa et al. 2007).

Case Example
A woman who had survived a plane crash in which the airplane was set on fire during landing was very frightened to fly again. For her work, she used to fly every week and she tried to continue to do this, but she panicked the moment the doors closed for take-off and urgently asked to get out. She spoke with pilots who were very understanding and said that they would never fly again if they had experienced what she had been through. This reinforced her fear of flying. Repeated exposure to the memory of what had happened and repeated focusing on the details of the worst moments of the crash in which she thought she was going to die reduced the anxiety that this memory evoked in her. This helped her overcome her fear of stepping into a plane, and she noticed that the panic reactions subsided after the take-off and after the landing.

3.3   Dual Representation Theory

Dual representation theory of PTSD (Brewin et al. 1996, 2010; Brewin 2008) assumes that there are two kinds of memory representations that play a role in PTSD. In this model, the flashbacks experienced by PTSD patients are assumed to be the consequence of the enhanced encoding of certain aspects of the traumatic event called sensation-near representations (S-reps). In earlier versions of the theory, these were called situationally accessible memory (SAM) to emphasize that these aspects can automatically be activated by triggers that the person encounters. This explains why a PTSD patient with flashbacks of being stabbed with a knife feels as if the trauma is occurring in the present, because the memory is primarily sensory and lacks a spatial and temporal context. This memory representation contains information that has not yet been processed by higher cognitive functions, but consists of information coming from lower perceptual processes and the direct autonomic and sensorimotor responses of the person. They are assumed to be processed in parts of the brain that are specialized for action in the environment, specifically the dorsal visual stream, insula, and amygdala. The information is closely and directly connected to the traumatic event itself and with the strong emotional reactions of the person when it happened. In case of the survivor of the stabbing incident, these memories would for instance be very much coupled to pain in the place where the knife once entered the survivor's body. Moreover, the model assumes that there is an impaired encoding of the material in parallel contextualized representations (C-reps). In earlier versions of the theory, these were termed the verbally accessible memory system (VAM) to indicate that the person had consciously processed these parts of information and could communicate about these with other people. Contextualized representations are assumed to be processed in the ventral visual stream and in the medial temporal lobe. Personal meanings, implications, and consequences of the traumatic event have been thought through, and an association has been made with previous and other experiences about which knowledge is present in the autobiographical memory. These representations could inhibit the re-experiencing symptoms but function poorly in PTSD. Retrieving material from the contextualized representations can be the result of a conscious search strategy ('where was I at the time of the stabbing incident, and with whom?') but also be automatically activated by cues that remind the person of an incident. Because attention is very focused on danger and survival in case of a traumatic event and because this coincides with high arousal, the contents of the contextualized representations will be limited.

According to Brewin (2008), this preferential encoding in PTSD may be a product of peri-traumatic dissociation reactions and the prefrontal cortex temporarily going 'off-line' in response to a level of stress that exceeds the person's coping. Flashbacks would then provide an initially adaptive pathway to natural recovery. They are an opportunity to encode the information that is lacking into contextualized representations and strengthen connections between C-reps and S-reps, to create a new memory representation of the traumatic event with a spatial and temporal context. The awareness that the trauma has happened in the past would then also decrease the need for sensory memories in response to trauma cues. Dual representation theory suggests that the process of re-encoding from S-reps to C-reps does not take place in PTSD, leading to persistent and intense flashbacks and nightmares and to a poorly functioning verbal memory.

Dual representation theory also offers explanations for how trauma-focused cognitive behavioural therapy could work (Brewin 2005). Brewin assumes that trauma treatment involves both the image-based S-reps and the more verbally oriented

C-reps. According to this theory, a form of imaginal exposure reduces re-experiencing symptoms, and cognitive restructuring techniques target beliefs that the person has about himself or herself and the world. When the trauma survivor deliberately maintains attention on the content of the flashbacks and no longer tries to avoid them, information that is only present in the S-reps is presumed to be re-encoded in C-reps, and connections between S-reps and C-reps are strengthened. Trauma survivors will then be able to place their memory in the past and to recognize that the threat is no longer present. This reduces the flashbacks and nightmares and thereby leads to PTSD symptom reduction. The different contents of memory representations and the re-encoding during treatment can be recognized in the following case example.

Case Example
A nurse was attacked by a patient at a mental health admission facility. The bathroom door of the patient's room had been left open by colleagues, but this had not been communicated to her. The access to the bathroom caused the psychotic patient to be within reach of an aftershave bottle, which he had destroyed. He used the broken bottle to stab her in the face when she entered his room to check on him. He entered into a fight with her. He was huge and she was not strong enough to resist him. She felt like she was left to her fate and that he would kill her. This incident had left a scar on her cheek and nose, which reminded her of the dangerous situation she had been in. In the exposure treatment, she remembered two parts of the trauma story again that she had forgotten about. One part was the moment that she was able to press her emergency pager. She realized that she had been able to actively cope with the situation and that this had made her colleagues rush to the room and prevent worse things from happening. The other part she remembered in an exposure session was the moment her colleagues gathered around her and she first realized what had happened. She remembered that one of her female colleagues held her and this made her cry in the session, which had not happened since the incident. Later, she also realized that the patient had a severe mental condition and that the attacker's victim could have been anyone; she was no specific target. This mitigated the pain she felt over the scars. When she was confronted with the patient in court, she realized that he was a normal-sized man contrary to what she thought she had seen before.

3.4 Cognitive Theory and 'Hotspots' in Trauma Narratives

3.4.1 Cognitive Theory of PTSD

Some emotional responses of trauma survivors depend on cognitive appraisal. Cognitive factors, such as expectancies and the individual's amount of control over the situation, have been elaborated by Ehlers and Clark (2000) in their model of PTSD. They propose that experiencing extreme stress, which depends on the person's appraisal of the threat, is an essential factor in the occurrence of acute stress reactions, which display emotional, behavioural, and biological effects. Failure to effectively regulate this acute reaction may result in an ongoing dysregulation, which may ultimately lead to posttraumatic stress symptoms. Ehlers and Clark describe that pathological responses to traumatic events occur when the trauma survivor processes the trauma in a way that produces a sense of current threat. This sense of current threat can be outward-focused to an external source of threat (for instance, that a trauma survivor feels that she cannot trust other people's actions) or inward-focused as an internal threat to the self and the future (e.g. when a trauma survivor feels that her body has been ruined forever by a sexual assault). Negative appraisals about danger, violations of boundaries, and loss are thought to be responsible for the range of emotions experienced by trauma survivors with PTSD.

Trauma survivors with PTSD can thus experience an ongoing sense of threat either because they fear that the trauma will recur or because they believe they are not able to cope with their emotions. Furthermore, the nature of the trauma memory itself is different from that of an ordinary memory. Therefore, another possible reason for the ongoing sense of threat is that the trauma memory is inadequately integrated with the person's broader autobiographical memories and beliefs. This means that the person has the feeling that a traumatic event will occur more frequently, that another robbery will take place or that another plane crash will occur. Situations that are in some respect similar to the traumatic event may evoke a strong sense of threat. This usually happens in an unintentional, cue-driven manner. Similarly to Brewin's dual representation theory, Ehlers and Clark describe that the memory of the trauma is poorly elaborated and does not have sufficient context in terms of time and place. An important distinction in Ehlers and Clark's theory is the difference between data-driven and conceptual processing. Data-driven processing is focused on sensory information, and conceptual processing on the meaning of the situation, organizing the information, and placing it in the appropriate context. According to Ehlers and Clark, conceptual processing facilitates integration of the trauma memory with autobiographical knowledge, whereas data-driven processing leads to perceptual priming and difficulty to retrieve the trauma memory intentionally. Flashbacks in this model are presumed to be the result of enhanced perceptual priming, which is a reduced perceptual threshold for trauma-related stimuli.

Ehlers and Clark also identified many coping strategies that play an important role in the onset and maintenance of PTSD. Behavioural coping strategies include active attempts to suppress unwanted thoughts, use of alcohol and medication to control one's feelings, seeking distraction, avoidance of trauma reminders, and adoption of safety behaviours. Cognitive coping strategies that play a role are persistent rumination, dissociation, and selective attention to threat cues.

Case Examples

- Several aspects of Ehlers and Clark's model can be illustrated by the example of politicians under terrorist threat who have to live under strict protective measures (Nijdam et al. 2008, 2010). Politicians who received death threats and viewed them as not serious or not dangerous were almost free from stress reactions, whereas the politicians who took them very seriously had more stress responses and were disturbed by their responses to the situation. Their own assessment of the danger or threat proved to be very important in whether stress reactions occurred or not. Experiencing the situation as high risk or being extremely alert to signals that could indicate danger reinforced their perception of being under threat. Furthermore, some politicians also indicated that they suddenly started suspecting that people with a certain appearance were planning a terrorist attack, without having any real evidence for such a suspicion.

- An explicit form of negative appraisal is the concept of mental defeat, defined by Ehlers and colleagues (2000) as 'the perceived loss of all autonomy, a state of giving up in one's own mind all efforts to retain one's identity as a human being with a will of one's own'. The inability to influence one's own fate is a risk factor for very negative self-appraisals. After several life-threatening car accidents with permanent damage to his back and knees and after the crib death of his daughter, a trauma survivor expressed that he now felt 'as if the system is broken'. He was afraid that the stress of these accidents had been too much for his body to bear and that he would totally break down. Stressful years at work and in private life added to this perception. When he was paged for his work in case of an emergent dike burst, this triggered recollections of the accidents. When he encountered the sentence 'It is not safe to live' in a book, he noticed that he completely agreed with this statement and this frightened him very much.

3.4.2 'Hotspots' in Trauma Narratives

Ehlers and Clark developed cognitive therapy for PTSD, which is a highly effective treatment (Bradley et al. 2005). In this therapy, negative appraisals and cognitions are investigated and replaced by appraisals and cognitions that are more adaptive. Ehlers and colleagues also continued to study intrusive memories and found that these mainly represented stimuli that were present shortly before the moments of the trauma with the greatest emotional impact (Ehlers et al. 2002). They called these stimuli 'warning signals', because they alert the person to danger if encountered again. These stimuli are logically connected with a sense of current threat and are often re-experienced. Ehlers and colleagues (2004) developed a therapeutic strategy in which the intrusions lead the therapist to the moments with the greatest emotional impact, also called 'hotspots'. In trauma-focused cognitive behavioural therapy, they assume that it is essential to focus on hotspots and change their meaning, in order to lead to a decrease in PTSD symptoms.

It is interesting to note that cognitive behavioural therapies of PTSD have seen this condition primarily as an anxiety disorder and much attention has been directed to optimal treatment of anxiety responses. The first case series on hotspots were important, because they showed that a range of emotions are often associated with these peak emotional moments in the trauma story. Anger, grief, shame, and guilt were shown to often be associated with hotspots (Grey et al. 2001, 2002), next to the typical emotional responses of anxiety, helplessness, or horror. This led Ehlers and colleagues (Ehlers et al. 2004) to believe that imaginal exposure functions not only to ensure emotional habituation but to identify the hotspots in the trauma story and use these as a starting point for cognitive restructuring. By this combination of techniques, new information can be added while reliving the trauma memory, which reduces the level of current threat. This technique was also elaborated by Grey and colleagues (2002), who, in an elegant way, combined imaginal exposure and cognitive restructuring for the broad spectrum of the emotions they found in hotspots. The way hotspots are addressed in imaginal exposure may be important for symptom reduction in trauma-focused psychotherapy (Nijdam et al. 2013).

3.5   Psychoanalytical Theory

Psychoanalytical theories on traumatic experiences have a long history. Already at the very beginning of psychoanalytic thinking about 120 years ago, Freud and his mentor Breuer (1895/1987) tried to reconstruct the essence of psychotrauma. They assumed that memories resisting abreaction by expression of the related emotions (catharsis) could not be further psychically processed. They considered two reasons responsible for such a development. In the first case, the nature of the traumatic event, social conditions, or a personal motive of the affected person stimulated repression of the event. In the second case, the event occurred during a hypnoid or dissociative state (e.g. paralysing affects, hypnagogic states, autohypnosis) hindering the person from adequate psychic reaction to the event. Here, the influence of the French school of Charcot and Janet is, of course, easily recognizable (c.f. Kudler 2012). As a consequence of these processes, the traumatic event resulted in isolated rather than integrated memory traces. Freud's later approach (1920/1955) was based on the psychophysiology of that time conceptualizing mental processes in energetic terms, a perspective that fascinated Freud throughout his life. He assumed that during trauma, large quantities of excitation originating from external stimuli overwhelm the psychic system. In order to stabilize, the psychic system would be forced to engage in potentially endless repetitive cycles until the trauma was successfully mastered.

Since that time, a vast number of psychoanalytic publications have complemented or changed the very early perspectives on trauma. It appears hardly possible to give a comprehensive summary of all relevant aspects. Neither are there a limited number of trauma theories which could be considered psychoanalytic mainstream.

Nevertheless, several key aspects can be identified. For the present purpose, we will highlight three central topics of psychodynamic reflection on psychotrauma:

- Trauma is not an event but a subjective experience.
- Parts of the personality shaped by previous interpersonal experiences may limit an individual's tolerance for processing potentially traumatic experiences.
- Trauma is a process with social dimensions.

3.5.1   Trauma as a Subjective Experience

Trauma refers to diverse and complex processes. This is already obvious from the different types of traumatic events trauma therapists are confronted with. However, the endless variety of possible traumatic events is only one reason for this complexity. A second factor lies within trait and state factors related to the trauma victim. Even if two persons would develop PTSD after the same event (e.g. an accident), their behaviours, thoughts, and feelings during the accident as well as later memories, ways of processing them, individual symptoms, and required steps for improvement may differ fundamentally.

Considering the interaction between event, personality, and current life context, it becomes evident why psychoanalysts stress that trauma may best be referred to not as an event, but rather as a subjective experience. As early as 1954, Mitscherlich (1954) emphasized the importance of dismantling the trauma of its 'false objectivity' (p. 565, own translation) and to put it into a dynamic relation with the injured being. This subjective approach requires clinicians not to be seduced by the striking traumatic nature of an event but to engage together with the patient into a detailed analysis of the meaning of the event. Clinical experience shows that the most harmful impact of an experience does not always coincide with the moment of highest objective danger or injury. For instance, the most painful memory of a child's sexual abuse by a stepfather may not refer to the moments of rape but to the discovery that the child's mother pretended not to notice anything. The traumatizing potential of an experience may not be rooted only in the event itself. Rather, the relation between the event and previous life experiences, current life topics, or values needs to be considered. Some examples may illustrate this:

- An experience of victimization by adolescent hooligans may exert its pathogenic impact not only through the injuries suffered or the momentary experience of helplessness alone. Rather, this event may become associated with earlier experiences of being bullied by schoolmates. The incidence might be interpreted as proving that the victim will never be able to be safe from hatred by social groups.
- Of course we all understand that surviving an accident during which one's partner was killed can cause posttraumatic stress and feelings of guilt. Such feelings could easily be understood as survivor guilt. However, in one case, an extensive analysis of the meaning of the event showed that the not yet communicated

decision to separate from this partner caused the feelings of guilt and prevented the patient from elaborating the trauma.

- Not having been able to prevent the death of one's child during a civil war may destroy the self-perception of being a reliable parent. Processes such as these were identified by Abraham (1920/1955) who described how trauma can destroy the illusory belief in one's invulnerability (compare Janoff-Bulman 1992, for a more recent comprehensive version of this theory).
- Even in one of the most extreme forms of trauma – torture – individual psycho-logical aspects appear to be of significance. For instance, Basoglu et al. (1997) reported that political activists suffered from lower degrees of posttraumatic stress and other psychopathology as compared to non-activists, even when they were more severely tortured.

In summary, trauma is not (only) an event but a subjective experience. In addition to the objective characteristics of an event, the subjective meaning of its experience can reveal clinically important information. The huge variability in the number of traumatic events necessary for an individual person to develop posttraumatic stress disorder (PTSD) is in line with this argument (e.g. Neuner et al. 2004).

3.5.2   Significance of the Personality in the Posttraumatic Process

Interpersonal experiences are a crucial factor influencing development of psychic structures and personality. Acquisition of language, meaning, or cultural stances takes place in interpersonal situations. All these interactions leave their traces. According to Kernberg (e.g. Clarkin et al. 2006) the building blocks of psychologi-cal structures include a self-representation, a representation of another person (called 'object representation'), and an affect linking the two of them. Due to their impact on the development of psychic structures and personality, consequences of interaction experiences are present throughout a person's entire life, even if their interpersonal nature may not be remembered. For instance, a person may have grown up in a family emphasizing excellent performance (e.g. only the best results in school, sports, etc.) as a condition for attention, confirmation, and love. In conse-quence, the person may hold ambition as a central and personal value. An underly-ing representation could be himself or herself after a low school grade and a contemptuous father, linked by the emotion of shame. The interpersonal experi-ences which led to his or her ambitious character may or may not be remembered. For the following, it is important to keep in mind that the psychic structures underly-ing personality represent interpersonal experiences. They influence later percep-tions, interpretations, and behaviours in interpersonal situations but are active also when one is alone.

One of the key features of PTSD is the oscillation between re-experiencing and avoidance of traumatic memories. The theory of Horowitz (1986) describes how trauma survivors can experience the need to integrate new information accompanying the traumatic experience, but at the same time, the information is warded off as provoking 'too much emotional response' (p. 100). This causes an alternating pattern between reliving (promoting the processing of the information) and avoiding (protecting the person by suppressing the threatening information). According to Horowitz, a stagnation of this process leads to persistent posttraumatic stress symptoms. Understanding why the processing of the traumatic memory is avoided is thus of importance. Here, the impact of the personality as shaped by interpersonal experiences needs to be considered. Why does this individual person I am working with in psychotherapy try to avoid remembering the trauma? On the first view, this may appear to be a trivial question with an obvious answer. For instance, a patient will describe fear of overwhelming emotions by answering 'Because it is painful and I can't bear so much pain'. This is, however, an answer from a one-person-psychology perspective (Gill 1982). Let us remember that interpersonal experiences have shaped this person and thus reconsider from a two-person-psychology perspective (Gill 1982).

Consider, for example, that a patient is retelling one part of the traumatic event but without any signs of emotions. And let us assume that this patient – if more involved – would become sad or angry. Are there interpersonal reasons that the patient does not start to cry or speak in an angry tone? In the history of this patient, there may have been experiences such as being rejected, punished, or ignored in response to such expressions. For instance, one patient was laughed at by her father and ignored by her mother when trying to make them aware of the violations by her uncle. Another patient mentioned that his older brothers made fun of him each time he showed any signs of weakness (e.g. crying). Although psychoanalysis assumes that the present situation is influenced by the consequences of such previous experiences, they are not necessarily the primary focus of treatment. Previous experiences are of therapeutic significance to the extent that they influence the here and now. They can be approached in the here and now by emphasizing the interpersonal character of the present situation. The therapist can offer himself or herself as the one hindering the perception or communication of the conflicting emotion. Identification of how the therapist is perceived by the patient is needed. For instance, the patient may expect not to be accepted as a 'real man' anymore when crying or as 'too dangerous' when showing aggressions. By re-establishing a two-person-psychology perspective on avoidance, relevant interpersonal patterns can be identified. The steps necessary for dissolving such patterns vary interindividually. Typically, joint identification of the pattern and consideration of its protective function for the therapeutic relationship (e.g. not experiencing/showing anger in order not to frighten the therapist who may otherwise abandon the patient) would be among the first steps.

Bowlby (1969/1982), the originator of attachment theory, proposed the idea that the first interpersonal relationship was the dyad between the child and caretaker which operated to keep the child safe and help him or her survive during the first precarious years of life. The child develops a cognitive-affective or psychic structure which Bowlby termed 'a working model' of the contingencies which kept the relationship with the caretaker going well and therefore the child 'safe'. Bowlby extended the concept of 'working models' as applicable to all important relationships including parents, peers, and spouses. The working model for each included assumptions about the emotions, behaviours, and interactions with the other person that are necessary to maintain the relationship. The models are used to guide behaviours in new situations or with new relationships and are particularly important and 'activated' in times of stress or trauma.

From an attachment point of view, the patient in the above examples is behaving with the therapist in a way consistent with a 'working model' from his past as means by which to keep the therapist engaged. The patient will not show anger in the belief that this is necessary to keep the therapist's attention. Alternatively, a patient will expect the therapist to ignore the importance of the event and may, therefore, himself dismiss its importance and talk little about it or with little affect. In this interpersonal model, part of recovery from trauma includes the therapist helping the patient realize that individuals in his present life will not necessarily have the same reactions to his pain as he is expecting based on his past experiences. In attachment-based interventions, the therapeutic task is not necessarily to dismiss the old 'working models' but rather to present to the patient the opportunity to create a new relational model where the patient can express alternative behaviours and emotions (anger, sadness) and where the relationship (in this particular case, with the therapist) will be maintained and the patient will survive and perhaps even thrive.

In order to adapt an interpersonal pattern to be more flexible, it may be necessary to work through it at many occasions during treatment and in daily life. Thus the therapeutic work includes the patients' expectations about how the therapist would react to their way of dealing with the trauma. One occasion for addressing this issue is when the patient's 'working model' becomes obvious by the difference between expected and actual reactions of the therapist. The therapist would then, for instance, acknowledge how difficult it must be to work through the trauma memory when he needs to be afraid of the therapist's reaction to any emotion he may show. Of course, the therapist could skip this work and convince a patient of the necessity to confront the memory, which may be a faster solution. However, doing this because the therapist as an expert told the person to do so may miss the opportunity for personal development or of recognizing and leaving behind repeated interpersonal patterns related to the traumatic experience. In one case, a patient got into a traumatic situation after listening to ill advice (to walk at night in a dangerous area because it was 'such a lovely night') against his own feelings. It turned out that this man expected others to tell him what to do, in the context of therapy as well as in other contexts. Any directive approach may be at risk to repeat the patient's working model which preceded the traumatic situation. The approach of loosening entrenched interpersonal patterns in order to enable the individual to confront the trauma in his or her way complements the repertoire for therapeutic decisions. The strong focus on personality development may also help to avoid future traumatization due to preventing behaviours related to the risk of re-traumatization or by enhancing the individual's resilience.

As mentioned above, emphasizing interindividual differences (e.g. developmental history, personality traits and current states, social environment) makes it hardly possible to develop one trauma definition covering all possible constellations. *One* possible definition derived from the preceding discussion could be: an event becomes traumatic when the trauma victim does not feel free to perceive and/or express the subjective experience as this would bring him or her into a position which needs to be avoided as judged on the basis of previous interaction experiences. Therefore, the memory or parts of it cannot be worked through and be integrated into general memory structures.

3.5.3 Trauma as a Process with Social Dimensions

One further psychoanalytic contribution relevant for clinical work with trauma survivors shall be mentioned. The psychoanalyst Keilson performed extensive clinical and scientific work with Dutch Jewish orphans whose parents had been killed in the Holocaust. His theory of sequential traumatization (Keilson 1992) differentiates between three phases in the trauma process: the beginning persecution and terror after the German occupation of the Netherlands, the acute direct persecution (e.g. deportation to a concentration camp), and the post-war period. He observed that experiences and conditions after the liberation from Nazi Germany strongly moderated the effect of the traumas sustained during the previous sequences. His concept has recently been further elaborated including the interaction of social trauma and migration by Becker (2007). From the concept of sequential trauma, we can learn that trauma is best conceptualized not as an event, but an open-ended process. In the case of social trauma, the concept gains an ethical dimension criticizing the replacement of societal responsibility by individual psychopathology by means of our current diagnostic approach (Becker 1995). But even independent of the framework of social trauma in which this concept was developed, it is important to remember that the process of traumatization does not end when the acute trauma phase is concluded. All later experiences in interpersonal contexts – be it on private or societal level, with clinical or legal instances – should not be separated from the trauma process. How others do or do not refer to the traumatic event, posttraumatic symptoms, or personality changes may be as meaningful as public/sociopolitical stances as, for example, conveyed by the media. The significance of the reactions of others in processing traumatic events has been repeatedly supported by empirical evidence (Mueller et al. 2008; Ullman et al. 2007). Furthermore, Belsher et al. (2011) showed that the relationship between social constraints and posttraumatic psychopathology may be partially mediated by negative posttraumatic cognitions. Another example of the application of the interpersonal perspective is the analysis of occurrence of posttraumatic repetitions in the example of dreams (Gardner and Orner 2009; Lansky 1995).

In a sample of severely traumatized inpatients, Lansky observed that posttraumatic nightmares may not occur randomly, but appeared to be related to current social experiences. During the day preceding the posttraumatic dream, '[…] posttraumatic vulnerability is intensified by a narcissistic wound (or many wounds) resulting from some interpersonal failures such as an inability to become emotionally involved or a dissociative episode. *It is from awareness of these interpersonal failures that shame arises as a signal that the patient is cut off from the possibility of meaningful bonding. These patients thus perceive themselves as different from other people and outside of, as well as unworthy of, meaningful attachments'* (Lansky 1995, p. 81, italics in the original). Lansky concludes that the emotion of shame resulting from such interpersonal experiences then triggers the posttraumatic nightmare where it is transformed into fear. This testable hypothesis integrates the perspectives that trauma is a process (rather than an event) with social dimensions which takes place in the present (rather than in the past).

3.6   PTSD from a Societal Perspective

As expressed in the above paragraph, it is important to consider the interpersonal and social perspective in which traumatic events and PTSD symptoms take place. Social comparisons with other people can be an important moderator in this respect as some individuals, for instance, express the opinion that they feel it as 'unfair' that they experienced so many traumatic events compared with others. Moreover, a lack of perceived social support has been demonstrated to increase the risk of developing PTSD after being exposed to a trauma (Ozer et al. 2003). The following case examples illustrate these phenomena:

• A police officer in training on his second day of work was confronted with an arrestee who had not been properly examined and shot himself through the head with a gun that he had hidden beneath his clothes. The police officer vividly remembers many parts of the incident, such as the moment that the arrestee aimed at him with the gun and the moment he shot himself. However, he cannot remember the face of the man, only his angry expression. He increasingly developed PTSD symptoms after this incident and was confronted with many other suicides during his training. His supervisor says that the PTSD symptoms cannot be work related, since he cannot remember the face of the arrestee and therefore doubts whether what he saw was traumatic. The supervisor assumes that the PTSD symptoms originate from earlier experiences in his youth.
• A young mother who has experienced emotional neglect and physical abuse during her childhood recovered from these experiences by means of trauma-focused psychotherapy. This treatment decreased the intrusions of the traumatic experiences considerably. She also noticed that she became more assertive and dared to defend herself and her daughter when being treated in an unfair way. However, her younger stepsister in her country of origin, whom she took care of while still a child, told her that she does not believe that the patient has experienced emotional and physical abuse in her youth. The pictures of the stepsister on Facebook are a continuing slideshow of all the things the patient did not have in her adolescence and that her stepsister takes for granted. This hinders her in her further recovery from her PTSD symptoms.

Recognition of the impact of traumatic events by important others is not only important for the individual trauma survivor but is also connected with the societal views on trauma and PTSD. In this respect, it is interesting to see which factors contributed to the recognition of PTSD in the diagnostic and statistical manual of mental disorders in 1980 (DSM-III; American Psychiatric Association 1980). Historically, much interest has been on soldiers deployed on mission, who dropped out of the deployment as a result of 'shell shock' (Myers 1940) or 'war neurosis' (Kardiner and Spiegel 1947). The symptoms these soldiers displayed bore much resemblance to PTSD symptoms. The recognition of PTSD in the post-Vietnam war era was remarkable, as battle dropout was less frequent than in earlier wars, but delayed stress responses were much more common (Lifton 1973; Figley 1978). A lack of social support may also have contributed to PTSD prevalence rates in Vietnam veterans (Oei et al. 1990), as veterans were often treated with disdain. Another societal development in the 1970s was the revelation of mental health symptoms after child sexual abuse. Feminists warned about the consequences of rape and incest. A third societal development contributing to the formalization of PTSD, especially in Europe and the United States, was the increasing number of people who suffered under the late sequelae of the Second World War (e.g. Withuis 2010). Symptoms resulting from war experiences proved to have important similarities to those resulting from other types of trauma.

Whereas the feminist emphasis on the consequences of unwanted sexual experiences contributed to the recognition of PTSD, the condition became more controversial by subsequent elaborations of this topic in the professional field. During the 1980s, therapists described that adult incest survivors were often reluctant to disclose their abuse to others (e.g. Miller 1997/1979), and toward the end of this decade, this shifted to the belief that many survivors were unable to remember their sexual abuse experiences (McNally 2003). Techniques such as hypnosis and guided imagery exercises were applied to help survivors recover their memories of the sexual experiences, but these methods proved to lead to 'false memories' while increasing the confidence in the survivor that they were genuine (Steblay and Bothwell 1994). McNally (2003) describes similar developments in daycare centres, where odd behaviours of children were seen as signs of sexual abuse, and suggestive interrogations were carried out until the children confessed their abuse. This led to unsubstantiated lawsuits and conviction of alleged abusers in both groups. Similar suggestive therapeutic techniques were applied to war or resistance experiences (e.g. Enning 2009). Professionals increasingly changed their view and left behind suggestive techniques when they became aware of these facts. The professional stance adopted by McNally (2003) and others in the trauma field is that although some traumatic events are only remembered years after their occurrence, events that are experienced as overwhelmingly traumatic rarely slip from awareness. Geraerts et al. (2009) express that some recovered memories of trauma, especially those that do not occur in the context of suggestive therapeutic practices, may be accurate. In a therapeutic context, therapists are not responsible for finding out the absolute truth as proven by evidence in lawsuits but to help patients to the best of their abilities to recover from their mental health conditions.

The sociologist Withuis (2010) describes the changes in ideas about health problems and highlights the importance of considering secondary benefits of symptoms and the concept of premorbidity. Directly after the Second World War, the societal opinion was that someone's health would deteriorate if the symptoms were given too much attention. Because the costs for shell shock patients after the First World War had been much larger than foreseen, European countries like England, France, Germany, Italy, and Austria were cautious about a new cohort of patients with psychogenic illnesses. From 1975 on, the societal opinion had completely turned around, and health problems were seen as arising from a lack of attention. This societal development facilitated recognition of PTSD in the early 1980s. Withuis defines secondary gain, or benefits, as the invalidating effect that results from treating people as ill and discharging them from their daily obligations. The concept of premorbidity refers to the influence of the mental health of the survivor *before* the traumatic experience on the consequences of the trauma later on. Many soldiers and resistance workers of the Second World War filed for a resistance or war pension in the 1970s and 1980s and were awarded the pension without taking into account whether traumatic experiences were causally related to their symptoms. The risk of thinking only in terms of traumatization, Withuis claims, is that it denies the association between person and mental health problem by attributing the cause of the mental health problem solely to the external stressor. In the decades that followed, it gave people an alibi to attribute all kinds of problems to traumatic experiences. Meanwhile, premorbid factors contributing to vulnerability for posttraumatic psychopathology and factors that enhance resilience are investigated in many studies and shape the clinical picture of PTSD. Including the possibility of secondary gains and the role of pre-trauma vulnerability factors in our clinical views remain important.

In sum, in the treatment of trauma survivors with PTSD, it is essential to integrate psychological theories about symptom development, maintenance, and recovery with important moderators in the context of close relationships and societal values. In their socio-interpersonal model of PTSD, Maercker and Horn (2013) distinguish the relevant processes in this respect at the individual level, the level of close relationships, and the distant social level. At the individual level, the social affective processes that occur as the individual interacts with others are specified, such as shame, guilt, and anger. At the second close relationships level, the social support or negative exchange between the trauma survivor and important others takes place. The distant social level of the cultural and societal context encompasses the societal acknowledgment of trauma, collective trauma experiences, and cultural values. Being aware of these processes and taking them into account in treatment, Maerker and Horn argue, will possibly enhance treatment outcome for patients with PTSD.

Conclusion

When trauma survivors develop PTSD, trauma memories are stored in a distinct way that hinders the individual in his or her daily life. Psychological theories have proposed different ways in which the mechanisms underlying the development of PTSD, natural recovery, and the improvement of symptoms during psychotherapy for PTSD can be explained. Some theories focus on fear as the primary emotional network involved, whereas others propose that emotions such as anger, grief, and guilt are equally important. Some theories emphasize the role of negative appraisals of traumatic events or stress responses; others focus on the role of different representations of the trauma memory. The social perspective is also important, as traumatic experiences happen in the context of responses of others and societal views on trauma, and these influence and shape the symptoms of the individual trauma survivor. One common concept in the psychological theories of PTSD is memory, with traumatic events from the past being remembered far too well and decreased concentration on, and capacity for, everyday tasks which do not involve danger. The activation of traumatic memory by trauma-related cues is closely linked to survival and therefore connected to fast stress responses initiated by the amygdala and the secretion of stress hormones, which will be described in detail in the next chapter.

References

Abraham, K. (1921). Symposium on psychoanalysis and the war neurosis held at the fifth international psycho-analytical congress Budapest, September 1918. The International Psycho-Analytical Library, 2, 22-29.

American Psychiatric Association (APA). (1980). *Diagnostic and statistical manual of mental disorders* (3rd ed.). Washington, DC: APA.

American Psychiatric Association (APA). (2013). *Diagnostic and statistical manual of mental disorders* (5th ed.). Washington, DC: APA.

Basoglu, M., Mineka, S., Paker, M., Aker, T., Livanou, M., & Gok, S. (1997). Psychological preparedness for trauma as a protective factor in survivors of torture. *Psychological Medicine, 27*(6), 1421–1433.

Becker, D. (1995). The deficiency of the concept of posttraumatic stress disorder when dealing with victims of human rights violations. In R. Kleber, C. Figley, & B. Gersons (Eds.), *Beyond trauma* (pp. 99–110). New York: Plenum Press.

Becker, D. (2007). *Die Erfindung des Traumas – Verflochtene Geschichten* [The invention of trauma – Twisted stories]. Berlin: Freitag Mediengesellschaft.

Belsher, B. E., Ruzek, J. I., Bongar, B. C., & Cordova, M. J. (2011). Social constraints, posttraumatic cognitions, and posttraumatic stress disorder in treatment-seeking trauma survivors: Evidence for a social-cognitive processing model. *Psychological Trauma: Theory, Research, Practice, and Policy, 2*, 8749. doi:10.3402/ejpt.v2i0.8749.

Bowlby, J. (1969/1982). *Attachment and loss* (Attachment 2nd ed., Vol. 1). New York: Basic Books.

Bradley, R., Greene, J., Russ, E., Dutra, L., & Westen, D. (2005). A multidimensional meta-analysis of psychotherapy for PTSD. *American Journal of Psychiatry, 162*, 214–227.

Brewin, C. R. (2003). *Posttraumatic stress disorder: Malady or myth?* New Haven: Yale University Press.

Brewin, C. R. (2005). Implications for psychological intervention. In J. J. Vasterling & C. R. Brewin (Eds.), *Neuropsychology of PTSD: Biological, cognitive and clinical perspectives* (pp. 271–291). New York: Guilford Press.

Brewin, C. R. (2008). What is it that a neurobiological model of PTSD must explain? *Progress in Brain Research, 167*, 217–228.

Brewin, C. R., & Holmes, E. A. (2003). Psychological theories of posttraumatic stress disorder. *Clinical Psychology Review, 23*, 339–376.

Brewin, C. R., Dalgleish, T., & Joseph, S. (1996). A dual representation theory of posttraumatic stress disorder. *Psychological Review, 103*, 670–686.

Brewin, C. R., Gregory, J. D., Lipton, M., & Burgess, N. (2010). Intrusive images in psychological disorders: Characteristics, neural mechanisms, and treatment implications. *Psychological Review, 117*, 210–232.

Clarkin, J. F., Yeomans, F. E., & Kernberg, O. F. (2006). *Psychotherapy for borderline personality: Focusing on object relations.* Arlington: American Psychiatric Publishing.

Crowder, R. G. (1976). *Principles of learning and memory.* Hillsdale: Erlbaum.

Ehlers, A., & Clark, D. M. (2000). A cognitive model of posttraumatic stress disorder. *Behaviour Research and Therapy, 38*, 319–345.

Ehlers, A., Maercker, A., & Boos, A. (2000). Posttraumatic stress disorder following political imprisonment: The role of mental defeat, alienation, and perceived permanent change. *Journal of Abnormal Psychology, 109*, 45–55.

Ehlers, A., Hackmann, A., Steil, R., Clohessy, S., Wenninger, K., & Winter, H. (2002). The nature of intrusive memories after trauma: The warning signal hypothesis. *Behaviour Research and Therapy, 40*, 995–1002.

Ehlers, A., Hackmann, A., & Michael, T. (2004). Intrusive re-experiencing in post-traumatic stress disorder: Phenomenology, theory and therapy. *Memory, 12*, 403–415.

Enning, B. (2009). *De oorlog van Bastiaans. De LSD-behandeling van het kampsyndroom* [Bastiaans' war. The LSD-treatment of the concentration camp syndrome]. Amsterdam: Augustus.

Figley, C. R. (1978). *Stress disorders among Vietnam veterans.* New York: Brunner/Mazel.

Foa, E. B., & Riggs, D. S. (1995). Posttraumatic stress disorder following assault: Theoretical considerations and empirical findings. *Current Directions in Psychological Science, 5*, 61–65.

Foa, E. B., & Rothbaum, B. O. (1998). *Treating the trauma of rape.* New York: Guilford Press.

Foa, E. B., & Street, G. P. (2001). Women and traumatic events. *Journal of Clinical Psychiatry, 62*, 29–34.

Foa, E. B., Steketee, G., & Rothbaum, B. O. (1989). Behavioral/cognitive conceptualisation of post-traumatic stress disorder. *Behavior Therapy, 20*, 155–176.

Foa, E. B., Hembree, E. A., & Rothbaum, B. O. (2007). *Prolonged exposure therapy for PTSD. Emotional processing of traumatic experiences.* New York: Oxford University Press.

Foa, E. B., Keane, T. M., Friedman, M. J., & Cohen, J. A. (2008). *Effective treatments for PTSD: Practice guidelines from the International Society for Traumatic Stress Studies* (2nd ed.). New York: Guilford Press.

Freud, S. (1920/1955). *Beyond the pleasure principle. The standard edition of the complete psychological works of Sigmund Freud* (Beyond the pleasure principle, group psychology and other works, Vol. XVIII (1920–1922), pp. 1–64). London: Hogarth Press and the Institute of Psycho-Analysis.

Freud, S., & Breuer, J. (1895/1987). *Studien über Hysterie* [Studies on hysteria]. Frankfurt a.M.: S. Fischer.

Gardner, S. E., & Orner, R. J. (2009). Searching for a new evidence base about repetitions. An exploratory survey of patients' experiences of traumatic dreams before, during and after therapy. *Counselling and Psychotherapy Research, 9*(1), 27–32.

Geraerts, E., Lindsay, D. S., Merckelbach, H., Jelicic, M., Raymaekers, L., Arnold, M. M., & Schooler, J. W. (2009). Cognitive mechanisms underlying recovered-memory experiences of childhood sexual abuse. *Psychological Science, 20*, 92–98.

Gill, M. M. (1982). *Analysis of transference* (Theory and technique, Vol. 1). New York: International Universities Press.

Grey, N., & Holmes, E. (2008). "Hotspots" in trauma memories in the treatment of post-traumatic stress disorder: A replication. *Memory, 16*, 788–796.

Grey, N., Holmes, E., & Brewin, C. (2001). Peritraumatic emotional 'hot spots' in memory. *Behavioural and Cognitive Psychotherapy, 29*, 367–372.

Grey, N., Young, K., & Holmes, E. (2002). Cognitive restructuring within reliving: A treatment for emotional 'hotspots' in posttraumatic stress disorder. *Behavioural and Cognitive Psychotherapy, 30*, 37–56.

Horowitz, M. J. (1986). *Stress response syndromes.* New York: Jason Aronson.

Janoff-Bulman, R. (1992). *Shattered assumptions. Towards a new psychology of trauma.* New York: Free Press.

Kardiner, A., & Spiegel, J. (1947). *War, stress, and neurotic illness*. New York: Hoeber.

Keane, T. M., Zimering, R. T., & Caddell, R. T. (1985). A behavioral formulation of PTSD in Vietnam veterans. *Behavior Therapist, 8*, 9–12.

Keilson, H. (1992). Sequential Traumatisation in Children. A clinical and statistical follow-up study on the fate of the Jewish war orphans in the Netherlands. Jerusalem: The Hebrew University Magnes Press.

Kudler, H. (2012). A psychodynamic conceptualization of retraumatization. In M. P. Duckworth & V. M. Follette (Eds.), *Retraumatization: Assessment, treatment, and prevention* (pp. 33–59). New York: Routledge.

Lang, P. J. (1979). A bio-informational theory of emotional imagery. *Journal of Psychophysiology, 16*, 495–512.

Lang, P. J. (1985). The cognitive psychophysiology of emotion: Fear and anxiety. In A. H. Tuma & J. Maser (Eds.), *Anxiety and the anxiety disorders*. Hillsdale: Lawrence Erlbaum Associates.

Lansky, M. R. (1995). *Posttraumatic nightmares: Psychodynamic explorations*. Hillsdale: Analytic Press.

Lifton, R. J. (1973). *Home from the war: Vietnam veterans: Neither victims nor executioners*. New York: Touchstone.

Maercker, A., & Horn, A. B. (2013). A socio-interpersonal perspective on PTSD: The case for environments and interpersonal processes. *Clinical Psychology and Psychotherapy, 20*, 465–481.

McNally, R. J. (2003). *Remembering trauma*. Cambridge, MA: The Belknap Press of Harvard University Press.

Miller, A. (1997/1979). *The drama of the gifted child: The search for the true self* (Rev. ed.). New York: Basic Books.

Mitscherlich, A. (1954). Zur psychoanalytischen Auffassung psychosomatischer Krankheitsentstehung [On the psychoanalytic understanding of psychosomatic pathogenesis]. *Psyche, 7*(10), 561–578.

Mowrer, O. H. (1960). *Learning theory and behavior*. New York: Wiley.

Mueller, J., Moergeli, H., & Maercker, A. (2008). Disclosure and social acknowledgement as predictors of recovery from posttraumatic stress: A longitudinal study in crime victims. *Canadian Journal of Psychiatry, 53*(3), 160–168.

Myers, C. S. (1940). *Shell shock in France*. Cambridge: Cambridge University Press.

National Collaborating Centre for Mental Health (NCCMH). (2005). *Post-traumatic stress disorder (PTSD): The management of PTSD in adults and children in primary and secondary care* (CG 26). http://www.nice.org.uk/guidance/cg26/resources/cg26-posttraumatic-stress-disorder-ptsd-full-guideline-including-appendices-1132.

Neuner, F., Schauer, M., Karunakara, U., Klaschik, C., Robert, C., & Elbert, T. (2004). Psychological trauma and evidence for enhanced vulnerability for posttraumatic stress disorder through previous trauma among West Nile refugees. *BMC Psychiatry, 4*, 34.

Nijdam, M. J., Olff, M., De Vries, M., Martens, W. J., & Gersons, B. P. R. (2008). *Psychosocial effects of threat and protection. Commissioned report for the National Coordinator of Counterterrorism (NCTb)*. Amsterdam: Center for Psychological Trauma, Academic Medical Center at the University of Amsterdam.

Nijdam, M. J., Gersons, B. P. R., & Olff, M. (2010). Dutch politicians' coping with terrorist threat. *British Journal of Psychiatry, 197*, 328–329.

Nijdam, M. J., Baas, M. A. M., Olff, M., & Gersons, B. P. R. (2013). Hotspots in trauma memories and their relationship to successful trauma-focused psychotherapy: A pilot study. *Journal of Traumatic Stress, 26*, 38–44.

Oei, T. P. S., Lim, B., & Hennessy, B. (1990). Psychological dysfunction in battle: Combat stress reactions and posttraumatic stress disorder. *Clinical Psychology Review, 10*, 355–388.

Ozer, E. J., Best, S. R., Lipsey, T. L., & Weiss, D. S. (2003). Predictors of posttraumatic stress disorder and symptoms in adults: A meta-analysis. *Psychological Bulletin, 129*, 52–73.

Steblay, N. M., & Bothwell, R. K. (1994). Evidence for hypnotically refreshed testimony: The view from the laboratory. *Law and Human Behavior, 18*, 635–651.

Ullman, S., Townsend, S., Filipas, H., & Starzynski, L. (2007). Structural models of the relations of assault severity, social support, avoidance coping, self-blame, and PTSD among sexual assault survivors. *Psychology of Women Quarterly, 31*(1), 23–37.

van der Kolk, B. A. (2007). The history of trauma in psychiatry. In M. J. Friedman, T. M. Keane, & P. A. Resick (Eds.), *Handbook of PTSD: Science and practice* (pp. 19–36). New York: Guilford Press.

Withuis, J. (2010). The management of victimhood: Long term health damage from asthenia to PTSD. In J. Withuis & A. Mooij (Eds.), *The politics of war trauma: The aftermath of World War II in eleven European countries*. Chicago: The University of Chicago Press.

Neurobiological Findings in Post-traumatic Stress Disorder

Iris-Tatjana Kolassa, Sonja Illek, Sarah Wilker,
Alexander Karabatsiakis, and Thomas Elbert

Studies on mass conflict, torture, or natural disasters have shown that survivors may develop a spectrum of clinical symptoms as a consequence of the experienced traumatic stress. Surprisingly, cross-cultural similarities and consistencies greatly outweigh cultural and ethnic differences (Elbert and Schauer 2002). Hence, there must be a common underlying neurobiological basis of post-traumatic stress disorder (PTSD) symptoms. In this chapter, we present a selection of findings on the underlying neurobiology of PTSD and the structure of traumatic memories in particular. The research findings are interpreted within the context of the fear network model, a theoretical model which explains the formation of traumatic memories and has been proven to be helpful to integrate the diverse findings on neurobiological alterations associated with PTSD.

We first summarize the most important risk factors for the formation of strong traumatic memories and the onset of PTSD, which are (1) cumulative trauma exposure as the strongest environmental factor and (2) genetic risk as an individual biological factor. This is supplemented by a section on epigenetic modifications (Sect. 4.3), which result from the interaction of the biological-genetic makeup and the sociocultural conditions. We continue by presenting evidence for structural and functional alterations in the brain of survivors with PTSD (Sect. 4.4), which might be either a consequence of the accumulation of traumatic stress or a predisposing risk factor for the disorder. Furthermore, we explain potential underlying molecular

I.-T. Kolassa (✉) • S. Illek • S. Wilker • A. Karabatsiakis
Clinical & Biological Psychology, Institute of Psychology & Education, University of Ulm,
Albert-Einstein-Allee 47, 89069 Ulm, Germany
e-mail: Iris.Kolassa@uni-ulm.de

T. Elbert
Clinical Psychology & Neuropsychology, University of Konstanz,
Universitätsstr. 10, 78457 Konstanz, Germany

© Springer International Publishing Switzerland 2015
U. Schnyder, M. Cloitre (eds.), *Evidence Based Treatments for Trauma-Related Psychological Disorders: A Practical Guide for Clinicians*,
DOI 10.1007/978-3-319-07109-1_4

mechanisms which might account for the adverse health consequences and premature aging often observed in PTSD (Sect. 4.5). This chapter concludes with a section on the potential reversibility of the adverse physiological effects of trauma by means of successful treatment with trauma-focused therapy (Sect. 4.6) and an outlook on neurobiological research on other trauma-related mental health disorders (Sect. 4.7).

4.1 Cumulative Trauma Exposure Forms Strong Traumatic Memories

Although the vast majority of people experience at least one traumatic event, lifetime prevalence of PTSD in adult Americans is estimated to be limited to 7–12 % (DiGangi et al. 2013; Kessler et al. 1995, 2005; Pace and Heim 2011). However, PTSD lifetime prevalence in populations with greater exposure to traumatic stressors is much higher, with, for instance, up to 58 % after combat exposure (Kessler et al. 1995) and 50 % in Sudanese refugees in Uganda (Neuner et al. 2004). Those numbers show that the development of PTSD is decisively influenced by the cumulative exposure to traumatic stress, which can best be operationalized as the number of different traumatic event types experienced and was termed *traumatic load* (Kolassa et al. 2010a, b; Neuner et al. 2004).

Cumulative trauma affects the severity of major depression and PTSD in a dose-response relationship even a decade after the traumatic event. All symptom categories of depression and PTSD, except for avoidance, correlate highly with cumulative trauma (Mollica et al. 1998). Neuner and colleagues (2004) assessed a sample of 3,371 refugees living in the West Nile region and found a positive correlation between traumatic load and PTSD prevalence as well as severity of PTSD symptoms. PTSD prevalence for participants reporting three or fewer traumatic event types was 23 %, while it reached 100 % for individuals who reported at least 28 events (Neuner et al. 2004). This *building block effect* (Schauer et al. 2003) was replicated and further specified multiple times (Eckart et al. 2009; Kolassa et al. 2010a, b, c). It suggests that there is no ultimate resilience for PTSD (Kolassa and Elbert 2007; Wilker and Kolassa 2013), i.e., any individual will develop PTSD when trauma exposure reaches extreme levels. Furthermore, traumatic load not only influences PTSD risk and severity but also the ability to spontaneously remit from PTSD over time, which means that the individuals which are most affected are those who are least likely to experience spontaneous remission without treatment (Kolassa et al. 2010b).

The fear network model established by the work group of Elbert (Elbert and Schauer 2002) as an extension of Lang (1979) and Foa and Kozak (1986) explains how the accumulation of traumatic stress can lead to intense fear memories. This model proposes that memories of traumatic events, similar to other memories, are stored in propositional networks which are configured by new learning experiences. When exposed to a traumatic stressor, sensory and perceptual information (e.g., the sight of blood, the sound of cries, the smell of fire) together with the cognitive (e.g., the thought "I will die"), affective (e.g., feelings of fear, horror, anger, disgust), and

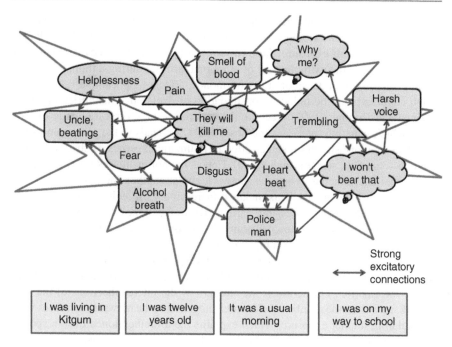

Fig. 4.1 The fear network in PTSD: sensory (*rectangles*), emotional (*circles*), cognitive (thought *bubbles*), and interoceptive (*triangles*) elements of the network are highly interconnected, as opposed to the autobiographical context information (*rectangles* below) which is stored separately (From Wilker and Kolassa (2013), reprinted with permission)

physiological responses (e.g., increase or decrease in heart rate, sweating, tense or weak legs) is stored in memory during a highly aroused state (cf. Fig. 4.1). The physiological response during a traumatic event prepares the individual for survival and can take the form of an alarm response: mind and body become extremely aroused and are braced for actions such as hiding, fighting, or escape. Another type of adaptive defensive responding, if fight or flight is not possible, is tonic or flaccid immobility including fainting (Schauer and Elbert 2010). Following the terminology first introduced by Metcalfe and Jacobs (1996), these sensory-perceptual, cognitive, affective, and physiological elements of the resulting memory network are termed "hot memories" and opposed to "cold memories," which store the context information (time and space) of a particular event.

Evidence not only from cognitive psychology but also from neuroscience confirms distinct neural bases to the abstract, flexible, contextualized representations (cold memory) and to the inflexible, sensory-bound representations (Brewin et al. 2010; Kolassa and Elbert 2007). The latter, part of the hot memory system, is thought to be supported primarily by areas of the brain directly involved in perception (e.g., representational cortex, amygdala, insula) rather than in higher-order cognitive control. By contrast, cold memories require the involvement of the hippocampus and surrounding medial temporal lobe structures (Brewin et al. 1996,

2010). For emotional experiences within the normal range, hot and cold information are well integrated and stored together in autobiographical memory. Yet, if PTSD develops after trauma exposure, these two forms of memory become dissociated for two reasons: first, the extreme state of emotional arousal during a traumatic event, accompanied by the release of stress hormones, affects hippocampal functioning, which could explain the reduced consolidation of declarative memories in PTSD (Elzinga and Bremner 2002). Second, the experience of several traumatic experiences, which generally precedes the onset of PTSD, leads to the activation of the same fear memory structure, since different traumatic experiences share common elements (e.g., fear, screams, and blood). Hence, the hot memories for several traumatic experiences merge in one fear network and strengthen the associative interconnections of its elements. This makes it increasingly difficult to disentangle the different traumatic experiences and, particularly, to recall the adequate corresponding context information. Following principles of associative learning, an interconnected fear network thus encompasses sensory, cognitive, physiological, and emotional experiences and includes the action disposition related to the experience (sensory representation, hot memory) but is detached from the autobiographical context information. Furthermore, the strength of the interconnections of the fear network, as well as the number of elements integrated in the network, increases with accumulating trauma exposure, which explains the aforementioned dose-response effect of traumatic load. Environmental stimuli (e.g., a smell or noise) and internal cues (e.g., a thought), usually in combination, can later activate this network at any given time. The ignition of only a few elements in the network is sufficient for activating the whole structure and leads to strong involuntary memories (intrusive symptoms). This may express itself as a flashback, a perception that one is back in the traumatic situation with its sounds of the harsh voice, smells of blood, feelings of fear, and thoughts of dying (cf. Fig. 4.1). Since the activation of the fear network serves as a frightening and painful recollection, many people suffering from trauma-related experiences learn to avoid cues that act as reminders of the traumatic event. They try to avoid thinking about any part represented in the fear/trauma network, not to talk about it, and to stay away from people and places that remind them of the frightening event.

The fear network model corresponds well with results of structural and functional alterations in the brain of trauma survivors with PTSD (see Sect. 4.4 in this chapter) and provides not only a neurobiological explanation of the development of PTSD symptoms in the aftermath of traumatic stress but also a rationale for trauma-focused therapy approaches (Kolassa and Elbert 2007). The reactivation of consolidated memories turns them into a labile state in which modification is possible (Nadel et al. 2012). Hence, the activation of the fear network during treatment allows the modification of the present memory structure through habituation and extinction learning (Ehlers et al. 2010). One example of such an exposure-based treatment is *Narrative Exposure Therapy* (NET; Schauer et al. 2011 see also Chap. 12 of this book) – a short-term treatment for traumatic stress disorders. By connecting the "hot" sensory, emotional, cognitive, and interoceptive memories of the trauma to the "cold" autobiographical memories, an activation of the fear network disconnected from context can be prevented and the client can achieve control over the distressing memories. The therapist further supports the client to work through the experienced traumatic experiences in a chronological order, which helps to disentangle the traumatic events which merge in the fear network. The effectiveness of NET supports the concept of a fear network in PTSD (see Robjant and Fazel 2010 for a review on evidence for the effectiveness of NET).

4.2   Genetic Factors in the Etiology, Symptomatology, and Treatment of PTSD

As summarized above, traumatic load increases the risk to develop PTSD in a dose-dependent manner. Yet, individual risk factors are known to interact with traumatic load and influence the likelihood of subsequent PTSD development. From a biological perspective, it is hence crucial to look at genetic and epigenetic risk factors for PTSD.

4.2.1   Heritability of PTSD

Family studies examining biological relatives of patients diagnosed with PTSD first indicated genetic risk factors in disorder etiology. For example, children of PTSD patients from different contexts (Holocaust survivors, Cambodian refugees) were found to be at greater risk for PTSD following trauma exposure (Sack et al. 1995; Yehuda et al. 2001). Given that families share genetic and environmental influences (e.g., observational learning and parental distress), twin studies are needed to examine the heritability of PTSD more closely. Comparing PTSD in identical or monozygotic (MZ) twin pairs with those in fraternal or dizygotic (DZ) twin pairs results in heritability estimates of PTSD around 30–40 % (Stein et al. 2002; True et al. 1993), a figure which corresponds with estimates for anxiety disorders (Hettema et al. 2003). However, caution is needed, as identical twins may share a more similar exposure to stressful experiences in comparison to fraternal twins.

Whereas twin studies are useful to estimate the heritability of a disorder or trait, association studies are needed to identify which genes and, hence, physiological mechanisms are involved in the etiology of a certain disorder. Candidate gene association studies compare the genotype frequencies of polymorphic regions of certain candidate genes between affected individuals and healthy controls. Polymorphic regions of the genome are defined as regions that vary naturally between individuals. The most commonly studied polymorphisms are single nucleotide polymorphisms (SNPs; variation in a single base pair) and variable number of tandem repeat polymorphisms (VNTRs; the number of repeats and, hence, the length of a repetitive region of the genome differ). As a consequence, both polymorphisms can lead to functional differences in the gene-expression product.

Since PTSD requires exposure to an environmental stressor to manifest, the standard case-control design is not adequate for PTSD research, since controls might also carry genetic risk factors which never had an impact because the individual was not sufficiently exposed to traumatic stressors. Therefore, to understand genetic susceptibility of PTSD, it is crucial to carefully assess traumatic load and include it in the subsequent genetic analyses (Cornelis et al. 2010; Wilker and Kolassa 2013).

4.2.2 Genetics of the Fear Network

According to the fear network model detailed above (Elbert and Schauer 2002; Kolassa and Elbert 2007), strongly interconnected, highly accessible emotional-sensory fear memories, which are detached from the corresponding autobiographical context information, lead to intrusive PTSD symptoms (Wilker and Kolassa 2013).

Accordingly, fear memory formation, and fear conditioning in particular, has been widely used as a model for PTSD development. Fear conditioning is a prominent paradigm in PTSD research, since it can be easily studied in animals and provides a sound explanation on how previously neutral stimuli (e.g., a policeman) can become triggers of fear due to a traumatic experience. The hippocampus, the medial prefrontal cortex (mPFC), and the amygdala (together termed *limbic-frontal neurocircuitry of fear*) were identified as the main areas involved in the acquisition and regulation of conditioned fear in animal studies. The interplay of these areas during (traumatic) stress is influenced by the neuromodulatory actions of neurotransmitters, such as serotonin, dopamine, and norepinephrine, as well as hormones, such as glucocorticoids (for reviews see, e.g., Ressler and Nemeroff 2000; Rodrigues et al. 2009; Shin and Liberzon 2009). Therefore, these systems have been targeted by candidate gene association studies on PTSD.

Whereas studies only comparing the prevalence of genetic risk alleles in PTSD patients and controls have yielded conflicting results, research which accounts for the aforementioned building block effect and, hence, investigates gene × environment interactions has brought converging evidence for several genetic risk factors which will be summarized in the following.

4.2.2.1 Modulators of the Serotonergic System

The neurotransmitter serotonin is known to influence emotional learning and memory through its inhibitory action on the amygdala (cf. Meneses and Liy-Salmeron 2012; Ressler and Nemeroff 2000). The serotonin transporter is responsible for the active clearance of serotonin from the synaptic cleft. Among candidate genes encoding proteins involved in the serotonergic system, there is convergent evidence indicating an influence of the serotonin transporter gene on the risk to develop PTSD subsequent to traumatic stress. A length polymorphism within the promoter region of the serotonin transporter gene (termed serotonin transporter gene-linked polymorphic region; 5-HTTLPR) influences its activity: in contrast to the long (l) allele, the short (s) allele is associated with lower gene transcription and, hence, lower serotonin transporter activity, higher amygdala reactivity to emotional stimulation, and enhanced fear conditioning (Greenberg et al. 1999; Heils et al. 1996; Lonsdorf et al. 2009; Munafò et al. 2008). Studies investigating gene × environment

Fig. 4.2 Fitted values of probability for lifetime PTSD plotted against the number of traumatic event types for different genotypes (From Kolassa et al. (2010a), reprinted with permission)

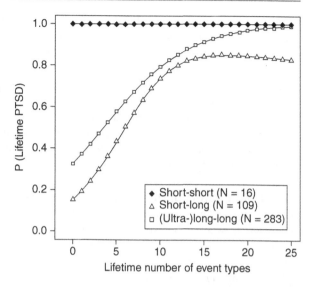

interactions consistently show that the short variant enhances PTSD susceptibility subsequent to traumatic stress (Kilpatrick et al. 2007; Kolassa et al. 2010a; Mercer 2012; Pietrzak et al. 2013; Xie et al. 2009, 2012). To give an example, in a sample of Rwandan genocide survivors, carriers of the long variant of the serotonin transporter polymorphism showed the typical building block effect: the more traumatic events experienced, the higher the prevalence of PTSD. Yet, this cumulative effect was not seen in individuals carrying two copies of the short alleles, who already developed PTSD at relatively low traumatic load (Kolassa et al. 2010a; cf. Fig. 4.2).

Interestingly, the short allele was also associated with higher risk of PTSD symptom relapse 6 months after the completion of an 8-week trauma-focused cognitive behavior therapy (Bryant et al. 2010), suggesting more persistent fear memories in carriers of this risk genotype. Furthermore, PTSD patients who were homozygous for the long allele showed higher responsiveness to a pharmacological PTSD treatment with sertraline as well as a lower dropout rate (Mushtaq et al. 2012). Whereas there are only few studies investigating the influence of genetic polymorphisms on PTSD treatment success, this first evidence might indicate the need of personalized treatments depending on individual biological risk factors.

4.2.2.2 Modulators of the Dopaminergic System

Dopamine is another neuromodulator of the neurocircuitry of fear. More precisely, dopaminergic influx in the amygdala is important for the consolidation of fear memories (Guarraci et al. 2000). Dopaminergic activity is modulated by the enzyme catechol-O-methyltransferase (COMT), which degrades and thereby deactivates dopamine and other catecholamines. A SNP in the *COMT* gene results in the integration of the amino acid methionine (Met) instead of valine (Val) in the resulting protein (*COMT* Val158Met polymorphism). On the functional level, the Met allele is associated with lower COMT enzyme activity and, therefore, higher extracellular dopamine levels (Lachman et al. 1996), as well as impaired fear extinction learning (Lonsdorf et al. 2009). Similarly, the Met allele has been found to interact with traumatic load to predict higher risk for the development of PTSD (Boscarino et al. 2011; Kolassa et al. 2010c). Furthermore, there is initial evidence that this polymorphism might influence therapeutic treatment success. To date, only one study has investigated the influence of *COMT* genotype on psychotherapeutic outcome in a sample of panic disorder patients and found that Met/Met carriers benefited less from the exposure-based elements of the treatment (Lonsdorf et al. 2010). Since effective PTSD treatments also require exposure to the traumatic experiences, it would be interesting to investigate whether these findings translate to PTSD.

4.2.2.3 Modulators of the Biological Stress Responses

During a stressful or traumatic experience, the body's alarm response is initiated by two major stress axes, the hypothalamus-pituitary-adrenal (HPA) axis and the locus coeruleus noradrenergic (LCNA) system. Their joint activity prepares the body for survival, e.g., by mobilizing glucose, increasing the heart rate and blood pressure, and enhancing muscle tension.

The HPA axis activation consists of three steps: initially, corticotropin-releasing hormone is released from the hypothalamus. This stimulates the pituitary gland to secrete adrenocorticotropic hormone, which leads to the release of cortisol from the adrenal glands. Whereas this stress response is initially adaptive, a prolonged HPA axis activity can lead to adverse health consequences. In order to avoid chronic HPA axis activation, the binding of cortisol to glucocorticoid receptors exerts negative feedback on the release of further corticotropin-releasing hormone and adrenocorticotropic hormone from the hypothalamus and pituitary, respectively. Elevated cortisol levels have been further found to increase the memorization of emotional experiences, rendering the glucocorticoid system an interesting target for candidate gene association studies on PTSD (see, e.g., Wolf 2009 for a review). Yet, studies investigating glucocorticoid receptor polymorphisms have yielded inconsistent results (Bachmann et al. 2005; Hauer et al. 2011). Another interesting candidate in the glucocorticoid system is the gene encoding co-chaperone FK506-binding protein 51 (*FKBP5*), which regulates cortisol-binding affinity of the glucocorticoid receptor. More precisely, when *FKBP5* binds to co-chaperone FK506, the resulting receptor complex decreases the binding capacity for cortisol (Binder 2009), resulting in reduced negative feedback and, hence, a prolonged stress reaction. So far, research consistently points towards an interaction of *FKBP5* risk alleles and adult or childhood trauma exposure in the risk to develop PTSD (Binder et al. 2008; Boscarino et al. 2011, 2012; Xie et al. 2010).

Stress or emotional arousal leads to the release of noradrenaline from the basolateral amygdala, and this noradrenergic neurotransmission is required to form memories of emotional experiences (e.g., McGaugh and Roozendaal 2002). PTSD is associated with both central and peripheral noradrenergic hyperactivity (Heim and Nemeroff 2009), yet few studies investigated genes involved in the noradrenergic system. One interesting exception is the work of de Quervain and coworkers (2007), who investigated a deletion variant in the gene *ADRA2B*, coding the alpha-2B-adrenergic receptor, which was associated with enhanced memory for emotionally arousing material in healthy volunteers and more pronounced intrusive memories in survivors of the Rwandan genocide (de Quervain et al. 2007).

In sum, reliable genetic associations were found with genes involved in the development of pathological memories. Understanding genetic risk factors relevant to the formation of intense fear memories is especially important, since those biological systems present a promising target for modifications through future treatment opportunities, especially on a pharmacological level.

Yet, despite increasing efforts and technological advances, only a small proportion of the estimated PTSD heritability can be explained by the identified genetic risk factors. Explanations for this "missing heritability" (Manolio et al. 2009) include the presence of complex multigene interactions and interactions between the individual environmental exposure with the genetic makeup of a person. Furthermore, research in the last decades has elucidated that environmental exposure can shape gene expression through epigenetic modification (Zhang and Meaney 2010). The next section will hence illuminate epigenetic mechanisms, which are essential to obtain a full understanding of the interaction of nature and nurture in PTSD etiology.

4.3 Epigenetic Alterations Associated with PTSD

The term epigenetics originates from the Greek syllable epi, meaning upon, and genetics. The epigenome can be viewed as a "second layer of information" (Zhang and Meaney 2010, p. 447) which consists of chemical modifications altering the accessibility of the DNA, without changing the sequence of nucleotides. More precisely, gene expression depends upon the binding of transcription factors to the promoter region of a gene, and different epigenetic mechanisms dynamically allow or prevent transcription factor binding. These mechanisms are crucial to cell differentiation: since the genome of mostly all cells in a given human individual is the same, the epigenetic profile allows the specialization regarding the cellular function (e.g., heart cell vs. neuron) by determining which genetic sequences are expressed as proteins. Furthermore, and of particular relevance in the context of PTSD, epigenetic alterations allow for the dynamic adaption of gene expression to challenging environmental demands (Zhang and Meaney 2010). In the last years, evidence suggesting that traumatic stress can influence the individual epigenetic profile has accumulated (Malan-Müller et al. 2013). At first, it was supposed that particularly early developmental adversity leads to alteration in the epigenome, which can be associated with higher stress vulnerability later in life. Thereafter, however, it was acknowledged that epigenetic modifications occur during the entire lifespan and are crucial to learning and memory (Zhang and Meaney 2010). Hence, on the one hand, early developmental stress can lead to stable epigenetic alterations which constitute a risk factor for later PTSD development. On the other hand, adult traumatic stress might also lead to epigenetic modifications which could in turn perpetuate the psychological symptoms and biological alterations associated with PTSD.

The three epigenetic mechanisms which may lead to an alteration of the transcriptional accessibility of genes without changing their structure are RNA-associated silencing, histone modification, and most prominently DNA methylation (Egger et al. 2004). The modifications can enhance or decrease gene expression and even "silence" the gene entirely (Sutherland and Costa 2003).

First evidence for the influence of early experiences on the epigenetic profile stems from animal studies which show that low versus high maternal care of rat mothers leads to differential DNA methylation in their offspring (Weaver et al. 2004). More precisely, low maternal care was associated with enhanced methylation of the glucocorticoid receptor gene (*GCCR*) promoter in the hippocampus and, hence, reduced GCCR expression. As indicated earlier, the GCCR is involved in negative regulatory feedback of the hypothalamic-pituitary-adrenal (HPA) axis. Increased *GCCR* promoter methylation can therefore reduce GCCR sensitivity, which might lead to a prolonged HPA activation under stress. Returning to the study by Weaver et al. (2004), these epigenetic changes, which may persist into adulthood, could be prevented by placing the rodents with rat mothers providing them with high maternal care – a finding that is of utmost importance for psychotherapy in the field of psychotrauma.

McGowan et al. (2009) showed comparable findings in humans: they found enhanced methylation in a neuron-specific glucocorticoid receptor gene (*NR3C1*, the human homolog of the site investigated in rats in the Weaver study) promoter in the hippocampi of suicide victims who had experienced childhood abuse, compared to suicide victims with no documented history of childhood abuse. The study implies a common effect of early stress experiences on the epigenetic regulation of hippocampal GCCR expression (McGowan et al. 2009). This was confirmed by a recent study (Mehta et al. 2013) comparing DNA methylation and gene expression between a sample of PTSD patients with childhood and adult trauma, a PTSD sample without childhood trauma, and a trauma-exposed control group without PTSD. The authors found distinct gene expression patterns in the two PTSD groups, indicating differential biological pathways involved in PTSD etiology depending on childhood trauma history. Furthermore, only in the childhood trauma group, differences in gene expression overall matched with epigenetic modifications of the corresponding gene loci, suggesting that childhood trauma leads to enduring epigenetic alterations which still influence gene expression in adulthood.

Likewise, Radtke et al. (2011) showed for the first time that prenatal stress – in particular intimate partner violence – experienced by mothers during pregnancy altered the methylation status of the *GCCR* of their offspring (assessed at age 10–19). Hence, this study provides a possible link between prenatal stress and psychopathology later in life (Radtke et al. 2011).

Indeed, recent studies provide initial evidence that epigenetic modifications influence the probability of PTSD development. For instance, Koenen and colleagues showed in a primarily African American sample from the Detroit Neighborhood Health Study that methylation level at the serotonin transporter promoter polymorphisms (5-HTTLPR) and traumatic load interacted to predict PTSD vulnerability (Koenen et al. 2011). Chang and colleagues investigated the dopamine transporter gene, another genetic locus previously found to be implicated in PTSD vulnerability (Drury et al. 2009; Segman et al. 2002; Valente et al. 2011; but see Bailey et al. 2010). They found the highest PTSD probability in carriers of the high-risk genotype, who also present with higher methylation levels at this locus (Chang et al. 2012). Moreover, it was recently suggested that the combination of an *FKBP5* risk genotype and early adversity leads to demethylation at the *FKBP5* locus, which may be associated with higher FKBP5 responsiveness and an augmented stress response later in life (Klengel et al. 2012). These studies provide first evidence that traumatic experiences, especially if they occur during early developmental windows, can shape the epigenetic profile, which in turn influences the vulnerability for PTSD in the case of subsequent trauma exposure. Furthermore, the work of Klengel and coworkers indicates that epigenetic alterations may be influenced by genotype. Consequently, we are confronted with a complex interaction of genetics, epigenetics, and early and late trauma exposure in the prediction of PTSD.

4.4 Structural and Functional Alterations in the Brain of Trauma Survivors with PTSD

Structural changes associated with PTSD such as hippocampal atrophy could be the cause for functional impairments and dysfunctions associated with PTSD (Sherin and Nemeroff 2011) but were also discussed as risk factors (Gilbertson et al. 2002).

Using brain-imaging methods, PTSD has been implicated with structural changes in the medial prefrontal cortex (mPFC), the amygdala, and the hippocampus (see Liberzon and Sripada 2008 for a review). The mPFC performs inhibitory control over stress responses through its connection to the amygdala, and it plays a major role in fear extinction (Heim and Nemeroff 2009). According to the neurocircuitry model of PTSD, regions of the ventral mPFC, which are supposed to inhibit the amygdala, are dysfunctional in patients suffering from the disorder. At the same time as the amygdala responses are amplified, the hippocampus shows deficits in explicit learning and memory and, therefore, fails to identify safe environments (Rauch et al. 2006). The hippocampus (Fig. 4.3) is especially important in the development of PTSD; it is crucial for controlling stress responses as well as declarative memory, and it plays a major role in contextual aspects of fear conditioning (Heim and Nemeroff 2009). Since this area of the brain is known for its high plasticity, studies investigating structural changes in the brain due to PTSD have mainly focused on volume changes in the hippocampus (Hughes and Shin 2011). Animal studies show that pathological stress can lead to hippocampal size reduction, possibly caused by adverse effects of stress hormones (Sapolsky et al. 1990). Several meta-analyses describe smaller hippocampal volumes in trauma-exposed individuals with and without PTSD, when compared to a non-exposed control group (Smith 2005; Woon et al. 2010), while others find hippocampal volume reduction only in PTSD patients but not in trauma-exposed and non-exposed control groups (Karl et al. 2006; Kitayama et al. 2005).

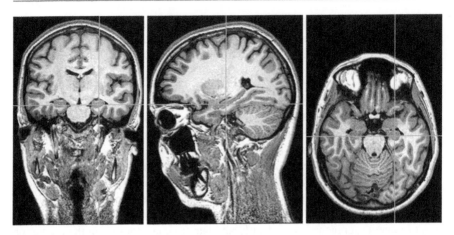

Fig. 4.3 Morphological alterations of the hippocampus have been repeatedly found in PTSD and might represent a risk factor or a consequence of the disorder

Gilbertson and colleagues (2002) conducted a study with twins; they compared war veterans with combat exposure to their twins without combat exposure. In accordance with previous studies, they also found smaller hippocampi in PTSD patients. However, the co-twins of the PTSD patients who neither suffered from PTSD nor had been exposed to combat also had smaller hippocampi compared to the non-PTSD control group (Gilbertson et al. 2002). This suggests smaller hippocampal volume to be a risk factor for PTSD rather than a consequence of the disorder. In a further study, configural processing performance was found to be significantly lower in PTSD patients in comparison to trauma-exposed controls. Nevertheless, the co-twins of the PTSD patients showed the same impairments which were related to hippocampal volume, even though they did not suffer from PTSD, nor were they trauma-exposed as adults (Gilbertson et al. 2002). However, a recent study of Teicher et al. (2012), which presents evidence that childhood adversity massively affects hippocampal development, provides an alternative explanation for the results of the Gilbertson work group. It is possible that those twins exposed to adversity during vulnerable childhood periods may have both a reduced hippocampal volume and a greater risk for developing PTSD when exposed to combat. Possibly such altered development of hippocampal organization may reduce contextualizing representations of stressful events and generalize fear. While this brain organization may be adaptive in dangerous environments, it also includes the risk of extending the fear network and eventually the maladaptive formation of PTSD.

Finally, another study found reduced hippocampal volume in current PTSD patients compared to a control group with remitted PTSD. Again, two alternative explanations could account for this finding: on the one hand, lower hippocampus volume could be a risk factor for a chronic pathology of PTSD. On the other hand, smaller hippocampus volume could be a consequence of PTSD, which might be reversible if the disorder remits (Apfel et al. 2011).

To conclude, the current state of research does not clearly support the notion that reduced hippocampus volume is a consequence of traumatic stress or a (genetic) risk factor for PTSD onset. Yet, an association of PTSD with reduced hippocampal volume is evident and corresponds well with the assumption of unreliable autobiographical context information of the fear network model.

Since the amygdala plays a central role in the neurocircuitry of fear in general, and the acquisition and expression of conditioned fear reactions in particular, several studies looked at structural alterations of the amygdala in survivors suffering from PTSD. Yet, in contrast to research on hippocampus volume, results are far from consistent. For instance, a meta-analysis from 2009 which summarized nine studies found no differences in left and right amygdala volume if PTSD patients were compared to trauma-exposed or unexposed control groups (Woon and Hedges 2009). More recent studies continue to provide inconsistent findings. Kuo and colleagues (2012) found enhanced total amygdala volumes in combat veterans with PTSD compared to trauma-exposed veterans without PTSD. Yet, another study also investigating trauma-exposed military veterans found reduced left and right amygdala volume in PTSD (Morey et al. 2012).

Finally, PTSD-associated structural alterations of the PFC, which plays a central role in fear inhibition and extinction learning through its inhibitory influence on the amygdala, have been investigated. A recent meta-analysis summarized the results of nine studies using voxel-based morphometry to assess gray matter volume in PTSD patients opposed to trauma-exposed controls and found significantly reduced volumes in several regions implicated in the neurocircuitry of fear, including the left hippocampus and the ventromedial PFC (Kühn and Gallinat 2013).

In addition to the identified structural alterations in the neurocircuitry of fear, it is also of interest to understand if the functioning or the interplay of these structures is altered in PTSD patients. A consistent body of research indicates that amygdala reactions to threatening cues are accelerated in PTSD. The common design to investigate amygdala reactivity is to compare brain activity while presenting neutral versus emotional stimuli. For instance, Brohawn and coworkers (2010) found significantly elevated amygdala reactivity in response to negative pictures in PTSD patients compared to trauma-exposed controls. These results were confirmed in numerous studies, revealing higher amygdala activity in response to fearful or aversive stimuli in PTSD patients versus controls (see Hayes et al. 2012 for a recent meta-analysis), as well as a positive correlation between current PTSD symptom severity and amygdala reactivity to these stimuli (Armony et al. 2005; Dickie et al. 2008, 2011). In addition, a recent study found enhanced spontaneous amygdala activity in PTSD, indicating that an increase in amygdala activity in PTSD is not only present during specific experimental provocations but can be a general condition in PTSD (Yan et al. 2013). Heightened amygdala activity is associated with decreased mPFC activity in response to aversive stimuli (Hayes et al. 2012). This is supplemented by recent evidence indicating that trauma survivors with PTSD show reduced functional connectivity between the amygdala and the mPFC in response to fearful stimuli, a finding that can further explain the failure of the mPFC to inhibit exaggerated amygdala responses in PTSD (Stevens et al. 2013).

Somewhat in contrast to the general finding of prefrontal hypoactivity in PTSD, Adenauer and colleagues found enhanced early activation in the right prefrontal cortex in response to aversive pictures in PTSD patients, compared to trauma-exposed individuals not suffering from PTSD and unexposed control subjects (Adenauer et al. 2010). Such early activity might be missed in functional magnetic resonance imaging studies, which have a lower time resolution than the magnetoencephalography (MEG) paradigm implemented in the Adenauer study. This early prefrontal activity might represent an acquired hypersensitivity to threatening stimuli in a traumatized brain, which constitutes one form of expression of a strong fear network that is prepared to rapidly detect danger (Rockstroh and Elbert 2010). This early adaptive activation is most likely followed by subsequent deactivation of prefrontal regions, a vigilance-avoidance pattern that was also described for other anxiety disorders (Adenauer et al. 2010).

4.5   The Effects of Psychological Trauma on Physical Health: Identifying Potential Molecular Modulators

PTSD has been associated with poor self-reported health and increased healthcare utilization (Schnurr and Jankowski 1999) but also unfavorable lifestyle factors such as physical inactivity and smoking (Zen et al. 2012). Psychological stress, particularly if it takes extreme (traumatic) forms, has been shown to enhance the risk for cardiovascular, cerebrovascular, respiratory, gastrointestinal, musculoskeletal, inflammatory, and autoimmune diseases, as well as other age-related diseases including even cancer (Boscarino 2004; Felitti et al. 1998; Fuller-Thomson and Brennenstuhl 2009; Glaesmer et al. 2011; Schnurr and Jankowski 1999). For more details, see Chap. 5.

Although traumatic experiences and PTSD have often been related to adverse health outcomes, the precise molecular mechanisms underlying this relationship warrant further investigation. The ongoing stress an individual is exposed to through adverse environments (traumatic stressors) seems to cause the immune system to age prematurely and to alter various molecular pathways. Sommershof et al. (2009) showed a relative reduction in naïve cytotoxic and regulatory T cells in the lymphocytes of PTSD patients as well as a relative increase in memory T cells due to more past infections and a higher wear and tear of the immune system. The reduction in naïve cytotoxic T cells might lead to a compromised immune response, which could then contribute to the enhanced susceptibility for infections. A similar effect is observed in elderly people, where the natural reduction of naïve T lymphocytes leads to a greater risk for diseases associated with aging (Shen et al. 1999). In addition, the reduction of regulatory T cells might put PTSD patients at risk for inflammatory and autoimmune diseases. Indeed, there is a high prevalence of autoimmune and inflammatory diseases in PTSD patients (Boscarino 2004). More interestingly, we observed in this study (Sommershof et al. 2009) and in an extension study (Morath et al. 2014a) that naïve cytotoxic T cells and regulatory T cells were also reduced in trauma-exposed individuals without a diagnosis of PTSD; this group took an intermediate position between PTSD patients and controls. As traumatized individuals with PTSD usually experienced more traumatic events than traumatized individuals without PTSD, this suggests a cumulative effect of traumatic stress on T-cell distribution independent of the diagnosis of PTSD (Sommershof et al. 2009).

Another potential link connecting PTSD to poor physical health is the increased pro-inflammatory status observed in individuals who experienced traumatic events or suffered from chronic stress. Gola et al. (2013) observed an augmented pro-inflammatory state in PTSD patients: peripheral blood mononuclear cells (PBMCs) exhibited an increased spontaneous secretion of pro-inflammatory cytokines (IL-1β, IL-6, and TNF-α). In addition, IL-6 and TNF-α were significantly positively associated with PTSD symptom severity. The enhanced spontaneous production of pro-inflammatory cytokines observed in PTSD patients indicates that traumatic stress leads to a preactivation of PBMCs (Gola et al. 2013). A chronic upregulation of pro-inflammatory cytokines might increase the risk for various physical diseases such as atherosclerosis, myocardial infarction, and stroke (Schnurr and Jankowski 1999). One mechanism by which a chronic inflammatory state leads to adverse health outcomes is the overproduction of free radicals. In low doses, free radicals serve to protect the body against pathogens; however, in higher concentrations, they can have detrimental consequences, including the impairment of functioning of DNA, proteins, and lipids. Together, the adverse consequences of free radical over-concentration are termed oxidative stress (Khansari et al. 2009). Chronic inflammation, and the resulting oxidative stress, has been associated with several types of cancer, pathological aging, and a wide range of age-related diseases such as diabetes, cardiovascular, and autoimmune disease (Hold and El-Omar 2008).

A biomarker that can be interpreted as a measure of physical age is the length of the telomeres of a cell (von Zglinicki and Martin-Ruiz 2005). Telomeres, which cap and protect the end of the chromosomes from damage and uncontrolled fusion with neighboring chromosomes, are essential for chromosome replication and stability. During cell division the telomeres are successively consumed and consequently shorten in length (Chan and Blackburn 2004). A shortening of the telomeres increases the risk for age-related diseases such as cardiovascular diseases but also cancer and cancer mortality (Epel et al. 2008; Willeit et al. 2010). Childhood maltreatment (Tyrka et al. 2010), childhood chronic or serious illness (Kananen et al. 2010), and psychological stress (Epel et al. 2004) have been associated with shorter telomeres. Moreover, Entringer et al. (2011) observed significantly shorter telomeres in the offspring of mothers who had been exposed to psychosocial stress during pregnancy. The study provides initial evidence for a transgenerational transmission of adverse health effects caused by stress exposure during pregnancy (Entringer et al. 2011).

Another biomarker measuring physiological aging is the N-glycan profile. N-glycosylation is the enzymatic attachment of a sugar molecule to a lipid or protein. N-glycans are secondary gene products which are not directly regulated by the genome and can be influenced by environmental stress (Varki 2008). The concentration of the nine different N-glycan structures in human plasma varies as a function of age. Particularly, N-glycan peak 1 increases with age, whereas N-glycan peak 6 decreases. The logarithmized ratio of the concentration of these two N-glycan structures has been established as a biomarker of physiological aging and was termed GlycoAgeTest. The test may even be used as a marker for general health in humans (Vanhooren et al. 2010).

Moreno-Villanueva et al. (2013) found significant alterations in the GlycoAgeTest for individuals with PTSD and trauma-exposed subjects in contrast to a low-stress control group. This alteration in N-glycosylation was equal to an acceleration of physiological aging by 15 years. The trauma-exposed subjects were positioned between the PTSD and the low-stress exposure group. In addition, a significant positive correlation of traumatic load with the GlycoAgeTest was observed, i.e., the more traumatic stress a person had experienced, the higher the GlycoAgeTest score and, therefore, the higher the person's physiological age (Moreno-Villanueva et al. 2013). In sum, the N-glycosylation profile strengthens the concept that traumatic stress causes an acceleration of physiological aging which might be mediated by a state of low-grade inflammation.

4.6 Reversibility of Immunological and Molecular Alterations in PTSD Through Psychotherapy

As described above (Sect. 4.5), experiencing traumatic stress can cause severe biological alterations. Fortunately, at least some of these biological modifications seem to be reversible through psychotherapy.

Morath et al. (2014a) showed in a recent study that the initial reduction of regulatory T cells in PTSD patients could be reversed to some extent through a treatment with Narrative Exposure Therapy (NET) in a 1-year follow-up. The positive effect on the patients' immunological level was not observed in the waiting list control group. Unfortunately, some of the alterations in the immunological profile could not be reversed by psychotherapy, in particular, the reduction of naïve and memory T lymphocytes (Morath et al. 2014a).

Furthermore, Morath et al. (2014b) found that basal DNA strand breaks were increased in PTSD patients when compared to a control group. Interestingly, treatment with NET led to a decrease in DNA strand breaks together with a PTSD symptom reduction (Morath et al. 2014b).

Moreover, treatment with trauma-focused cognitive-behavioral therapy (TF-CBT) was found to be correlated with reduced stress symptoms on the biological level, including a declined heart rate, blood pressure, and electromyogram (EMG) reactivity. Implying that TF-CBT leads to those alterations in physiological reactivity, these findings can explain the modified stress response achieved through psychotherapy (for a review see Zantvoord et al. 2013).

Correspondingly, Adenauer et al. (2011) found not only decreased PTSD and depressive symptom severity after treatment with NET but also enhanced parietal and occipital activity in the brains of trauma survivors when exposed to adverse, threatening stimuli. Those activity changes point towards a cortical top-down regulation of attention which may be caused by NET and enable the patient to reevaluate threatening stimuli detached from their original trauma (Adenauer et al. 2011). Hence, this study demonstrates that the modification of a fear memory network through effective trauma-focused therapy is associated with corresponding changes in cortical activity.

These initial findings show that psychotherapy, in this case NET, can be effective even on a molecular level and is able to reverse some of the severe biological changes in individuals suffering from trauma-associated psychopathology. Consequently, those studies underscore the importance of adequate psychological treatment for trauma survivors.

4.7 Future Promising Directions of Neurobiological Research in Trauma-Related Disorders

This chapter focused on neurobiological findings in PTSD, one of the most commonly observed psychological disorders in the aftermath of trauma exposure. Yet, the psychological impact of trauma is not limited to the onset of PTSD but may also lead to profound alterations of the survivor's personality. As LeDoux (2003) indicates in his concept of the "synaptic self," personality is formed by an interaction of genetic makeup and environmental experiences which manifest in the formation of memories (i.e., the establishment of new synaptic connections). Emotional arousal enhances the consolidation of memories, which explains the detrimental influence of traumatic experiences. Furthermore, if strong emotional experiences occur during sensitive developmental periods, their impact on personality building is even higher, explaining the strong impact of childhood abuse and maltreatment (LeDoux 2003). There are several concepts which try to acknowledge the long-lasting impact of (early) traumatization on individual development. These concepts include the suggested new diagnoses "developmental trauma disorder" (van der Kolk 2005) as well as "complex PTSD" (Maercker et al. 2013).

The literature on epigenetic alterations in response to early adversity reviewed earlier further highlights the high impact of childhood experiences on neurobiological development and hence the establishment of the synaptic self. For instance, Klengel and colleagues showed that childhood but not adult trauma exposure was associated with allele-specific demethylation at the FKBP5 locus which may lead to enduring alterations of the stress system (Klengel et al. 2012). While research on the influence of early adversity on neurobiological alterations (especially epigenetics) is accumulating, the literature on distinct neurobiological signatures of complex PTSD or developmental trauma disorder is still relatively sparse. In the future, it would be interesting to investigate whether these diagnostic categories are at least partly reflected by distinct underlying biomolecular processes (cf. Miller 2010). Recent technological advances enable the assessment and computational analysis of large biological data sets with high coverage in the fields of genetics, epigenetics, or proteomics (Patti et al. 2012) and may hence allow identifying both distinct and shared biological pathways of trauma-related psychological disorders. Once the identification of distinct neurobiological signatures of the aforementioned trauma-related disorders becomes possible, this may point to novel treatment opportunities directed at these more complex reactions to trauma.

References

Adenauer, H., Pinösch, S., Catani, C., Gola, H., Keil, J., Kissler, J., & Neuner, F. (2010). Early processing of threat cues in posttraumatic stress disorder-evidence for a cortical vigilance-avoidance reaction. *Biological Psychiatry, 68*(5), 451–458.

Adenauer, H., Catani, C., Gola, H., Keil, J., Ruf, M., Schauer, M., & Neuner, F. (2011). Narrative exposure therapy for PTSD increases top-down processing of aversive stimuli – Evidence from a randomized controlled treatment trial. *BMC Neuroscience, 12*(1), 127.

Apfel, B. A., Ross, J., Hlavin, J., Meyerhoff, D. J., Metzler, T. J., Marmar, C. R., et al. (2011). Hippocampal volume differences in Gulf War veterans with current versus lifetime posttraumatic stress disorder symptoms. *Biological Psychiatry, 69*(6), 541–548.

Armony, J. L., Corbo, V., Clément, M.-H., & Brunet, A. (2005). Amygdala response in patients with acute PTSD to masked and unmasked emotional facial expressions. *The American Journal of Psychiatry, 162*(10), 1961–1963.

Bachmann, A. W., Sedgley, T. L., Jackson, R. V., Gibson, J. N., Young, R. M., & Torpy, D. J. (2005). Glucocorticoid receptor polymorphisms and post-traumatic stress disorder. *Psychoneuroendocrinology, 30*(3), 297–306.

Bailey, J. N., Goenjian, A. K., Noble, E. P., Walling, D. P., Ritchie, T., & Goenjian, H. A. (2010). PTSD and dopaminergic genes, DRD2 and DAT, in multigenerational families exposed to the Spitak earthquake. *Psychiatry Research, 178*(3), 507–510.

Binder, E. B. (2009). The role of FKBP5, a co-chaperone of the glucocorticoid receptor in the pathogenesis and therapy of affective and anxiety disorders. *Psychoneuroendocrinology, 34*(Suppl 1), S186–S195.

Binder, E. B., Bradley, R. G., Liu, W., Epstein, M. P., Deveau, T. C., Mercer, K. B., et al. (2008). Association of FKBP5 polymorphisms and childhood abuse with risk of posttraumatic stress disorder symptoms in adults. *JAMA, the Journal of the American Medical Association, 299*(11), 1291–1305.

Boscarino, J. A. (2004). Posttraumatic stress disorder and physical illness: Results from clinical and epidemiologic studies. *Annals of the New York Academy of Sciences, 1032*, 141–153.

Boscarino, J. A., Erlich, P. M., Hoffman, S. N., Rukstalis, M., & Stewart, W. F. (2011). Association of FKBP5, COMT and CHRNA5 polymorphisms with PTSD among outpatients at risk for PTSD. *Psychiatry Research, 188*(1), 173–174.

Boscarino, J., Erlich, P. M., Hoffman, S. N., & Zhang, X. (2012). Higher FKBP5, COMT, CHRNA5, and CRHR1 allele burdens are associated with PTSD and interact with trauma exposure: Implications for neuropsychiatric research and treatment. *Neuropsychiatric Disease and Treatment, 8*, 131–139.

Brewin, C. R., Dalgleish, T., & Joseph, S. (1996). A dual representation theory of posttraumatic stress disorder. *Psychological Review, 103*(4), 670–686.

Brewin, C. R., Gregory, J. D., Lipton, M., & Burgess, N. (2010). Intrusive images in psychological disorders: Characteristics, neural mechanisms, and treatment implications. *Psychological Review, 117*(1), 210–232.

Brohawn, K. H., Offringa, R., Pfaff, D. L., Hughes, K. C., & Shin, L. M. (2010). The neural correlates of emotional memory in posttraumatic stress disorder. *Biological Psychiatry, 68*(11), 1023–1030.

Bryant, R. A., Felmingham, K. L., Falconer, E. M., Pe Benito, L., Dobson-Stone, C., Pierce, K. D., & Schofield, P. R. (2010). Preliminary evidence of the short allele of the serotonin transporter gene predicting poor response to cognitive behavior therapy in posttraumatic stress disorder. *Biological Psychiatry, 67*(12), 1217–1219.

Chan, S. R. W. L., & Blackburn, E. H. (2004). Telomeres and telomerase. *Philosophical Transactions of the Royal Society, B: Biological Sciences, 359*(1441), 109–122.

Chang, S.-C., Koenen, K. C., Galea, S., Aiello, A. E., Soliven, R., Wildman, D. E., et al. (2012). Molecular variation at the SLC6A3 locus predicts lifetime risk of PTSD in the Detroit Neighborhood Health Study. *PLoS ONE, 7*(6), e39184.

Cornelis, M. C., Nugent, N. R., Amstadter, A. B., & Koenen, K. C. (2010). Genetics of post-traumatic stress disorder: Review and recommendations for genome-wide association studies. *Current Psychiatry Reports, 12*(4), 313–326.

de Quervain, D. J.-F., Kolassa, I.-T., Ertl, V., Onyut, P. L., Neuner, F., Elbert, T., & Papassotiropoulos, A. (2007). A deletion variant of the α2b-adrenoceptor is related to emotional memory in Europeans and Africans. *Nature Neuroscience, 10*(9), 1137–1139.

Dickie, E. W., Brunet, A., Akerib, V., & Armony, J. L. (2008). An fMRI investigation of memory encoding in PTSD: Influence of symptom severity. *Neuropsychologia, 46*(5), 1522–1531.

Dickie, E. W., Brunet, A., Akerib, V., & Armony, J. L. (2011). Neural correlates of recovery from post-traumatic stress disorder: A longitudinal fMRI investigation of memory encoding. *Neuropsychologia, 49*(7), 1771–1778.

DiGangi, J., Guffanti, G., McLaughlin, K. A., & Koenen, K. C. (2013). Considering trauma exposure in the context of genetics studies of posttraumatic stress disorder: A systematic review. *Biology of Mood & Anxiety Disorders, 3*(1), 2.

Drury, S. S., Theall, K. P., Keats, B. J. B., & Scheeringa, M. (2009). The role of the dopamine transporter (DAT) in the development of PTSD in preschool children. *Journal of Traumatic Stress, 22*(6), 534–539.

Eckart, C., Engler, H., Riether, C., Kolassa, S., Elbert, T., & Kolassa, I.-T. (2009). No PTSD-related differences in diurnal cortisol profiles of genocide survivors. *Psychoneuroendocrinology, 34*(4), 523–531.

Egger, G., Liang, G., Aparicio, A., & Jones, P. A. (2004). Epigenetics in human disease and prospects for epigenetic therapy. *Nature, 429*(6990), 457–463.

Ehlers, A., Bisson, J., Clark, D. M., Creamer, M., Pilling, S., Richards, D., et al. (2010). Do all psychological treatments really work the same in posttraumatic stress disorder? *Clinical Psychology Review, 30*(2), 269–276.

Elbert, T., & Schauer, M. (2002). Burnt into memory – Psychological trauma. *Nature, 419*, 883.

Elzinga, B. M., & Bremner, J. D. (2002). Are the neural substrates of memory the final common pathway in posttraumatic stress disorder (PTSD)? *Journal of Affective Disorders, 70*(1), 1–17.

Entringer, S., Epel, E. S., Kumsta, R., Lin, J., Hellhammer, D. H., Blackburn, E. H., et al. (2011). Stress exposure in intrauterine life is associated with shorter telomere length in young adulthood. *Proceedings of the National Academy of Sciences of the United States of America, 108*(33), E513–E518.

Epel, E. S., Blackburn, E. H., Lin, J., Dhabhar, F. S., Adler, N. E., Morrow, J. D., & Cawthon, R. M. (2004). Accelerated telomere shortening in response to life stress. *Proceedings of the National Academy of Sciences of the United States of America, 101*(49), 17312–17315.

Epel, E., Merkin, S., Cawthon, R., Blackburn, E., Adler, N., & Pletcher, M. (2008). The rate of leukocyte telomere shortening predicts mortality from cardiovascular disease in elderly men. *Aging (Albany NY), 1*, 81–88.

Felitti, V. J., Anda, R. F., Nordenberg, D., Williamson, D. F., Spitz, A. M., Edwards, V., et al. (1998). Relationship of childhood abuse and household dysfunction to many of the leading causes of death in adults. The Adverse Childhood Experiences (ACE) Study. *American Journal of Preventive Medicine, 14*(4), 245–258.

Foa, E. B., & Kozak, M. J. (1986). Emotional processing of fear: Exposure to corrective information. *Psychological Bulletin, 99*(1), 20–35.

Fuller-Thomson, E., & Brennenstuhl, S. (2009). Making a link between childhood physical abuse and cancer: Results from a regional representative survey. *Cancer, 115*(14), 3341–3350.

Gilbertson, M. W., Shenton, M. E., Ciszewski, A., Kasai, K., Lasko, N. B., Orr, S. P., & Pitman, R. K. (2002). Smaller hippocampal volume predicts pathologic vulnerability to psychological trauma. *Nature Neuroscience, 5*(11), 1242–1247.

Glaesmer, H., Brähler, E., Gündel, H., & Riedel-Heller, S. G. (2011). The association of traumatic experiences and posttraumatic stress disorder with physical morbidity in old age: A German population-based study. *Psychosomatic Medicine, 73*(5), 401–406.

Gola, H., Engler, H., Sommershof, A., Adenauer, H., Kolassa, S., Schedlowski, M., et al. (2013). Posttraumatic stress disorder is associated with an enhanced spontaneous production of pro-inflammatory cytokines by peripheral blood mononuclear cells. *BMC Psychiatry, 13*(1), 40.

Greenberg, B. D., Tolliver, T. J., Huang, S. J., Li, Q., Bengel, D., & Murphy, D. L. (1999). Genetic variation in the serotonin transporter promoter region affects serotonin uptake in human blood platelets. *American Journal of Medical Genetics, 88*(1), 83–87.

Guarraci, F. A., Frohardt, R. J., Falls, W. A., & Kapp, B. S. (2000). The effects of intra-amygdaloid infusions of a D2 dopamine receptor antagonist on Pavlovian fear conditioning. *Behavioral Neuroscience, 114*(3), 647–651.

Hauer, D., Weis, F., Papassotiropoulos, A., Schmoeckel, M., Beiras-Fernandez, A., Lieke, J., et al. (2011). Relationship of a common polymorphism of the glucocorticoid receptor gene to traumatic memories and posttraumatic stress disorder in patients after intensive care therapy. *Critical Care Medicine, 39*(4), 643–650.

Hayes, J. P., Hayes, S. M., & Mikedis, A. M. (2012). Quantitative meta-analysis of neural activity in posttraumatic stress disorder. *Biology of Mood & Anxiety Disorders, 2*(1), 9.

Heils, A., Teufel, A., Petri, S., Stöber, G., Riederer, P., Bengel, D., & Lesch, K. P. (1996). Allelic variation of human serotonin transporter gene expression. *Journal of Neurochemistry, 66*(6), 2621–2624.

Heim, C., & Nemeroff, C. (2009). Neurobiology of posttraumatic stress disorder. *CNS Spectrums, 14*, 13–24.

Hettema, J. M., Annas, P., Neale, M. C., Kendler, K. S., & Fredrikson, M. (2003). A twin study of the genetics of fear conditioning. *Archives of General Psychiatry, 60*(7), 702–708.

Hold, G. L., & El-Omar, E. M. (2008). Genetic aspects of inflammation and cancer. *The Biochemical Journal, 410*(2), 225–235.

Hughes, K. C., & Shin, L. M. (2011). Functional neuroimaging studies of post-traumatic stress disorder. *Expert Review of Neurotherapeutics, 11*(2), 275–285.

Kananen, L., Surakka, I., Pirkola, S., Suvisaari, J., Lönnqvist, J., Peltonen, L., et al. (2010). Childhood adversities are associated with shorter telomere length at adult age both in individuals with an anxiety disorder and controls. *PLoS ONE, 5*(5), e10826.

Karl, A., Schaefer, M., Malta, L. S., Dörfel, D., Rohleder, N., & Werner, A. (2006). A meta-analysis of structural brain abnormalities in PTSD. *Neuroscience and Biobehavioral Reviews, 30*(7), 1004–1031.

Kessler, R. C., Sonnega, A., Bromet, E., Hughes, M., & Nelson, C. B. (1995). Posttraumatic stress disorder in the National Comorbidity Survey. *Archives of General Psychiatry, 52*(12), 1048–1060.

Kessler, R. C., Berglund, P., Demler, O., Jin, R., Merikangas, K. R., & Walters, E. E. (2005). Lifetime prevalence and age-of-onset distributions of DSM-IV disorders in the National Comorbidity Survey Replication. *Archives of General Psychiatry, 62*(6), 593–602.

Khansari, N., Shakiba, Y., & Mahmoudi, M. (2009). Chronic inflammation and oxidative stress as a major cause of age-related diseases and cancer. *Recent Patents on Inflammation & Allergy Drug Discovery, 3*(1), 73–80.

Kilpatrick, D. G., Koenen, K. C., Ruggiero, K. J., Acierno, R., Galea, S., Resnick, H. S., et al. (2007). The serotonin transporter genotype and social support and moderation of posttraumatic stress disorder and depression in hurricane-exposed adults. *The American Journal of Psychiatry, 164*(11), 1693–1699.

Kitayama, N., Vaccarino, V., Kutner, M., Weiss, P., & Bremner, J. D. (2005). Magnetic resonance imaging (MRI) measurement of hippocampal volume in posttraumatic stress disorder: A meta-analysis. *Journal of Affective Disorders, 88*(1), 79–86.

Klengel, T., Mehta, D., Anacker, C., Rex-Haffner, M., Pruessner, J. C., Pariante, C. M., et al. (2012). Allele-specific FKBP5 DNA demethylation mediates gene–childhood trauma interactions. *Nature Neuroscience, 16*(1), 33–41.

Koenen, K. C., Uddin, M., Chang, S.-C., Aiello, A. E., Wildman, D. E., Goldmann, E., & Galea, S. (2011). SLC6A4 methylation modifies the effect of the number of traumatic events on risk for posttraumatic stress disorder. *Depression and Anxiety, 28*(8), 639–647.

Kolassa, I.-T., & Elbert, T. (2007). Structural and functional neuroplasticity in relation to traumatic stress. *Current Directions in Psychological Science, 16*(6), 321–325.

Kolassa, I.-T., Ertl, V., Eckart, C., Glöckner, F., Kolassa, S., Papassotiropoulos, A., et al. (2010a). Association study of trauma load and SLC6A4 promoter polymorphism in posttraumatic stress disorder: Evidence from survivors of the Rwandan genocide: Trauma load, genetics and risk for PTSD [Somatosensory evoked potentials in the acute phase of focal cerebral ischemia]. *The Journal of Clinical Psychiatry, 71*(5), 543–547.

Kolassa, I.-T., Ertl, V., Eckart, C., Kolassa, S., Onyut, L. P., & Elbert, T. (2010b). Spontaneous remission from PTSD depends on the number of traumatic event types experienced. *Psychological Trauma: Theory, Research, Practice, and Policy, 2*(3), 169–174.

Kolassa, I.-T., Kolassa, S., Ertl, V., Papassotiropoulos, A., & de Quervain, D. J.-F. (2010c). The risk of posttraumatic stress disorder after trauma depends on traumatic load and the catechol-o-methyltransferase Val158Met polymorphism. *Biological Psychiatry, 67*(4), 304–308.

Kühn, S., & Gallinat, J. (2013). Gray matter correlates of posttraumatic stress disorder: A quantitative meta-analysis. *Biological Psychiatry, 73*(1), 70–74.

Kuo, J. R., Kaloupek, D. G., & Woodward, S. H. (2012). Amygdala volume in combat-exposed veterans with and without posttraumatic stress disorder. *Archives of General Psychiatry, 69*(10), 1080.

Lachman, H. M., Papolos, D. F., Saito, T., Yu, Y. M., Szumlanski, C. L., & Weinshilboum, R. M. (1996). Human catechol-O-methyltransferase pharmacogenetics: Description of a functional polymorphism and its potential application to neuropsychiatric disorders. *Pharmacogenetics, 6*(3), 243–250.

Lang, P. J. (1979). A bio-informational theory of emotional imagery. *Psychophysiology, 16*(6), 495–512.

LeDoux, J. (2003). The self: Clues from the brain. *Annals of the New York Academy of Sciences, 1001*, 295–304.

Liberzon, I., & Sripada, C. S. (2008). The functional neuroanatomy of PTSD: A critical review. *Progress in Brain Research, 167*, 151–169.

Lonsdorf, T. B., Weike, A. I., Nikamo, P., Schalling, M., Hamm, A. O., & Ohman, A. (2009). Genetic gating of human fear learning and extinction: Possible implications for gene-environment interaction in anxiety disorder. *Psychological Science, 20*(2), 198–206.

Lonsdorf, T. B., Ruck, C., Bergstrom, J., Andersson, G., Ohman, A., Lindefors, N., et al. (2010). The COMTval158met polymorphism is associated with symptom relief during exposure-based cognitive-behavioral treatment in panic disorder. *BMC Psychiatry, 10*, 99.

Maercker, A., Brewin, C. R., Bryant, R. A., Cloitre, M., van Ommeren, M., Jones, L. M., Humayan, A., Kagee, A., Llosa, A. E., Rousseau, C., Somasundaram, D. J., Souza, R., Suzuki, Y., Weissbecker, I., Wesseley, S. C., First, M. B., & Reed, G. M. (2013). Diagnosis and classification of disorders specifically associated with stress: Proposals for ICD-11. *World Psychiatry : Official Journal of the World Psychiatric Association (WPA), 12*(3), 198–206.

Malan-Müller, S., Seedat, S., & Hemmings, S. M. J. (2013). Understanding posttraumatic stress disorder: Insights from the methylome. *Genes, Brain and Behavior, 13*(1), 52–68.

Manolio, T. A., Collins, F. S., Cox, N. J., Goldstein, D. B., Hindorff, L. A., Hunter, D. J., et al. (2009). Finding the missing heritability of complex diseases. *Nature, 461*(7265), 747–753.

McGaugh, J. L., & Roozendaal, B. (2002). Role of adrenal stress hormones in forming lasting memories in the brain. *Current Opinion in Neurobiology, 12*(2), 205–210.

McGowan, P. O., Sasaki, A., D'Alessio, A. C., Dymov, S., Labonté, B., Szyf, M., et al. (2009). Epigenetic regulation of the glucocorticoid receptor in human brain associates with childhood abuse. *Nature Neuroscience, 12*(3), 342–348.

Mehta, D., Klengel, T., Conneely, K. N., Smith, A. K., Altmann, A., Pace, T. W., et al. (2013). Childhood maltreatment is associated with distinct genomic and epigenetic profiles in posttraumatic stress disorder. *Proceedings of the National Academy of Sciences of the United States of America, 110*(20), 8302–8307.

Meneses, A., & Liy-Salmeron, G. (2012). Serotonin and emotion, learning and memory. *Reviews in the Neurosciences, 23*(5–6), 543–553.

Mercer, K. B. (2012). Acute and posttraumatic stress symptoms in a prospective gene×environment study of a university campus shooting. *Archives of General Psychiatry, 69*(1), 89.

Metcalfe, J., & Jacobs, W. (1996). A "hot-system/cool-system" view of memory under stress. *PTSD Research Quarterly, 1996*(7), 1–3.

Miller, G. (2010). Psychiatry. Beyond DSM: Seeking a brain-based classification of mental illness. *Science, 327*(5972), 1437.

Mollica, R. F., McInnes, K., Poole, C., & Tor, S. (1998). Dose-effect relationships of trauma to symptoms of depression and post-traumatic stress disorder among Cambodian survivors of mass violence. *The British Journal of Psychiatry, 173*(6), 482–488.

Morath, J., Gola, H., Sommershof, A., Hamuni, G., Kolassa, S., Catani, C., et al. (2014a). The effect of trauma-focused therapy on the altered T cell distribution in individuals with PTSD: Evidence from a randomized controlled trial. *Journal of Psychiatric Research, 54*, 1–10.

Morath, J., Moreno-Villanueva, M., Hamuni, G., Kolassa, S., Ruf-Leuschner, M., Schauer, M., et al. (2014b). Effects of psychotherapy on DNA strand break accumulation originating from traumatic stress. *Psychotherapy and Psychosomatics, 83*(5), 289–297.

Moreno-Villanueva, M., Morath, J., Vanhooren, V., Elbert, T., Kolassa, S., Libert, C., et al. (2013). N-glycosylation profiling of plasma provides evidence for accelerated physiological aging in post-traumatic stress disorder. *Translational Psychiatry, 3*(10), e320.

Morey, R. A., Gold, A. L., LaBar, K. S., Beall, S. K., Brown, V. M., Haswell, C. C., et al. (2012). Amygdala volume changes in posttraumatic stress disorder in a large case-controlled veterans group. *Archives of General Psychiatry, 69*(11), 1169.

Munafò, M. R., Brown, S. M., & Hariri, A. R. (2008). Serotonin transporter (5-HTTLPR) genotype and amygdala activation: A meta-analysis. *Biological Psychiatry, 63*(9), 852–857.

Mushtaq, D., Ali, A., Margoob, M. A., Murtaza, I., & Andrade, C. (2012). Association between serotonin transporter gene promoter-region polymorphism and 4- and 12-week treatment response to sertraline in posttraumatic stress disorder. *Journal of Affective Disorders, 136*(3), 955–962.

Nadel, L., Hupbach, A., Gomez, R., & Newman-Smith, K. (2012). Memory formation, consolidation and transformation. *Neuroscience & Biobehavioral Reviews, 36*(7), 1640–1645.

Neuner, F., Schauer, M., Karunakara, U., Klaschik, C., Robert, C., & Elbert, T. (2004). Psychological trauma and evidence for enhanced vulnerability for posttraumatic stress disorder through previous trauma among West Nile refugees. *BMC Psychiatry, 4*(1), 34.

Pace, T. W., & Heim, C. M. (2011). A short review on the psychoneuroimmunology of posttraumatic stress disorder: From risk factors to medical comorbidities. *Brain, Behavior, and Immunity, 25*(1), 6–13.

Patti, G. J., Yanes, O., & Siuzdak, G. (2012). Innovation: Metabolomics: The apogee of the omics trilogy. *Nature Reviews Molecular Cell Biology, 13*(4), 263–269.

Pietrzak, R. H., Galea, S., Southwick, S. M., & Gelernter, J. (2013). Examining the relation between the serotonin transporter 5-HTTPLR genotype x trauma exposure interaction on a contemporary phenotypic model of posttraumatic stress symptomatology: A pilot study. *Journal of Affective Disorders, 148*(1), 123–128.

Radtke, K. M., Ruf, M., Gunter, H. M., Dohrmann, K., Schauer, M., Meyer, A., & Elbert, T. (2011). Transgenerational impact of intimate partner violence on methylation in the promoter of the glucocorticoid receptor. *Translational Psychiatry, 1*(7), e21.

Rauch, S. L., Shin, L. M., & Phelps, E. A. (2006). Neurocircuitry models of posttraumatic stress disorder and extinction: Human neuroimaging research–past, present, and future. *Biological Psychiatry, 60*(4), 376–382.

Ressler, K. J., & Nemeroff, C. B. (2000). Role of serotonergic and noradrenergic systems in the pathophysiology of depression and anxiety disorders. *Depression and Anxiety, 12*(Suppl 1), 2–19.

Robjant, K., & Fazel, M. (2010). The emerging evidence for Narrative Exposure Therapy: A review. *Clinical Psychology Review, 30*(8), 1030–1039.

Rockstroh, B., & Elbert, T. (2010). Traces of fear in the neural web – Magnetoencephalographic responding to arousing pictorial stimuli. *International Journal of Psychophysiology: Official Journal of the International Organization of Psychophysiology, 78*(1), 14–19.

Rodrigues, S. M., LeDoux, J. E., & Sapolsky, R. M. (2009). The influence of stress hormones on fear circuitry. *Annual Review of Neuroscience, 32*, 289–313.

Sack, W. H., Clarke, G. N., & Seeley, J. (1995). Posttraumatic stress disorder across two generations of Cambodian refugees. *Journal of the American Academy of Child and Adolescent Psychiatry, 34*(9), 1160–1166.

Sapolsky, R. M., Uno, H., Rebert, C. S., & Finch, C. E. (1990). Hippocampal damage associated with prolonged glucocorticoid exposure in primates. *The Journal of Neuroscience: The Official Journal of the Society for Neuroscience, 10*(9), 2897–2902.

Schauer, M., & Elbert, T. (2010). Dissociation following traumatic stress. Etiology and treatment. *Journal of Psychology, 218*(2), 109–127.

Schauer, M., Neuner, F., Karunakara, U., Klaschik, C., Robert, C., & Elbert, T. (2003). PTSD and the "building block" effect of psychological trauma among West Nile Africans. *European Society for Traumatic Stress Studies Bulletin, 10*(2), 5–6.

Schauer, M., Elbert, T., & Neuner, F. (2011). *Narrative exposure therapy: A short-term treatment for traumatic stress disorders* (2nd ed.). Cambridge, MA: Hogrefe.

Schnurr, P. P., & Jankowski, M. K. (1999). Physical health and post-traumatic stress disorder: Review and synthesis. *Seminars in Clinical Neuropsychiatry, 4*(4), 295–304.

Segman, R. H., Cooper-Kazaz, R., Macciardi, F., Goltser, T., Halfon, Y., Dobroborski, T., & Shalev, A. Y. (2002). Association between the dopamine transporter gene and posttraumatic stress disorder. *Molecular Psychiatry, 7*(8), 903–907.

Shen, S. S., Kim, J. S., & Weksler, M. E. (1999). Effect of age on thymic development, T cell immunity, and helper T cell function. *Reviews of Physiology, Biochemistry and Pharmacology, 139*, 123–139.

Sherin, J. E., & Nemeroff, C. B. (2011). Post-traumatic stress disorder: The neurobiological impact of psychological trauma. *Dialogues in Clinical Neuroscience, 13*(3), 263–278.

Shin, L. M., & Liberzon, I. (2009). The neurocircuitry of fear, stress, and anxiety disorders. *Neuropsychopharmacology, 35*(1), 169–191.

Smith, M. E. (2005). Bilateral hippocampal volume reduction in adults with post-traumatic stress disorder: A meta-analysis of structural MRI studies. *Hippocampus, 15*(6), 798–807.

Sommershof, A., Aichinger, H., Engler, H., Adenauer, H., Catani, C., Boneberg, E.-M., et al. (2009). Substantial reduction of naïve and regulatory T cells following traumatic stress. *Brain, Behavior, and Immunity, 23*(8), 1117–1124.

Stein, M. B., Jang, K. L., Taylor, S., Vernon, P. A., & Livesley, W. J. (2002). Genetic and environmental influences on trauma exposure and posttraumatic stress disorder symptoms: A twin study. *The American Journal of Psychiatry, 159*(10), 1675–1681.

Stevens, J. S., Jovanovic, T., Fani, N., Ely, T. D., Glover, E. M., Bradley, B., & Ressler, K. J. (2013). Disrupted amygdala-prefrontal functional connectivity in civilian women with post-traumatic stress disorder. *Journal of Psychiatric Research, 47*(10), 1469–1478.

Sutherland, J. E., & Costa, M. (2003). Epigenetics and the environment. *Annals of the New York Academy of Sciences, 983*, 151–160.

Teicher, M. H., Anderson, C. M., & Polcari, A. (2012). Childhood maltreatment is associated with reduced volume in the hippocampal subfields CA3, dentate gyrus, and subiculum. *Proceedings of the National Academy of Sciences of the United States of America, 109*(9), E563–E572.

True, W. R., Rice, J., Eisen, S. A., Heath, A. C., Goldberg, J., Lyons, M. J., et al. (1993). A twin study of genetic and environmental contributions to liability for posttraumatic stress symptoms. *Archives of General Psychiatry, 50*, 257–264.

Tyrka, A. R., Price, L. H., Kao, H.-T., Porton, B., Marsella, S. A., & Carpenter, L. L. (2010). Childhood maltreatment and telomere shortening: Preliminary support for an effect of early stress on cellular aging. *Biological Psychiatry, 67*(6), 531–534.

Valente, N. L. M., Vallada, H., Cordeiro, Q., Bressan, R. A., Andreoli, S. B., Mari, J. J., & Mello, M. F. (2011). Catechol-O-methyltransferase (COMT) val158met polymorphism as a risk factor for PTSD after urban violence. *Journal of Molecular Neuroscience, 43*(3), 516–523.

van der Kolk, B. (2005). Developmental Trauma Disorder: Toward a rational diagnosis for children with complex trauma histories. *Psychiatric Annals, 35*(5), 401–408.

Vanhooren, V., Dewaele, S., Libert, C., Engelborghs, S., de Deyn, P. P., Toussaint, O., et al. (2010). Serum N-glycan profile shift during human ageing. *Experimental Gerontology, 45*(10), 738–743.

Varki, A. (Ed.). (2008). *Essentials of glycobiology* (2nd ed.). Cold Spring Harbor: Cold Spring Harbor Laboratory Press.

von Zglinicki, T., & Martin-Ruiz, C. M. (2005). Telomeres as biomarkers for ageing and age-related diseases. *Current Molecular Medicine, 5*(2), 197–203.

Weaver, I. C. G., Cervoni, N., Champagne, F. A., D'Alessio, A. C., Sharma, S., Seckl, J. R., et al. (2004). Epigenetic programming by maternal behavior. *Nature Neuroscience, 7*(8), 847–854.

Wilker, S., & Kolassa, I.-T. (2013). The formation of a neural fear network in posttraumatic stress disorder: Insights from molecular genetics. *Clinical Psychological Science, 1*(4), 452–469.

Willeit, P., Willeit, J., Mayr, A., Weger, S., Oberhollenzer, F., Brandstätter, A., et al. (2010). Telomere length and risk of incident cancer and cancer mortality. *JAMA: The Journal of the American Medical Association, 304*(1), 69–75.

Wolf, O. T. (2009). Stress and memory in humans: Twelve years of progress? *Brain Research, 1293*, 142–154.

Woon, F. L., & Hedges, D. W. (2009). Amygdala volume in adults with posttraumatic stress disorder: A meta-analysis. *The Journal of Neuropsychiatry and Clinical Neurosciences, 21*(1), 5–12.

Woon, F. L., Sood, S., & Hedges, D. W. (2010). Hippocampal volume deficits associated with exposure to psychological trauma and posttraumatic stress disorder: A meta-analysis. *Progress in Neuro-Psychopharmacology & Biological Psychiatry, 34*(7), 1181–1188.

Xie, P., Kranzler, H. R., Poling, J., Stein, M. B., Anton, R. F., Brady, K., et al. (2009). Interactive effect of stressful life events and the serotonin transporter 5-HTTLPR genotype on posttraumatic stress disorder diagnosis in 2 independent populations. *Archives of General Psychiatry, 66*(11), 1201.

Xie, P., Kranzler, H. R., Poling, J., Stein, M. B., Anton, R. F., Farrer, L. A., & Gelernter, J. (2010). Interaction of FKBP5 with childhood adversity on risk for post-traumatic stress disorder. *Neuropsychopharmacology, 35*(8), 1684–92.

Xie, P., Kranzler, H. R., Farrer, L., & Gelernter, J. (2012). Serotonin transporter 5-HTTLPR genotype moderates the effects of childhood adversity on posttraumatic stress disorder risk: A replication study. *American Journal of Medical Genetics Part B: Neuropsychiatric Genetics, 159*(6), 644–652.

Yan, X., Brown, A. D., Lazar, M., Cressman, V. L., Henn-Haase, C., Neylan, T. C., et al. (2013). Spontaneous brain activity in combat related PTSD. *Neuroscience Letters, 547*, 1–5.

Yehuda, R., Halligan, S. L., & Bierer, L. M. (2001). Relationship of parental trauma exposure and PTSD to PTSD, depressive and anxiety disorders in offspring. *Journal of Psychiatric Research, 35*(5), 261–270.

Zantvoord, J. B., Diehle, J., & Lindauer, R. J. (2013). Using neurobiological measures to predict and assess treatment outcome of psychotherapy in posttraumatic stress disorder: Systematic review. *Psychotherapy and Psychosomatics, 82*(3), 142–151.

Zen, A. L., Whooley, M. A., Zhao, S., & Cohen, B. E. (2012). Post-traumatic stress disorder is associated with poor health behaviors: Findings from the Heart and Soul Study. *Health Psychology, 31*(2), 194–201.

Zhang, T.-Y., & Meaney, M. J. (2010). Epigenetics and the environmental regulation of the genome and its function. *Annual Review of Psychology, 61*, 439–466, C1–3.

Understanding Pathways from Traumatic Exposure to Physical Health

Paula P. Schnurr

Although most research on the effects of traumatic exposure has focused on symptoms and functioning, a number of studies have shown that exposure to a traumatic event can have negative effects on physical health as well. For example, Felitti and colleagues (1998) investigated the effects of childhood trauma on adults in a large healthcare maintenance organization in the USA. For almost every disease category, individuals who had a higher number of traumatic events in childhood also had a higher likelihood of serious chronic diseases in adulthood, including cardiovascular, metabolic, endocrine, and respiratory systems. Although the investigators did not explicitly examine potential mechanisms for their findings, one explanation was suggested by evidence that childhood trauma was related to increased likelihood of poor health behaviors such as smoking and drinking.

However, behavioral factors alone do not account for the relationship between traumatic exposure and poor health. Instead, the most consistent factor is the development of posttraumatic stress disorder (PTSD). This chapter reviews the evidence on the physical health consequences of traumatic exposure by using a model that conceptualizes PTSD as the primary mediator through which exposure affects physical health (Friedman and Schnurr 1995; Schnurr and Jankowski 1999; Schnurr and Green 2004; Schnurr et al. 2007b; Schnurr et al. in press).

P.P. Schnurr
National Center for PTSD and Geisel School of Medicine at Dartmouth,
White River Junction, VT, USA

Department of Psychiatry, Geisel School of Medicine at Dartmouth,
Hanover, NH, USA

© Springer International Publishing Switzerland 2015
U. Schnyder, M. Cloitre (eds.), *Evidence Based Treatments for Trauma-Related Psychological Disorders: A Practical Guide for Clinicians,*
DOI 10.1007/978-3-319-07109-1_5

5.1 Defining and Measuring Physical Health

Understanding the relationship between traumatic exposure and physical health requires understanding of what is meant by "health" itself. The World Health Organization (WHO) defines health as "a state of complete physical, mental, and social well-being and not merely the absence of disease or infirmity" (http://www.who.int/about/definition/en/print.html, accessed 10/11/2013). This definition, reflecting a contemporary biopsychosocial perspective, actually appears in the preamble to the WHO constitution written in 1946. Recognition of health as a complex state thus has a long history.

Wilson and Cleary (1995) describe health as a continuum of increasing complexity, beginning with biological and physiological variables that represent disease or changes to physical systems. Next are symptoms, followed by functional status, health perceptions, and health-related quality of life. These elements influence each other but are not perfectly correlated and can be influenced by personal and environmental factors, e.g., two individuals with the same degree of pain may function very differently due to differences in temperament, social support, and physical exercise.

Both objective and subjective measures are needed in order to fully capture the continuum of physical health. These include not only laboratory tests, clinical exams, and archival records, but also self-reports. One concern about the use of self-reported measures of physical health is the influence of psychological factors such as negative affectivity (Watson and Pennebaker 1989) on how physical health is reported. In fact, comparisons between archival sources and self-reports usually find that self-reports are valid but not perfect substitutes for objective measures of variables such as utilization and diagnosis (Edwards et al. 1994; Sjahid et al. 1998; Wallihan et al. 1999). However, archival records are not necessarily perfect indicators either because they may be incomplete or inaccurate. Furthermore, although self-reports do not always agree with more objective indicators, an individual's perspective is needed to obtain information about all parts of the health continuum except for biological and physical variables.

5.2 A Conceptual Framework for Understanding How Traumatic Exposure Affects Physical Health

Traumatic exposure is linked to adverse outcomes across the continuum of health outcomes: self-reported health problems and functioning (e.g., Glaesmer et al. 2011; Paras et al. 2009; Scott et al. 2011; Spitzer et al. 2009), biological indicators of morbidity (e.g., Sibai et al. 1989; Spitzer et al. 2011), service utilization (Dube et al. 2009; Walker et al. 1999), and mortality (e.g., Boehmer et al. 2004; Sibai et al. 2001).

In order to understand how exposure to a traumatic event could adversely affect physical health, it is necessary to consider what happens following the exposure. Direct effects of trauma are not the answer in most cases. It appears that relatively few trauma survivors are injured or made ill as a result of their exposure; even in a sample of combat veterans who were seeking care for a variety of problems, only

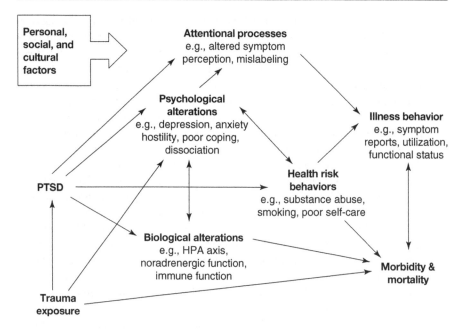

Fig. 5.1 A model relating traumatic exposure and PTSD to physical health outcomes (From Schnurr and Green (2004, p. 248). In the public domain)

21 % had sustained physical injuries in combat (Moeller-Bertram et al. 2013). Also, the types of health problems that emerge—e.g., cardiovascular morbidity and mortality in civilians exposed to war (Sibai et al. 1989, 2001)—typically are not linked to the type of trauma experienced.

So if the traumatic event typically does not lead to direct physical harm, how does the exposure affect physical heath? Schnurr and Green (2004), building on prior work (Friedman and Schnurr 1995; Schnurr and Jankowski 1999), proposed that the answer is severe and persistent distress resulting from traumatic exposure—primarily PTSD but also other mental disorders (Fig. 5.1). The distress is necessary to engage psychological, biological, behavioral, and attentional mechanisms that can lead to poor health. This chapter focuses on PTSD because very few studies have examined the effects of disorders other than PTSD on physical health in trauma survivors. The focus also is on health problems that are not a direct result of a traumatic event.

Psychological mechanisms include comorbid problems often associated with PTSD that have been linked to poor health. Depression, for example, is associated with increased risk of cardiovascular disease and factors such as greater platelet activation, decreased heart rate variability, and greater likelihood of hypertension that could explain the association (Ford 2004). Biological alterations that are associated with PTSD offer additional mechanisms, e.g., increased activation of the locus coeruleus/norepinephrine-sympathetic system and dysregulation of the hypothalamic-pituitary-adrenal system (see Friedman and McEwen 2004).

Behavioral mechanisms are health risk behaviors associated with PTSD, such as smoking, substance abuse, poor self-care, and lack of adherence to medical regimens (Rheingold et al. 2004; Zen et al. 2012). Attentional mechanisms could affect both health perceptions and illness behavior; for example, Pennebaker (2000) suggested that avoidance of thinking about a trauma and then mislabeling the physical and emotional consequences of the avoidance could heighten perceived symptoms. A distinctive aspect of the model is that factors such as smoking and depression, which are often treated as confounding variables to be controlled, are mechanisms through which PTSD can adversely affect health (Schnurr and Green 2004).

Schnurr and Green's (2004) model uses the concept of allostatic load to explain how these mechanisms could lead to disease. Allostatic load is defined as "the strain on the body produced by repeated up and downs of physiologic response, as well as the elevated activity of physiologic systems under challenge, and the changes in metabolism and wear and tear on a number of organs and tissues" (McEwen and Stellar 1993, p. 2094). Because load is defined by cumulative changes, over time and across biological systems, it explains how changes in PTSD that are too subtle to produce disease by themselves could lead to disease (Friedman and McEwen 2004; Schnurr and Green 2004; Schnurr and Jankowski 1999). Schnurr and Jankowski (1999) gave the example of hyperarousal and hyperreactivity in PTSD in combination with the physical effects of substance abuse and smoking and suggested that allostatic load might be greater in PTSD relative to other mental disorders. This hypothesis remains to be tested, but one study found that allostatic load was higher in individuals with PTSD than in traumatized controls (Glover et al. 2006).

5.3   Review of the Literature

There is abundant evidence linking PTSD with poor physical health across a range of outcomes (Friedman and Schnurr 1995; Green and Kimerling 2004; Schnurr and Jankowski 1999). In terms of self-reports, PTSD is associated with poor general health, more physical symptoms and number of chronic health conditions, and lower physical functioning (e.g., Boscarino 1997; Cohen et al. 2009a; Löwe et al. 2010; O'Toole and Catts 2008; Vasterling et al. 2008). For example, in a large national probability sample of US adults, PTSD was associated with increased odds of neurological, vascular, gastrointestinal, metabolic or autoimmune, and bone or joint conditions (Sareen et al. 2005). Most of the findings are from cross-sectional studies, but some evidence comes from longitudinal studies that have found initial PTSD to predict poorer health at a subsequent follow-up (Boyko et al. 2010; Engelhard et al. 2009; Vasterling et al. 2008). A recent meta-analysis of 62 studies, most of which were based on self-reported physical health or other nonobjective indicators, found significant effects of PTSD on health ranging from $r = .17$ for cardiorespiratory health to $r = .48$ for general physical symptoms (Pacella et al. 2013).

PTSD also is associated with poor health measured by objective indicators such as physician-diagnosed disease in both cross-sectional (e.g., Agyemang et al. 2012; Andersen et al. 2010; Nazarian et al. 2012; Seng et al. 2006) and longitudinal studies (e.g., Dirkzwager et al. 2007; Kimerling et al. 1999). The range of outcomes is striking. One cross-sectional study of a large sample of women who were receiving public healthcare in the USA found that women who had PTSD were more likely than women with another mental disorder to have syndromes such as chronic fatigue, irritable bowel, and fibromyalgia as well as disorders with more defined etiology, such as cancer and circulatory, endocrine, and respiratory disease (Seng et al. 2006). A longitudinal study found that PTSD symptoms were associated with greater incidence of physician-diagnosed arterial, musculoskeletal, gastrointestinal, and dermatological disorders in a sample of older male veterans (Schnurr et al. 2000b), even after statistical adjustment for age, smoking, body mass index, and alcohol use.

Cardiovascular outcomes have been a particular focus in this literature. Prospective studies have shown that PTSD is associated with increased risk of coronary heart disease in older male veterans (Kubzansky et al. 2007), male Vietnam veterans (Boscarino and Chang 1999; Kang et al. 2006; Vaccarino et al. 2013), and civilian women (Kubzansky et al. 2009). Pain is another area of particular focus, spanning both self-reported and physician-diagnosed measures. Individuals with PTSD report higher levels of chronic pain that is not related to traumatic injury such as rheumatoid arthritis (e.g., Mikuls et al. 2013) and have an increased likelihood of pain syndromes such as chronic pelvic pain and fibromyalgia (e.g., Seng et al. 2006).

Evidence on the relationship between PTSD and utilization of medical services is somewhat mixed. Some studies have found that PTSD is associated only with greater use of mental health services or emergency care (e.g., Possemato et al. 2010). However, the majority of studies have found that PTSD is associated with greater use of medical care services (e.g., Gill et al. 2009; Glaesmer et al. 2011; O'Toole and Catts 2008; Schnurr et al. 2000a). Few studies have examined cost implications, but there is some evidence that PTSD is associated with higher healthcare costs (e.g., Walker et al. 2004).

All of the studies on PTSD and mortality have been conducted using military veteran samples. Some of these studies have found that PTSD is associated with excess mortality (e.g., Boscarino 2006; Kasprow and Rosenheck 2000; see Abrams et al. 2011; O'Toole et al. 2010, for exceptions). Other studies have found that PTSD is associated with mortality due only to external causes or diseases related to substance abuse (e.g., Bullman and Kang 1994; Drescher et al. 2003). A recent study found that PTSD was associated with all-cause mortality, but not after statistical adjustment for demographic, behavioral, and clinical factors (Chwastiak et al. 2010).

5.3.1 Explicit Tests of PTSD as a Mediator of the Relationship Between Traumatic Exposure and Physical Health

Evidence that PTSD mediates the effects of traumatic exposure on physical health comes from several types of analyses: (a) multiple regression analyses in which a statistically significant association between exposure and physical health is reduced or eliminated when PTSD is added to the model; (b) structural equation modeling, a more formal version of (a); and (c) comparisons involving individuals with PTSD, traumatized controls, and nontraumatized controls. Most of these studies have examined self-reported health outcomes (e.g., Campbell et al. 2008; Löwe et al. 2010; Norman et al. 2006; Schuster-Wachen et al. 2013; Tansill et al. 2012; Wolfe et al. 1994), with few exceptions (e.g., Glaesmer et al. 2011; Schnurr et al. 2000b). The effects can be substantial. For example, a study of 900 older male veterans found that PTSD mediated 90 % of the effect of combat exposure on health (Schnurr and Spiro 1999).

However, the effects also may differ across populations and outcomes. A study of Vietnam Veterans found that PTSD mediated 58 % of the effect of warzone exposure on self-reported health in men but only 35 % of the effect in women (Taft et al. 1999). A study of PTSD and self-reported health in primary care patients also found the effects of mediation to be larger in men (Norman et al. 2006). Although trauma exposure was related to digestive disease and cancer in women, PTSD did not mediate these relationships. Exposure was related to arthritis and diabetes in men, but PTSD mediated only the association between trauma and arthritis. In another study showing differential mediation across outcomes, combat exposure predicted increased incidence of physician-diagnosed arterial, pulmonary, and upper gastrointestinal disorders and other heart disorders over a 30-year interval in older veterans, yet PTSD mediated only the effect of exposure on arterial disorders (Schnurr et al. 2000b).

5.3.2 Evidence on Potential Mechanisms Through Which PTSD Affects Physical Health

To date, no study has simultaneously examined the psychological, biological, behavioral, and attentional factors Schnurr and Green (2004) hypothesized to mediate the relationship between PTSD and health. Instead, studies have focused on specific domains or individual factors.

Of all the potential psychological mediators, depression is arguably the most important because it has well-documented associations with a range of physical health problems (Ford 2004). The data on depression are generally consistent with its hypothesized role as a mediator of the relationship between PTSD and health. For example, in one study, controlling for depression significantly reduced the association between PTSD and somatic symptoms, which is consistent with the idea that depression is a mediator of the relationship (Löwe et al. 2010). In another study, depression fully mediated the relationship between PTSD and pain (Poundja et al. 2006). Depression also may mediate the relationship between PTSD and other mediators. Zen et al. (2012) found that depression mediated the relationship between PTSD and both physical inactivity and medication nonadherence.

The data on health behaviors are mixed. Some studies have found that health behaviors are partial mediators of the relationship between PTSD and health (e.g., Crawford et al. 2009; Flood et al. 2009). Other studies have failed to find that health behaviors mediate the relationship (e.g., Del Gaizo et al. 2011; Schnurr and Spiro 1999). Although it makes sense that health behaviors would at least partially mediate the relationship between PTSD and physical health, these behaviors do not appear to account for a substantial amount of the effect. Furthermore, many studies have controlled for these factors and still find that PTSD is related to poor health (e.g., Boscarino 1997; O'Toole and Catts 2008; Schnurr et al. 2000b).

In terms of biological mediators, the most substantial evidence comes from studies of risk factors for cardiovascular disease. Individuals with PTSD are more likely than individuals with depression or with no mental disorder to have hypertension (e.g., Kibler et al. 2008). A recent study found that PTSD symptoms were associated with increased risk of developing obesity in a group of normal-weight nurses who were followed over a 16-year interval (Kubzansky et al. 2013). Another recent study found that male and female veterans with PTSD were at increased risk of obesity, as well as smoking, hypertension, diabetes, and dyslipidemia (Cohen et al. 2009b). PTSD also is associated with low-grade inflammation, an additional risk factor for cardiovascular disease (Guo et al. 2012; Pace et al. 2012; Spitzer et al. 2010).

Friedman and McEwan (2004) had suggested that PTSD would be associated with risk of metabolic syndrome, a constellation of risk factors including obesity, hyperlipidemia, hyperglycemia, and hypertension. Recent studies have found this to be the case and have shown that the association between PTSD and metabolic syndrome is independent of other risk factors such as demographic characteristics, health risk behaviors, and depression (Heppner et al. 2009; Jin et al. 2009; Weiss et al. 2011).

Metabolic syndrome illustrates one of the key features of allostatic load, which is the combined effect of multiple risk factors. The studies linking PTSD with metabolic syndrome therefore provide support for the possibility that higher allostatic load is a key mechanism through which PTSD affects physical health.

5.3.3 Evidence on Whether Treating PTSD Improves Physical Health

Despite the evidence suggesting that PTSD leads to poor health, there is only limited information on the question of whether treating PTSD improves health. The best evidence comes from studies that have used measures of self-reported physical symptoms and physical functioning, but the evidence is not consistent. Recent studies have found that symptoms (Galovksi et al. 2009; Rauch et al. 2009) and functioning (Beck et al. 2009; Dunne et al. 2012; Neuner et al. 2008) improved following cognitive behavioral therapy for PTSD. For example, Dunne et al. (2012) found that cognitive behavioral therapy for PTSD in patients with chronic whiplash disorders led to reductions in neck disability and improvements in physical functioning. In contrast, other studies have failed to find improvements in physical functioning following treatment with fluoxetine (Malik et al. 1999) or cognitive behavioral therapy (Schnurr et al. 2007a).

There has been very little research on the effects of PTSD treatment on physician-diagnosed disorder or other objective indicators of morbidity. Whether treating PTSD can improve a disorder such as coronary artery disease or diabetes thus is unknown and even uncertain given the mixed evidence from trials on the treatment of depression (e.g., Bogner et al. 2007; Writing Committee for the ENRICHD Investigators 2003). Even though PTSD may have increased the likelihood of an individual developing a given disorder, the biological mechanisms through which this has occurred may become independent of PTSD and nonreversible through the reduction of PTSD symptoms alone. Consider the case of metabolic syndrome. It is plausible that reduced hyperarousal following successful treatment could lead to reductions in hypertension. However, the majority of people with hypertension do not suffer from PTSD or any mental disorder (e.g., Hamer et al. 2010), so simply reducing the hyperarousal may not be sufficient in order to treat the hypertension. Furthermore, it is less plausible that obesity, hyperlipidemia, and hyperglycemia would improve without behavioral changes such as better diet and exercise and compliance with medical regimens to control these factors.

5.4   Implications for Research

Schnurr and Green (2004) proposed a research agenda that included both methodological and content issues to be addressed. In terms of methodological issues, they called for studies based on large representative samples and on populations outside the USA, and with measures of PTSD and other posttraumatic reactions and not only measures of traumatic exposure. They also called for studies that were based on biological measures of morbidity. In terms of treatment issues, Schnurr and Green (2004) called for studies that provide more definitive information about which health problems are, and are not, associated with PTSD and other posttraumatic reactions and for measures of physical health to be added to studies of the biological correlates of PTSD. They also called for studies on reactions to traumatic exposure other than PTSD and for research on the effects of PTSD treatment on physical health, including system-level interventions designed to integrate mental and physical healthcare.

Although the evidence showing that traumatic exposure is associated with adverse physical health has grown substantially, there are still key gaps in all of these methodological and content issues. One is the lack of research on significant posttraumatic reactions in the absence of PTSD, especially depression. PTSD appears to have effects that are distinctive from the effects of comorbid disorders, but it would be helpful to delineate for which disorders PTSD has unique effects. Another key gap is the use of biological measures of morbidity. Much of the increase in this area has focused on cardiovascular disease, with less focus on other disease categories such as endocrine and immunological disorders. Studies of mechanism are critically needed, in particular, studies that examine allostatic load as a mechanism linking PTSD (and potentially, other disorders) to physical health. Further study of health outcomes in PTSD treatments trials is important, but specific efforts should be made to focus on populations with physician-diagnosed disorders. It would be useful to examine conditions that could respond to behavioral and psychological change, such as diabetes. It also would be useful to evaluate integrated efforts to reduce health risk behaviors in PTSD patients. A study by McFall et al. (2010), showing the benefits of integrating smoking cessation into PTSD treatment, is an excellent example of the latter and also of interventions that target systems of care.

There are important analytical issues to consider too. When studying events that are likely to cause injury or illness (such as accidents, combat, or torture), analyses need to delineate the direct effects of trauma from the indirect effects caused by PTSD or other reactions. Another analytic issue is how psychological and behavioral correlates of PTSD such as depression and smoking are handled. Statistically adjusting for these factors is appropriate if the goal is to determine whether PTSD has independent effects on health. If the goal is to examine these factors as mechanisms, methods such as hierarchical regression, path analysis, and structural equation modeling are more appropriate.

5.5 Implications for Clinical Practice

The effects of PTSD on physical health have implications for clinical practice. Patients with PTSD may be dealing with physical health burden in addition to PTSD: medical disorders, reduced physical functioning, and simply not feeling well. A holistic, patient-centered approach to care requires that mental health providers may need to address physical health problems, particularly if these problems interfere with treatment adherence or treatment response. Kilpatrick et al. (1997) emphasized the importance of psychoeducation to help patients understand how their trauma-related symptoms may be related to their physical problems and how addressing both physical and mental health problems could enhance recovery.

Many providers are familiar with addressing substance use disorders when treating trauma survivors. Providers may need to address additional health risk behaviors as well and make necessary referrals. Some providers may be reluctant to address smoking in particular out of a concern that patients who use smoking to help manage PTSD symptoms may find it difficult to stay engaged in intensive trauma-focused work if this coping strategy is taken away. However, McFall and colleagues (2010), who found that integrating smoking cessation treatment into outpatient PTSD care was effective for reducing smoking, also found that PTSD symptoms did not increase as a result of smoking cessation. Integrating medical care into a mental healthcare setting also may be helpful, particularly for patients who have significant psychiatric problems (Druss et al. 2001).

Because PTSD is associated with increased utilization of medical services (e.g., Gill et al. 2009; Glaesmer et al. 2011; Schnurr et al. 2000b), providers in medical care settings may need to increase efforts to address PTSD. Many patients with PTSD seek care only in medical settings—typically primary care, where their PTSD may go unrecognized (Liebschutz et al. 2007; Magruder and Yeager 2008; Samson et al. 1999). Providers in these settings may need to more routinely screen for PTSD and engage in strategies to help patients receive care for their PTSD symptoms. There are a variety of strategies for integrating medical and mental healthcare that have been shown to work in mental health disorders other than PTSD (Bower et al.

2006; Roy-Byrne et al. 2010), but very little research has examined these strategies in PTSD. One recent randomized clinical trial found that collaborative care using a telephone care manager was not more effective than usual care for veterans with PTSD (Schnurr et al. 2013), but further study is needed to make definitive conclusions about the optimal strategies for addressing PTSD in primary and specialty care medical settings. At a minimum, more education for patients and providers is needed (Green et al. 2011).

5.6   Implications for Society

The increased risk of poor health associated with exposure to traumatic events has important implications for society. One is that some disease may be prevented by either reducing the risk of exposure or by reducing the risk of PTSD and other significant posttraumatic disorders. The health benefits of reducing the risk of preventable exposures such as accidents and physical and sexual assault are obvious (and for reasons in addition to those specific to trauma). However, there could be important population health benefits of preventing posttraumatic symptomatology by interrupting the cascade of biological, psychological, behavioral, and attentional changes that may emerge when a traumatized individual fails to recover. There also could be important monetary benefits of prevention given that PTSD is associated with increased financial costs (Marshall et al. 2000; Marciniak et al. 2005; Walker et al. 2004).

Increased awareness of traumatic exposure and its consequences is key from a public health perspective. The greater likelihood of health risk behaviors associated with traumatic exposure, and especially with PTSD, suggests that recognition and management of posttraumatic reactions could enhance public health campaigns for problems such as smoking and obesity and the importance of engaging in preventive healthcare to improve population health. Increased awareness of the effects of traumatic exposure and PTSD on physical health is needed at a global health level as well, particularly in countries with recent or ongoing conflict or disasters and in third world countries with limited healthcare and mental healthcare infrastructure.

The relationship between traumatic exposure and poor physical health also has implications for legal and compensation systems. Should individuals with PTSD receive compensation for physical health problems? It makes sense that an individual who developed PTSD and sustained permanent knee damage as a result of a life-threatening accident at work would receive compensation for both conditions. But should the same individual receive additional compensation after developing coronary artery disease or diabetes? The scientific evidence at this point is not conclusive enough to support the burden of proof necessary to determine causality. Furthermore, there are no established scientific methods for determining whether such disease in a given individual is due to posttraumatic symptoms or other factors. This is an extremely complicated question to answer because physical disorders are typically influenced by multiple factors, including genetics, demographic characteristics, pretraumatic health, and posttraumatic factors unrelated to the trauma.

Conclusions

There is substantial evidence showing that individuals who are exposed to a traumatic event have increased risk of poor health. This chapter is based on a model in which PTSD and other significant distress reactions are the mechanism(s) through which exposure affects health (Schnurr and Green 2004). Biological, psychological, behavioral, and attentional changes associated with PTSD are the proposed mechanisms through which PTSD could affect physical health, with the concept of allostatic load (McEwen and Stellar 1993) as an explanation for how even subtle changes could combine to adversely affect health. The literature showing that PTSD is associated with poor health is highly consistent across self-reported and objective indicators, although there is relatively less evidence on objective indicators of morbidity other than cardiovascular disease and on mortality. Nevertheless, recognizing the physical health effects of traumatic exposure has important implications for research, practice, and society as a whole.

References

Abrams, T. E., Vaughan-Sarrazin, M., & Vander Weg, M. W. (2011). Acute exacerbations of chronic obstructive pulmonary disease and the effect of existing psychiatric comorbidity on subsequent mortality. *Psychosomatics, 52*, 441–449. doi:10.1016/j.psym.2011.03.005.

Agyemang, C., Goosen, S., Anujuo, K., & Ogedegbe, G. (2012). Relationship between posttraumatic stress disorder and diabetes among 105,180 asylum seekers in the Netherlands. *European Journal of Public Health, 22*, 658–662. doi:10.1093/eurpub/ckr138.

Andersen, J., Wade, M., Possemato, K., & Ouimette, P. (2010). Association between posttraumatic stress disorder and primary care provider-diagnosed disease among Iraq and Afghanistan veterans. *Psychosomatic Medicine, 72*, 498–504. doi:10.1097/PSY.0b013e3181d969a1.

Beck, J. G., Coffey, S. F., Foy, D. W., Keane, T. M., & Blanchard, E. B. (2009). Group cognitive behavior therapy for chronic posttraumatic stress disorder: An initial randomized pilot study. *Behavior Therapy, 40*, 82–92. doi:10.1016/j.beth.2008.01.003.

Boehmer, T. K. C., Flanders, D., McGeehin, M. A., Boyle, C., & Barrett, D. H. (2004). Postservice mortality in Vietnam veterans: 30-year follow-up. *Archives of Internal Medicine, 164*, 1908–1916. doi:10.1001/archinte.164.17.1908.

Bogner, H. R., Morales, K. H., Post, E. P., & Bruce, M. L. (2007). Diabetes, depression, and death: A randomized controlled trial of a depression treatment program for older adults based in primary care (PROSPECT). *Diabetes Care, 30*, 3005–3010. doi:10.2337/dc07-0974.

Boscarino, J. A. (1997). Diseases among men 20 years after exposure to severe stress: Implications for clinical research and medical care. *Psychosomatic Medicine, 59*, 605–614.

Boscarino, J. (2006). Posttraumatic stress disorder among U.S. Army veterans 30 years after military service. *Annals of Epidemiology, 16*, 248–256. doi:10.1016/j.annepidem.2005.03.009.

Boscarino, J. A., & Chang, J. (1999). Electrocardiogram abnormalities among men with stress-related psychiatric disorders: Implications for coronary heart disease and clinical research. *Annals of Behavioral Medicine, 21*, 227–234. doi:10.1007/BF02884839.

Bower, P., Gilbody, S., Richards, D., Fletcher, J., & Sutton, A. (2006). Collaborative care for depression in primary care: Making sense of a complex intervention: Systematic review and meta-regression. *British Journal of Psychiatry, 189*, 484–493. doi:10.1192/bjp.bp.106.023655.

Boyko, E. J., Jacobson, I. G., Smith, B., Ryan, M. A. K., Hooper, T. I., Amoroso, P. J., Gackstetter, G. D., Barrett-Connor, E., & Smith, T. C. (2010). Risk of diabetes in U.S. military service members in relation to combat deployment and mental health. *Diabetes Care, 33*, 1771–1777. doi:10.2337/dc10-0296.

Bullman, T. A., & Kang, H. K. (1994). Posttraumatic stress disorder and the risk of traumatic deaths among Vietnam veterans. *Journal of Nervous and Mental Disease, 182*, 604–610.

Campbell, R., Greeson, M. R., Bybee, D., & Raja, S. (2008). The co-occurrence of childhood sexual abuse, adult sexual assault, intimate partner violence, and sexual harassment: A meditational model of posttraumatic stress disorder and physical health outcomes. *Journal of Consulting and Clinical Psychology, 76*, 194–207. doi:10.1037/0022-006X.76.2.194.

Chwastiak, L. A., Rosenheck, R. A., Desai, R., & Kasis, L. E. (2010). Association of psychiatric illness and all-cause mortality in the national Department of Veterans Affairs health care system. *Psychosomatic Medicine, 72*, 817–822. doi:10.1097/PSY.0b013e3181eb33e9.

Cohen, B. E., Marmar, C., Neylan, T. C., Schiller, N. B., Ali, S., & Wholley, M. A. (2009a). Posttraumatic stress disorder and health-related quality of life in patients with coronary heart disease. *Archives of General Psychiatry, 66*, 1214–1220. doi:10.1001/archgenpsychiatry.2009.149.

Cohen, B. E., Marmar, C., Ren, L., Bertenthal, D., & Seal, K. H. (2009b). Association of cardiovascular risk factors with mental health diagnoses in Iraq and Afghanistan War veterans using VA health care. *JAMA, 302*, 489–491. doi:10.1001/jama.2009.1084.

Crawford, E. F., Drescher, K. D., & Rosen, C. S. (2009). Predicting mortality in veterans with posttraumatic stress disorder thirty years after Vietnam. *Journal of Nervous and Mental Disease, 197*, 260–265. doi:10.1097/NMD.0b013e31819dbfce.

Del Gaizo, A. L., Elhai, J. D., & Weaver, T. L. (2011). Posttraumatic stress disorder, poor physical health, and substance use behaviors in a national trauma-exposure sample. *Psychiatry Research, 188*, 390–395. doi:10.1016/j.psychres.2011.03.016.

Dirkzwager, A. J. E., van der Velden, P. G., Grievink, L., & Yzermans, J. (2007). Disaster-related posttraumatic stress disorder and physical health. *Psychosomatic Medicine, 69*, 435–440. doi:10.1097/PSY.0b013e318052e20a.

Drescher, K. D., Rosen, C. S., Burling, T. A., & Foy, D. W. (2003). Causes of death among male veterans who received residential treatment for PTSD. *Journal of Traumatic Stress, 16*, 535–543. doi:10.1023/B:JOTS.0000004076.62793.79.

Druss, B. G., Rohrbaugh, R. M., Levinson, C. M., & Rosenheck, R. A. (2001). Integrated medical care for patients with serious psychiatric illness: A randomized trial. *Archives of General Psychiatry, 58*, 861–868. doi:10.1001/archpsyc.58.9.861.

Dube, S. R., Fairewather, D., Pearson, W. S., Felitti, V. J., Anda, R. F., & Croft, J. B. (2009). Cumulative childhood stress and autoimmune diseases in adults. *Psychosomatic Medicine, 71*, 243–250. doi:10.1097/PSY.0b013e3181907888.

Dunne, R. L., Kenardy, J., & Sterling, M. (2012). A randomized controlled trial of cognitive-behavioral therapy for the treatment of PTSD in the context of chronic whiplash. *Clinical Journal of Pain, 28*, 755–765. doi:10.1097/AJP.0b013e318243e16b.

Edwards, W. S., Winn, D. M., Kurlantzick, V., Sheridan, J., Berk, M. L., Retchin, S., et al. (1994). *Evaluation of National Health Interview Survey diagnostic reporting*. Hyattsville: National Center for Health Statistics.

Engelhard, I. M., van den Hout, M. A., Weerts, J., Hox, J. J., & vanDoornen, L. J. P. (2009). A prospective study of the relation between posttraumatic stress and physical health symptoms. *International Journal of Clinical and Health Psychology, 9*, 365–372.

Felitti, V. J., Anda, R. F., Norenberg, D., Williamson, D. F., Spitz, A. M., Edwards, V., Koss, M. P., & Marks, J. S. (1998). Relationship of childhood abuse and household dysfunction to many of the leading causes of death in adults. *American Journal of Preventative Medicine, 14*, 245–258. doi:10.1016/S0749-3797(98)00017-8.

Flood, A. M., McDevitt-Murphy, M. E., Weathers, F. W., Eakin, D. E., & Benson, T. A. (2009). Substance use behaviors as a mediator between posttraumatic stress disorder and physical health in trauma-exposed college students. *Journal of Behavioral Medicine, 32*, 234–243. doi:10.1007/s10865-008-9195-y.

Ford, D. (2004). Depression, trauma, and cardiovascular health. In P. P. Schnurr & B. L. Green (Eds.), *Trauma and health: Physical health consequences of exposure to extreme stress* (pp. 73–97). Washington, DC: American Psychological Association.

Friedman, M. J., & McEwen, B. S. (2004). Posttraumatic stress disorder, allostatic load, and medical illness. In P. P. Schnurr & B. L. Green (Eds.), *Trauma and health: Physical health consequences of exposure to extreme stress* (pp. 157–188). Washington, DC: American Psychological Association.

Friedman, M. J., & Schnurr, P. P. (1995). The relationship between PTSD, trauma, and physical health. In M. J. Friedman, D. S. Charney, & A. Y. Deutch (Eds.), *Neurobiological and clinical consequences of stress: From normal adaptation to PTSD* (pp. 507–527). Philadelphia: Lippincott-Raven.

Galovksi, T. E., Monson, C., Bruce, S. E., & Resick, P. A. (2009). Does cognitive-behavioral therapy for PTSD improve perceived health and sleep impairment? *Journal of Traumatic Stress, 22*, 197–204. doi:10.1002/jts.20418.

Gill, J. M., Szanton, S., Taylor, T. J., Page, G. G., & Campbell, J. C. (2009). Medical conditions and symptoms associated with posttraumatic stress disorder in low-income urban women. *Journal of Women's Health, 18*, 261–267. doi:10.1089/jwh.2008.0914.

Glaesmer, H., Brahler, E., Gundel, H., & Riedel-Heller, S. G. (2011). The association of traumatic experiences and posttraumatic stress disorder with physical morbidity in old age: A German population-based study. *Psychosomatic Medicine, 73*, 401–406. doi:10.1097/PSY.0b013e31821b47e8.

Glover, D. A., Stuber, M., & Poland, R. E. (2006). Allostatic load in women with and without PTSD symptoms. *Psychiatry, 69*, 191–203. doi:10.1521/psyc.2006.69.3.191.

Green, B. L., & Kimerling, R. (2004). Trauma, posttraumatic stress disorder, and health status. In P. P. Schnurr & B. L. Green (Eds.), *Trauma and health: Physical health consequences of exposure to extreme stress* (pp. 13–42). Washington, DC: American Psychological Association.

Green, B. L., Kaltman, S., Frank, L., Glennie, M., Subramanian, A., Fritts-Wilson, M., Neptune, D., & Chung, J. (2011). Primary care providers' experiences with trauma patients: A qualitative study. *Psychological Trauma: Theory, Research, Practice, and Policy, 3*, 37–41. doi:10.1037/a0020097.

Guo, M., Liu, T., Guo, J.-C., Jiang, X.-L., Chen, F., & Gao, Y.-S. (2012). Study on serum cytokine levels in posttraumatic stress disorder patients. *Asian Pacific Journal of Tropical Medicine, 5*, 323–325. doi:10.1016/S1995-7645(12)60048-0.

Hamer, M., Batty, G. D., Stamatakis, E., & Kivimaki, M. (2010). The combined influence of hypertension and common mental disorder on all-cause and cardiovascular disease mortality. *Journal of Hypertension, 28*, 2401–2406. doi:10.1097/HJH.0b013e32833e9d7c.

Heppner, P. S., Crawford, E. F., Haji, U., Afari, N., Hauger, R. L., Dashevsky, B. A., Horn, P. S., Nunnink, S. E., & Baker, D. G. (2009). The association of posttraumatic stress disorder and metabolic syndrome: A study of increased health risk in veterans. *BMC Medicine, 7*, 1–8. doi:10.1186/1741-7015-7-1.

Jin, H., Lanouette, N. M., Mudaliar, S., Henry, R., Folsom, D. P., Khandrika, S., Glorioso, D. K., & Jeste, D. (2009). Association of posttraumatic stress disorder with increased prevalence of metabolic syndrome. *Journal of Clinical Psychopharmacology, 29*, 210–215. doi:10.1097/JCP.0b013e3181a45ed0.

Kang, H. K., Bullman, T. A., & Taylor, J. T. (2006). Risk of selected cardiovascular diseases and posttraumatic stress disorder among former World War II prisoners of war. *Annals of Epidemiology, 16*, 381–386. doi:10.1016/j.annepidem.2005.03.004.

Kasprow, W. J., & Rosenheck, R. (2000). Mortality among homeless and nonhomeless mentally ill veterans. *Journal of Nervous and Mental Disease, 188*, 141–147. doi:10.1097/00005053-200003000-00003.

Kibler, J. L., Joshi, K., & Ma, M. (2008). Hypertension in relation to posttraumatic stress disorder and depression in the US National Comorbidity Survey. *Behavioral Medicine, 34*, 125–131. doi:10.3200/BMED. 34.4.125-132.

Kilpatrick, D. G., Resnick, H., & Acierno, R. (1997). Health impact of interpersonal violence 3: Implications for clinical practice and public policy. *Behavioral Medicine, 23*, 79–85. doi:10.1080/08964289709596731.

Kimerling, R., Calhoun, K. S., Forehand, R., Armistead, L., Morse, E., Morse, P., Clark, R., & Clark, L. (1999). Traumatic stress in HIV-infected women. *AIDS Education and Prevention, 11*, 321–330.

Kubzansky, L. D., Koenen, K. C., Spiro, A., Vokonas, P. S., & Sparrow, D. (2007). Prospective study of posttraumatic stress disorder symptoms and coronary heart disease in the Normative Aging Study. *Archives of General Psychiatry, 64*, 109–116. doi:10.1001/archpsyc.64.1.109.

Kubzansky, L. D., Koenen, K. C., Jones, C., & Eaton, W. W. (2009). A prospective study of posttraumatic stress disorder symptoms and coronary heart disease in women. *Health Psychology, 28*, 125–130. doi:10.1037/0278-6133.28.1.125.

Kubzansky, L. D., Bordelois, P., Hee, J. J., Robert, A. L., Cerda, M., Bluestone, N., & Koenen, K. C. (2013). The weight of traumatic stress: A prospective study of posttraumatic stress disorder symptoms and weight status in women. *JAMA Psychiatry*. doi:10.1001/jamapsychiatry.2013.2798.

Liebschutz, J., Saitz, R., Brower, V., Keane, T. M., Lloyd-Travaglini, C., Averbuch, T., & Samet, J. H. (2007). PTSD in urban primary care: High prevalence and low physician recognition. *Journal of General Internal Medicine, 22*, 719–726. doi:10.1007/s11606-007-0161-0.

Löwe, B., Kroenke, K., Spitzer, R. L., Williams, J. B. W., Mussell, M., Rose, M., Wingenfeld, K., Sauer, N., & Spitzer, C. (2010). Trauma exposure and posttraumatic stress disorder in primary care patients: Cross-sectional criterion standard study. *Journal of Clinical Psychiatry, 72*, 304–312. doi:10.4088/JCP.09m05290blu.

Magruder, K. M., & Yeager, D. E. (2008). Patient factors relating to detection of posttraumatic stress disorder in Department of Veterans Affairs primary care settings. *Journal of Rehabilitation Research & Development, 45*, 371–382. doi:10.1682/JRRD.2007.06.0091.

Malik, M. L., Connor, K. M., Sutherland, S. M., Smith, R. D., Davison, R. M., & Davidson, J. R. T. (1999). Quality of life and posttraumatic stress disorder: A pilot study assessing changes in SF-36 scores before and after treatment in a placebo-controlled trial of fluoxetine. *Journal of Traumatic Stress, 12*, 387–393. doi:10.1023/A:1024745030140.

Marciniak, M. D., Lage, M. J., Dunayevich, E., Russell, J. M., Bowman, L., Landbloom, R. P., & Levine, L. R. (2005). The cost of treating anxiety: the medical and demographic correlates that impact total medical costs. *Depression and Anxiety, 12*, 178–184. doi:10.1002/da.20074.

Marshall, R. P., Jorm, A. F., Grayson, D. A., & O'Toole, B. I. (2000). Medical-care costs associated with posttraumatic stress disorder in Vietnam veterans. *Australian and New Zealand Journal of Psychiatry, 34*, 954–962. doi:10.1046/j.1440-1614.2000.00831.x.

McEwen, B. S., & Stellar, E. (1993). Stress and the individual: Mechanisms leading to disease. *Archives of Internal Medicine, 153*, 2093–2101. doi:10.1001/archinte.1993.00410180039004.

McFall, M., Saxon, A. J., Malte, C. A., Chow, B., Bailey, S., Baker, D. G., Beckham, J. C., Boardman, K. D., Carmody, T. P., Joseph, A. M., Smith, M. W., Shih, M. C., Lu, Y., Holodniy, M., Lavori, P. W., & CSP 519 Study Team. (2010). Integrating tobacco cessation into mental health care for posttraumatic stress disorder: A randomized controlled trial. *JAMA, 304*, 2485–2493. doi:10.1001/jama.2010.1769.

Mikuls, T. R., Padala, P. R., Sayles, H. R., Yu, F., Michaud, K., Caplan, L., Kerr, G. S., Reimold, A., Cannon, G. W., Richards, J. S., Lazaro, D., Thiele, G. M., & Boscarino, J. (2013). Prospective study of posttraumatic stress disorder and disease activity outcome sin US veterans with rheumatoid arthritis. *Arthritis Care & Research, 65*, 227–234. doi:10.1002/acr.21778.

Moeller-Bertram, T., Afari, N., Mostoufi, S., Fink, D. S., Johnson Wright, L., & Baker, D. G. (2013). Specific pain complaints in Iraq and Afghanistan veterans screening positive for posttraumatic stress disorder. *Psychosomatics*. doi:10.1016/j.psym.2013.01.011.

Nazarian, D., Kimerling, R., & Frayne, S. M. (2012). Posttraumatic stress disorder, substance use disorders, and medical comorbidity among returning U.S. veterans. *Journal of Traumatic Stress, 25*, 220–225. doi:10.1001/archinte.1993.00410180039004.

Neuner, F., Lamaro Onyut, P., Ertl, V., Odenwald, M., Schauer, E., & Elbert, T. (2008). Treatment of posttraumatic stress disorder by trained lay counselors in an African refugee settlement: A randomized controlled trial. *Journal of Consulting and Clinical Psychology, 76*, 686–694. doi:10.1037/0022-006X.76.4.686.

Norman, S. B., Means-Christensen, A. J., Craske, M. G., Sherbourne, C. D., Roy-Byrne, P. P., & Stein, M. B. (2006). Associations between psychological trauma and physical illness in primary care. *Journal of Traumatic Stress, 19*, 461–470. doi:10.1002/jts.20129.

O'Toole, B. I., & Catts, S. V. (2008). Trauma, PTSD, and physical health: An epidemiological study of Australian Vietnam veterans. *Journal of Psychosomatic Research, 64*, 33–40. doi:10.1016/j.jpsychores.2007.07.006.

O'Toole, B. I., Catts, S. V., Outram, S., Pierse, K. R., & Cockburn, J. (2010). Factors associated with civilian mortality in Australian Vietnam veterans three decades after the war. *Military Medicine, 175*, 88–95. doi:10.1093/aje/kwp146.

Pace, T. W., Wingenfeld, K., Schmidt, I. M., Meinlschmidt, G., Hellhammer, D. H., & Heim, C. M. (2012). Increased peripheral NF-κB pathway activity in women with childhood abuse-related posttraumatic stress disorder. *Brain, Behavior, and Immunity, 26*, 13–17. doi:10.1016/j.bbi.2011.07.232.

Pacella, M. L., Hruska, B., & Delahanty, D. L. (2013). The physical health consequences of PTSD and PTSD symptoms: A meta-analytic review. *Journal of Anxiety Disorder, 27*, 33–46. doi:10.1016/j.janxdis.2012.08.004.

Paras, M. L., Murad, M. H., Chen, L. P., Goranson, E. N., Sattler, A. L., Colbenson, K. M., Elamin, M. B., Seime, R. J., Prokop, L. J., & Zirakzadeh, A. (2009). Sexual abuse and lifetime diagnosis of somatic disorders: A systematic review and meta-analysis. *JAMA, 302*, 550–561. doi:10.1001/jama.2009.1091.

Pennebaker, J. (2000). Psychological factors influencing the reporting of physical symptoms. In A. A. Stone, J. S. Turkkan, C. A. Bachrach, J. B. Jobe, H. S. Kurtzman, & V. S. Cain (Eds.), *The science of self-report: Implications for research and practice* (pp. 299–315). Mahwah: Erlbaum.

Possemato, K., Wade, M., Andersen, J., & Ouimette, P. (2010). The impact of PTSD, depression, and substance use disorders on disease burden and health care utilization among OEF/OIF veterans. *Psychological Trauma: Theory, Research, Practice, and Policy, 2*, 218–223. doi:10.1037/a0019236.

Poundja, J., Fikretoglu, D., & Brunet, A. (2006). The co-occurrence of posttraumatic stress disorder symptoms and pain: Is depression a mediator? *Journal of Traumatic Stress, 19*, 747–751. doi:10.1002/jts.20151.

Rauch, S. A. M., Grunfeld, T. E. E., Yadin, E., Cahill, S. P., Hembree, E., & Foa, E. B. (2009). Changes in reported physical health symptoms and social function with Prolonged Exposure therapy for chronic posttraumatic stress disorder. *Depression and Anxiety, 26*, 732–738.

Rheingold, A. A., Acierno, R., & Resnick, H. S. (2004). Trauma, posttraumatic stress disorder, and health risk behaviors. In P. P. Schnurr & B. L. Green (Eds.), *Trauma and health: Physical health consequences of exposure to extreme stress* (pp. 217–243). Washington, DC: American Psychological Association.

Roy-Byrne, P., Craske, M. G., Sullivan, G., Rose, R. D., Edlund, M. J., Lang, A. J., Bystritsky, A., Welch, S. S., Chavira, D. A., Golinelli, D., Campbell-Sills, L., Sherbourne, C. D., & Stein, M. B. (2010). Delivery of evidence-based treatment for multiple anxiety disorders in primary care: A randomized controlled trial. *JAMA, 303*, 1921–1928. doi:10.1001/jama.2010.608.

Samson, A. Y., Bensen, S., Beck, A., Price, D., & Nimmer, C. (1999). Posttraumatic stress disorder in primary care. *Journal of Family Practice, 48*, 222–227.

Sareen, J., Cox, B. J., Clara, I., & Asmundson, G. J. G. (2005). The relationship between anxiety disorders and physical disorders in the U.S. National Comorbidity Survey. *Depression and Anxiety, 21*, 193–202. doi:10.1002/da.20072.

Schnurr, P. P., & Green, B. L. (2004). Understanding relationships among trauma, posttraumatic stress disorder, and health outcomes. In P. P. Schnurr & B. L. Green (Eds.), *Trauma and health: Physical health consequences of exposure to extreme stress* (pp. 247–275). Washington, DC: American Psychological Association.

Schnurr, P. P., & Jankowski, M. K. (1999). Physical health and post-traumatic stress disorder: Review and synthesis. *Seminars in Clinical Neuropsychiatry, 4*, 295–304.

Schnurr, P. P., & Spiro, A. (1999). Combat exposure, posttraumatic stress disorder symptoms, and health behaviors as predictors of self-reported physical health in older veterans. *Journal of Nervous and Mental Disease, 187*, 353–359. doi:10.1097/00005053-199906000-00004.

Schnurr, P. P., Friedman, M. J., Sengupta, A., Jankowski, M. K., & Holmes, T. (2000a). PTSD and utilization of medical treatment services among male Vietnam veterans. *Journal of Nervous and Mental Disease, 188*, 496–504.

Schnurr, P. P., Spiro, A., & Paris, A. H. (2000b). Physician-diagnosed medical disorders in relation to PTSD symptoms in older male military veterans. *Health Psychology, 19*, 91–97. doi:10.1037/0278-6133.19.1.91.

Schnurr, P. P., Friedman, M. J., Engel, C. C., Foa, E. B., Shea, M. T., Chow, B. K., Resick, P. A., Thurston, V., Orsillo, S. M., Haug, R., Turner, C., & Bernardy, N. (2007a). Cognitive-behavioral therapy for posttraumatic stress disorder in women: A randomized controlled trial. *JAMA, 297*, 820–830. doi:10.1001/jama.297.8.820.

Schnurr, P. P., Green, B. L., & Kaltman, S. (2007b). Trauma exposure and physical health. In M. J. Friedman, T. M. Keane, & P. A. Resick (Eds.), *Handbook of PTSD: Science and practice* (pp. 406–424). New York: Guilford.

Schnurr, P. P., Friedman, M. J., Oxman, T. E., Dietrich, A. J., Smith, M. W., Shiner, B., Forshay, E., Gui, J., & Thurston, V. (2013). RESPECT-PTSD: Re-engineering systems for the primary care treatment of PTSD, a randomized controlled trial. *Journal of General Internal Medicine, 28*, 32–40. doi:10.1007/s11606-012-2166-6.

Schnurr, P. P., Schuster-Wachen, J., Green, B. L., & Kaltman, S. (in press). Trauma exposure and physical health. In M. J. Friedman, T. M. Keane, & P. A. Resick (Eds.), *Handbook of PTSD: Science and practice* (2nd edition). New York: Guilford.

Schuster-Wachen, J., Shipherd, J. C., Suvak, M., Vogt, D., King, L. A., & King, D. W. (2013). Posttraumatic stress symptomatology as a mediator of the relationship between warzone exposure and physical health symptoms in men and women. *Journal of Traumatic Stress, 26*, 319–328. doi:10.1002/jts.21818.

Scott, K. M., Von Korff, M., Angermeyer, M. C., Benjet, C., Bruffaerts, R., de Girolamo, G., & Kessler, R. C. (2011). Association of childhood adversities and early-onset mental disorders with adult-onset chronic physical conditions. *Archives of General Psychiatry, 68*, 838–844. doi:10.1001/archgenpsychiatry.2011.77.

Seng, J. S., Clark, M. K., McCarthy, A., & Ronis, D. L. (2006). PTSD and physical comorbidity among women receiving Medicaid: Results from service use data. *Journal of Traumatic Stress, 19*, 45–56. doi:10.1002/jts.20097.

Sibai, A. M., Armenian, H. K., & Alam, S. (1989). Wartime determinants of arteriographically confirmed coronary artery disease in Beirut. *American Journal of Epidemiology, 130*, 623–631.

Sibai, A. M., Fletcher, A., & Armenian, H. K. (2001). Variations in the impact of long-term wartime stressors on mortality among the middle-aged and older population in Beirut, Lebanon, 1983–1993. *American Journal of Epidemiology, 154*, 128–137. doi:10.1093/aje/154.2.128.

Sjahid, S. I., van der Linden, P. D., & Stricker, B. H. C. (1998). Agreement between the pharmacy medication history and patient interview for cardiovascular drugs: The Rotterdam elderly study. *British Journal of Clinical Pharmacology, 45*, 591–595. doi:10.1046/j.1365-2125.1998.00716.x.

Spitzer, C., Barnow, S., Volzke, H., John, U., Freyberger, H. J., & Grabe, H. J. (2009). Trauma, posttraumatic stress disorder, and physical illness: Findings from the general population. *Psychosomatic Medicine, 71*, 1012–1017.

Spitzer, C., Barnow, S., Volzke, H., Wallaschofski, H., John, U., Freyberger, H. J., Löwe, B., & Grabe, H. J. (2010). Association of posttraumatic stress disorder with low-grade elevation of C-reactive protein: Evidence from the general population. *Journal of Psychiatric Research, 44*, 15–21. doi:10.1016/j.jpsychires.2009.06.002.

Spitzer, C., Koch, B., Grabe, H. J., Ewert, R., Barnow, S., Felix, S. B., Ittermann, T., Obst, A., Völzke, H., Gläser, S., & Schaper, C. (2011). Association of airflow limitation with trauma exposure and posttraumatic stress disorder. *European Respiratory Journal, 37*, 1068–1075. doi:10.1097/PSY.0b013e3181bc76b5.

Taft, C. T., Stern, A. S., King, L. A., & King, D. W. (1999). Modeling physical health and functional health status: The role of combat exposure, posttraumatic stress disorder, and personal resource attributes. *Journal of Traumatic Stress, 12*, 3–23. doi:10.1023/A:1024786030358.

Tansill, E. C., Edwards, K. M., Kearns, M. C., Gidycz, C. A., & Calhoun, K. S. (2012). The mediating role of trauma-related symptoms in the relationship between sexual victimization and physical health symptomatology in undergraduate women. *Journal of Traumatic Stress, 25*, 79–85. doi:10.1002/jts.21666.

Vaccarino, V., Goldberg, J., Rooks, C., Shah, A. J., Veledar, E., Faber, T. L., Votaw, J. R., Forsberg, C. W., & Bremner, J. D. (2013). Posttraumatic stress disorder and incidence of coronary heart disease: A twin study. *Journal of the American College of Cardiology, 62*, 970–978. doi:10.1016/j.jacc.2013.04.085.

Vasterling, J. J., Schumm, J., Proctor, S. P., Gentry, E., King, D. W., & King, L. A. (2008). Posttraumatic stress disorder and health functioning in a non-treatment-seeking sample of Iraq war veterans: A prospective analysis. *Journal of Rehabilitation Research and Development, 45*, 347–358. doi:10.1682/JRRD.2007.05.0077.

Walker, E. A., Gelfand, A. N., Katon, W. J., Koss, M. P., Von Korff, M., Bernstein, D. E., & Russo, J. (1999). Adult health status of women with histories of childhood abuse and neglect. *American Journal of Medicine, 107*, 332–339. doi:10.1016/S0002-9343(99)00235-1.

Walker, E. A., Newman, E., & Koss, M. P. (2004). Costs and health care utilization associated with traumatic experiences. In P. P. Schnurr & B. L. Green (Eds.), *Trauma and health: Physical health consequences of exposure to extreme stress* (pp. 43–69). Washington, DC: American Psychological Association.

Wallihan, D. B., Stump, T. E., & Callahan, C. M. (1999). Accuracy of self-reported health service use and patterns of self-care among urban older adults. *Medical Care, 37*, 662–670.

Watson, D., & Pennebaker, J. W. (1989). Health complaints, stress, and distress: Exploring the central role of negative affectivity. *Psychological Review, 96*, 234–254. doi:10.1037/0033-295X.96.2.234.

Weiss, T., Skelton, K., Phifer, J., Jovanovic, T., Gillespie, C. F., Smith, A., Umpierrez, G., Bradley, B., & Ressler, K. J. (2011). Posttraumatic stress disorder is a risk factor for metabolic syndrome in an impoverished urban population. *General Hospital Psychiatry, 33*, 135–142. doi:10.1016/j.genhosppsych.2011.01.002.

Wilson, I. B., & Cleary, P. D. (1995). Linking clinical variables with health-related quality of life. *JAMA, 273*, 59–65. doi:10.1001/jama.1995.03520250075037.

Wolfe, J., Schnurr, P. P., Brown, P. J., & Furey, J. (1994). Posttraumatic stress disorder and war-zone exposure as correlates of perceived health in female Vietnam War veterans. *Journal of Consulting and Clinical Psychology, 62*, 1235–1240. doi:10.1037/0022-006X.62.6.1235.

Writing Committee for the ENRICHD Investigators. (2003). Effect of treating depression and low perceived social support on clinical events after myocardial infarction: The Enhancing Recovery in Coronary Heart Disease Patients (ENRICHD) randomized trial. *JAMA, 289*, 3106–3116. doi:10.1001/jama.289.23.3106.

Zen, A. L., Whooley, M. A., Zhao, S., & Cohen, B. E. (2012). Posttraumatic stress disorder is associated with poor health behaviors: Findings from the Heart and Soul Study. *Health Psychology, 31*, 194–201. doi:10.1037/a0025989.

Part II

Stress and Trauma Related Disorders

The Diagnostic Spectrum of Trauma-Related Disorders

6

Richard A. Bryant

6.1 Introduction

Classifying mental disorders, including traumatic stress disorders, in psychiatry has often been difficult because of the need to discriminate between normal and abnormal states. This situation is particularly difficult in the context of posttraumatic presentations because stress responses are common, and it raises issues of where a line should be drawn between normative reaction and disorder. This chapter reviews the current status of diagnostic systems for describing posttraumatic stress conditions. There has been much activity in this space in recent years because the major diagnostic systems have been undergoing significant reviews and modifications. In this context, this chapter reviews the current status of the major conditions, including posttraumatic stress disorder (PTSD), complex PTSD, acute stress disorder (ASD), acute stress reaction (ASR) and prolonged grief disorder.

6.2 History of DSM

The American Psychiatric Association's diagnostic recognition of stress-related conditions can be traced back to the origins of the *Diagnostic and Statistical Manual for Mental Disorders* (DSM). In the initial iteration, DSM-I (American Psychiatric Association 1952) identified 'gross stress reactions', which was a loosely defined classification aimed to describe those affected by traumatic exposure. Arguably influenced by military conceptualizations that stress reactions were typically transient, this conceptualization was based on the premise that these reactions were temporary. In

R.A. Bryant, PhD
School of Psychology, University of New South Wales, Sydney, NSW 2052, Australia
e-mail: r.bryant@unsw.edu.au

© Springer International Publishing Switzerland 2015
U. Schnyder, M. Cloitre (eds.), *Evidence Based Treatments for Trauma-Related Psychological Disorders: A Practical Guide for Clinicians*,
DOI 10.1007/978-3-319-07109-1_6

DSM-II (American Psychiatric Association 1968), this diagnosis was removed and replaced by 'situational reaction', which described reactions to the full range of severe and mild aversive experiences. The first significant recognition of posttraumatic stress reactions came in 1980 with the publication of DSM-III (American Psychiatric Association 1980). Strongly influenced by the need to formally recognize the mental health needs of Vietnam veterans, this diagnosis encompassed 17 symptoms that fell into three clusters: re-experiencing, avoidance and hyperarousal. This formulation remained for many years and set the framework by which PTSD has been understood since 1980. In DSM-IV (American Psychiatric Association 1994), it underwent minor revisions but essentially kept to the same formula as set by DSM-III. DSM-IV defined PTSD as having been exposed to or witnessing a severely threatening experience and responding with fear, horror or helplessness. This was the gatekeeper to the diagnosis because only if these experiences were present could one then consider the re-experiencing, avoidance and arousal symptoms.

6.3   History of ICD

The World Health Organization has traditionally recognized stress-related conditions in its International Classification of Diseases (ICD). ICD-8 described 'transient situational disturbance' that was a broad category that comprised adjustment problems, severe stress reactions and combat neurosis (World Health Organization 1965). In the next revision (ICD-9), acute stress reaction (ASR) and adjustment reaction (AR) were introduced, and another two were noted in ICD-10 (World Health Organization 1994): posttraumatic stress disorder (PTSD) and enduring personality change after catastrophic experiences (EPACE). The latter two disorders marked important changes from prior diagnoses, which had been conceptualized as transient reactions which normally subside after a period of time had elapsed since the trauma. It is worth noting that the ICD approach has often been influenced by military psychiatry and so an emphasis was placed on the temporary nature of stress reactions. It is also worth noting an important difference between ICD and DSM in terms of their missions. Whereas DSM is understandably focused on US health-care agendas, ICD is more globally focused and aims to address the mental health needs of people across the rest of the world. This focus has resulted in ICD diagnoses being more attuned to the needs of low-resource settings and those affected by conflict, disaster and war. Accordingly, an explicit goal of ICD has been to place the emphasis on practical applications, which includes having diagnoses that are (a) consistent with clinicians' usual classifications, (b) simple diagnoses with minimal symptoms and (c) useful to allow distinctive decisions about treatment between conditions (Reed 2010).

6.4   Classification in DSM-5

There were a number of core changes in DSM-5. One of the fundamental shifts was the location of trauma-related disorders in DSM. Traditionally, PTSD and ASD were classified with anxiety disorders because of the common phenomenology and presumed mechanisms. Leading up to DSM-5, there was considerable debate about creation of a fear circuitry section that would comprise PTSD, ASD, panic disorder, agoraphobia, social phobia and specific phobia (Andrews et al. 2009). This proposal rests on the notion that there is a common aetiology and neural circuitry underpinning these disorders. Building on fear conditioning models, it was proposed that these disorders commence when stimuli are paired with an inherently aversive event; subsequent exposure to the conditioned stimuli signals threat and results in anxiety (Milad et al. 2006). Although PTSD is the classic example of a disorder commencing after a conditioned aversive experience, there is also evidence that aversive experiences can precede onset of panic disorder (Faravelli 1985; Manfro et al. 1996) and social phobia (McCabe et al. 2003). In terms of neural circuitry, fear circuitry disorders tend to be characterized by excessive amygdala reactivity and, to a lesser extent, impaired regulation of that response by the medial prefrontal cortex (Rauch and Drevets 2009; Shin and Liberzon 2010), whereas different neural networks appear to be involved in non-fear circuitry anxiety disorders (Cannistraro et al. 2004; Rauch et al. 2007). This is supported by evidence that following trauma, fear circuitry disorders are characterized by elevated heart rate but non-fear circuitry disorders are not (Bryant et al. 2011a). Despite this overlap between PTSD and other fear circuitry disorders, other arguments were put forward to challenge the view that trauma-related disorders should be understood as anxiety disorders. First, the evidence that aversive experiences precipitate most fear circuitry disorders is mixed (Rapee et al. 1990, 2009). Second, many symptoms of PTSD can be found in other disorders; numbing, withdrawal and disinterest are common in depression (Blanchard and Penk 1998). Third, fear conditioning models cannot readily explain the guilt, anger and shame that often characterize PTSD, and so it is argued that this weakens the argument that PTSD is exclusively a fear circuitry disorder (Horowitz 2007). On this basis, the decision was made to include PTSD, ASD, adjustment disorder and dissociative disorders into a category of *trauma and stressor-related disorders*. The decision to not conceptualize PTSD as an anxiety disorder has been controversial, especially considering that the treatments for PTSD overlap very strongly with those for other fear circuitry disorders.

6.5   PTSD

6.5.1   DSM-5

A number of reasonably significant changes were introduced in the DSM-5 definition of PTSD (see Table 6.1). The major change to the entry point to the diagnosis was that the subjective aspect of the stressor (A2: 'fear, horror or helplessness') was removed. This had been initially introduced, in part, to ensure that minor reactions to events would not qualify for a PTSD diagnosis (Friedman et al. 2011). Studies indicate that this qualification to the stressor definition is poorly predictive of PTSD (Brewin et al. 2000) and that some people who would otherwise meet criteria for PTSD were excluded from the diagnosis (O'Donnell et al. 2010; Rizvi et al. 2008).

DSM-5 has few changes to the re-experiencing cluster. In contrast, the avoidance conceptualization has been markedly altered. Whereas DSM-IV presumed PTSD

Table 6.1 Posttraumatic stress disorder definitions in DSM-5 and proposed for ICD-11

DSM-5	ICD-11
A. *Exposed to death/threatened death*	A. *Exposure to threat*
Experienced/witnessed threat to life	B. *Re-experiencing* (at least 1 of):
Learning events occur to close other person	Intrusive memories
B. *Re-experiencing* (at least 1 of):	Flashbacks
Intrusive memories	Nightmares
Nightmares	C. *Avoidance* (at least 1 of):
Flashbacks	Thoughts
Distress to reminders	Situations
Physiological reactivity	D. *Perceived threat* (at least 1 of):
C. *Avoidance* (at least 1 of):	Hypervigilance
Avoid thoughts/feelings	Startle response
Avoid situations	E. *Duration* (at least several weeks)
D. *Negative alterations in cognition/mood* (at least 3 of):	F. Impairment
Dissociative amnesia	
Negative expectations of self/world	
Distorted blame	
Negative emotional state	
Diminished interest	
Detachment	
Emotional numbing	
E. *Hyperarousal* (at least 2 of):	
Reckless/self-destructive behaviour	
Hypervigilance	
Startle response	
Concentration deficits	
Sleep problems	
F. Minimum 1 month after trauma	
G. Impairment	
Specifier: with dissociative symptoms	
Specifier: with delayed expression	

comprised three factors, multiple factor analytic studies have indicated that the construct is better explained by four factors: re-experiencing, active avoidance, passive avoidance (including numbing) and arousal (Asmundson et al. 2000; King et al. 1998; Marshall 2004). Accordingly, DSM-5 now has a separate cluster that requires the person to satisfy at least one of two active avoidance symptoms (of either internal or external reminders). The major change has been the addition of a new cluster, termed *negative alterations in cognitions and mood*. This cluster recognizes that numbing is distinct from active avoidance, but also notes the importance of exaggerated negative appraisals about the trauma and the range of emotional responses that can be experienced in PTSD. This has led to the addition of new symptoms. On the basis that many people with PTSD blame themselves and feel guilty (Feiring and Cleland 2007), self-blame has been added to this new cluster. Given the abundant evidence that people with PTSD have negative evaluations about themselves and the world (e.g. 'I am a bad person') and that they will not enjoy positive future experiences ('Nothing will ever work for me') (Ehring et al. 2008), the DSM-IV symptom of foreshortened future has been replaced by a symptom that involves exaggerated negative appraisals about oneself and the world. Evidence that PTSD can also exist in association with diverse negative mood states, including anger, shame and guilt (Leskela et al. 2002; Orth and Wieland 2006), led to the inclusion of a symptom of pervasive negative mood states. The arousal cluster has remained largely the same in DSM-5 as it was in DSM-IV, with a few exceptions. Based on evidence that reckless or self-destructive behaviour has been observed in a range of PTSD populations (Fear et al. 2008), this has been added as an additional symptom to the arousal cluster. The only further modification to this cluster was altering irritable mood to aggressive behaviour because this is seen as more indicative of PTSD (Jakupcak et al. 2007).

What is the impact of the altered PTSD definition in DSM-5? One study of traumatic injury survivors found comparable rates of PTSD across both DSM-5 (6.7 %) and DSM-IV (5.9 %) definitions (O'Donnell et al. 2014). Further, this study found that comorbidity with depression was comparable across both DSM-5 and DSM-IV definitions (67 % vs. 69 %). One interesting outcome of the DSM-5 modifications is that it has greatly expanded the possible number of permutations by which PTSD can now be diagnosed; whereas in DSM-IV there were 79,794 possible combinations, the added cluster and the new symptoms in DSM-5 have resulted in 636,120 possible clinical presentations of PTSD (Galatzer-Levy and Bryant 2013). It is premature to cast judgement on how the DSM-5 definition is faring relative to the DSM-IV iteration of the condition because it will require multiple studies conducted in different settings to answer this question.

6.5.2 ICD-11

As noted above, ICD-11, which is expected to be published in 2017, proposes a considerably simpler definition than DSM-5 – and this is exemplified in the proposed definition of PTSD (see Table 6.1). It has been noted that PTSD was more readily diagnosed in ICD-10 than DSM-IV and that ICD-10 required an impairment requirement to raise the threshold for diagnostic criterion (Peters et al. 1999). ICD-11 is also introducing a formal stressor criterion to tighten the entry for the diagnosis (Maercker et al. 2013a). Arguably the biggest difference between DSM-5 and ICD-11 is the latter's emphasis on re-experiencing symptoms. In an attempt to reduce comorbidity and focus PTSD on its core element (i.e. a memory-based disorder characterized by reliving of the traumatic experience), considerable weight was placed on the role of the distinctive types of memory for the trauma evident in PTSD (Maercker et al. 2013b). Specifically, whereas intrusive memories are evident across many disorders, the sense of reliving of a trauma is apparently distinctive to PTSD (Brewin et al. 2010; Bryant et al. 2011c). Accordingly, ICD-11 defines *re-experiencing the traumatic event(s) in the present*, reflected by either vivid intrusive memories, flashbacks or nightmares, accompanied by fear or horror; in this definition, flashbacks can range from transient experiences to a complete disconnection from one's current state of awareness (Maercker et al. 2013b). ICD-11 also stresses avoidance of re-experiencing symptoms, which includes effortful avoiding of internal (e.g. thoughts, emotions) and external (e.g. situations) reminders. The third emphasis is an excessive sense of current threat, which can be reflected in hypervigilance or by exaggerated startle.

Overall, the ICD-11 definition is intended to simplify the diagnosis for clinicians and allow diagnosis to be made on the basis of satisfying two symptoms of each of the three central features of PTSD. This definition is clearly much simpler than the DSM-5 criteria and leads to much fewer potential permutations by which the diagnosis can be made. Some initial evidence has emerged about the relative performances of the DSM-5 and ICD-11 definitions of PTSD. In one study of 510 traumatically injured patients, PTSD current prevalence using DSM-5 criteria was markedly higher than the ICD-11 definition (6.7 % vs. 3.3 %), and ICD-11 tended to have lower comorbidity with depression (O'Donnell et al. 2014).

6.6 Acute Stress Disorder

DSM-5 and ICD-11 have two very different conceptualizations of acute stress responses, and they do not match onto each other. They are based on different premises, have very different timeframes and consequently are operationally defined in very distinct ways. In fact, ASD only exists in DSM and has never been a diagnosis in ICD, which instead has a construct termed acute stress reaction.

6.6.1 DSM-5

ASD was first introduced in DSM-IV for two stated reasons: (a) to describe severe acute stress reactions that predated the PTSD diagnosis (which can only be recognized 1 month after trauma exposure) and (b) as a means to identify people who are at high risk for developing subsequent PTSD (Spiegel et al. 1996). In DSM-IV, to meet criteria for ASD, one needed to experience a traumatic event and respond with fear, horror or helplessness (criterion A), and also dissociative (criterion B), re-experiencing (criterion C), avoidance (criterion D) and arousal (criterion E) symptom clusters. Whereas most clusters were similar to those in PTSD, although more loosely defined (Bryant and Harvey 1997), the exception was the dissociative cluster which required at least three of five possible symptoms (emotional numbing, derealization, depersonalization, reduced awareness of surroundings or dissociative amnesia). This emphasis resulted from arguments at the time that dissociative responses were central to posttraumatic response because they impeded emotional processing of the experience, and therefore were predictive of PTSD (Harvey and Bryant 2002).

In preparing the ASD diagnosis for DSM-5, a core question was: How well was ASD predicting PTSD? Longitudinal studies that indexed the relationship between ASD and later PTSD display a convergent pattern. Whereas the majority of individuals with a diagnosis of ASD do subsequently develop PTSD, most people who eventually experience PTSD do *not* initially display ASD (Bryant 2011). That is, although ASD is performing adequately in terms of most people who meet criteria are high risk for PTSD, it is performing poorly by not identifying most people who are high risk. For this reason, it was decided in DSM-5 that the ASD diagnosis should not be aiming to predict PTSD but rather simply describe severe stress reactions in the initial month (Bryant et al. 2011b). A driving reason for retaining the diagnosis was that a major utility of the ASD diagnosis is that within the US healthcare system having a diagnosis can facilitate access to mental health services.

Recognizing that the requirement of dissociative symptoms was arguably too prescriptive in the DSM-IV definition and precluded many distressed people from being identified (Bryant et al. 2008; Dalgleish et al. 2008), the DSM-5 definition was modified such that to meet criteria one needs to satisfy at least 9 out of possible 14 symptoms without regard to any specific clusters (American Psychiatric Association 2013) (see Table 6.2). Although the diagnosis is structured in a way that does not require any specific symptoms or clusters, to meet criteria one nonetheless must display re-experiencing and/or avoidance symptoms. This retains the essential core of ASD as being comparable to PTSD. One study has reported that the DSM-5 (14 %) identifies more distressed people than the DSM-IV (8 %) definition (Bryant et al. in press). Interestingly, this study also reported that the DSM-5 definition also identified more participants who developed PTSD than DSM-IV criteria.

6.6.2 ICD-11

Acute stress reactions (ASR) have always been conceptualized in ICD as transient responses that are not necessarily psychopathological (Table 6.2). It is a category that is meant to capture the initial distress that is commonly experienced after traumatic exposure, and it was expected that these reactions would subside within a week or soon after the threat has eased (Isserlin et al. 2008). In this way, ASR is qualitatively different from DSM-5's ASD because it is neither a mental disorder in its own right nor a predictor of subsequent disorder. It is also worth noting that in ICD-11 there is no minimal time in which PTSD can be diagnosed, and so the issue of having a diagnostic 'gap' to describe posttraumatic stress responses (which existed in DSM prior to DSM-IV) does not apply to ICD.

In terms of its definition, ASR has never been limited to strict PTSD definitions because it is intended to encompass the broader array of reactions that can occur in the initial aftermath of trauma. Motivated by the need to be applicable to emergency workers, military personnel and disaster agencies who respond initially to trauma, especially large-scale events, the described symptoms are intentionally very broad and non-prescriptive. The symptoms may include shock, sense of confusion, sadness, anxiety, anger, despair, overactivity, stupor and social withdrawal. Underscoring

Table 6.2 DSM-5 criteria for acute stress disorder and proposed ICD-11 criteria for acute stress reaction

DSM-5	ICD-11
A. *Exposed to death/threatened death*	A. *Exposure to threat*
Witnessed death/threat	B. Transient emotional, somatic cognitive or behavioural symptoms
Learning events occur to close other person	C. Normal response to severe stressor
B. *Presence of at least 9 of:*	D. Symptoms appear within days
Intrusive memories	E. Symptoms subside within 1 week or removal of stressor
Nightmares	F. Symptoms do not meet criteria for mental disorder
Flashbacks	
Psychological/ physiological reactivity	
Numbing/detachment	
Derealization/depersonalization	
Dissociative amnesia	
Avoidance of thoughts/feelings	
Avoidance of situations	
Hypervigilance	
Irritable/aggressive behaviour	
Startle response	
Sleep problems	
Concentration deficits	
C. Symptoms lasts at least 3 days to 1 month after trauma	
D. Impairment	
E. Not due to substance or medical causes	

the intent that ASR is not a mental disorder, it is coded as a 'Z' code, distinguishing it from mental disorders. ICD-11 proposes that if the symptoms of ASR persist beyond a week, one should consider a diagnosis of adjustment disorder or PTSD.

6.7 Complex PTSD

Perhaps the most difficult traumatic stress condition to categorize over the past 20 years has been the notion of complex PTSD. Dating back to the early 1990s, the notion of more complicated PTSD responses has been discussed at length, typically in the context of describing the more complex reactions suffered by survivors of prolonged, and often childhood, trauma. It was argued that those who had suffered sustained and severe trauma, such as childhood abuse, torture or domestic violence, can experience marked problems with their sense of identity and organization of emotions (Herman 1992). Termed disorders of extreme distress not otherwise specified (DESNOS), it was never well defined and accordingly not systematically studied.

In more recent years, the field has moved towards the construct of complex PTSD, which has enjoyed a tighter definition. This is a proposed condition that requires the PTSD symptoms noted above but also reflects the impact that trauma can have on systems of self-organization, specifically in affective, self-concept and relational domains. Unlike the PTSD symptoms in which reactions of fear or horror are tied to trauma-related stimuli, these three latter types of disturbances are pervasive and persistent and occur across various contexts and relationships regardless of proximity to traumatic reminders. Specifically, the construct has evolved to comprise three major sets of disturbances in addition to the core PTSD responses: affective regulation, self-construct and interpersonal. These have been identified both from studies of patients (Roth et al. 1997) and expert clinicians (Cloitre et al. 2011). Though not defined by exposure to prolonged trauma, this constellation of reactions is typically associated with very prolonged and severe traumatic experiences (van der Kolk et al. 2005).

6.7.1   DSM-5

The possibility of introducing complex PTSD in DSM-5 was debated; however, it was rejected. It was decided to not consider complex PTSD as a separate entity because in the DSM-IV field trials, only 8 % of those who displayed DESNOS did not also have PTSD; thus, it was suggested that it could only be considered as a subtype (Friedman et al. 2011). It was argued that it was premature to introduce this subtype because it had not been adequately defined, insufficient data existed to warrant its distinction from other disorders (including Borderline Personality Disorder), and there was no evidence that people with this presentation respond differentially to treatments that work effectively with PTSD (Resick et al. 2012). In contrast, DSM-5 did introduce a dissociative subtype of PTSD which was regarded as a viable alternative to complex PTSD. This subtype builds on evidence of two types of presentation of PTSD: one characterized by elevated arousal and one by blunting/dissociative responses. This division is largely based on some evidence that people who present with dissociative symptoms show less reactivity at both peripheral (Griffin et al. 1997) and neural (Felmingham et al. 2008; Lanius et al. 2012) levels relative to those with non-dissociative symptoms. Although other studies have reported that there is no difference in reactivity in dissociative and non-dissociative presentations of PTSD (Kaufman et al. 2002; Nixon et al. 2005), this subtype was nonetheless introduced into DSM-5 in recognition that it was a valid sub-entity.

6.7.2   ICD-11

It appears that a different approach is being taken in ICD-11. ICD has a different organizational structure than DSM, and so if accepted, complex PTSD may be a 'sibling' disorder to PTSD rather than a subtype. The proposal being put forward for ICD-11 is based on the core PTSD symptoms with the addition of affective, self

Table 6.3 Proposed ICD-11 criteria for complex PTSD

1. Exposure to extreme/prolonged trauma
2. Core symptoms of PTSD (re-experiencing, avoidance, perceptions of threat)
3. Pervasive problems with:
(a) Affect regulation
(b) Sense of self as diminished, defeated or worthless
(c) Difficulties in sustaining relationships

and relational disturbance (see Table 6.3). Affective disturbances include emotional reactivity, extreme outbursts, self-destructive behaviour and potentially dissociative states. Disturbances in self may include the sense of worthlessness, or of being defeated or diminished. Difficulties in relations often involve deficits in maintaining a sense of intimacy with others, disinterest in social relations or oscillating between intimate relations and estrangement. Initial evidence supporting this proposal comes from a latent profile analysis that showed patients with affective, self and relational disturbances comprised a distinct class from PTSD patients who were low on these symptoms; further, the former class were more likely to have suffered chronic rather than discrete traumas (Cloitre et al. 2013). Further evidence for the complex PTSD construct has come from other studies that have found supporting confirmatory factor analyses of the proposed structure, and higher rates of the proposed symptoms in survivors of childhood abuse (Knefel and Lueger-Schuster 2013), as well as from other studies using latent class analysis indicating a distinct class of complex PTSD (Elkit et al. 2014). Whether complex PTSD is introduced into ICD-11 is yet to be determined, and if it is, what form it will ultimately take remains to be seen. At this stage, it is gathering more support than it received in DSM-5, arguably because the several years delay in production of DSM-5 and ICD-11 means the latter can benefit from targeted research that is developing a broader evidence base to influence the final decision.

6.8 Prolonged Grief Disorder

6.8.1 DSM-5

One of the vehemently debated diagnoses in DSM-5 was the issue of introducing a diagnosis describing complicated grief reactions. DSM has traditionally not recognized grief as a mental disorder because it is concerned about pathologizing a normal response to bereavement. Much work has focused on the condition over the past decade, resulting in a much greater body of evidence than previously existed. Although most normative grief reactions subside after the initial period of mourning, this condition refers to the proportion of grief reactions that persist. There are mixed opinions about the optimal term for the condition. Whereas some prefer the term 'complicated grief' to reflect the fact that the symptoms are qualitatively different from normal grief reactions (Shear et al. 2011), others support the term 'prolonged

Table 6.4 Proposed ICD-11 criteria for prolonged grief disorder

1. Experienced bereavement of close other person
2. Severe yearning/emotional pain persisting for greater than 6 months since death
3. Grief impedes formal functioning
4. Grief reaction is beyond normative cultural/religious context
5. Associated features may include preoccupation with circumstances of death, bitterness about death, guilt, blame, difficulty accepting loss, reduced sense of self, oscillating between preoccupation and avoidance, difficulty progressing with activities or friendships, withdrawal, perception that life is meaningless, emotional numbing

grief' in recognition of the condition being a persistence of the same symptoms observed in the acute bereavement phase (Prigerson et al. 2009). Although there is disagreement about the finer details, the generally accepted definition involves intense yearning or emotional pain that persists beyond 6 months after the death and potentially having difficulty accepting the death, anger over the loss, a diminished sense of one's identity, feeling that life is empty and problems in engaging in new relationships or activities (Bryant 2012). Studies estimate that 10–15 % of bereaved people may suffer this condition, depending on the nature of the death and the relationship to the person (Shear et al. 2011). It was finally decided to not introduce the diagnosis on the basis that insufficient evidence exists to warrant its introduction as a separate diagnosis, instead relegating it to the Appendix as an area for future study.

6.8.2   ICD-11

Again, in contrast to DSM-5 a different approach appears to be taken in ICD-11. Termed prolonged grief disorder, it has been proposed that a new diagnosis be introduced to recognize the disabling nature of severe and persistent grief reactions (see Table 6.4). This disorder would be defined as severe and persisting yearning for the deceased or a persistent preoccupation with the deceased; this reaction may be compounded by difficulty accepting the death, feelings of loss of a part of oneself, anger about the loss, guilt or blame regarding the death or difficulty in engaging with new social or other activities. The diagnosis can only be made if the symptoms are impairing functioning and persist for over 6 months since the death (Maercker et al. 2013b). The evidence put forward to support this initiative includes multiple studies attesting to persistent yearning being central to the condition in adults (Simon et al. 2011) and children (Melhem et al. 2011). The disorder is distinct from anxiety and depression (Boelen and van den Bout 2005; Golden and Dalgleish 2010), and it contributes to a range of psychological, behavioural, medical and functional problems (Boelen and Prigerson 2007; Bonanno et al. 2007; Simon et al. 2007). From an ICD-11 perspective, it is important that these patterns have been observed across western and non-western cultures (Fujisawa et al. 2010; Morina et al. 2010). Further support for the ICD-11 diagnosis comes from evidence that targeted treatments for prolonged grief are effective relative to those that have shown efficacy for depression (Shear et al. 2005).

Once again, it remains to be seen whether ICD-11 introduces prolonged grief disorder as a new diagnosis. The decision by DSM-5 to not formally recognize this condition as a disorder raises the possibility that many bereaved patients who suffer ongoing and disabling distress may be misdiagnosed with depression or anxiety, and not directed to the optimal intervention. Of course, the ICD-11 does bring a degree of risk of overdiagnosis of grief responses because some grief responses may take longer than 6 months to resolve (Wakefield 2013). ICD-11 will emphasize that the diagnosis can only be made when the response is beyond what is culturally normative because it is sensitive to the problems of inappropriately prescribing a diagnosis across cultural contexts.

6.9   Summary

Posttraumatic psychiatric diagnoses have evolved significantly since they were introduced decades ago. Interesting distinctions are developing between the two major systems currently available. Whereas DSM is moving towards more complex and broader conceptualizations of PTSD, ICD in contrast is shifting towards a simpler and more focused definition. Beyond PTSD, ICD appears to be adopting a more lateral approach by considering complex PTSD and prolonged grief disorder. This is understandable as the different diagnostic systems have distinct agendas that they are addressing, guided by the respective needs of the American Psychiatric Association and the World Health Organization. With different nomenclatures operating across the world, there is the possibility of confusion and discrepancies in how traumatic stress is operationalized across the world. Time will tell how these respective systems will serve the field, facilitate identification of conditions and lead affected people to appropriate treatments.

References

American Psychiatric Association. (1952). *Diagnostic and Statistical Manual of Mental Disorders (DSM I)*. Washington, DC: American Psychiatric Association.

American Psychiatric Association. (1968). *Diagnostic and statistical manual of mental disorders* (2nd ed.). Washington, DC: American Psychiatric Association.

American Psychiatric Association. (1980). *Diagnostic and statistical manual of mental disorders* (3rd ed.). Washington, DC: American Psychiatric Association.

American Psychiatric Association. (1994). *Diagnostic and statistical manual of mental disorders* (4th ed.). Washington, DC: American Psychiatric Association.

American Psychiatric Association. (2013). *Diagnostic and statistical manual for mental disorders* (5th ed.). Washington, DC: American Psychiatric Association.

Andrews, G., Charney, D. S., Sirovatka, P. J., & Regier, D. A. (Eds.). (2009). *Stress-induced and fear circuitry disorders: Refining the research agenda for DSM-V*. Arlington: American Psychiatric Association.

Asmundson, G. J., Frombach, I., McQuaid, J., Pedrelli, P., Lenox, R., & Stein, M. B. (2000). Dimensionality of posttraumatic stress symptoms: A confirmatory factor analysis of DSM-IV symptom clusters and other symptom models. *Behaviour Research and Therapy, 38*(2), 203–214.

Blanchard, E. B., & Penk, W. E. (1998). Posttraumatic stress disorder and comorbid major depression: Is the correlation an illusion? *Journal of Anxiety Disorders, 12*(1), 21–37.

Boelen, P. A., & Prigerson, H. G. (2007). The influence of symptoms of prolonged grief disorder, depression, and anxiety on quality of life among bereaved adults: A prospective study. *European Archives of Psychiatry and Clinical Neuroscience, 257*(8), 444–452.

Boelen, P. A., & van den Bout, J. (2005). Complicated grief, depression, and anxiety as distinct post loss syndromes: A confirmatory factor analysis study. *American Journal of Psychiatry, 162*(11), 2175–2177.

Bonanno, G. A., Neria, Y., Mancini, A., Coifman, K. G., Litz, B., & Insel, B. (2007). Is there more to complicated grief than depression and posttraumatic stress disorder? A test of incremental validity. *Journal of Abnormal Psychology, 116*(2), 342–351.

Brewin, C. R., Andrews, B., & Rose, S. (2000). Fear, helplessness, and horror in posttraumatic stress disorder: Investigating DSM-IV criterion A2 in victims of violent crime. *Journal of Traumatic Stress, 13*(3), 499–509.

Brewin, C. R., Gregory, J. D., Lipton, M., & Burgess, N. (2010). Intrusive images in psychological disorders: Characteristics, neural mechanisms, and treatment implications. *Psychological Review, 117*(1), 210–232.

Bryant, R. A. (2011). Acute stress disorder as a predictor of posttraumatic stress disorder: A systematic review. *Journal of Clinical Psychiatry, 72,* 233–239.

Bryant, R. A. (2012). Grief as a psychiatric disorder. *British Journal of Psychiatry, 201,* 9–10.

Bryant, R. A., & Harvey, A. G. (1997). Acute stress disorder: A critical review of diagnostic issues. *Clinical Psychology Review, 17*(7), 757–773.

Bryant, R. A., Creamer, M., O'Donnell, M. L., Silove, D., & McFarlane, A. C. (2008). A multisite study of the capacity of acute stress disorder diagnosis to predict posttraumatic stress disorder. *Journal of Clinical Psychiatry, 69*(6), 923–929.

Bryant, R. A., Creamer, M., O'Donnell, M., Silove, D., & McFarlane, A. C. (2011a). Heart rate after trauma and the specificity of fear circuitry disorders. *Psychological Medicine, 41,* 2573–2580.

Bryant, R. A., Friedman, M. J., Spiegel, D., Ursano, R., & Strain, J. (2011b). A review of acute stress disorder in DSM-5. *Depression and Anxiety, 28*(9), 802–817.

Bryant, R. A., O'Donnell, M. L., Creamer, M., McFarlane, A. C., & Silove, D. (2011c). Posttraumatic intrusive symptoms across psychiatric disorders. *Journal of Psychiatric Research, 45*(6), 842–847.

Bryant, R. A., Creamer, M., O'Donnell, M., Silove, D., McFarlane, A.C., & Forbes, D. (in press). A comparison of the capacity of DSM-IV and DSM-5 acute stress disorder definitions to predict posttraumatic stress disorder. *Journal of Clinical Psychiatry.*

Cannistraro, P. A., Wright, C. I., Wedig, M. M., Martis, B., Shin, L. M., Wilhelm, S., & Rauch, S. L. (2004). Amygdala responses to human faces in obsessive-compulsive disorder. *Biological Psychiatry, 56*(12), 916–920.

Cloitre, M., Courtois, C. A., Charuvastra, A., Carapezza, R., Stolbach, B. C., & Green, B. L. (2011). Treatment of complex PTSD: Results of the ISTSS expert clinician survey on best practices. *Journal of Traumatic Stress, 24*(6), 615–627.

Cloitre, M., Garvert, D., Brewin, C.R., Bryatn, R.A., & Maercker, A. (2013). Evidence for ICD-11 PTSD and complex PTSD: A latent profile analysis. *European Journal of Psychotraumatology, 4,* 20706. http://dx.doi.org/10.3402/ejpt.v4i0.20706

Dalgleish, T., Meiser-Stedman, R., Kassam-Adams, N., Ehlers, A., Winston, F., Smith, P., et al. (2008). Predictive validity of acute stress disorder in children and adolescents. *British Journal of Psychiatry, 192*(5), 392–393.

Ehring, T., Ehlers, A., & Glucksman, E. (2008). Do cognitive models help in predicting the severity of posttraumatic stress disorder, phobia, and depression after motor vehicle accidents? A prospective longitudinal study. *Journal of Consulting and Clinical Psychology, 76*(2), 219–230.

Elkit, A., Hyland, P. Shevlin, M. (2014). Evidence of symptom profiles consistent with posttraumatic stress disorder and complex posttraumatic stress disorder in different trauma samples. *European Journal of Psychotraumatology, 5,* 24221. http://dx.doi.org/10.3402/ejpt. v5.24221

Faravelli, C. (1985). Life events preceding the onset of panic disorder. *Journal of Affective Disorders, 9*(1), 103–105.

Fear, N. T., Iversen, A. C., Chatterjee, A., Jones, M., Greenberg, N., Hull, L., et al. (2008). Risky driving among regular armed forces personnel from the United Kingdom. *American Journal of Preventative Medicine, 35*(3), 230–236.

Feiring, C., & Cleland, C. (2007). Childhood sexual abuse and abuse-specific attributions of blame over 6 years following discovery. *Child Abuse and Neglect, 31*(11–12), 1169–1186.

Felmingham, K., Kemp, A. H., Williams, L., Falconer, E., Olivieri, G., Peduto, A., et al. (2008). Dissociative responses to conscious and non-conscious fear impact underlying brain function in post-traumatic stress disorder. *Psychological Medicine, 38*(12), 1771–1780.

Friedman, M. J., Resick, P. A., Bryant, R. A., & Brewin, C. R. (2011). Considering PTSD for DSM-5. *Depression and Anxiety, 28,* 750–769.

Fujisawa, D., Miyashita, M., Nakajima, S., Ito, M., Kato, M., & Kim, Y. (2010). Prevalence and determinants of complicated grief in general population. *Journal of Affective Disorders, 127*(1–3), 352–358.

Galatzer-Levy, I., & Bryant, R. A. (2013). 636,120 ways to have posttraumatic stress disorder: The relative merits of categorical and dimensional approaches to posttraumatic stress. *Perspectives in Psychological Science, 8,* 651–662.

Golden, A.-M., & Dalgleish, T. (2010). Is prolonged grief distinct from bereavement-related posttraumatic stress? *Psychiatry Research, 178,* 336–341.

Griffin, M. G., Resick, P. A., & Mechanic, M. B. (1997). Objective assessment of peritraumatic dissociation: Psychophysiological indicators. *American Journal of Psychiatry, 154*(8), 1081–1088.

Harvey, A. G., & Bryant, R. A. (2002). Acute stress disorder: A synthesis and critique. *Psychological Bulletin, 128*(6), 886–902.

Herman, J. L. (1992). Complex PTSD: A syndrome in survivors of prolonged and repeated trauma. *Journal of Traumatic Stress, 5*(3), 377–391.

Horowitz, M. J. (2007). Understanding and ameliorating revenge fantasies in psychotherapy. *American Journal of Psychiatry, 164*(1), 24–27.

Isserlin, L., Zerach, G., & Solomon, Z. (2008). Acute stress responses: A review and synthesis of ASD, ASR, and CSR. *American Journal of Orthopsychiatry, 78*(4), 423–429.

Jakupcak, M., Conybeare, D., Phelps, L., Hunt, S., Holmes, H. A., Felker, B., et al. (2007). Anger, hostility, and aggression among Iraq and Afghanistan war veterans reporting PTSD and subthreshold PTSD. *Journal of Traumatic Stress, 20*(6), 945–954.

Kaufman, M. L., Kimble, M. O., Kaloupek, D. G., McTeague, L. M., Bachrach, P., Forti, A. M., et al. (2002). Peritraumatic dissociation and physiological response to trauma-relevant stimuli in Vietnam combat veterans with posttraumatic stress disorder. *The Journal of Nervous and Mental Disease, 190*(3), 167–174.

King, D. W., Leskin, G. A., King, L. A., & Weathers, F. W. (1998). Confirmatory factor analysis of the clinician-administered PTSD Scale: Evidence for the dimensionality of posttraumatic stress disorder. *Psychological Assessment, 10*(2), 90–96.

Knefel, M., & Lueger-Schuster, B. (2013). An evaluation of ICD-11 PTSD and complex PTSD criteria in a sample of adult survivors of childhood institutional abuse. *European Journal of Psychotraumatology, 4,* 22608. http://dx.doi.org/10.3402/ejpt.v4i0.22608

Lanius, R. A., Brand, B., Vermetten, E., Frewen, P. A., & Spiegel, D. (2012). The dissociative subtype of posttraumatic stress disorder: Rationale, clinical and neurobiological evidence, and implications. *Depression and Anxiety, 29*(8), 701–708.

Leskela, J., Dieperink, M., & Thuras, P. (2002). Shame and posttraumatic stress disorder. *Journal of Traumatic Stress, 15*(3), 223–226.

Maercker, A., Brewin, C. R., Bryant, R. A., Cloitre, M., Reed, G. M., van Ommeren, M., et al. (2013a). Proposals for mental disorders specifically associated with stress in the International Classification of Diseases-11. *Lancet, 381*(9878), 1683–1685.

Maercker, A., Brewin, C. R., Bryant, R. A., Cloitre, M., van Ommeren, M., Jones, L. M., et al. (2013b). Diagnosis and classification of disorders specifically associated with stress: Proposals for ICD-11. *World Psychiatry, 12*(3), 198–206.

Manfro, G. G., Otto, M. W., McArdle, E. T., Worthington, J. J., 3rd, Rosenbaum, J. F., & Pollack, M. H. (1996). Relationship of antecedent stressful life events to childhood and family history of anxiety and the course of panic disorder. *Journal of Affective Disorders, 41*(2), 135–139.

Marshall, G. N. (2004). Posttraumatic stress disorder symptom checklist: Factor structure and English-Spanish measurement invariance. *Journal of Traumatic Stress, 17*(3), 223–230.

McCabe, R. E., Antony, M. M., Summerfeldt, L. J., Liss, A., & Swinson, R. P. (2003). Preliminary examination of the relationship between anxiety disorders in adults and self-reported history of teasing or bullying experiences. *Cognitive Behavior Therapy, 32*(4), 187–193.

Melhem, N. M., Porta, G., Shamseddeen, W., Payne, M. W., & Brent, D. A. (2011). Grief in children and adolescents bereaved by sudden parental death. *Archives of General Psychiatry, 68*, 911–919.

Milad, M. R., Rauch, S. L., Pitman, R. K., & Quirk, G. J. (2006). Fear extinction in rats: Implications for human brain imaging and anxiety disorders. *Biological Psychology, 73*(1), 61–71.

Morina, N., Rudari, V., Bleichhardt, G., & Prigerson, H. G. (2010). Prolonged grief disorder, depression, and posttraumatic stress disorder among bereaved Kosovar civilian war survivors: A preliminary investigation. *International Journal of Social Psychiatry, 56*(3), 288–297.

Nixon, R. D. V., Bryant, R. A., Moulds, M. L., Felmingham, K. L., & Mastrodomenico, J. A. (2005). Physiological arousal and dissociation in acute trauma victims during trauma narratives. *Journal of Traumatic Stress, 18*(2), 107–113.

O'Donnell, M. L., Creamer, M., McFarlane, A., Silove, D., & Bryant, R. A. (2010). Should A2 be a diagnostic requirement for posttraumatic stress disorder in DSM-V? *Psychiatry Research, 176*, 257–260.

O'Donnell, M. L., Alkemade, N., Nickerson, A., Creamer, M., McFarlane, A. C., Silove, D., Bryant, R. A., & Forbes, D. (2014). The impact of the diagnostic changes to posttraumatic stress disorder for DSM-5 and the proposed changes to ICD-11. *British Journal of Psychiatry, 205*, 230–235.

Orth, U., & Wieland, E. (2006). Anger, hostility, and posttraumatic stress disorder in trauma-exposed adults: A meta-analysis. *Journal of Consulting and Clinical Psychology, 74*(4), 698–706.

Peters, L., Slade, T., & Andrews, G. (1999). A comparison of ICD-10 and DSM-IV criteria for posttraumatic stress disorder. *Journal of Traumatic Stress, 12*(2), 335–343.

Prigerson, H. G., Horowitz, M. J., Jacobs, S. C., Parkes, C. M., Aslan, M., Goodkin, K., et al. (2009). Prolonged grief disorder: Psychometric validation of criteria proposed for DSM-V and ICD-11. *PLoS Medicine, 6*(8), e1000121. doi:10.1371/journal.pmed.1000121.

Rapee, R. M., Litwin, E. M., & Barlow, D. H. (1990). Impact of life events on subjects with panic disorder and on comparison subjects. *American Journal of Psychiatry, 147*(5), 640–644.

Rapee, R. M., & Bryant, R. A. (2009). Stress and psychosocial factors in onset of fear circuitry disorders. In G. Andrews, D. S. Charney, P. J. Sirovatka, & D. A. Regier (Eds.), *Stress-induced and fear circuitry disorders: Advancing the research agenda for DSM-V* (pp. 195–214). Arlington: American Psychiatric Publishing, Inc.

Rauch, S. L., & Drevets, W. C. (2009). Neuroimaging and neuroanatomy of stress-induced and fear circuitry disorders. In G. Andrews, D. S. Charney, P. J. Sirovatka, & D. A. Regier (Eds.), *Stress-induced and fear circuitry disorders: Refining the research agenda for DSM-V* (pp. 215–254). Arlington: American Psychiatric Association.

Rauch, S. L., Wedig, M. M., Wright, C. I., Martis, B., McMullin, K. G., Shin, L. M., & Wilhelm, S. (2007). Functional magnetic resonance imaging study of regional brain activation during implicit sequence learning in obsessive-compulsive disorder. *Biological Psychiatry, 61*(3), 330–336.

Reed, G. M. (2010). Toward ICD-11: Improving the clinical utility of WHO's International Classification of Mental Disorders. *Professional Psychology: Research and Practice, 41*, 457–464.

Resick, P. A., Bovin, M. J., Calloway, A. L., Dick, A. M., King, M. W., Mitchell, K. S., & Wolf, E. J. (2012). A critical evaluation of the complex PTSD literature: Implications for DSM-5. *Journal of Traumatic Stress, 25*(3), 241–251.

Rizvi, S. L., Kaysen, D., Gutner, C. A., Griffin, M. G., & Resick, P. A. (2008). Beyond fear: The role of peritraumatic responses in posttraumatic stress and depressive symptoms among female crime victims. *Journal of Interpersonal Violence, 23*(6), 853–868.

Roth, S., Newman, E., Pelcovitz, D., van der Kolk, B., & Mandel, F. S. (1997). Complex PTSD in victims exposed to sexual and physical abuse: Results from the DSM-IV field trial for posttraumatic stress disorder. *Journal of Traumatic Stress, 10*(4), 539–555.

Shear, K., Frank, E., Houck, P. R., & Reynolds, C. F., 3rd. (2005). Treatment of complicated grief: A randomized controlled trial. *Journal of the American Medical Association, 293*(21), 2601–2608.

Shear, M. K., Simon, N., Wall, M., Zisook, S., Neimeyer, R., Duan, N., et al. (2011). Complicated grief and related bereavement issues for DSM-5. *Depression and Anxiety, 28*(2), 103–117.

Shin, L. M., & Liberzon, I. (2010). The neurocircuitry of fear, stress, and anxiety disorders. *Neuropsychopharmacology, 35*(1), 169–191.

Simon, N. M., Shear, K. M., Thompson, E. H., Zalta, A. K., Perlman, C., Reynolds, C. F., et al. (2007). The prevalence and correlates of psychiatric comorbidity in individuals with complicated grief. *Comprehensive Psychiatry, 48*(5), 395–399.

Simon, N. M., Wall, M. M., Keshaviah, A., Dryman, M. T., Leblanc, N. J., & Shear, M. K. (2011). Informing the symptom profile of complicated grief. *Depression and Anxiety, 28*(2), 118–126.

Spiegel, D., Koopmen, C., Cardeña, C., & Classen, C. (1996). Dissociative symptoms in the diagnosis of acute stress disorder. In L. K. Michelson & W. J. Ray (Eds.), *Handbook of dissociation* (pp. 367–380). New York: Plenum Press.

van der Kolk, B. A., Roth, S., Pelcovitz, D., Sunday, S., & Spinazzola, J. (2005). Disorders of extreme stress: The empirical foundation of a complex adaptation to trauma. *Journal of Traumatic Stress, 18*(5), 389–399.

Wakefield, J. C. (2013). The DSM-5 debate over the bereavement exclusion: Psychiatric diagnosis and the future of empirically supported treatment. *Clinical Psychology Review, 33*(7), 825–845.

World Health Organization, W. H. (1965). *International statistical classification of diseases, injuries, and causes of death* (8th ed.). Geneva: World Health Organization.

World Health Organization, W. H. (1994). *International statistical classification of diseases, injuries, and causes of death* (8th ed.). Geneva: World Health Organization.

Part III

Psychotherapy

Early Intervention After Trauma

7

Richard A. Bryant

7.1 Introduction

The personal, social, and economic costs of posttraumatic stress disorder (PTSD) have stimulated enormous efforts over the past several decades into developing better strategies to reduce the adverse psychological effects of trauma. Much of this energy has been devoted to early intervention strategies. By early intervention, we mean interventions that are implemented in the initial hours, days, or weeks after trauma exposure. The goals of these approaches are variably to reduce the acute stress or to achieve secondary prevention to avert subsequent PTSD. In this chapter I will review the current strategies for early intervention, the evidence for these strategies, and the challenges that are facing the field.

7.2 Providing Early Interventions to All Survivors

Over the past three decades, there has been a very common trend to provide immediate psychological response to all survivors of trauma. This approach has been driven by the perception that all people are vulnerable to adverse effects of trauma, and if we do not provide interventions shortly after the trauma exposure, dire results will occur. However, this presumption of vulnerability has been shown to be wrong. Most people are highly resilient and do not require formal mental health interventions. People are able to adjust to the experience once the immediate threat passes and use their own resources or social networks to adapt successfully.

R.A. Bryant, PhD
School of Psychology, University of New South Wales, Sydney,
NSW 2052, Australia
e-mail: r.bryant@unsw.edu.au

© Springer International Publishing Switzerland 2015
U. Schnyder, M. Cloitre (eds.), *Evidence Based Treatments for Trauma-Related Psychological Disorders: A Practical Guide for Clinicians*,
DOI 10.1007/978-3-319-07109-1_7

Despite this pattern, perhaps early interventions may facilitate adaptation or perhaps assist people who would otherwise develop psychiatric problems to avert these outcomes. Although there have been variants of early interventions for 100 years (Shephard 2000), including interventions provided to soldiers in the immediate aftermath of combat, they have been most popular since the 1980s. These interventions are most commonly referred to as 'psychological debriefing', and there are numerous iterations of them. The simplest means of evaluating the role of psychological debriefing is to review the history and efficacy of its most popular variant: Critical Incident Stress Debriefing (CISD). This programme was initiated in the 1980s by a firefighter, Jeffrey Mitchell, who argued that it could 'generally alleviate the acute stress responses which appear at the scene and immediately afterwards and will eliminate, or at least inhibit, delayed stress reactions' (Mitchell 1983, p. 36). CISD typically consists of a single debriefing session and is usually administered within several days of the trauma exposure. The session typically lasts between 3 and 4 h (Everly and Mitchell 1999). It formally comprises seven phases. The introduction phase introduces the format and clarifies that it is not intended to be psychotherapy. The fact phase asks participants to recount their accounts of the traumatic incident. The cognitive phase invites participants to describe their cognitive responses to the experience, with encouragement to be aware of initial thoughts about what occurred. Next, in the reaction phase, participants are encouraged to express emotional responses they have about the experience. In the symptom phase, the participants are asked to notice symptoms or reactions with the view of identifying stress reactions. The teaching phase involves normalising stress reactions. Finally, in the re-entry phase, a summary is provided of the debriefing session and any necessary referrals are offered. Although CISD was initially targeted toward emergency responders, it has subsequently expanded to encompass a much broader audience. Summarising the growth of CISD by the end of the 1990s, the authors wrote, 'Mitchell's CISD model of psychological debriefing is generally recognized as the most widely used in the world and is used across the greatest diversity of settings and operational applications' (Everly and Mitchell 1999, p. 84).

Does CISD help people? There are many reports in the literature of CISD being well received and participants finding it helpful (Adler et al. 2008; Carlier et al. 2000). This does not amount to evidence, however. Numerous trials have been conducted that have assessed people who have and have not received CISD (or variants of it) and compared their functioning (typically in terms of PTSD levels) at subsequent follow-up assessments (for a review, see McNally et al. 2003). Overall, these studies indicate that CISD and related debriefing interventions do not result in reduced levels of posttraumatic stress relative to not receiving the intervention (Bisson et al. 2007).

Can debriefing do harm? This is a critical issue because it may be important to respect people's natural adaption processes, and it can be unwise to interfere with these mechanisms. This issue has become particularly relevant in the light of some evidence that CISD may be harmful; this conclusion emerges from studies that found that those (particularly those who display marked PTSD symptoms initially following trauma) who received debriefing had worse PTSD than those who did not receive it (Bisson et al. 1997; Mayou et al. 2000). Another controlled study found that emotional debriefing led to a delayed recovery relative to educational input (Sijbrandij et al. 2006). Although these studies are limited by methodological flaws, it nonetheless raises concerns that global interventions may not be warranted. It has been suggested that activating trauma memories for a brief period after which the person is not seen repeatedly may not be helpful and may even further consolidate trauma memories (Bisson and Andrew 2007). Debriefing may also be harmful because it typically occurs without prior assessment, and so it involves a standard intervention for all regardless of individual differences in premorbid vulnerability, distress severity, or social context. Accordingly, treatment guidelines around the world generally recommend against this intervention (Foa et al. 2009).

If psychological debriefing, such as CISD, is out of fashion, then what is the preferred alternative? In light of evidence that a single-session intervention is not preventative of subsequent adaptation, more recent approaches simply aim at helping people cope with the acute response. The most common new approach is psychological first aid (PFA; Brymer et al. 2006). It is not really accurate to describe PFA as new because it actually contains many of the components of CISD and other forms of debriefing. It has tried to retain fundamental strategies without encouraging steps that may be unhelpful, such as encouraging emotional catharsis in the acute setting. PFA involves suggested strategies to provide safety, information, emotional support, and access to services, heighten expectancy of recovery, encourage utilisation of social support, and promote self-care. Like other forms of universal intervention, PFA does not commence with a formal assessment. This approach is now promoted in practice guidelines (Inter-Agency Standing Committee 2007), which is questionable since there is no evidence that it is beneficial. When one scrutinises PFA, it is difficult to determine how to evaluate its efficacy because it does not have clear and explicit goals that are readily tested. Whereas CISD explicitly aimed to reduce PTSD severity – which could be tested through trials – the PFA approach is somewhat unfalsifiable because assisting people to cope in the acute phase is difficult to operationalise.

7.3   Who Should Receive Early Intervention

In contrast to approaches that provide universal intervention to all trauma survivors, other approaches have adopted a targeted strategy that intends to focus on trauma survivors who are at high risk for subsequent PTSD. This framework presumes that we can identify people in the acute phase who will subsequently develop PTSD. Over the past several decades, much work has focused on acute predictors of longer-term PTSD – and in that time the enthusiasm for how confidently we can predict chronic PTSD has tempered a lot.

The main challenge for our field in this regard has been the recognition that acute stress reactions are not linearly related to PTSD reactions at subsequent points in time. Earlier work indicated that the initial spike in traumatic stress in the weeks after trauma exposure remitted markedly in the following months; this was shown in cohorts of survivors of rape (Rothbaum et al. 1992), nonsexual assault (Riggs et al. 1995), motor vehicle accidents (Blanchard et al. 1996), disasters (van Griensven et al. 2006), and terrorist attacks (Galea et al. 2003). This raised a challenge for early identification of trauma survivors at risk of developing PTSD because how do we disentangle transient stress reactions from the early reactions that are precursors of subsequent PTSD?

The problem of early identification is highlighted when we consider more recent research on the longitudinal course of posttraumatic stress reactions, which has underscored the complicated trajectories of posttraumatic response. Of course the most salient example of this is delayed-onset PTSD, which has traditionally been recognised as PTSD that develops at least 6 months after trauma exposure. Systematic reviews of the available evidence attest to the frequency of delayed-onset PTSD, with approximately 25 % of PTSD cases being delayed onset, with particular frequency in military populations following deployment (Smid et al. 2009). Increasing evidence tells us that the changing course of posttraumatic stress reactions can be influenced by ongoing stressors, appraisals people make, social factors, or health issues (Bryant et al. 2013). For example, in a study of survivors of Hurricane Katrina, rates of PTSD generally increased over the initial 2 years following the hurricane, which has been attributed to the ongoing stressors in the region arising from lack of infrastructure, poor housing, and lack of other necessary community resources (Kessler et al. 2008). This issue has been further highlighted by a body of evidence that has used latent growth mixture modelling to map the different trajectories that trauma survivors experience. This statistical strategy classifies homogenous groups in a population to identify class of variation over time, and rather than assuming that all people belong to a homogenous population, it tracks *heterogenous* patterns of response. Across a number of studies, four major trajectories have been noted: (a) a resilient class with consistently few PTSD symptoms, (b) a recovery class with initial distress then gradual remission, (c) a delayed-reaction class with initial low symptom levels but increased symptoms over time, and (d) a chronic distress class with consistently high PTSD levels. These trajectories have been noted in a range of trauma survivors, including traumatic injury (deRoon-Cassini et al. 2010), disaster (Pietrzak et al. 2013), and military personnel deployed to the Middle East (Bonanno et al. 2012). This highlights that it is not a straightforward task to identify who will eventually develop PTSD after trauma, and attempts at early intervention need to recognise that not all high-risk trauma survivors can be identified in the acute phase.

7.4 Trauma-Focused Cognitive Behaviour Therapy

As distinct from universal interventions, more recent studies have focused on treating people with severe stress reactions. These have focused primarily on people with ASD, although some studies have treated acute PTSD. Early interventions can be divided into psychological and biological strategies. Much more work has been done in psychological interventions, arguably because of the substantial success of trauma-focused psychotherapies in treating chronic PTSD. Without doubt the front-line treatment of PTSD is exposure-based therapies, which is reflected in international treatment guidelines (Foa et al. 2009). Meta-analyses support these conclusions (Bradley et al. 2005; Roberts et al. 2009).

Early intervention following trauma has generally abridged standard CBT approaches by shortening them to five or six sessions while retaining the core content. The key commonality of these approaches is that they usually have a trauma-focused exposure as the centrepiece of treatment. Therapy usually commences with psychoeducation about the trauma responses and then focuses on anxiety management, exposure, and cognitive restructuring. Anxiety management techniques aim to reduce anxiety through a variety of techniques, including breathing retraining or relaxation skills or self-talk. Therapy usually gives most attention to prolonged exposure, which involves both imaginal and in vivo exposure. During imaginal exposure the patient is asked to vividly imagine their traumatic experience for prolonged periods, usually for at least 30 min. The therapist asks the patient to provide a narrative of their traumatic experience in a way that emphasises all sensory, cognitive, and affective details. In vivo exposure involves graded exposure to feared and avoided situations in which the patient is asked to stay in close proximity to fearful reminders of the trauma; this begins with minimally fearful situations and then increasing to more frightening situations. This approach is thought to be effective via a number of mechanisms, including extinction of initially conditioned fear responses, integration of corrective information, and self-mastery through management of exposure itself (Rothbaum and Mellman 2001; Rothbaum and Schwartz 2002). Cognitive restructuring is usually conducted following exposure and identifies the evidence for maladaptive automatic thoughts about the trauma, the person, and their future. This approach is based on much work showing that excessively negative appraisals in the acute period after trauma are strongly predictive of subsequent PTSD (Ehring et al. 2008).

Although there were some earlier attempts at early intervention (Frank et al. 1988; Kilpatrick and Veronen 1984), possibly the first study that attempted abridged forms of trauma-focused exposure approaches in the framework of early intervention was a study in which Edna Foa's team provided brief CBT to sexual and nonsexual assault victims shortly after the assault (Foa et al. 1995). Participants received four sessions of CBT, and their responses were compared with matched participants who had received repeated assessments; although at posttreatment the CBT participants had less PTSD than those in the matched condition, this difference dissipated at 5-month follow-up. It should be noted that those receiving CBT had less depression and re-experiencing symptoms than the control participants.

One potential limitation of this study is that it focused on all trauma survivors who had symptoms severe enough to meet PTSD criteria (without the 1-month duration requirement), and we have seen that many people who are initially distressed may subsequently adapt regardless of intervention. In an attempt to address this issue, other studies have focused on people who meet criteria for ASD because of some evidence that most people who do display ASD are more at risk for subsequent PTSD (Bryant 2011). In an initial study adopting this approach, Bryant and colleagues randomised motor vehicle accident or nonsexual assault survivors with ASD to either CBT or nondirective supportive counselling (SC) (Bryant et al. 1998). Both interventions consisted of five 1½-h-weekly individual sessions. Emphasis in therapy was placed on imaginal and in vivo exposure and cognitive restructuring. Six months after treatment, there were fewer participants in the CBT group (20 %) who met criteria for PTSD relative to supportive counselling participants (67 %). A later study by the same group dismantled CBT by allocating ASD participants to five sessions of either (a) CBT (prolonged exposure, cognitive therapy, anxiety management), (b) prolonged exposure combined with cognitive therapy, or (c) supportive counselling (Bryant et al. 1999). This study found that at 6-month follow-up, PTSD was observed in approximately 20 % of both active treatment groups compared to 67 % of those receiving supportive counselling. A follow-up of participants who completed these two treatment studies indicated that the treatment gains of those who received CBT were maintained 4 years after treatment (Bryant et al. 2003a).

Since these early studies, a range of studies have followed that have essentially replicated these findings. One study randomised civilian trauma survivors ($N=89$) with ASD to either CBT, CBT associated with hypnosis, or SC (Bryant et al. 2005). Hypnosis was employed because some theories posit that hypnosis may facilitate emotional processing in a condition that is characterised by dissociative symptoms (i.e. ASD) (Spiegel et al. 1996). Individuals with ASD have been shown to be particularly skilled at using hypnosis (Bryant et al. 2001), and so this study used hypnosis immediately prior to imaginal exposure with the suggestion to facilitate processing of trauma memories. All participants received the same number of sessions and identical length of exposure, with the exception that some participants received the hypnotic induction prior to the exposure exercise. Regarding those who completed treatment, more participants who received SC (57 %) had PTSD criteria at 6-month follow-up than those who received CBT (21 %) or CBT+hypnosis (22 %). Participants in the CBT+hypnosis condition did have fewer re-experiencing symptoms at posttreatment than those in the CBT condition, suggesting that the hypnosis may have facilitated the exposure component. Another study of ASD participants ($N=24$) who sustained mild traumatic brain injury compared the relative efficacies of CBT and SC in people who lost consciousness as result of their traumatic injury (Bryant et al. 2003a). Fewer participants receiving CBT (8 %) met criteria for PTSD at 6-month follow-up than those receiving supportive counselling (58 %). In the largest study of ASD to date, Bryant and colleagues randomly allocated 90 civilian trauma survivors to either (a) imaginal and in vivo exposure, (b) cognitive restructuring, or (c) assessment only (Bryant et al. 2008b). Exposure therapy led to lower levels of PTSD, depression, and anxiety at 6-month follow-up compared to other conditions.

It is important to be aware that other teams have also demonstrated the utility of early intervention using trauma-focused interventions. Jon Bisson and his team randomised 152 injury survivors to receive four sessions of CBT or no intervention in the first 3 weeks after the trauma (Bisson et al. 2004). Those who received the active intervention had lower PTSD symptoms at 13-month follow-up. This approach focused on severe acute PTSD symptoms, rather than ASD, which is more consistent with the DSM-5 definition of ASD by not requiring the specific clusters of ASD symptoms. Similarly, early provision of CBT has been shown to be beneficial in other studies that have targeted trauma survivors with elevated PTSD levels (Lindauer et al. 2005).

Rather than using a prolonged exposure approach, several studies have focused on more cognitively oriented approaches. Echeburua and colleagues provided 20 participants with acute posttraumatic stress with either cognitive restructuring and coping skills training or progressive relaxation training (Echeburua et al. 1996). There were no differences between conditions at posttreatment; however, cognitive restructuring led to less severe PTSD symptoms 12 months later. An Israeli study provided two sessions of SC or CBT that aimed to promote memory reconstruction to facilitate recovery in 17 survivors of road accidents (Gidron et al. 2001). This study used an entry criterion of a resting heart rate higher than 94 beats per minute at admission to the emergency room (on the basis that elevated heart rate in the acute phase is predictive of PTSD; Bryant et al. 2008a; Shalev et al. 1998). Treatment was delivered by the telephone 1–3 days after the accident. Patients who received the CBT intervention had less PTSD 3–4 months after the trauma than did those who received SC.

In an important study that compared early and later intervention, Shalev randomised 242 patients who were admitted to an emergency department and met criteria for either full or subsyndromal ASD. Participants were allocated to either prolonged exposure, cognitive restructuring, wait list (who were subsequently randomised to exposure or cognitive restructuring after 12 weeks), escitalopram (SSRI), or placebo (Shalev et al. 2012). At 9-month follow-up, PTSD outcomes did not differ between prolonged exposure (21 %) and restructuring (22 %) conditions; in contrast, there were higher rates in the SSRI (42 %) and placebo (47 %) conditions. There were *no* longer-term differences between participants who received the early or later therapy. One important implication of this study is that early intervention is not essential for optimal outcome and one can provide therapy some time later and achieve the same outcomes in the long run. This is not to minimise the benefit of early intervention, however, because there are clear advantages in reducing the stress (and associated problems) that can occur in the intermediate phase after trauma.

Another study commenced exposure therapy very soon after trauma by administering it in the emergency room for trauma patients and then repeating it weekly over the following 2 weeks (Rothbaum et al. 2012). Compared to an assessment-only comparison condition, patients who received exposure therapy had reduced PTSD at the 3-month follow-up. The interesting implication that emerges from this study is that it indicates that exposure therapy can be safely commenced very soon after trauma exposure.

Other controlled trials that have applied CBT to acute PTSD have recruited patients within 3 months of the trauma and therefore not provided therapy in the very acute phase after trauma. These studies also point to the utility of early intervention using exposure-based approaches. Each of these studies shows moderate to large effect sizes of PTSD symptom reduction (Ehlers et al. 2003; Sijbrandij et al. 2007).

Notably, not all studies have reported beneficial effects of trauma-focused early intervention. One large study randomised 90 female assault survivors who had acute PTSD symptoms to either prolonged exposure, SC, or a repeated assessment within 4 weeks of trauma (Foa et al. 2006). Nine months after treatment, all participants had made similar gains in terms of reducing PTSD; this finding did not change when only those who met ASD criteria were included. Another null finding was found in a study that used a writing paradigm, in which 67 traumatic injury patients were randomised to either a trauma writing intervention group or an information control group (Bugg et al. 2009). There were no differences between the groups at either posttreatment or follow-up assessments.

In summary, early provision of trauma-focused therapies, and particularly those that encourage emotional processing, appears to be efficacious in preventing subsequent PTSD. This conclusion is supported by systematic review of the available evidence (Ponniah and Hollon 2009). It is important to qualify this claim, however, by noting that a substantive proportion of people do not respond to early intervention, and so it should not be regarded as a panacea for posttraumatic problems.

Case Study: Trauma-Focused Cognitive Behaviour Therapy

Lou presented for treatment following a severe truck accident. He was a professional truck driver who had not had a serious road accident in over 20 years of driving long-haul trucks. Two weeks prior to presentation, he was driving his truck on an interstate highway when a motorcyclist riding in the opposite direction lost control of her motorcycle, skidded across the road, and slid up the wheels of Lou's truck. Lou immediately tried to assist the girl; however, she was partly crushed under one of the wheels. It transpired that he interacted with her briefly until she died while Lou was holding her head in his hands, waiting for paramedics to arrive.

Therapy commenced with a thorough assessment, which revealed that Lou had no prior psychological problems, had a supportive wife, and was a devout Catholic who believed it was extremely sinful to ever take a life. He expressed this view very strongly in the initial session, expressing great blame for (a) not averting the accident and (b) not saving the girl. He described severe re-experiencing symptoms, including frequent nightmares of the girl's bloodied face. He also reported often having intrusive memories of the experience, including seeing the motorcycle slide under his truck. Lou was engaging in pervasive avoidance of any reminders of the accident, including discussing it with his wife, thinking about it, or being exposed to situational reminders. Although it was his only source of income, Lou refused to drive since the accident. In terms of DSM-5 criteria, Lou satisfied the definition of ASD.

Following education about the rationale for processing the trauma memory to allow Lou the opportunity to understand what had occurred (previously precluded by his avoidance of thinking or talking about the experience), therapy commenced with prolonged exposure of the accident. Consistent with most forms of prolonged exposure (Bryant and Harvey 2000; Foa and Rothbaum 1998), this involved close engagement of the memory by asking Lou to relive what occurred in a subjectively compelling way. He found this highly distressing and was only able to narrate the trauma to the point of seeing the girl under the truck. The goal of exposure therapy in the initial sessions is to engage and master the anxiety, not necessarily to ensure that all aspects of the trauma are encompassed. This can be done in subsequent exposure sessions. In the initial session, Lou repeated the exposure to the accident three times to ensure that he was doing it for 30 min. He found this extremely distressing but was able to master the distress adequately.

Prolonged exposure was continued for four additional sessions. In the third session, Lou was strongly encouraged to focus on the 'hotspot' of the feature of the accident that he was avoiding – interacting with the girl as she lay under the truck. He was asked to slow down his narrative at this point and to stay with what was occurring at this time. He became very distressed during this reliving, during which he recounted that she disclosed to him that she was pregnant. This became a pivotal moment in Lou's memory of the trauma because he felt that he was responsible for the death of the unborn child, which was the source of extreme guilt. Considerable time was spent using cognitive restructuring techniques that challenged Lou to consider what alternative action he could have taken to (a) avert the accident, (b) save the girl, or (c) save the unborn child. The reliving was an important aspect for Lou to admit the guilt he felt about the deaths and allowed him to then realistically challenge his thoughts that he was responsible for either death. From the second therapy session, Lou was also instructed to commence a graded in vivo exposure programme in which he and his wife drove their family car for an hour twice a day. This commenced with quiet streets, gradually building up to busy roads, and then the freeway. Within 4 weeks, Lou was able to drive his truck again on the freeway.

Lou received a total of six therapy sessions, which is common for people with ASD. By the time he completed therapy, he still had some recurrent dreams, but these diminished to weekly rather than multiple times a night. He was not engaging in avoidance, was discussing the incident with his wife and other drivers, and had accepted that the accident was not his fault. Importantly, Lou understood the need to continue practising exposure every few days and to challenge any thoughts that he identified as being unrealistic about the trauma.

7.5   Pharmacological Approaches

Apart from psychological interventions, a handful of studies have also explored the potential for early provision of pharmacological interventions. Most of these approaches are rooted in fear conditioning models in the weeks after trauma as key mechanisms that lead to PTSD (Rauch et al. 2006). These models posit that when a traumatic event (unconditioned stimulus) occurs, people respond with fear (unconditioned response); this elevated fear leads to strong associative conditioning between the fear response and the stimuli associated with the trauma. Reminders of the trauma (conditioned stimuli) can then trigger fear reactions (conditioned response), including re-experiencing symptoms. This strong response to the traumatic event involves the release of stress neurochemicals (including norepinephrine and epinephrine) into the cortex, leading to an overconsolidation of trauma memories. Sensitisation can occur from repetitive distress, which elevates sensitivity of limbic networks, and this leads to increasing reactivity to trauma-related stimuli (Post et al. 1995).

One of the earlier studies was conducted by Roger Pitman's team, who attempted to prevent PTSD by reducing the level of noradrenergic response in the very immediate phase after trauma. The study administered propranolol (a β-adrenergic blocker) or placebo within 6 h of trauma exposure (Pitman et al. 2002). Although propranolol did not reduce PTSD relative to placebo at the 3-month follow-up, patients receiving propranolol did display less reactivity to trauma reminders 3 months later. Another study, albeit an uncontrolled one, administered propranolol immediately after trauma reduced PTSD severity 2 months after the trauma (Vaiva et al. 2003). Another controlled trial found that it had no preventative effect, but this study administered propranolol within 48 h after trauma, which may have been too late to achieve the desired effect (Stein et al. 2007). The impact of propranolol may be complex. Just as gender has been shown to influence outcomes of psychotherapy (Felmingham and Bryant 2012), another study reported gender-specific effects for the impact of propranolol on PTSD in children (Nugent et al. 2010).

Another possibility for preventing PTSD via reduction of norepinephrine levels in the acute phase is the use of opioids, such as morphine. Norepinephrine is inhibited by morphine, which is reflected in the impact of morphine on conditioning. For example, morphine injections into the amygdala of rats impair their level of fear conditioning (Clark et al. 1972) and cause amnesia for fear conditioning (McNally and Westbrook 2003). Extending this work to humans, uncontrolled studies have shown that administering morphine in the immediate hours after trauma has been associated with lower subsequent PTSD levels (Bryant et al. 2009; Holbrook et al. 2010; Saxe et al. 2001). These studies have been naturalistic and observational rather than controlled trials (it is difficult to randomise injured patients to receive morphine or an alternative comparator!), and so we cannot place much emphasis on this evidence at the current time.

In terms of other pharmacological agents, considerably fewer controlled trials have been conducted relative to psychotherapy trials. As mentioned earlier, Shalev and colleagues compared escitalopram with placebo and psychotherapies (Shalev et al. 2012); SSRIs have been shown to decrease firing of noradrenergic neurons (Szabo et al. 1999), and so it is possible that escitalopram could have a preventative effect in the acute phase. This study found that the SSRI was no more effective than placebo in preventing PTSD and less effective than CBT (Shalev et al. 2012). Another randomised trial found that 7 days of treatment with imipramine was more effective in treating symptoms of ASD in 25 child and adolescent burn victims than chloral hydrate (Robert et al. 1999).

The glucocorticoid system is another means by which secondary prevention may be achieved. We have evidence from animal studies that hydrocortisone administration after a stressor leads to less fear behaviour than placebo (Cohen et al. 2008). Similarly in human participants, cortisol administered shortly after trauma exposure leads to fewer traumatic memories (Schelling et al. 2004). There is very little initial support favouring the utility of cortisol as a means of early intervention: one study found that high-dose hydrocortisone within hours of trauma exposure led to reduced subsequent PTSD compared to placebo (Zohar et al. 2011). Although tentative, this evidence does point to the possibility that acute cortisol administration may play some beneficial role in preventing subsequent PTSD.

7.6   Stepped Care

As mentioned earlier, arguably the most difficult challenge is to determine who should receive early intervention. Our identification of people who require assistance will never be perfect because the relationship between acute and chronic stress reactions is complex and predicted by multiple factors that cannot be indexed in the acute phase. Complicating this issue further is the problem that many people immediately after trauma exposure may not want intervention. The problems caused by pain, income loss, and job or family interruption or the social chaos that often accompanies a traumatic event may distract the person from being receptive to offers for intervention. Only a small proportion of acutely traumatised people actually accept offers for treatment (Shalev et al. 2012). This has led many commentators to emphasise the need for ongoing monitoring of some subgroups after trauma rather than placing the full emphasis on early intervention.

In an attempt to do this, stepped care models of intervention have strived to integrate early intervention with monitoring and appropriate care as the need becomes apparent. Several models exist to achieve this. O'Donnell reported a study in which traumatically injured patients are (a) screened in the acute phase for high risk of PTSD development, (b) subsequently screened 4 weeks later to determine if high-risk status has maintained, and (c) then offered trauma-focused psychotherapy for those who indicate high risk (O'Donnell et al. 2012). Patients who had persistently high posttraumatic stress were randomised to CBT or treatment as usual; a 12-month follow-up indicated that those receiving CBT enjoyed lower PTSD levels than those who received usual treatment. In a similar vein, Doug Zatzick has conducted a series of trials in which traumatically injured patients are identified through initial screening and then provided with collaborative care – this involves case management and is integrated into the patient's overall medical recovery. A case manager oversees the patient's progress and may offer pharmacotherapy, psychosocial interventions, and CBT. A major aim of this framework is that it intends to reduce the likelihood that the patient will not be identified and treated within the health system. Across several controlled trials, this approach has been shown to be effective relative to treatment as usual in reducing PTSD and enhancing functioning (Zatzick et al. 2004, 2013). Applying this framework in the post-disaster setting, Brewin reports on a screen-and-treat approach that was implemented within weeks of the 2005 London bombings (Brewin et al. 2008). In this programme, people were screened 2 months after the bombings, and those who screened positive were provided with fuller assessments – identified cases were then treated with CBT or EMDR. This approach resulted in increased identification of people requiring care and also robust response rates to treatment (Brewin et al. 2010).

7.7   Placing Early Intervention in Context

Building on the stepped care approach, recent models have responded to disaster scenarios by contextualising early intervention in relation to interventions that may occur subsequent to the acute phase. For example, following major bushfires in Australia in 2009, a three-tiered model was initiated to address the different stages of trauma response (Forbes 2009). In the initial period (days) after the fires, PFA was administered to all survivors who were affected by the disaster. This intervention was provided by many providers who received rapid training in PFA and was intended to disseminate PFA to as many people as possible. In recognition that many disaster survivors do not access formal mental health services, this programme trained government employees, health providers, local primary care physicians, and volunteer agency workers who were most likely to be dealing with the disasters in the acute period.

A second tier of intervention was based on Skills for Psychological Recovery (SPR), which was a transdiagnostic intervention developed after Hurricane Katrina (Brymer et al. 2006). This intervention is based on the evidence of the core strategies that can address common problems following disasters: assessment and problem formulation, behavioural activation, cognitive reframing, anxiety management, increasing social support, and problem-solving. Although PFA contains some elements of these strategies, such as facilitating social support and cognitive reframing, SPR is qualitatively distinct from PFA insofar as the former commences with a personal assessment, is highly structured, devotes multiple sessions to targeting problems identified by the survivor, and is intentionally focused on addressing a presenting problem rather than representing a generic preventative function. Instead of treating established mental disorders, SPR attempts to address many of the subsyndromal problems that arise after trauma. This approach may be provided in the weeks (or even months) after trauma exposure and is intended to be delivered by health providers who are not necessarily highly qualified mental health specialists. These strategies have been applied in different settings after disasters and are generally perceived well by non-specialist providers (Forbes et al. 2010). At the third tier, those people who still suffer clinical disorders are treated by specialist mental health providers in evidence-based interventions. The advantage of this approach is that it recognises that not all problems can be identified in the acute phase, that new problems may emerge as time elapses after the trauma, and that suitable resources can be appropriately allocated to needs as they arise.

7.8 Challenges for Early Intervention

We have already seen that there are significant challenges for early intervention, including difficulty identifying those at high risk for subsequent PTSD, the fluctuating nature of problems that arise throughout the recovery period, and reluctance to seek care in the acute period. Additional challenges exist. Many early intervention models are predicated on the notion that trauma has a discrete onset and offset and early intervention occurs in the period after this. Whereas this is appropriate in many cases (e.g. motor vehicle accidents, assaults, etc.), there are many other examples where the traumatic experience is very protracted and it is difficult to determine when early intervention is appropriate. For example, disasters can involve very prolonged stressors that include fear for one's safety, loss of housing, food and water shortages, and illness. Similarly, people living in war zones may experience long periods of trauma exposure punctuated by periods of respite. In these cases, it is probably not suitable to conceptualise intervention as early versus later. Instead it is more appropriate to implement interventions according to the needs of the individual, the resources that are available, and the capacity of the person to undertake the intervention. Conceptualised in this way, intervention can be planned in a more flexible framework that can be provided at various time points and can accommodate the distinctive needs of a person at different points in the adaptation period.

7.9 Concluding Comment

There is no doubt that early interventions for PTSD have made enormous progress in the last two decades. We have moved beyond simplistic notions of universal intervention for all trauma survivors as a goal for preventing subsequent mental health problems. Exemplifying the current state of knowledge is the recent TENTS consensus statement that incorporated experts throughout Europe, who used a Delphi process to identify core principles of trauma response (Bisson et al. 2010; Witteveen et al. 2012). This process determined against universal debriefing or screening for all trauma-exposed people, as was the decision to not recommend pharmacological interventions. The TENTS project did endorse education, social support, and stepped care frameworks that utilise evidence-based trauma-focused psychotherapy for people with severe acute stress responses.

Our field has become more knowledgeable about the complexities of trauma response. Associated with the awareness that there is not a linear relationship between acute response and long-term outcome is the realisation that early intervention is not a panacea to later problems. Several challenges remain. First, screening is a poorly developed science in terms of early detection of posttraumatic response, and more subtle indices are required, as well as the capacity to conduct ongoing monitoring of high-risk individuals. Second, front-line treatments do not achieve optimal levels of success, and it is important to identify how to improve treatment outcomes in those who access care. Developing treatments that aim to overcome obstacles to treatment success is key to this endeavour. Third, most people do not seek care in the acute period, and too often this results in lengthy delays in ever seeking treatment. Overcoming barriers to care is a major challenge that public health agencies need to address if early intervention is to function at a truly effective level.

References

Adler, A. B., Litz, B. T., Castro, C. A., Suvak, M., Thomas, J. L., Burrell, L., et al. (2008). A group randomized trial of critical incident stress debriefing provided to U.S. peacekeepers. *Journal of Traumatic Stress, 21,* 253–263.

Bisson, J., & Andrew, M. (2007). Psychological treatment of post-traumatic stress disorder (PTSD). *Cochrane Database System Review,* (3), CD003388.

Bisson, J. I., Jenkins, P. L., Alexander, J., & Bannister, C. (1997). Randomised controlled trial of psychological debriefing for victims of acute burn trauma. *British Journal of Psychiatry, 171,* 78–81.

Bisson, J. I., Shepherd, J. P., Joy, D., Probert, R., & Newcombe, R. G. (2004). Early cognitive-behavioural therapy for post-traumatic stress symptoms after physical injury. Randomised controlled trial. [see comment]. *British Journal of Psychiatry, 184,* 63–69.

Bisson, J. I., Brayne, M., Ochberg, F. M., & Everly, G. S. (2007). Early psychosocial intervention following traumatic events. *American Journal of Psychiatry, 164*(7), 1016–1019.

Bisson, J. I., Tavakoly, B., Witteveen, A. B., Ajdukovic, D., Jehel, L., Johansen, V. J., Nordanger, D., Orengo Garcia, F., Punamaki, R. L., Schnyder, U., Sezgin, A. U., Wittmann, L., & Olff, M. (2010). TENTS guidelines: Development of post-disaster psychosocial care guidelines through a Delphi process. *British Journal of Psychiatry, 196*(1), 69–74.

Blanchard, E. B., Hickling, E. J., Barton, K. A., & Taylor, A. E. (1996). One-year prospective follow-up of motor vehicle accident victims. *Behaviour Research and Therapy, 34*(10), 775–786.

Bonanno, G. A., Mancini, A. D., Horton, J. L., Powell, T. M., Leardmann, C. A., Boyko, E. J., et al. (2012). Trajectories of trauma symptoms and resilience in deployed U.S. military service members: Prospective cohort study. *British Journal of Psychiatry, 200*(4), 317–323.

Bradley, R., Greene, J., Russ, E., Dutra, L., & Westen, D. (2005). A multidimensional meta-analysis of psychotherapy for PTSD. *American Journal of Psychiatry, 162*(2), 214–227.

Brewin, C. R., Scragg, P., Robertson, M., Thompson, M., d'Ardenne, P., & Ehlers, A. (2008). Promoting mental health following the London bombings: A screen and treat approach. *Journal of Traumatic Stress, 21*(1), 3–8.

Brewin, C. R., Fuchkan, N., Huntley, Z., Robertson, M., Thompson, M., Scragg, P., d'Ardenne, P., & Ehlers, A. (2010). Outreach and screening following the 2005 London bombings: Usage and outcomes. *Psychological Medicine, 40*(12), 2049–2057.

Bryant, R. A. (2011). Acute stress disorder as a predictor of posttraumatic stress disorder: A systematic review. *Journal of Clinical Psychiatry, 72*(2), 233–239.

Bryant, R. A., & Harvey, A. G. (2000). *Acute stress disorder: A handbook of theory, assessment, and treatment.* Washington, DC: American Psychological Association.

Bryant, R. A., Harvey, A. G., Dang, S. T., Sackville, T., & Basten, C. (1998). Treatment of acute stress disorder: A comparison of cognitive-behavioral therapy and supportive counseling. *Journal of Consulting and Clinical Psychology, 66*(5), 862–866.

Bryant, R. A., Sackville, T., Dang, S. T., Moulds, M., & Guthrie, R. (1999). Treating acute stress disorder: An evaluation of cognitive behavior therapy and supportive counseling techniques. *American Journal of Psychiatry, 156*(11), 1780–1786.

Bryant, R. A., Guthrie, R. M., & Moulds, M. L. (2001). Hypnotizability in acute stress disorder. *American Journal of Psychiatry, 158*(4), 600–604.

Bryant, R. A., Moulds, M., Guthrie, R., & Nixon, R. D. (2003a). Treating acute stress disorder following mild traumatic brain injury. *American Journal of Psychiatry, 160*(3), 585–587.

Bryant, R. A., Moulds, M. L., & Nixon, R. V. (2003b). Cognitive behaviour therapy of acute stress disorder: A four-year follow-up. *Behaviour Research and Therapy, 41*(4), 489–494.

Bryant, R. A., Moulds, M. L., Guthrie, R. M., & Nixon, R. D. (2005). The additive benefit of hypnosis and cognitive-behavioral therapy in treating acute stress disorder. *Journal of Consulting and Clinical Psychology, 73*(2), 334–340.

Bryant, R. A., Creamer, M., O'Donnell, M., Silove, D., & McFarlane, A. C. (2008a). A multisite study of initial respiration rate and heart rate as predictors of posttraumatic stress disorder. *Journal of Clinical Psychiatry, 69*(11), 1694–1701.

Bryant, R. A., Mastrodomenico, J., Felmingham, K. L., Hopwood, S., Kenny, L., Kandris, E., et al. (2008b). Treatment of acute stress disorder: A randomized controlled trial. *Archives of General Psychiatry, 65*(6), 659–667.

Bryant, R. A., Creamer, M., O'Donnell, M., Silove, D., & McFarlane, A. C. (2009). A study of the protective function of acute morphine administration on subsequent posttraumatic stress disorder. *Biological Psychiatry, 65*(5), 438–440.

Bryant, R. A., O'Donnell, M., Creamer, M., McFarlane, A. C., & Silove, D. (2013). A multi-site analysis of the fluctuating course of posttraumatic stress disorder. *JAMA Psychiatry, 70*, 839–846.

Brymer, M., Layne, C., Pynoos, R., Ruzek, J. I., Steinberg, A., Vernberg, E., & Watson, P. J. (2006). *Psychological first aid; field operations guide.* Washington, DC: US Department of Health and Human Services.

Bugg, A., Turpin, G., Mason, S., & Scholes, C. (2009). A randomised controlled trial of the effectiveness of writing as a self-help intervention for traumatic injury patients at risk of developing post-traumatic stress disorder. *Behaviour Research and Therapy, 47*(1), 6–12.

Carlier, I. V., Voerman, A. E., & Gersons, B. P. (2000). The influence of occupational debriefing on post-traumatic stress symptomatology in traumatized police officers. *British Journal of Medical Psychology, 73*(Pt 1), 87–98.

Clark, A. G., Jovic, R., Ornellas, M. R., & Weller, M. (1972). Brain microsomal protein kinase in the chronically morphinized rat. *Biochemical Pharmacology, 21*(14), 1989–1990.

Cohen, H., Matar, M. A., Buskila, D., Kaplan, Z., & Zohar, J. (2008). Early post-stressor intervention with high-dose corticosterone attenuates posttraumatic stress response in an animal model of posttraumatic stress disorder. *Biological Psychiatry, 64*(8), 708–717.

deRoon-Cassini, T. A., Mancini, A. D., Rusch, M. D., & Bonanno, G. A. (2010). Psychopathology and resilience following traumatic injury: A latent growth mixture model analysis. *Rehabilitation Psychology, 55*(1), 1–11.

Echeburua, E., de Corral, P., Sarasua, B., & Zubizarreta, I. (1996). Treatment of acute posttraumatic stress disorder in rape victims: An experimental study. *Journal of Anxiety Disorders, 10*(3), 185–199.

Ehlers, A., Clark, D. M., Hackmann, A., McManus, F., Fennell, M., Herbert, C., & Mayou, R. (2003). A randomized controlled trial of cognitive therapy, a self-help booklet, and repeated assessments as early interventions for posttraumatic stress disorder. *Archives of General Psychiatry, 60*(10), 1024–1032.

Ehring, T., Ehlers, A., & Glucksman, E. (2008). Do cognitive models help in predicting the severity of posttraumatic stress disorder, phobia, and depression after motor vehicle accidents? A prospective longitudinal study. *Journal of Consulting and Clinical Psychology, 76*(2), 219–230.

Everly, G. S., Jr., & Mitchell, J. T. (1999). *Critical Incident Stress Management (CISM): A new era and standard of care in crisis intervention* (2nd ed.). Ellicott City: Chevron.

Felmingham, K. L., & Bryant, R. A. (2012). Gender differences in the maintenance of response to cognitive behavior therapy for posttraumatic stress disorder. *Journal of Consulting and Clinical Psychology, 80*(2), 196–200.

Foa, E. B., & Rothbaum, B. O. (1998). *Treating the trauma of rape: Cognitive-behavioral therapy for PTSD.* New York: Guilford Press.

Foa, E. B., Hearst Ikeda, D., & Perry, K. J. (1995). Evaluation of a brief cognitive-behavioral program for the prevention of chronic PTSD in recent assault victims. *Journal of Consulting and Clinical Psychology, 63*(6), 948–955.

Foa, E. B., Zoellner, L. A., & Feeny, N. C. (2006). An evaluation of three brief programs for facilitating recovery after assault. *Journal of Traumatic Stress, 19*(1), 29–43.

Foa, E. B., Keane, T. M., Friedman, M. J., & Cohen, J. A. (Eds.). (2009). *Effective treatments for PTSD: Practice guidelines from the International Society of Traumatic Stress Studies* (2nd ed.). New York: Guilford.

Forbes, D. (2009). Psychological support and treatment for victims of Victoria's bushfires. *InPsych, 4*, 10–11.

Forbes, D., Fletcher, S., Wolfgang, B., Varker, T., Creamer, M., Brymer, M. J., et al. (2010). Practitioner perceptions of skills for psychological recovery: A training programme for health practitioners in the aftermath of the Victorian bushfires. *Australian and New Zealand Journal of Psychiatry, 44*(12), 1105–1111.

Frank, E., Anderson, B., Stewart, B. D., Dancu, C., Hughes, C., & West, D. (1988). Efficacy of cognitive behavior therapy and systematic desensitization in the treatment of rape trauma. *Behavior Therapy, 19*, 403–420.

Galea, S., Vlahov, D., Resnick, H., Ahern, J., Susser, E., Gold, J., et al. (2003). Trends of probable post-traumatic stress disorder in New York City after the September 11 terrorist attacks. *American Journal of Epidemiology, 158*(6), 514–524.

Gidron, Y., Gal, R., Freedman, S., Twiser, I., Lauden, A., Snir, Y., & Benjamin, J. (2001). Translating research findings to PTSD prevention: Results of a randomized-controlled pilot study. *Journal of Traumatic Stress, 14*(4), 773–780.

Holbrook, T. L., Galarneau, M. R., Dye, J. L., Quinn, K., & Dougherty, A. L. (2010). Morphine use after combat injury in Iraq and post-traumatic stress disorder. *New England Journal of Medicine, 362*, 110–117.

Inter-Agency Standing Committee. (2007). *IASC guidelines on mental health and psychosocial support in emergency settings*. Geneva: IASC.

Kessler, R. C., Galea, S., Gruber, M. J., Sampson, N. A., Ursano, R. J., & Wessely, S. (2008). Trends in mental illness and suicidality after Hurricane Katrina. *Molecular Psychiatry, 13*(4), 374–384.

Kilpatrick, D. G., & Veronen, L. J. (1984). Treatment for rape-related problems: Crisis intervention is not enough. In W. L. Claiborn, L. H. Cohen, & C. A. Spector (Eds.), *Crisis intervention* (2nd ed., pp. 165–185). New York: Human Sciences Press.

Lindauer, R. J. L., Gersons, B. P. R., van Meijel, E. P. M., Blom, K., Carlier, I. V. E., Vrijlandt, I., & Olff, M. (2005). Effects of brief eclectic psychotherapy in patients with posttraumatic stress disorder: Randomized clinical trial. *Journal of Traumatic Stress, 18*(3), 205–212.

Mayou, R. A., Ehlers, A., & Hobbs, M. (2000). Psychological debriefing for road traffic accident victims: Three-year follow-up of a randomised controlled trial. *British Journal of Psychiatry, 176*, 589–593.

McNally, G. P., & Westbrook, R. F. (2003). Anterograde amnesia for Pavlovian fear conditioning and the role of one-trial overshadowing: Effects of preconditioning exposures to morphine in the rat. *Journal of Experimental Psychology: Animal Behavior Processes, 29*(3), 222–232.

McNally, R. J., Bryant, R. A., & Ehlers, A. (2003). Does early psychological intervention promote recovery from posttraumatic stress? *Psychological Science in the Public Interest, 4*, 45–79.

Mitchell, J. T. (1983). When disaster strikes: The critical incident stress debriefing process. *Journal of Emergency Medical Services, 8*, 36–39.

Nugent, N. R., Christopher, N. C., Crow, J. P., Browne, L., Ostrowski, S., & Delahanty, D. L. (2010). The efficacy of early propranolol administration at reducing PTSD symptoms in pediatric injury patients: A pilot study. *Journal of Traumatic Stress, 23*(2), 282–287.

O'Donnell, M. L., Lau, W., Tipping, S., Holmes, A. C., Ellen, S., Judson, R., et al. (2012). Stepped early psychological intervention for posttraumatic stress disorder, other anxiety disorders, and depression following serious injury. *Journal of Traumatic Stress, 25*(2), 125–133.

Pietrzak, R. H., Van Ness, P. H., Fried, T. R., Galea, S., & Norris, F. H. (2013). Trajectories of posttraumatic stress symptomatology in older persons affected by a large-magnitude disaster. *Journal of Psychiatric Research, 47*, 520–526.

Pitman, R. K., Sanders, K. M., Zusman, R. M., Healy, A. R., Cheema, F., Lasko, N. B., et al. (2002). Pilot study of secondary prevention of posttraumatic stress disorder with propranolol. *Biological Psychiatry, 51*(2), 189–192.

Ponniah, K., & Hollon, S. D. (2009). Empirically supported psychological treatments for adult acute stress disorder and posttraumatic stress disorder: A review. *Depression and Anxiety, 26*(12), 1086–1109.

Post, R. M., Weiss, S. R. B., & Smith, M. A. (1995). Sensitization and kindling. Implications for the evolving neural substrates of post-traumatic stress disorder. In M. J. Friedman, D. S. Charney, & A. Y. Deutch (Eds.), *Neurobiological and clinical consequences of stress: From normal adaptation to PTSD* (pp. 203–224). Philadelphia: Lipincott-Raven.

Rauch, S. L., Shin, L. M., & Phelps, E. A. (2006). Neurocircuitry models of posttraumatic stress disorder and extinction: Human neuroimaging research-past, present, and future. *Biological Psychiatry, 60*(4), 376–382.

Riggs, D. S., Rothbaum, B. O., & Foa, E. B. (1995). A prospective examination of symptoms of posttraumatic stress disorder in victims of nonsexual assault. *Journal of Interpersonal Violence, 10*(2), 201–214.

Robert, R., Blakeney, P. E., Villarreal, C., Rosenberg, L., & Meyer, W. J., III. (1999). Imipramine treatment in pediatric burn patients with symptoms of acute stress disorder: A pilot study. *Journal of the American Academy of Child and Adolescent Psychiatry, 38*(7), 873–882.

Roberts, N. P., Kitchiner, N. J., Kenardy, J., & Bisson, J. I. (2009). Systematic review and meta-analysis of multiple-session early interventions following traumatic events. *American Journal of Psychiatry, 166*(3), 293–301.

Rothbaum, B. O., & Mellman, T. A. (2001). Dreams and exposure therapy in PTSD. *Journal of Traumatic Stress, 14*(3), 481–490.

Rothbaum, B. O., & Schwartz, A. C. (2002). Exposure therapy for posttraumatic stress disorder. *American Journal of Psychotherapy, 56*(1), 59–75.

Rothbaum, B. O., Foa, E. B., Riggs, D. S., Murdock, T., & Walsh, W. (1992). A prospective examination of post-traumatic stress disorder in rape victims. *Journal of Traumatic Stress, 5*(3), 455–475.

Rothbaum, B. O., Kearns, M. C., Price, M., Malcoun, E., Davis, M., Ressler, K. J., et al. (2012). Early intervention may prevent the development of posttraumatic stress disorder: A randomized pilot civilian study with modified prolonged exposure. *Biological Psychiatry, 72*(11), 957–963.

Saxe, G., Stoddard, F., Courtney, D., Cunningham, K., Chawla, N., Sheridan, R., et al. (2001). Relationship between acute morphine and the course of PTSD in children with burns. *Journal of the American Academy of Child & Adolescent Psychiatry, 40*(8), 915–921.

Schelling, G., Kilger, E., Roozendaal, B., de Quervain, D. J. F., Briegel, J., Dagge, A., Kapfhammer, H. P., et al. (2004). Stress doses of hydrocortisone, traumatic memories, and symptoms of post-traumatic stress disorder in patients after cardiac surgery: A randomized study. *Biological Psychiatry, 55*(6), 627–633.

Shalev, A. Y., Sahar, T., Freedman, S., Peri, T., Glick, N., Brandes, D., et al. (1998). A prospective study of heart rate response following trauma and the subsequent development of posttraumatic stress disorder. *Archives of General Psychiatry, 55*(6), 553–559.

Shalev, A. Y., Ankri, Y., Israeli-Shalev, Y., Peleg, T., Adessky, R., & Freedman, S. (2012). Prevention of posttraumatic stress disorder by early treatment: Results from the Jerusalem trauma outreach and prevention study. *Archives of General Psychiatry, 69*(2), 166–176.

Shephard, B. (2000). *A war of nerves: Soldiers and psychiatrists in the twentieth century.* London: Johnathan Cape.

Sijbrandij, M., Olff, M., Reitsma, J. B., Carlier, I. V. E., & Gersons, B. P. R. (2006). Emotional or educational debriefing after psychological trauma: Randomised controlled trial. *British Journal of Psychiatry, 189*, 150–155.

Sijbrandij, M., Olff, M., Reitsma, J. B., Carlier, I. V. E., de Vries, M. H., & Gersons, B. P. R. (2007). Treatment of acute posttraumatic stress disorder with brief cognitive behavioral therapy: A randomized controlled trial. *American Journal of Psychiatry, 164*(1), 82–90.

Smid, G. E., Mooren, T. T., van der Mast, R. C., Gersons, B. P., & Kleber, R. J. (2009). Delayed posttraumatic stress disorder: Systematic review, meta-analysis, and meta-regression analysis of prospective studies. *Journal of Clinical Psychiatry, 70*(11), 1572–1582.

Spiegel, D., Koopmen, C., Cardeña, C., & Classen, C. (1996). Dissociative symptoms in the diagnosis of acute stress disorder. In L. K. Michelson & W. J. Ray (Eds.), *Handbook of dissociation* (pp. 367–380). New York: Plenum Press.

Stein, M. B., Kerridge, C., Dimsdale, J. E., & Hoyt, D. B. (2007). Pharmacotherapy to prevent PTSD: Results from a randomized controlled proof-of-concept trial in physically injured patients. *Journal of Traumatic Stress, 20*(6), 923–932.

Szabo, S. T., de Montigny, C., & Blier, P. (1999). Modulation of noradrenergic neuronal firing by selective serotonin reuptake blockers. *British Journal of Pharmacology, 126*, 568–571.

Vaiva, G., Ducrocq, F., Jezequel, K., Averland, B., Lestavel, P., Brunet, A., & Marmar, C. R. (2003). Immediate treatment with propranolol decreases posttraumatic stress disorder two months after trauma. *Biological Psychiatry, 54*(9), 947–949.

van Griensven, F., Chakkraband, M. L. S., Thienkrua, W., Pengjuntr, W., Cardozo, B. L., Tantipiwatanaskul, P., et al. (2006). Mental health problems among adults in tsunami-affected areas in southern Thailand. *Journal of the American Medical Association, 296*(5), 537–548.

Witteveen, A. B., Bisson, J. I., Ajdukovic, D., Arnberg, F. K., Bergh Johannesson, K., Bolding, H. B., Elklit, A., Jehel, L., Johansen, V. A., Lis-Turlejska, M., Nordanger, D. O., Orengo-García, F., Polak, A. R., Punamaki, R. L., Schnyder, U., Wittmann, L., & Olff, M. (2012). Post-disaster psychosocial services across Europe: The TENTS project. *Social Science and Medicine, 75*(9), 1708–1714.

Zatzick, D. F., Roy-Byrne, P., Russo, J., Rivara, F., Droesch, R., Wagner, A., et al. (2004). A randomized effectiveness trial of stepped collaborative care for acutely injured trauma survivors. *Archives of General Psychiatry, 61*(5), 498–506.

Zatzick, D., Jurkovich, G., Rivara, F. P., Russo, J., Wagner, A., Wang, J., et al. (2013). A randomized stepped care intervention trial targeting posttraumatic stress disorder for surgically hospitalized injury survivors. *Annals of Surgery, 257*(3), 390–399.

Zohar, J., Yahalom, H., Kozlovsky, N., Cwikel-Hamzany, S., Matar, M. A., Kaplan, Z., et al. (2011). High dose hydrocortisone immediately after trauma may alter the trajectory of PTSD: Interplay between clinical and animal studies. *European Neuropsychopharmacology, 21*(11), 796–809.

Prolonged Exposure Therapy

8

Carmen P. McLean, Anu Asnaani, and Edna B. Foa

Prolonged exposure (PE) is an efficacious and effective treatment for PTSD that has been studied extensively and disseminated around the world. The theoretical underpinning of PE is emotional processing theory (EPT; Foa and Kozak 1985, 1986), an influential theory of pathological anxiety and therapeutic recovery. In this chapter, we briefly review EPT's account of the development and treatment of PTSD. We then describe the structure and key components of PE and illustrate its delivery using a case example. Next we provide an overview of the most common challenges faced by therapists delivering PE and discuss ways of overcoming these obstacles to maximize benefit from PE. We end our discussion with a summary of the extensive evidence supporting the efficacy and effectiveness of PE for a wide range of PTSD sufferers.

8.1 Theoretical Basis for Prolonged Exposure

Prolonged exposure (PE) therapy is based on emotional processing theory (EPT; Foa and Kozak 1985, 1986) which provides a comprehensive model for understanding the psychopathology and treatment of anxiety disorders. Foa and Cahill (2001) expanded EPT to provide a theoretical account for the development of chronic PTSD, the mechanisms involved in natural recovery after a traumatic event

C.P. McLean, PhD (✉)
Department of Psychiatry, Center for the Treatment and Study of Anxiety,
University of Pennsylvania, 3535 Market Street, 6th Floor, Philadelphia,
PA 19104, USA
e-mail: mcleanca@mail.med.upenn.edu

A. Asnaani, PhD • E.B. Foa, PhD
Department of Psychiatry, University of Pennsylvania, Philadelphia, PA USA

© Springer International Publishing Switzerland 2015
U. Schnyder, M. Cloitre (eds.), *Evidence Based Treatments for Trauma-Related Psychological Disorders: A Practical Guide for Clinicians*,
DOI 10.1007/978-3-319-07109-1_8

and in PE with chronic PTSD. A central premise of EPT is that emotions, including fear, are represented in memory as cognitive networks that include representations of the distressing stimuli, emotional responses, and their meaning. An emotional structure is activated when a person confronts information that matches some of the representations in the structure. In normal (nonpathological) emotional structures, the associations among the stimuli, responses, and meaning representation correspond to reality (e.g., house fires mean danger); activation of normal structures then is adaptive because they help avoid danger. In contrast, pathological emotional structures involve erroneous associations (e.g., crowded stores are dangerous, being raped is my fault). In PTSD, the traumatic memory is represented as a pathological emotional network that includes erroneous associations among representations of stimuli, responses, and their meaning. At present, the structure of fear has been delineated more clearly than other emotions (such as guilt, shame, and anger); therefore, we will focus on the structure of this emotion in this chapter.

For example, an individual with PTSD who has experienced a life-threatening motor vehicular accident may have a fear structure that includes representations of stimuli such as smells of gasoline and representations of responses such as increased respiration, quicker heart beating, and sweating. Of particular importance is the meaning assigned to the stimuli, such as the meaning of a gasoline smell as "danger" or the meaning of physiological symptoms as "I am afraid." Input matching some representations in the fear structure will activate the entire structure. Thus, smelling the scent of gasoline will activate the person's fear structure of cars.

According to EPT, the two mechanisms involved in both natural recovery and symptom reduction after therapy (Foa and Cahill 2001; Cahill and Foa 2007) are activation of the fear (emotional) structure and incorporation of information that disconfirms the pathological association in the structure. Specifically, natural recovery from trauma occurs via trauma-related erroneous perceptions, thoughts, and feelings being disconfirmed via thinking and talking about the trauma and/or approaching trauma reminders in daily life and by realizing that thinking and confronting trauma reminders do not result in the anticipated harm ("being attacked again" or "falling apart"). In contrast, persistent avoidance of trauma-related situations, objects, memories, thoughts, and feelings constitutes risk factors for developing PTSD because avoidance prevents the activation of the emotional structure and incorporation of information that disconfirms the unrealistically expected harm (e.g., being attacked in a crowded store) (Foa et al. 2006). It follows that effective treatment for PTSD should help patients confront safely trauma-related thoughts, images, objects, situations, and activities in order to promote activation of the traumatic structure and disconfirmation of distressing, harmful outcomes.

The two central therapeutic techniques in PE are (1) imaginal exposure, i.e., revisiting, by recounting aloud, the patient's memory of the trauma followed by processing of the experience, and (2) in vivo exposure, i.e., approaching safely situations and objects that the patient avoids because they are reminders of the trauma and hence cause distress. Once the negative emotion (e.g., fear) is activated in a safe setting, corrective learning occurs through integration of information that disconfirms the anticipated harm. Imaginal exposure corrects several inaccurate perceptions. First, it helps the patient organize the traumatic memory and gain a new perspective about what happened during the traumatic experience (e.g., "I did the best I could under the circumstances" instead of "I could have saved my friend if I were more competent"). Second, the repeated revisiting and recounting of the traumatic memory helps the patient distinguish between remembering the trauma and being traumatized again. Third, it helps the patient realize that the emotional distress associated with revisiting does not persist indefinitely and that remembering the trauma does not result in "falling apart." In vivo exposure helps to correct erroneous perceptions (1) by helping to break the patient's habit of terminating distress by avoiding or escaping the distressing situation, (2) by correcting the exaggerated probability estimates of harm by activating the fear structure in the absence of feared outcomes (e.g., realizing that being out after dark does not result in another rape), and (3) by letting the patient realize that he or she can tolerate distress without relying on escape. As a result of these processes, patients are able to change their negative trauma-related cognitions about themselves and the world (e.g., I am totally incompetent, the world is completely dangerous) which, according to EPT, are the core psychopathological features of PTSD (Foa and Rothbaum 1998).

8.2   Implementing Prolonged Exposure Therapy

Prolonged exposure (PE) is a specific exposure therapy program designed to help PTSD sufferers to emotionally process their traumatic experiences through the main two PE procedures: (a) in vivo exposure typically as homework, i.e., gradual approach to trauma-related, safe situations that the person avoids because these are trauma reminders, and (b) imaginal exposure to the memory of the traumatic event, by having patients recount their trauma memories out loud followed by processing of the experience in session and then by listening to a recording of their account for homework. PE also includes two minor procedures: (a) psychoeducation about the nature of trauma and trauma reactions, which incorporates the presentation of a clear rationale for the use of exposure therapy to patients, and (b) training in controlled breathing.

The current PE program for treatment of PTSD consists of 8–15 individual 90-min sessions. In the first meeting, the clinician provides a detailed rationale for PE and explains that PTSD is maintained by two key factors. The first factor is avoidance of thoughts and images related to the trauma and avoidance of trauma reminders. The clinician explains that although avoidance is effective in reducing anxiety in the short term, it maintains PTSD by preventing opportunities to emotionally process and digest the trauma memory. The second factor is unhelpful and often erroneous perceptions and beliefs that have developed in the wake of the trauma: "the world is extremely dangerous" and "I (the survivor) am completely incompetent." PE aims to alter these erroneous perceptions by providing opportunities to obtain corrective information that disconfirms these perceptions or beliefs via imaginal and in vivo exposure.

Case Example

Nancy is a 29-year-old single Latina woman currently pursuing a graduate degree. She sought treatment at the University of Pennsylvania's Center for the Treatment and Study of Anxiety (CTSA) and presented with symptoms of PTSD and major depressive disorder (MDD). Nancy's baseline score on the posttraumatic stress symptom inventory (PSS-I) was 34, indicating severe PTSD symptoms. Her baseline score of the Beck Depression Inventory (BDI) was 28, indicating moderate depression. She reported daily reexperiencing symptoms regarding the trauma, vivid nightmares, insomnia, and autonomic hyperarousal.

The Traumatic Event Currently Causing the Most Distress (Index Event)

Nancy reported that on July 4th 10 years ago, she agreed to spend time with the man she had been dating but recently broke up with. She reported that she knew she shouldn't trust him but agreed to go out to a party with him and some friends anyway. After watching her ex-boyfriend become increasingly intoxicated and belligerent, she tried to leave the bar and go home. This reportedly made her ex-boyfriend very angry and he broke a glass on the table and slashed her, cutting her face, shoulder, and lower neck, before running out of the bar. Bar staff and patrons brought Nancy to a back room and provided aid to her while waiting for emergency workers to arrive. She was taken to the hospital and was told that she needed surgery immediately. At one point, she was left alone, which was very upsetting to her as she was under the impression that she might die. Nancy survived the incident with no permanent medical complications; she has a visible scar on her shoulder and chin.

Case Formulation

Nancy's PTSD symptoms were maintained by her avoidance of external cues (e.g., men, crowds) and internal cues (e.g., emotions, memories) associated with the trauma. This avoidance blocked opportunities to disconfirm beliefs about the danger inherent to these cues and her ability to cope with the distress associated with exposure to them. Nancy's avoidance also functioned to maintain the more general dysfunctional perceptions and beliefs about others (e.g., "all men are dangerous") and herself (e.g., "I always make bad decisions"). These beliefs, in turn, helped maintain several of Nancy's PTSD and depressive symptoms, including her hyperarousal, anger, social withdrawal, and feelings of being disconnected from others. Nancy reported feeling invalidated by some of her friends and family, who reportedly suggested that Nancy "just get over it" and that she should "be grateful she is alive." Nancy internalized these comments in the form of self-criticism, and she experienced marked shame about her PTSD symptoms.

Course of Treatment

In the first session, the therapist and patient typically clarify which trauma will be focused on during imaginal exposure. For patients who have a history of multiple traumas, this "index trauma" is selected by determining which event is currently causing the greatest distress and dysfunction for the patient. Often, this will be the event that is associated with the most frequent and upsetting reexperiencing symptoms. The index trauma is identified during the first session as part of the trauma history interview. Nancy had experienced physical and verbal abuse in previous romantic relationships; however, the most recent traumatic event noted above was described as the most distressing event she had experienced. This index trauma served as the focus of the imaginal exposure. The beginning and end of the traumatic memory was also identified during this discussion.

Treatment began with the therapist providing an overview of the program and a rationale for exposure therapy. Nancy's therapist explained that PTSD symptoms are maintained by two factors: (1) avoidance of thoughts and feelings related to the trauma and avoidance of trauma reminders and (2) the presence of unhelpful, dysfunctional beliefs such as "the world is extremely dangerous" and "I am extremely incompetent." He then explained that PE alters these negative, dysfunctional perceptions by providing opportunities for disconfirming these perceptions through in vivo and imaginal exposure.

The first session also involved teaching the patient a slow-breathing relaxation technique that they are encouraged to practice on a daily basis to reduce daily stress. With her therapist's guidance, Nancy practiced the slow-breathing technique in session and agreed to continue to practice at home for homework.

The second session involved a brief discussion of common reactions to trauma in order to provide Nancy with a framework for understanding her symptoms. Nancy was forthcoming in describing the difficulties that she has experienced since the trauma. She reported that she didn't realize that some of her difficulties, such as difficulty concentrating and emotional numbing, were recognized as PTSD symptoms, and she expressed relief upon learning that PE is geared towards alleviating these symptoms. Next, Nancy's therapist introduced in vivo exposure which refers to confronting avoided places, people, and objects that reminded Nancy of the trauma. Nancy and her therapist collaboratively constructed an in vivo hierarchy of trauma-related situations that Nancy had been avoiding. Then, these situations were rank ordered based on how distressed Nancy expected to be if she confronted the situation. Distress ratings were collected using SUDS (subjective units of distress scale) from 0 (no distress) to 100 (intense distress). Nancy was able to identify a good range of situations for her hierarchy, with some that were associated with mild distress (e.g., going to the grocery store alone when it's not crowded), moderate distress (e.g., looking at photos of her ex-boyfriend/perpetrator), and high distress (e.g., going to a busy restaurant on a date). In vivo exposure was conducted in a stepwise fashion, beginning with situations that provoke moderate anxiety and gradually progressing to more challenging situations. After creating the in vivo hierarchy, Nancy and her therapist agreed on specific in vivo assignments that she would work on for homework that week. To simultaneously address Nancy's depression, the in vivo assignments were broadened to include behavioral activation items (e.g., watching movies; joining study groups). This focus was applied to "rebuilding life" tasks later in therapy, including joining a gym, making new friends, and reestablishing relationships with family.

In the beginning of the third session, Nancy reported that she had practiced the breathing retraining occasionally, and she thought it was helpful. She had completed most of the in vivo homework exercises and cited her busy school schedule as the reason she did not go to a coffee shop as planned. Nancy's therapist presented a detailed rationale for imaginal exposure. Nancy expressed some hesitation regarding imaginal exposure (e.g., "what if it doesn't work?") but also expressed considerable motivation and hope. Nancy's therapist reminded her of the traumatic memory that was identified as the most distressing during session 1 as well as the beginning and the end of the trauma. The therapist then asked Nancy to close her eyes and describe aloud what happened during that trauma, while visualizing the event as vividly as possible. Nancy was encouraged to recount the trauma in as much detail as possible, including the thoughts, feelings, and physical sensations that occurred during the traumatic event. Imaginal exposure was continued for a prolonged period (usually 30–45 min) and included multiple repetitions of Nancy's memory. Nancy was emotionally engaged with the traumatic memory during the imaginal exposure as evidenced by tearfulness and reported SUDS (30 at pre, 90 at peak, and 60 at post), and afterwards she reported that the image was very vivid for her. Imaginal exposure was followed immediately by 15–20 min of processing, which aims to help patients integrate new information and insights into their memory thereby promoting a more realistic perspective. During processing, Nancy described feeling guilty about the trauma (e.g., "I had a bad feeling early on. If I had listened to my gut it wouldn't have happened"). However, she also noted that revisiting the memory helped her realize that her ex-boyfriend was pleasant when he invited her to join him and his friends and she could not have predicted that he would be so violent, therefore she could not have prevented the attack. She even stated that in some ways she had acted quite bravely. Homework in vivo exposure exercises for the coming week were assigned at the end of the session. Nancy was also asked to listen to the audio recording of the entire session once and to listen to the imaginal exposure narrative daily.

The remainder of treatment (sessions 4–10) followed a standard agenda that began with reviewing the preceding week's homework. Nancy was generally adherent with the in vivo exposure homework; she always listened to the imaginal exposure audio but often completed only part of the in vivo exposure exercises. The avoided tasks were behavioral activation assignments (e.g., physical exercises) and were therefore arguably less critical to her recovery from PTSD than homework aimed at confrontation of avoided trauma-related situations.

During imaginal exposure, Nancy's peak SUDS rating decreased exponentially over the course of treatment. She often commented after the imaginal exposure that it was "getting easier" and that it felt more and more "like a memory." In session 7, the therapist introduced "hot spots," which he explained to Nancy as moments of the trauma memory that were causing the most distress. Nancy identified two hot spots: the first was when her ex-boyfriend smashed the glass and slashed her and the second was when she had been left alone in an emergency room. These hot spots were the focus of the imaginal exposure for session 7–9. During the processing, Nancy and her therapist discussed her feelings of guilt about the trauma. At baseline, Nancy was quite convinced that she was responsible for what happened to her because she "should have known better." However, as therapy progressed she began to articulate a new perspective, one in which her actions were not culpable but were instead reasonable, in light of the information she had at the time. Revisiting the memory again and again helped Nancy realize that there wasn't anything she could have done differently and that it could have happened to anyone. Being able to tolerate her distress during the first several weeks of in vivo and imaginal exposures, until the distress began to subside, helped Nancy change her view that she was incompetent in dealing with life and instead realize that she was a strong person who was able to cope successfully with difficult situations. Towards the end of treatment, she even expressed feeling that her decision to spend time with her ex-boyfriend was a reflection of her forgiving and kind nature, rather than an indicator that she has poor judgment.

During the final treatment session, the therapist and Nancy reviewed progress, discussed lessons learned, and made a plan for how Nancy could maintain the gains made during treatment. At the end of treatment, Nancy's PTSD symptoms had decreased significantly (PSS-I = 4, indicating minimal PTSD symptoms) as had her depressive symptoms (BDI = 6 indicating minimal depression). Nancy reported feeling that she was a worthy person, who had much to offer. While she did not feel ready to start dating, she agreed to work towards this goal slowly on her own, beginning with creating an online dating profile for herself. In contrast to the guilt feelings she described at the beginning of treatment, at the end of treatment Nancy recognized that she had done the best she could in a "crazy" situation. Nancy had shifted her approach to managing PTSD symptoms from avoidance, which maintains fear, to confrontation of trauma reminders, which promotes recovery and mastery.

8.3 Special Challenges to Implementing Prolonged Exposure Therapy

Patients rarely present with PTSD in the absence of additional psychiatric and/or physical health problems. In fact, comorbid disorders and associated problems are the rule rather than the exception among PTSD sufferers. Fortunately, as reviewed below, evidence is accumulating that PE is effective for PTSD sufferers with many commonly co-occurring disorders with little or no modification needed. We note that not all patients receiving PE do well, and unfortunately little is known about how to minimize nonresponse to treatment or premature dropout from treatment. Finally, we discuss some guidelines for when PE might be contraindicated.

8.3.1 Comorbid Depression

We now have considerable evidence that PE can effectively reduce PTSD symptoms among patients with comorbid depression. To illustrate, one study found that comorbid depression was unrelated to decrease in PTSD symptoms; those with current major depression, past major depression, and no history of major depression all benefitted equally from PE (Hagenaars et al. 2010). Interestingly, another study showed that patients with higher levels of depression pretreatment who received either cognitive processing therapy (CPT) or PE showed greater improvement in PTSD symptoms from pre- to posttreatment than those with lower depression (Rizvi et al. 2009).

Symptoms of PTSD and depression are closely linked, which may explain why reductions in PTSD severity tend to be associated with reductions in depressive symptoms as well. Not only has PE been found effective in reducing PTSD severity among those with comorbid depression, but it has also been found to significantly reduce depressive symptoms (Foa et al. 1991, 1999a; Marks et al. 1998; Paunovic and Ost 2001). It follows that among patients in which the primary presenting disorder is PTSD, comorbid depression should not be considered a contraindication for receiving PE. Depending on the patient's level of depression, therapists may want to incorporate more behavioral activation exercises when planning the in vivo hierarchy as recommended in the PE manual (Foa et al. 2007). In cases where major depression is the primary disorder or where the patient is deemed at a high risk for suicide, therapists should first provide crisis management and containment and/or an evidence-based treatment for depression prior to implementing PE.

8.3.2 Comorbid Substance Use

Traditionally, PTSD treatment studies have excluded patients with comorbid substance use disorders (Foa et al. 2005; Resick et al. 2008) based on the notion that PTSD treatment would be ineffective for patients with comorbid substance use or, worse, that it would exacerbate patients' substance use. More recently, however, studies have shown that PTSD and comorbid substance use can be treated successfully at the same time. For example, PE has now been found effective in reducing PTSD symptoms among patients with PTSD and comorbid alcohol dependence (Foa et al. 2013) and among those with comorbid cocaine dependence (Brady et al. 2001). Importantly, PE was not associated with an increase in substance use or craving in either of the aforementioned studies. Interestingly, Foa and colleagues found that patients who received PE were also more likely to maintain reductions in drinking 6 months after treatment termination (Foa et al. 2013). In summary, PE is effective and can be safely implemented in patients with PTSD and comorbid substance who are receiving concurrent substance use treatment.

As with comorbid depression, substance use and PTSD symptoms can be closely linked. In fact, it is commonly held that PTSD patients use substances, in part, to self-medicate their PTSD symptoms (e.g., Leeies et al. 2010; Nishith et al. 2001). Thus, by encouraging patients to approach trauma-related stimuli and process the traumatic memories, PE leads to decreased substance use indirectly by reducing PTSD symptoms. Therapists should carefully assess for substance use before implementing PE. Patients who have substance abuse/dependence should be referred for concurrent substance use treatment. Even patients who do not meet criteria for abuse or dependence may be using the substance as a subtle avoidance strategy, and this should be addressed in the context of PE (see also Chap. 16).

8.3.3 Comorbid Traumatic Brain Injury

Traumatic brain injury (TBI) is increasingly common among PTSD patients, especially among active military personnel and veterans who often suffer head injuries during traumatic experiences. Fortunately, there are some data showing that TBI, at least when either mild to moderate in severity, does not interfere with PTSD treatment. For example, a recent study of veterans with PTSD found that PE was as effective for individuals with and without a history of TBI (Sripada et al. 2013). The results of this research provide promising evidence that PE can be helpful for individuals with PTSD and comorbid TBI, and additional research is currently underway to further examine the effect of TBI on response to PE. In fact, because the PE protocol is relatively simple and easy to individualize to each patient, it may be particularly well suited for adaptation to comorbid PTSD and TBI. Therapists should be sure to screen for and assess cognitive impairment in patients reporting a history of TBI and should adapt the PE protocol (e.g., incorporating homework reminders, enlisting help from the patient's partner, shorter sessions) as needed.

8.3.4 Comorbid Borderline Personality Disorder

Borderline personality disorder (BPD) with frequent self-injurious behaviors is another condition that has been a rule out in some studies on PTSD treatment (Clarke et al. 2008; Feeny et al. 2002; Mueser et al. 2008). The concern has been that comorbid personality disorders, and perhaps BPD in particular, may interfere with PTSD treatment (Merrill and Strauman 2004). However, two studies indicate that individuals with comorbid BPD or BPD symptoms can also benefit from PTSD treatment. In the first study, Feeny et al. (2002) reanalyzed data of patients who received PE, stress inoculation training (SIT), or their combination and found that women with BPD symptoms benefited as much from PE treatment as those without

BPD symptoms. Although this study was not comprised of patients who met full diagnostic criteria for BPD, it shows that the presence of BPD symptoms did not impact treatment outcomes for PTSD symptoms, PTSD diagnostic status, depression, anxiety, and improving social functioning averaged across PE, SIT, and PE/ SIT.

Similar results were found in a study that examined women with full DSM-IV criteria for BPD and PTSD and who reported recent and/or imminent serious intentional self-injury (Harned et al. 2012). In this open trial study, 13 patients received dialectical behavior therapy (DBT) for a period of at least 2 months when they had stopped engaging in self-injurious behavior followed by PE once weekly while continuing DBT. While it is necessary to be cautious when comparing results across studies, Harned et al. (2012) reported that percentage of self-injurious behavior in patients receiving DBT-PE was distinctly lower than that reported in a trial examining the efficacy of DBT only (Linehan et al. 2006) who received DBT alone for up to 12 months. The authors concluded that "there was no evidence that the DBT-PE protocol increased intentional self-injury urges or behaviors, PTSD, treatment dropout, or crisis service use." These results have been replicated in a larger, randomized study of DBT versus DBT-PE (Harned et al. 2014).

In summary, PE can be effective for patients with PTSD and comorbid BPD when delivered after and then concurrently with DBT. When working with this population, therapists should carefully assess the presence and severity of self-injurious behavior and suicidality on an ongoing basis and coordinate care with the DBT therapist (see also Chap. 17).

8.3.5 Symptoms Associated with PTSD

Related to the concern about comorbid BPD, there has been a long-held concern that patients with high levels of dissociative symptoms are not good candidates for PE because dissociation would reduce the efficacy of treatment by limiting emotional engagement. However, several studies have shown that pretreatment levels of trait/state dissociation, depersonalization, and numbing are not related to PTSD symptom improvement or dropout from PE (Harned et al. 2012; Jaycox and Foa 1996; Shalev et al. 1996). That is, patients with high levels of dissociative symptoms showed a similarly large reduction in PTSD severity as patients with low levels of dissociative phenomena. However, one of the studies showing equivalent symptom improvement/dropout from PE with high and low dissociation found that individuals with high levels of dissociation were significantly more likely to meet criteria for PTSD (69 %) at follow-up than those with low dissociative symptoms (10 %) (Hagenaars et al. 2010). When working with patients who dissociate when distressed, therapists should discuss the issue with the patient, explain why dissociation is unhelpful for recovery, and agree upon ways to help support and ground the patient when needed. The PE protocol offers a number of suggestions for promoting optimal engagement (and hence minimizing the probability of dissociation) that should be considered in such cases. Among women with high dissociation whose PTSD was related to sexual abuse, Cloitre et al. (2012) found that providing emotional regulations skills training increased the benefit of modified prolonged exposure.

PE has also been found to ameliorate general anxiety (Foa et al. 2005), trauma-related guilt (Resick et al. 2002), and state anger (Cahill et al. 2003) and to improve social adjustment and functioning (Foa et al. 2005). Moreover, PE, with or without the addition of cognitive restructuring, was shown to significantly decrease reported physical health difficulties compared to wait list, and these improvements persisted at 1-year posttreatment (Rauch et al. 2009). In sum, PE can have a broad impact on the lives of PTSD sufferers by reducing both PTSD severity and associated symptoms and improving overall functioning.

8.3.6 Dropout

Although PE is often associated with rapid reductions in PTSD severity, it is important to note that some patients drop out of treatment or do not achieve a good response. A dropout rate of approximately 20–26 % has been found for CBT, both exposure and nonexposure treatments (Hembree et al. 2003), with dropout rates being lower in counseling or wait-list controls. For example, Schnurr et al. (2007) found that 38 % of those who received a combined treatment of PE with cognitive restructuring dropped out of treatment versus 21 % given present-centered therapy. On the other hand, in a recent study with adolescents (Foa et al. 2013), dropout from PE (10 %) was similar to the rate in client-centered counseling (17 %). Similarly, in a study examining efficacy of PE in individuals with comorbid alcohol dependence and PTSD, dropout rates were statistically equivalent across PE (37 %) and supportive counseling (29 %) (Foa et al. 2013). In a large-scale study by Resick and colleagues (2002), there was an equivalent dropout rate between those patients receiving CPT and PE (27 %). Thus, empirical studies indicate that PE does not have more dropout than other CBT treatments or control conditions.

Currently, very little is known about factors that predict treatment dropout. One study found that younger age, lower intelligence, and less education were associated with higher dropout from PE or CPT (Rizvi et al. 2009). In general, however, there are few factors that have been consistently identified as predicting dropout.

8.3.7 Contraindications

Like any treatment, there are contraindications to implementing PE. When considering whether or not to use PE, therapists should consider the following: first, PTSD must be the primary presenting issue. PE is the treatment for PTSD; therefore, a history of trauma in the absence of clinically significant PTSD symptoms is not sufficient to indicate PE. Second, there must be no safety issues such as imminent risk of suicide or homicide or current self-harm behavior. If present, PE should be withheld until the safety issues are addressed through crisis management or containment. Third, there must be no comorbid disorders that might interfere with treatment including unmanaged bipolar disorder or active psychosis. Although two recent studies suggest that PE can reduce PTSD symptoms among individuals with psychosis and recent suicidal behavior (van Minnen et al. 2012; Harned et al. 2014), more studies should be done with these patient populations. Finally, benzodiazepine use has been found to interfere with exposure therapy for PTSD (Davidson 2004), perhaps because they limit emotional activation and interfere with extinction learning (see Otto et al. 2005). Therefore, patients presenting for PTSD treatment who are already taking a benzodiazepine should be encouraged to work with their prescribing physician to discontinue this medication. Patients who are unwilling to discontinue the benzodiazepine should, at the very least, be asked to not use this medication prior to or during in vivo or imaginal exposures. Concurrent pharmacotherapy with newer and safer medications such as the selective serotonin reuptake inhibitors and the serotonin-norepinephrine reuptake inhibitors is not a contraindication to PE; however, as a general rule it is best if medication dosage remains stable during therapy so that the patient and therapist can accurately gauge the efficacy of therapy. (See also Chap. 26.)

8.4 Evidence Supporting Prolonged Exposure Therapy

A large number of randomized controlled trials indicate that PE is effective in reducing PTSD symptoms (see McLean and Foa 2011) and is associated with rapid change and maintenance of treatment gains over time, up to 5 years posttreatment (Foa et al. 2005; Powers et al. 2010; Taylor et al. 2003). PE has been found to be effective across a wide variety of trauma types and has been examined by independent research groups around the world (e.g., Israel: Nacasch et al. 2007, Japan: Asukai et al. 2008, Australia: Bryant et al. 2008, Netherlands: Hagenaars et al. 2010). As noted above, PE has demonstrated efficacy for PTSD sufferers with a number of common comorbid disorders (Foa et al. 2013; Harned et al. 2011; Hagenaars et al. 2010). PE has also been found to have a positive effect on associated symptoms of PTSD, including depression, general anxiety, guilt, anger, and anxiety sensitivity, and social functioning and health (Keane et al. 2006; Rauch et al. 2010).

PE is more effective than wait list (Foa et al. 1991, 1999a; Keane et al. 1989; Resick et al. 2002; Cahill et al. 2009; Difede et al. 2007), supportive counseling (Bryant et al. 2003; Schnurr et al. 2007), relaxation (Marks et al. 1998; Taylor et al. 2003; Vaughan et al. 1994), and treatment as usual (Asukai et al. 2008; Boudewyns and Hyer 1990; Cooper and Clum 1989; Nacasch et al. 2011). In addition, a meta-analysis pooling the findings across these numerous studies found that PE was associated with large effect sizes compared to control conditions at posttreatment and at follow-up (Powers et al. 2010). Other meta-analyses examining the efficacy of exposure therapy in general have revealed that exposure therapy is superior in symptom reduction to wait-list control or supportive therapy (Hofmann et al. 2012; Bradley et al. 2005). While research indicates that PE is superior to nontrauma-focused treatments or wait-list/control conditions, studies have found few differences among specific exposure therapies in the reduction of PTSD symptoms (Seidler and Wagner 2006; Bisson and Andrew 2007; Bisson et al. 2007).

Overall, the evidence in support of the efficacy of exposure therapy in general, and PE specifically, is extensive. Indeed, given this large evidence base for its efficacy, PE was identified in the joint Veterans Affairs-Department of Defense Clinical Practice Guideline for PTSD (VA/DoD Clinical Practice Guideline Working Group 2010) as "strongly recommended" for use with veterans with PTSD. Further, a 2008 report issued by the Institute of Medicine (IOM) concluded that exposure therapy was the sole treatment for PTSD with sufficient evidence for its efficacy. This conclusion led to its inclusion in practice guidelines for major key organizations providing care to trauma-exposed populations, namely, the American Psychiatric Association (2004), the Departments of Veterans Affairs and Defense (2004), and Foa et al. (2009).

As noted above, despite the impressive track record of PE, not all patients respond or complete treatment. There is room for improvement. Several studies have therefore explored whether the effects of PE can be bolstered or augmented. Specifically, cognitive enhancers hypothesized to boost extinction learning (e.g., D-cycloserine, methylene blue) have been receiving more attention as the field searches for ways to improve response and shorten treatment duration (Hofmann et al. 2011). Generally, these augmentation agents, while shown to be effective to varying degrees in several anxiety disorders, have had less support in the treatment of PTSD when using a component of PE (i.e., in session imaginal exposure only with no in vivo or imaginal homework; Litz et al. 2012). However, a recent pilot study found that individuals receiving virtual reality exposure therapy with d-cycloserine had significantly higher remission rates (46 %) than those receiving exposure therapy with placebo (8 %) (Difede et al. 2014). However, the rate of 8 % remission is much lower than was found in other PE studies (e.g., Foa et al. 2005; Schnurr et al. 2007). This inconsistency may be due to Difede et al. using a different treatment protocol than in PE studies. More investigation into the utility of cognitive enhancement with treatments for PTSD is needed. Other researchers have focused on the incorporation of supplemental psychological techniques with the hope that this may serve as significant adjuncts to PE. However, empirical evidence does not support the inclusion of these additional psychotherapy techniques (e.g., stress inoculation training: Foa et al. 1999a, b; cognitive restructuring: Foa et al. 2005; Marks et al. 1998). Outcome with the addition of these techniques is not better than PE alone, which suggests that all efficacious treatments modify the same dysfunctional cognitions underlying PTSD (Foa et al. 1999b). A number of studies have found benefit to incorporating skills training in emotional and social functioning with elements of PE for PTSD and related problems (Beidel et al. 2011; Cloitre et al. 2002, 2010; Turner et al. 2005). However, these studies have used only some components of PE; therefore, the utility of adding such treatment components to the full PE program is unclear. Research is underway to determine the mechanisms by which PE and other evidence-based treatments for PE work as our field moves towards the examination of neural circuits underlying changes in PTSD severity after treatment.

References

Asukai, N., Saito, A., Tsuruta, N., Ogami, R., & Kishimoto, J. (2008). Pilot study on prolonged exposure of Japanese patients with posttraumatic stress disorder due to mixed traumatic events. *Journal of Traumatic Stress, 21,* 340–343.

Beidel, D. C., Frueh, B. C., Uhde, T. W., Wong, N., & Mentrikoski, J. M. (2011). Multicomponent behavioral treatment for chronic combat-related posttraumatic stress disorder: A randomized controlled trial. *Journal of Anxiety Disorders, 25,* 224–231.

Bisson, J., & Andrew, M. (2007). Psychological treatment of post-traumatic stress disorder. *Cochrane Database of Systematic Reviews,* 8(2).

Bisson, J. I., Ehlers, A., Matthews, R., Pilling, S., Richards, D., & Turner, S. (2007b). Psychological treatments for chronic post-traumatic stress disorder – Systematic review and meta-analysis. *British Journal of Psychiatry, 190,* 97–104.

Boudewyns, P. A., & Hyer, L. (1990). Physiological response to combat memories and preliminary treatment outcome in Vietnam veteran PTSD patients treated with direct therapeutic exposure. *Behavior Therapy, 21,* 63–87.

Bradley, R., Greene, J., Russ, E., Dutra, L., & Westen, D. (2005). A multidimensional meta-analysis of psychotherapy for PTSD. *American Journal of Psychiatry, 162,* 214–227.

Brady, K. T., Dansky, B. S., Back, S. E., Foa, E. B., & Carroll, K. M. (2001). Exposure therapy in the treatment of PTSD among cocaine-dependent individuals: Preliminary findings. *Journal of Substance Abuse Treatment, 21,* 47–54.

Bryant, R. A., Moulds, M. L., Guthrie, R. M., Dang, S. T., & Nixon, R. D. V. (2003). Imaginal exposure alone and imaginal exposure with cognitive restructuring in treatment of posttraumatic stress disorder. *Journal of Consulting and Clinical Psychology, 71,* 706–712.

Bryant, R. A., Moulds, M. L., Guthrie, R. M., Dang, S. T., Mastrodomenico, J., Nixon, R. D. V., Felmingham, K. L., Hopwood, S., & Creamer, M. (2008). A randomized controlled trial of exposure therapy and cognitive restructuring for posttraumatic stress disorder. *Journal of Consulting and Clinical Psychology, 76,* 695–703.

Cahill, S. P., & Foa, E. B. (2007). Psychological theories of PTSD. In M. J. Friedman, T. M. Keane, & P. A. Resick (Eds.), *Handbook of PTSD: Science and practice.* New York: The Guilford Press.

Cahill, S. P., Rauch, S. A., Hembree, E. A., & Foa, E. B. (2003). Effect of cognitive-behavioral treatments for PTSD on anger. *Journal of Cognitive Psychotherapy, 17,* 113–131.

Cahill, S. P., Rothbaum, B. O., Resick, P. A., & Follette, V. (2009). Cognitive-behavioral therapy for adults. In *Effective treatments for PTSD: Practice guidelines from the International Society for Traumatic Stress Studies* (2nd ed.). New York: Guilford Press.

Clarke, S. B., Rizvi, S. L., & Resick, P. A. (2008). Borderline personality characteristics and treatment outcome in cognitive-behavioral treatments for PTSD in female rape victims. *Behavior Therapy, 39,* 72–78.

Cloitre, M., Koenen, K. C., Cohen, L. R., & Han, H. (2002). Skills training in affective and interpersonal regulation followed by exposure: A phase-based treatment for PTSD related to childhood abuse. *Journal of Consulting and Clinical Psychology, 70,* 1067–1074.

Cloitre, M., Stovall-Mcclough, K. C., Nooner, K., Zorbas, P., Cherry, S., Jackson, C. L., Gan, W., & Petkova, E. (2010). Treatment for PTSD Related to Childhood Abuse: A Randomized Controlled Trial. *American Journal of Psychiatry, 167,* 915–924.

Cloitre, M., Petkova, E., Wang, J., & Lu Lassell, F. (2012). An examination of the influence of a sequential treatment on the course and impact of dissociation among women with PTSD related to childhood abuse. *Depression and Anxiety, 29,* 709–717.

Cooper, N. A., & Clum, G. A. (1989). Imaginal flooding as a supplementary treatment for PTSD in combat veterans – A controlled study. *Behavior Therapy, 20,* 381–391.

Davidson, J. R. (2004). Use of benzodiazepines in social anxiety disorder, generalized anxiety disorder, and posttraumatic stress disorder. *Journal of Clinical Psychiatry, 65*(Suppl 5), 29–33.

Difede, J., Malta, L. S., Best, S., Henn-Haase, C., Metzler, T., Bryant, R., & Marmar, C. (2007). A randomized controlled clinical treatment trial for World Trade Center attack-related PTSD in disaster workers. *Journal of Nervous and Mental Disease, 195,* 861–865.

Difede, J., Cukor, J., Wyka, K., Olden, M., Hoffman, H., Lee, F. S., & Altemus, M. (2014). D-cycloserine augmentation of exposure therapy for post-traumatic stress disorder: A pilot randomized clinical trial. *Neuropsychopharmacology, 39*, 1052–1058.

Feeny, N. C., Zoellner, L. A., & Foa, E. B. (2002). Treatment outcome for chronic PTSD among female assault victims with borderline personality characteristics: A preliminary examination. *Journal of Personality Disorders, 16*, 30–40.

Foa, E. B., & Cahill, S. P. (2001). Psychological therapies: Emotional processing. In N. J. Smelser & P. B. Bates (Eds.), *International encyclopedia of social and behavioral sciences*. Oxford: Elsevier.

Foa, E. B., & Kozak, M. J. (1985). Treatment of anxiety disorders: Implications for psychopathology. In A. H. Tuma & J. D. Maser (Eds.), *Anxiety and the anxiety disorders*. Hillsdale: Erlbaum.

Foa, E. B., & Kozak, M. J. (1986). Emotional processing of fear – Exposure to corrective information. *Psychological Bulletin, 99*, 20–35.

Foa, E. B., & Rothbaum, B. O. (1998). *Treating the trauma of rape: A cognitive behavioral therapy for PTSD*. New York: Guilford.

Foa, E. B., Rothbaum, B. O., Riggs, D. S., & Murdock, T. B. (1991). Treatment of posttraumatic stress disorder in rape victims – A comparison between cognitive behavioral procedures and counseling. *Journal of Consulting and Clinical Psychology, 59*, 715–723.

Foa, E. B., Dancu, C. V., Hembree, E. A., Jaycox, L. H., Meadows, E. A., & Street, G. P. (1999a). A comparison of exposure therapy, stress inoculation training, and their combination for reducing posttraumatic stress disorder in female assault victims. *Journal of Consulting and Clinical Psychology, 67*, 194–200.

Foa, E. B., Ehlers, A., Clark, D. M., Tolin, D. F., & Orsillo, S. M. (1999b). The Posttraumatic Cognitions Inventory (PTCI): Development and validation. *Psychological Assessment, 11*, 303–314.

Foa, E. B., Hembree, E. A., Cahill, S. P., Rauch, S. A. M., Riggs, D. S., Feeny, N. C., & Yadin, E. (2005). Randomized trial of prolonged exposure for posttraumatic stress disorder with and without cognitive restructuring: Outcome at academic and community clinics. *Journal of Consulting and Clinical Psychology, 73*, 953–964.

Foa, E. B., Huppert, J. D., & Cahill, S. P. (2006). Emotional processing theory: An update. In *Pathological anxiety: Emotional processing in etiology and treatment*. New York: Guilford Press.

Foa, E. B., Hembree, E., & Rothbaum, B. O. (2007). *Prolonged exposure therapy for PTSD: Emotional processing of traumatic experiences therapist guide (treatments that work)*. New York: Oxford University Press.

Foa, E. B., Keane, T. M., Friedman, M., & Cohen, J. (2009). *Effective treatments for PTSD: Practice guidelines from the International Society for Traumatic Stress Studies*. New York: Guilford Press.

Foa, E. B., Yusko, D. A., Mclean, C. P., et al. (2013). Concurrent naltrexone and prolonged exposure therapy for patients with comorbid alcohol dependence and PTSD: A randomized clinical trial. *JAMA, 310*, 488–495.

Hagenaars, M. A., van Minnen, A., & Hoogduin, K. A. L. (2010). The impact of dissociation and depression on the efficacy of prolonged exposure treatment for PTSD. *Behaviour Research and Therapy, 48*, 19–27.

Harned, M. S., Pantalone, D. W., Ward-Ciesielski, E. F., Lynch, T. R., & Linehan, M. M. (2011). The prevalence and correlates of sexual risk behaviors and sexually transmitted infections in outpatients with borderline personality disorder. *Journal of Nervous and Mental Disease, 199*, 832–838.

Harned, M. S., Korslund, K. E., Foa, E. B., & Linehan, M. M. (2012). Treating PTSD in suicidal and self-injuring women with borderline personality disorder: Development and preliminary evaluation of a Dialectical Behavior Therapy Prolonged Exposure Protocol. *Behaviour Research and Therapy, 50*, 381–386.

Harned, M. S., Korslund, K. E., & Linehan, M. M. (2014). A pilot randomized controlled trial of Dialectical Behavior Therapy with and without the Dialectical Behavior Therapy Prolonged Exposure protocol for suicidal and self-injuring women with borderline personality disorder and PTSD. *Behaviour Research and Therapy, 55*, 7–17.

Hembree, E. A., Foa, E. B., Dorfan, N. M., Street, G. P., Kowalski, J., & Tu, X. (2003). Do patients drop out prematurely from exposure therapy for PTSD? *Journal of Traumatic Stress, 16*, 555–562.

Hofmann, S. G., Smits, J. A., Asnaani, A., Gutner, C. A., & Otto, M. W. (2011). Cognitive enhancers for anxiety disorders. *Pharmacology, Biochemistry and Behavior, 99*, 275–284.

Hofmann, S. G., Asnaani, A., Vonk, I. J., Sawyer, A. T., & Fang, A. (2012). The efficacy of cognitive behavioral therapy: A review of meta-analyses. *Cognitive Therapy Research, 36*, 427–440.

Institute of Medicine. (2008). *Treatment of posttraumatic stress disorder: An assessment of the evidence*. Washington, DC: The National Academies Press.

Jaycox, L. H., & Foa, E. B. (1996). Obstacles in implementing exposure therapy for PTSD: Case discussions and practical solutions. *Clinical Psychology & Psychotherapy, 3*, 176–184.

Keane, T. M., Fairbank, J. A., Caddell, J. M., & Zimering, R. T. (1989). Implosive (flooding) therapy reduces symptoms of PTSD in Vietnam combat veterans. *Behavior Therapy, 20*, 245–260.

Keane, T. M., Marshall, A. D., & Taft, C. T. (2006). Posttraumatic stress disorder: etiology, epidemiology, and treatment outcome. *Annual Review of Clinical Psychology, 2*, 161–197.

Leeies, M., Pagura, J., Sareen, J., & Bolton, J. M. (2010). The use of alcohol and drugs to self-medicate symptoms of posttraumatic stress disorder. *Depression and Anxiety, 27*, 731–736.

Linehan, M. M., Comtois, K. A., Murray, A. M., Brown, M. Z., Gallop, R. J., Heard, H. L., Korslund, K. E., Tutek, D. A., Reynolds, S. K., & Lindenboim, N. (2006). Two-year randomized controlled trial and follow-up of dialectical behavior therapy vs therapy by experts for suicidal behaviors and borderline personality disorder. *Archives of General Psychiatry, 63*, 757–766.

Litz, B. T., Salters-Pedneault, K., Steenkamp, M. M., Hermos, J. A., Bryant, R. A., Otto, M. W., & Hofmann, S. G. (2012). A randomized placebo-controlled trial of D-cycloserine and exposure therapy for posttraumatic stress disorder. *Journal of Psychiatric Research, 46*, 1184–1190.

Management of Post-Traumatic Stress Working Group. VA/DoD clinical practice guideline for management of post-traumatic stress. Washington (DC): Veterans Health Administration, Department of Defense; 2010. 251 p.

Marks, I., Lovell, K., Noshirvani, H., & Livanou, M. (1998). Treatment of posttraumatic stress disorder by exposure and/or cognitive restructuring – A controlled study. *Archives of General Psychiatry, 55*, 317–325.

Mclean, C. P., & Foa, E. B. (2011). Prolonged exposure therapy for post-traumatic stress disorder: A review of evidence and dissemination. *Expert Review of Neurotherapeutics, 11*, 1151–1163.

Merrill, K. A., & Strauman, T. J. (2004). The role of personality in cognitive-behavioral therapies. *Behavior Therapy, 35*, 131–146.

Mueser, K. T., Rosenberg, S. D., Xie, H., Jankowski, M. K., Bolton, E. E., Lu, W., Hamblen, J. L., Rosenberg, H. J., Mchugo, G. J., & Wolfe, R. (2008). A randomized controlled trial of cognitive-behavioral treatment for posttraumatic stress disorder in severe mental illness. *Journal of Consulting and Clinical Psychology, 76*, 259–271.

Nacasch, N., Foa, E. B., Fostick, L., Polliack, M., Dinstein, Y., Tzur, D., Levy, P., & Zohar, J. (2007). Prolonged exposure therapy for chronic combat-related PTSD: A case report of five veterans. *CNS Spectrums, 12*, 690–695.

Nacasch, N., Foa, E. B., Huppert, J. D., Tzur, D., Fostick, L., Dinstein, Y., Polliack, M., & Zohar, J. (2011). Prolonged exposure therapy for combat- and terror-related posttraumatic stress disorder: A randomized control comparison with treatment as usual. *Journal of Clinical Psychiatry, 72*, 1174–1180.

Nishith, P., Resick, P. A., & Mueser, K. T. (2001). Sleep difficulties and alcohol use motives in female rape victims with posttraumatic stress disorder. *Journal of Traumatic Stress, 14*, 469–479.

Otto, M. W., Bruce, S. E., & Deckersbach, T. (2005). Benzodiazepine use, cognitive impairment, and cognitive-behavioral therapy for anxiety disorders: Issues in the treatment of a patient in need. *Journal of Clinical Psychiatry, 66*(Suppl 2), 34–38.

Paunovic, N., & Ost, L. G. (2001). Cognitive-behavior therapy vs exposure therapy in the treatment of PTSD in refugees. *Behaviour Research and Therapy, 39*, 1183–1197.

Powers, M. B., Halpern, J. M., Ferenschak, M. P., Gillihan, S. J., & Foa, E. B. (2010). A meta-analytic review of prolonged exposure for posttraumatic stress disorder. *Clinical Psychology Review, 30*, 635–641.

Rauch, S. A. M., Defever, E., Favorite, T., Duroe, A., Garrity, C., Martis, B., & Liberzon, I. (2009). Prolonged exposure for PTSD in a Veterans Health Administration PTSD clinic. *Journal of Traumatic Stress, 22*, 60–64.

Rauch, S. A., Favorite, T., Giardino, N., Porcari, C., Defever, E., & Liberzon, I. (2010). Relationship between anxiety, depression, and health satisfaction among veterans with PTSD. *Journal of Affective Disorders, 121*, 165–168.

Resick, P. A., Nishith, P., Weaver, T. L., Astin, M. C., & Feuer, C. A. (2002). A comparison of cognitive-processing therapy with prolonged exposure and a waiting condition for the treatment of chronic posttraumatic stress disorder in female rape victims. *Journal of Consulting and Clinical Psychology, 70*, 867–879.

Resick, P. A., Galovski, T. E., Uhlmansiek, M. O. B., Scher, C. D., Clum, G. A., & Young-Xu, Y. (2008). A Randomized clinical trial to dismantle components of cognitive processing therapy for posttraumatic stress disorder in female victims of interpersonal violence. *Journal of Consulting and Clinical Psychology, 76*, 243–258.

Rizvi, S. L., Vogt, D. S., & Resick, P. A. (2009). Cognitive and affective predictors of treatment outcome in cognitive processing therapy and prolonged exposure for posttraumatic stress disorder. *Behaviour Research and Therapy, 47*, 737–743.

Schnurr, P. P., Friedman, M. J., Engel, C. C., Foa, E. B., Shea, M. T., Chow, B. K., Resick, P. A., Thurston, V., Orsillo, S. M., Haug, R., Turner, C., & Bernardy, N. (2007). Cognitive behavioral therapy for posttraumatic stress disorder in women – A randomized controlled trial. *Journal of the American Medical Association, 297*, 820–830.

Seidler, G. H., & Wagner, F. E. (2006). Comparing the efficacy of EMDR and trauma-focused cognitive-behavioral therapy in the treatment of PTSD: A meta-analytic study. *Psychological Medicine, 36*, 1515–1522.

Shalev, A. Y., Bonne, O., & Eth, S. (1996). Treatment of posttraumatic stress disorder: A review. *Psychosomatic Medicine, 58*(2),165–182.

Sripada, R. K., Rauch, S. A., Tuerk, P. W., Smith, E., Defever, A. M., Mayer, R. A., Messina, M., & Venners, M. (2013). Mild traumatic brain injury and treatment response in prolonged exposure for PTSD. *Journal of Traumatic Stress, 26*, 369–375.

Taylor, S., Thordarson, D. S., Maxfield, L., Fedoroff, I. C., Lovell, K., & Ogrodniczuk, J. (2003). Comparative efficacy, speed, and adverse effects of three PTSD treatments: Exposure therapy, EMDR, and relaxation training. *Journal of Consulting and Clinical Psychology, 71*, 330–338.

Turner, S. M., Beidel, D. C., & Frueh, B. C. (2005). Multicomponent behavioral treatment for chronic combat-related posttraumatic stress disorder: Trauma management therapy. *Behavior Modification, 29*, 39–69.

van Minnen, A., Harned, M. S., Zoellner, L., & Mills, K. (2012). Examining potential contraindications for prolonged exposure therapy for PTSD. *European Journal of Psychotraumatology, 3*. http://www.ncbi.nlm.nih.gov/pmc/articles/PMC3406222/

Vaughan, K., Armstrong, M. S., Gold, R., O'connor, N., Jenneke, W., & Tarrier, N. (1994). A trial of eye movement desensitization compared to image habituation training and applied muscle relaxation in post-traumatic stress disorder. *Journal of Behavior Therapy and Experimental Psychiatry, 25*, 283–291.

Cognitive Therapy for PTSD: Updating Memories and Meanings of Trauma

9

Anke Ehlers and Jennifer Wild

9.1 Understanding PTSD from a Cognitive Perspective

In the initial days and weeks after a traumatic event, most people will experience at least some symptoms of posttraumatic stress disorder (PTSD) such as intrusive memories, sleep disturbance, feeling emotionally numb, or being easily startled (Rothbaum et al. 1992). Most people will recover in the ensuing months, but for some the symptoms persist, often for years. What prevents these people from recovering? A lesson that we learned in treating and interviewing many trauma survivors is that what people find *most* distressing about a traumatic event varies greatly from person to person. Understanding the *personal* meanings of trauma and their relationship with *features of trauma memories* appears key to helping people with PTSD.

9.1.1 A Cognitive Model of PTSD

Ehlers and Clark (2000) suggested a cognitive model that explains why persistent PTSD develops. It guides the individual case conceptualization in the corresponding treatment approach, cognitive therapy for PTSD (CT-PTSD). This model suggests that PTSD develops if individuals process the traumatic experience in a way that produces a sense of a *serious current threat*. Once activated, the perception of current threat is accompanied by reexperiencing and arousal symptoms and strong emotions such as anxiety, anger, shame, or sadness. It is proposed that two key

A. Ehlers (✉) • J. Wild
Department of Experimental Psychology,
University of Oxford,
Oxford, UK
e-mail: anke.ehlers@psy.ox.ac.uk

© Springer International Publishing Switzerland 2015
U. Schnyder, M. Cloitre (eds.), *Evidence Based Treatments for Trauma-Related Psychological Disorders: A Practical Guide for Clinicians*,
DOI 10.1007/978-3-319-07109-1_9

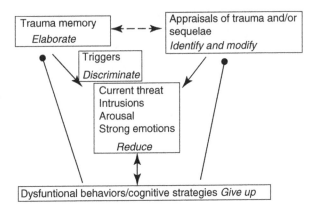

Fig. 9.1 Treatment goals in cognitive therapy for PTSD (Ehlers and Clark 2000). *Pointed arrows* stand for "leads to." *Round arrows* stand for "prevents a change in." *Dashed arrows* stand for "influences"

processes lead to a sense of current threat (see Fig. 9.1), namely, personal meanings of the trauma and the way traumatic experiences are laid down in memory.

First, it is suggested that individual differences in the personal meaning (appraisal) of the trauma and/or its sequelae (e.g., reactions of other people, initial PTSD symptoms, physical consequences of the trauma) determine whether persistent PTSD develops. For people with PTSD, the trauma and its aftermath have highly threatening personal meanings that go beyond what other people would find horrific about the situation. The perceived threat can be external or internal and leads to a range of negative emotions that are meaningfully linked with the type of appraisal. Perceived external threat can result from appraisals about impending danger (e.g., "I will be assaulted again"; "I cannot trust anyone"), leading to excessive fear, or a preoccupation with the unfairness of the trauma or its aftermath (e.g., "I will never be able to accept that the perpetrator got away with a minor sentence"), leading to persistent anger. Perceived internal threat often relates to negative appraisals of one's behavior, emotions, or reactions during the trauma and may lead to guilt (e.g., "It was my fault," "I should have prevented it") or shame (e.g., "I am inferior," "I am a bad person"). A common negative appraisal of consequences of the trauma in PTSD is perceived permanent change (e.g., "I have permanently changed to the worse," "My life is ruined"), which can lead to sadness and hopelessness.

Second, it is suggested that the worst moments of the trauma are poorly elaborated in memory, namely, inadequately integrated into their context (both within the event and within the context of previous and subsequent experiences/ information). This has the effect that people with PTSD remember the trauma in a disjointed way. While they recall the worst moments, it may be difficult for them to access other information that could correct impressions they had or predictions they made at the time. In other words, the memory for these moments has not been updated with what the person knows now. This has the effect that the threat they experienced during these moments is reexperienced as if it were happening right now rather than being a memory from the past. For example, when

John[1] nearly drowned during a ferry disaster, he thought that he would never see his children again. Whenever he recalled this particularly distressing moment, he was not able to access the fact that he still lived with his children and reexperienced the overwhelming sadness he had experienced at that moment again and again.

Ehlers and Clark (2000) also noted that intrusive trauma memories are easily triggered in PTSD by sensory cues that overlap perceptually with those occurring during trauma, for example, a similar sound, color, smell, shape, movement, or bodily sensation. They suggested that cognitive processing that focuses on perceptual features of the experience (data-driven processing) leads to strong perceptual priming (a reduced threshold for perception) for stimuli (and their sensory features) that occurred at the time of the traumatic event. Through learned associations, the stimuli also become associated with strong affective responses. This increases the chances that similar cues evoke distressing reexperiencing symptoms after the trauma.

In line with a role of associative learning, reexperiencing includes strong affective responses that are clearly related to the trauma, without the person recognizing that a trauma memory has been triggered (*affect without recollection*). For example, Anna, whose trauma involved being chased by a bull, felt an overwhelming urge that she had to "get out of here" when going for a walk in the country and jumped into an icy river. She was unaware of what had triggered this urge. Her partner spotted that she had responded to a cow grazing at a distance. Together, the proposed memory processes (poor elaboration, priming, and associative learning) explain why trauma memories remain so threatening in people with PTSD and why parts of these memories can be easily triggered by sensory reminders.

Why do the negative appraisals and the problematic nature of trauma memories persist in PTSD? Ehlers and Clark proposed that the negative appraisals and emotions prompt dysfunctional cognitive and behavioral responses that have the short-term aim of reducing distress but have the long-term consequence of preventing cognitive change and therefore maintain the disorder. Common examples include rumination about the trauma, avoidance of trauma reminders, suppression of trauma memories, excessive precautions (safety behaviors), substance use, and hypervigilance.

These maintain PTSD in three ways. First, some behaviors directly lead to increases in symptoms, for example, suppression of trauma memories leads to paradoxical increases in intrusion frequency. Second, other behaviors prevent changes in the problematic appraisals, for example, constantly checking one's rear mirror (a safety behavior) after a car accident prevents change in the appraisal that another accident will happen if one does not check the mirror. Third, other behaviors prevent elaboration of the trauma memory and its link to other experiences. For example, avoiding thinking about the event prevents people from updating the memory of

---

[1] Names and some details are changed in case examples to preserve anonymity.

the worst moments with information that could make them less threatening, for example, that they did not die or are not paralyzed.

9.1.2 Empirical Studies Testing the Proposed Factors

Studies have (1) compared trauma survivors with and without PTSD on the factors specified in Ehlers and Clark's (2000) model, (2) measured these factors soon after trauma and tested whether they predict PTSD later, and (3) tested them experimentally.

9.1.2.1 Negative Appraisals
Several studies have found strong empirical support for a relationship between PTSD and negative personal meanings (appraisals). Trauma survivors with PTSD endorsed negative appraisals of the trauma and its aftermath more strongly than those without PTSD (e.g., Foa et al. 1999). Negative appraisals correlate highly with the severity of PTSD symptoms. It is noteworthy that negative appraisals about the self (e.g., "What happened showed that I am a bad person," "My reactions since the event show that I am going crazy") correlate more strongly with PTSD severity than those about external danger (e.g., "The world is unsafe") (e.g., Duffy et al. 2013). Negative appraisals also help identify who is at risk of chronic PTSD after trauma. Several prospective studies recruited trauma survivors soon after their trauma and found that early negative appraisals strongly predicted PTSD 6 months or 1 year later (e.g., Dunmore et al. 2001; Ehring et al. 2008). Again, negative appraisals about the self were the most predictive.

9.1.2.2 Memory Processes
There is evidence from prospective studies of trauma survivors that a predominance *of data-driven processing* during trauma (as opposed to conceptual processing) predicts subsequent PTSD (e.g., Ehring et al. 2008; Halligan et al. 2003). Similar results were found in studies that experimentally induced intrusive memories of analogue traumatic pictures in healthy volunteers (e.g., Sündermann et al. 2013). Bourne et al. (2010) showed that performing a distracting verbal task that interfered with conceptual processing of a trauma film predicted poor intentional recall, but more frequent unintentional retrieval, similar to the pattern of memory retrieval observed in PTSD.

The hypothesis that cues are strongly *primed* during trauma and therefore more easily spotted afterwards has also gained empirical support. In a series of experiments, volunteers saw unpleasant picture stories that included some neutral objects that were unrelated to the content of the stories and parallel neutral stories. When participants were later asked to identify blurred pictures, they were better at identifying neutral objects that they had previously seen during a trauma story than those that they had seen in a neutral story (for reviews see Brewin 2014; Ehlers et al. 2012). Similarly, Kleim et al. (2012b) found that accident and assault survivors with PTSD identified blurred trauma-related pictures, but not general threat pictures, with greater likelihood than neutral pictures. The lower perceptual threshold in identifying trauma-related pictures also predicted PTSD 6 months later.

There is some evidence that PTSD is related to slow extinction learning of *conditioned associations* between neutral stimuli and fear responses and poor discrimination learning. Individual differences in the degree to with which such learned associations generalize to related stimuli also seems to play a role in the persistence of PTSD symptoms (for a review see Ehlers et al. 2012).

The nature of trauma memories has been a matter of considerable debate (see Ehlers 2015, for a review). There is some evidence from questionnaire studies and analyses of trauma narratives that people with PTSD recall the trauma in a disorganized and incoherent way, for example, gaps in memory and/or problems remembering the temporal order of events (e.g., Halligan et al. 2003; Jelinek et al. 2009). Five prospective longitudinal studies showed that objective measures of trauma memory disorganization taken in the initial weeks after the trauma predicted the severity of PTSD symptoms at follow-up (see Ehlers 2015, for a review). It is less clear whether the observed memory disorganization is specific to trauma narratives in PTSD, as some studies found that people with PTSD also recall other events in a disorganized way.

Some of the inconsistencies in the literature may be due to the fact that not all parts of the trauma memory are equally disorganized. The hypothesis that trauma memories are disjointed from other autobiographical information concerns moments of the trauma that are reexperienced (Ehlers et al. 2004). There is indeed some evidence that the memory for the worst moments of trauma is particularly disorganized (e.g., Evans et al. 2007). People with PTSD experienced intrusive memories to a greater extent as more disconnected from their context than those without PTSD (e.g., Michael et al. 2005). In an experimental study, assault survivors PTSD took longer than those without PTSD to retrieve autobiographical information when imagining the worst moment of their trauma, but not another negative life event (Kleim et al. 2008).

9.1.2.3 Behaviors and Cognitive Responses That Maintain PTSD

Several studies found that the maintaining behaviors and cognitive responses highlighted in Ehlers and Clark's model strongly correlate with PTSD (e.g., Duffy et al. 2013). Several prospective studies of trauma survivors found that rumination, suppression of trauma memories, and safety behaviors predicted chronic PTSD over and above what could be predicted from initial symptom levels (e.g., Dunmore et al. 2001; Ehring et al. 2008; Halligan et al. 2003; Kleim et al. 2012a).

Experimental studies investigated whether suppression of trauma memories and rumination play a causal role in maintaining PTSD symptoms. Most of the results are consistent with this hypothesis (for a review see Ehlers et al. 2012).

9.2   How to Do Cognitive Therapy for PTSD

9.2.1   Theory-Informed Individual Case Formulation

One of the basic ideas of cognitive therapy is that patients' symptoms and behavior make sense if one understands how they perceive themselves and the world and what they make of it. Therapists need to "get into the patient's head" (i.e., understand how patients perceive and interpret the world around them, what they think about themselves, and what beliefs motivate their behavior) before beginning the process of changing these cognitions. Cognitive therapy is a formulation-driven treatment. Treatment is tailored to the individual formulation and focuses on changing cognitions and cognitive processes that are directly relevant to the individual's problems. In CT-PTSD, Ehlers and Clark's cognitive model (2000) serves as the framework for an individualized formulation of the patient's problems and treatment. This model suggests three treatment goals that are targeted in treatment (Fig. 9.1):

- *To modify excessively negative appraisals of the trauma and its sequelae*
- *To reduce reexperiencing by elaboration of the trauma memories and discrimination of triggers*
- To *reduce behaviors and cognitive strategies that maintain the sense of current threat*

Therapist and patient collaboratively develop an individualized version of the model, which serves as the case formulation to be tested and revised in therapy. The maintaining factors are addressed with the procedures described below. The relative weight given to different treatment procedures differs from patient to patient, depending on the case formulation.

9.2.2 Therapeutic Style

Guided Discovery is central to the therapeutic style in cognitive therapy. Patient and therapist can be compared to a team of detectives that set out to *test* how well the patient's perceptions and ideas match up with reality. Together, they consider the patient's cognitions like hypotheses, exploring the evidence the patient has for and against them. A commonly used treatment technique is *Socratic questioning*. The therapist gently steers the patient towards considering a wider range of evidence or alternative interpretations by asking questions that help the patient consider the problem from different perspectives, with the aim to generate a less threatening alternative interpretation. For example, after being assaulted, Derek believed that he looked weak and was likely to be attacked again. In therapy, he considered the alternative hypothesis that his flashbacks gave him the impression that another assault was likely. Generating an alternative interpretation (insight) is usually not sufficient to generate a large emotional shift. A crucial, but sometimes neglected, step in therapy is therefore to test the patient's appraisals in behavioral experiments, which create *experiential* new evidence against the patient's threatening interpretations.

CT-PTSD follows these general principles, with some modifications. Therapists need to take extra care to establish a good therapeutic relationship with the patient (as many patients with PTSD feel they can no longer trust people) and make sure the patient feels safe in the therapeutic setting (as subtle trauma reminders can make the patient feel unsafe in many situations). CT-PTSD is a focused intervention that concentrates on changing cognitions that induce a *sense of current threat* after trauma. Careful assessment of the relevant appraisals is necessary. Patients may have other unhelpful negative thoughts that are not relevant to their sense of current threat and thus do not need to be addressed in treating their PTSD, unless they hinder the patient's engagement and progress in therapy.

Importantly, the main problematic appraisals that induce a sense of current threat are usually linked to particular moments during the trauma. The patient's evidence for their problematic appraisals typically stem from what they remember about their trauma. Disjointed recall makes it difficult to assess the problematic meanings by simply talking about the trauma and has the effect that insights from cognitive restructuring may be insufficient to produce a large shift in affect. Thus, work on appraisals of the trauma is closely integrated with work on the trauma memory in CT-PTSD.

9.2.3 Individual Case Formulation and Treatment Rationale

At the start of treatment, therapist and patient discuss the patient's symptoms and treatment goals. The therapist normalizes the PTSD symptoms as common reactions to an extremely stressful, overwhelming event and explains that many of the symptoms are a sign that the memory for the trauma is not fully processed yet.

The therapist asks the patient to give a brief account of the trauma and starts exploring the personal meanings ("What was the worst thing about the trauma?" "What were the worst moments and what did they mean to you?"). The *Posttraumatic Cognitions Inventory* (PTCI, Foa et al. 1999) can help with identifying cognitive themes that will need to be addressed in treatment. The therapist also asks the patient about the content of their intrusive memories and their meaning, as the moments that are reexperienced are often omitted from trauma narratives and the intrusions point to moments that are important for understanding the sense of current threat.

The therapist asks the patient what strategies they have used so far to cope with their distressing memories. Suppression of memories, avoidance, and numbing of emotions (including substance use) are commonly mentioned, as well as rumination (dwelling on the memories). The therapist then uses a *thought suppression experiment* (asking the patient to try hard not to think about an image such as a green rabbit or a black and white cat sitting on the therapist's shoulder) to demonstrate that suppressing mental images has paradoxical effects. After discussing this experience, the therapist encourages the patient to try to experiment with letting intrusive memories come and go during the next week (an exception to this homework assignment are patients who spend much time ruminating about the trauma, as they need to learn the distinction between intrusive memories and rumination first).

The therapist then uses the information gathered so far to develop an individual case formulation with the patient. This formulation contains the following core messages (in individualized form, using the patient's words as much as possible):

1. Many of the patient's current symptoms are caused by problems in the trauma memory. Therapy will help the patient in getting the memory in a shape where it

no longer pops up as frequent unwanted memories and feels like a memory of the past rather than something that is happening now.

2. The memory of the trauma and what happened in its aftermath influences the patients' current view of themselves and the world. The patient perceives a threat; a threat from the outside world, a threat to their view of themselves, or both. In therapy, the therapist and patient will discuss whether these conclusions are fair representations of reality and consider the possibility that the trauma memory colors their perception of reality.

3. Some of the strategies that the patient has used so far to control the symptoms and threat are understandable but counterproductive and maintain the problem. In therapy, the patient will experiment with replacing these strategies with other behaviors that may be more helpful.

The graphic presentation of the treatment model shown in Fig. 9.1 is usually not presented to the patient, as it is quite complex. Instead, different parts of the model, such as the vicious circle between intrusive memories and memory suppression, or the relationship between beliefs about future danger, safety behaviors, and hypervigilance may be drawn out for the patient to illustrate particular maintenance cycles that the patient is trying to change.

9.2.4 Modifying Excessively Negative Appraisals of the Trauma and Its Sequelae

9.2.4.1 Reclaiming Your Life Assignments

People with PTSD often feel that they have permanently changed for the worse and have become a different person since the trauma (e.g., Dunmore et al. 2001). Related to this perceived permanent change, patients with PTSD often give up activities and relationships that used to be important to them. This usually goes beyond avoidance of reminders of the traumatic event and may include activities that were previously a very significant part of the patient's life. Some activities may not have been possible in the immediate aftermath of the event and have just dropped out of the patient's repertoire. Giving up these activities maintains the perception of permanent change by providing confirmation that they have become a different person and that their life is less worthwhile since the trauma.

Each treatment session contains a discussion of what the patient can do to reclaim their life and corresponding homework assignments are agreed. In the first session, the rationale for these assignments is introduced. If patients have lost much of their former lives since the trauma, it is best to refer to "rebuilding your life." The therapist refers to the patient's treatment goals, which usually include an improvement in their ability to work and to have satisfying relationships. The initial discussion aims to map the areas where patients would like to reclaim their lives and to agree on an achievable first step in one of these areas, and the first homework is agreed. This intervention helps install hope that therapy will help the patient get back on track. It is also helpful for the therapist to get an idea of the patient's life and personality before the trauma so that they can build on their previous strengths and interests.

9.2.4.2 Changing Meanings of Trauma by Updating Trauma Memories

CT-PTSD uses a special procedure to shift problematic meanings (appraisals) of the trauma, termed *updating trauma memories*. This involves three steps:

Step 1: Identifying threatening personal meanings. To access the personal meanings of the trauma that generate a sense of current threat, the moments during the trauma that create the greatest distress and sense of "nowness" during recall (hot spots, Foa and Rothbaum 1998) are identified through *imaginal reliving* (Foa and Rothbaum 1998) or *narrative writing* (Resick and Schnicke 1993) and discussion of the content of intrusive memories. The personal meaning of these moments is explored through careful questioning (e.g., "What was the worst thing about this?" "What did you think was going to happen?" "What did this mean to you at the time?" "What does this mean to you now?" "What would it mean if your worst fear did happen?"). It is important to ask direct questions about patients' worst expected outcome, including their fears about dying, to elicit the underlying meanings, as this guides what information is needed to update their trauma memory.

Imaginal reliving and narrative writing both have particular strengths in working with trauma memories, and the relative weight given to each in CT-PTSD depends on the patient's level of engagement with the trauma memory and the length of the event. In *imaginal reliving* (Foa and Rothbaum 1998), patients visualize the traumatic event (usually with their eyes closed), starting with the first perception that something was wrong and ending at a point when they were safe again (e.g., the assailant left; being told in hospital that they were not paralyzed after an accident). Patients describe (usually in the present tense) moment by moment what is happening in the visualized event, including what they are feeling and thinking. This technique is particularly powerful in facilitating emotional engagement with the memory and accessing details of the memory (including emotions and sensory components). In our experience, it usually takes about 2 to 3 imaginal relivings of the traumatic event to access the hot spots sufficiently to assess their problematic meanings, although it may take longer if patients suppress their reactions or skip over difficult moments because, for example, they are ashamed about what happened.

Writing a narrative (Resick and Schnicke 1993) is particularly useful when the traumatic event lasted for an extended period of time and reliving the whole event would not be possible. The narrative covers the whole period and is then used to identify the moments or events with the greatest emotional significance so that their meaning can be explored further. Narrative writing is also particularly helpful for patients who dissociate and lose contact with the present situation when remembering the trauma or those who show very strong physical reactions when remembering the trauma (e.g., patients who were unconscious during parts of the trauma may feel very faint). Writing a narrative on a white-board or computer screen with the support of the therapist can help introduce the necessary distance for the patient to take in that they are looking back at the trauma rather than reliving it. Narrative writing is also especially helpful when aspects of what happened or the order of events are unclear, as it can be easily interwoven with a discussion about possible scenarios. Reconstructing the event with diagrams and models and a visit to the site of the trauma (which provides many retrieval cues) can be of further assistance in such instances. The narrative is useful for considering the event as a whole and for identifying information from different moments that have implications for the problematic meanings of the trauma and for updating the memory (see steps 2 and 3). After therapy, patients at times find it helpful to refer back to their updated narrative when memories are triggered, for example, around anniversaries of the trauma.

In our clinic, the majority of patients start with a few imaginal relivings, and the information generated during reliving is then used to write a narrative. The remaining patients only write a narrative with the help of the therapist and do not do reliving, for the reasons stated above.

Step 2. Identifying updating information. The next step is to identify information that provides evidence against the problematic meanings of each hot spot (updating information). It is important to remember that some of the updating information may be about what happened in the trauma. It can be something that the patient was already aware of, but has not yet been linked to the meaning of this particular moment in their memory, or something the patients has remembered during imaginal reliving or narrative writing. Examples include knowledge that the outcome of the traumatic event was better than expected (e.g., the patient did not die, is not paralyzed); information that explained the patient's or other people's behavior (e.g., the patient complied with the perpetrator's instructions because he had threatened to kill him; other people did not help because they were in shock); the realization that an impression or perception during the trauma was not true (e.g., the perpetrator had a toy gun rather than a real gun); or explanations from experts of what happened (e.g., explanations about medical procedures).

For other appraisals, cognitive restructuring is necessary, for example, for appraisals such as "I am a bad person," "It was my fault," "My actions were disgraceful," or "I attract disaster." Cognitive therapy techniques such as Socratic questioning, systematic discussion of evidence for and against the appraisals, behavioral experiments, discussing of hindsight bias, pie charts, or surveys are helpful. Imagery techniques can also be helpful in widening the patient's awareness of other factors that contributed to the event or in considering the value of alternative actions. For example, assault survivors who blame themselves for not fighting back during the trauma may visualize what would have happened if they had. This usually leads them to realize that they may have escalated the violence further and the assailant may have hurt them even more.

Step 3. Active incorporation of the updating information into the hot spots. Once updating information that the patient finds compelling has been identified, it is actively incorporated into the relevant hot spot. Patients are asked to bring the hot spot to mind (either through imaginal reliving or reading the corresponding part of the narrative) and to then remind themselves (prompted by the therapist) of the updating information either (a) by verbally (e.g., "I know now that …"), (b) by imagery (e.g., visualizing how one's wounds have healed; visualizing the perpetrator in prison; looking at a recent photo of the family or of oneself), (c) by performing movements or actions that are incompatible with the original meaning of this moment (e.g., moving about or jumping up and down for hot spots that involved predictions about dying or being paralyzed), or (d) through incompatible sensations (e.g., touching a healed arm). To summarize the updating process, a written narrative is created that includes and highlights the new meanings in a different font or color (e.g., "I know now that it was not my fault").

9.2.4.3 Changing Appraisals of Trauma Sequelae

For some patients, a main source of current threat comes from threatening appraisals of the aftermath of the traumatic event. For example, some patients believe that intrusive memories are a sign they are going crazy (e.g., Ehlers et al. 1998). Their failed attempts to control the intrusions are seen as further confirmation of their appraisals. Others interpret some people's responses after the event as signs that no one cares for them or understands them or that other people see them as inferior (e.g., Dunmore et al. 2001). Such appraisals are modified by the provision of information, Socratic questioning, and behavioral experiments.

9.2.5 Memory Work to Reduce Reexperiencing

9.2.5.1 Imaginal Reliving and Narrative Writing

The *updating trauma memories* procedure described above helps elaborate the trauma memory. Retrieving the memory and talking about it helps making it appear less vivid and intrusive. Patients may describe that some of the sensory impressions from the trauma fade away (e.g., colors or taste fading). When the hot spots have been successfully updated, patients usually experience a large reduction in reexperiencing symptoms and improvement in sleep.

9.2.5.2 Identification and Discrimination of Triggers of Reexperiencing Symptoms

Patients with PTSD often report that intrusive memories and other reexperiencing symptoms occur "out of the blue" in a wide range of situations. Careful detective work usually identifies sensory triggers that patients have not been aware of (e.g., particular colors, sounds, smells, tastes, touch). To identify these subtle triggers, patient and therapist carefully analyze where and when reexperiencing symptoms occur. Systematic observation in the session (by the patient and the therapist) and as homework is usually necessary to identify all triggers. Once a trigger has been identified, the next aim is to break the link between the trigger and the trauma memory.

This involves several steps. First, the patient learns to distinguish between "Then" versus "Now," that is, to focus on how the present triggers and their context ("Now") are different from the trauma ("Then"). This leads them to realize that there are more differences than similarities and that they are responding to a memory, not to current reality.

Second, intrusions are intentionally triggered in therapy so that the patient can learn to apply the "Then" versus "Now" discrimination. For example, traffic accident survivors may listen to sounds that remind them of the crash such as brakes screeching, collisions, glass breaking, or sirens. People who were attacked with a knife may look at a range of metal objects. People who were shot may listen to the sounds of gunfire generated on a computer. Survivors of bombings or fires may look at smoke produced by a smoke machine. People who saw a lot of blood during the trauma may look at red fluids. The "Then" versus "Now" discrimination can be facilitated by carrying out actions that were not possible during the trauma (e.g., movements that were not possible in the trauma, touching objects or looking at photos that remind them of their present life).

Third, patients apply these strategies in their natural environment. When reexperiencing symptoms occur, they remind themselves that they are responding to a memory. They focus their attention on how the present situation is different from the trauma and may carry out actions that were not possible during the trauma.

9.2.5.3 Site Visit
A visit to the site of the trauma completes the memory work. Visiting the site can help correct remaining problematic appraisals as the site provides many retrieval cues and helps access further information to update the appraisals. The site visit also helps complete the stimulus discrimination work. Patients realize that the "Now" is very different from the "Then," which helps place the trauma in the past.

9.2.5.4 Imagery Work
If reexperiencing symptoms persist after successful updating of the patient's hot spots and discrimination of triggers, imagery transformation techniques can be useful. The patient transforms the trauma image into a new image that signifies that the trauma is over. Transformed images can provide compelling evidence that the intrusions are a product of the patient's mind rather than perceptions of current reality. Image transformation is also particularly helpful with intrusions that represent images of things that did not actually happen during the trauma.

9.2.6   Dropping Dysfunctional Behaviors and Cognitive Strategies

The first step in addressing behaviors and cognitive strategies that maintain PTSD is usually to discuss their problematic consequences. Sometimes these can be demonstrated directly by a behavioral experiment. For example, the effects of selective attention to danger cues can be demonstrated by asking the patient to attend to possible signs of danger unrelated to the trauma. For example, an assault survivor may be asked to stand by a busy road for a few minutes and attend to signs of potentially risky driving. Patients find that this exercise makes them more aware of possible dangers. They then reflect on what this means for their own efforts to scan for signs of danger and consider the possibility that the world may not be as dangerous as they assumed. In other instances, a discussion of advantages and disadvantages is helpful, for example, when addressing rumination. The next step involves dropping or reversing the problematic strategy, usually in a behavioral experiment.

9.2.7 Duration of Treatment

CT-PTSD is usually delivered in up to 12 weekly sessions that last between 60 and 90 min and up to 3 optional monthly booster sessions. The mean number of sessions is around 10. Note that sessions that include work on the trauma memory such as imaginal reliving, updating memories, or the site visit, the therapist needs to allow sufficient time for the memory to be processed. Before going home, the patient needs sufficient time to refocus on current reality and their further plans for the day. These sessions would usually last around 90 min. Variations of the treatment are also effective. We have recently found that a 7-day intensive version of the treatment (delivered over 7 consecutive working days, with 2 to 4 hours of treatment per day, plus a few booster sessions; Ehlers et al. 2014) and a self-study assisted brief treatment are similarly effective (Ehlers et al. 2014).

Case Example
Paul was a 45-year-old paramedic of mixed ethnic background. He was referred for therapy by his family doctor as he felt very depressed and had problems sleeping. He felt also very worried that his family could be harmed in an accident or act of violence. He had quit work and spent most of the day at home.

The assessment showed that Paul suffered from PTSD and major depression. The symptoms had started about 2 years ago after a particularly distressing incident at work that involved a teenager being killed in a gang-related stabbing. Symptoms included frequent unwanted images of the dying teenager and other distressing incidents he had encountered at work; nightmares about his son or wife being in danger, harmed, or dying; avoiding work colleagues and social activities; feeling uninterested in things he used to enjoy; feeling emotionally numb; being hypervigilant for danger; and problems concentrating and sleeping. He sometimes thought about ending his life but would not do it because of his family. He used cannabis to cope with his distressing memories, but was not dependent. He agreed that he would not use cannabis on the days of his treatment sessions.

Paul's treatment goals were (a) to sleep better, without nightmares and at least 6 h per night, (b) to enjoy activities with his family again, and (c) to be able to work again.

Case Formulation

The cognitive assessment revealed the following factors that contributed to Paul's sense of current threat.

Appraisals

Paul blamed himself for not being able to save the teenager's life. He believed that he was a failure (belief rating: 100 %) and that the teenager's family would permanently suffer and never again feel close to their son (100 %). Paul also believed that his son and wife were in danger of being harmed either in an attack or an accident (90 %). He believed he was never going to be able to work again (70 %).

Trauma Memories

Paul's main reexperiencing symptoms included two images that he experienced daily. The first was an image of the dying teenager trying to say something to him. To Paul, this image meant that he was a failure, as he believed that if he had understood what the teenager was saying, he could have saved him. It also meant that he was responsible for the permanent suffering of the teenager's family as they would never again feel close to their son. The second intrusive image was of a body bag. When he had seen the body bag, Paul had immediately thought of his son and thought that he would not survive if his son died.

Paul also had intrusive memories of other distressing incidents he had encountered at work such as suicide and cot death, but he did not think he needed help with those memories.

When Paul described in the first session how he tried to help the dying teenager, he became distressed and tearful. He remembered most of what happened quite clearly but was unclear about some aspects that bothered him. He was unsure whether the teenager had actually spoken and why he could not understand him. He was also unsure whether he had followed the procedures correctly.

Paul had noticed that the intrusive images and physical symptoms were sometimes triggered when he saw teenagers or his own son. But he also experienced them "out of the blue," suggesting that there were other triggers that Paul had not spotted yet.

Maintaining Behaviors and Cognitive Strategies

Several behaviors and cognitive strategies that contributed to the maintenance of Paul's PTSD were identified:

- Rumination and worry
- Safety behaviors and hypervigilance
- Withdrawal from social life and other activities
- Cannabis use

Paul ruminated, sometimes for hours at a time, about what he should have done differently to prevent the teenager's death. He also ruminated about what would happen to his family if he could never work again. He spent a lot of time worrying about bad things that could happen to his family, including vivid images of his son or wife being hurt.

Paul took many unnecessary precautions to keep his family safe (safety behaviors). For example, he did not allow his teenage son to go to school or other places unaccompanied. When his son was at school, he frequently called him to make sure he was OK. This had led to tensions with his son. At night, he often checked whether his son and wife were still breathing. At home, he was hypervigilant for sounds that could indicate possible intruders, and outside his home, he scrutinized teenagers he saw for signs that they may be carrying knives.

Paul had given up his job and had lost touch with his friends, many of whom were work colleagues. He believed that his former colleagues now looked down on him because they knew he was a failure. He had also given up other activities he used to enjoy such as running.

Paul regularly tried to calm himself down by using cannabis, which he believed helped him "stop worrying" and fall asleep.

Comorbid Conditions

The cognitive assessment further suggested that Paul's comorbid depression was closely linked with many of the above factors, namely, his appraisal that he was a failure, his rumination, his social withdrawal, his lack of exercise, his restricted lifestyle (staying at home most of the time), and his inability to work. It was also likely that his cannabis use was a maintaining factor. Paul felt hopeless about his symptoms ("I will never get better," "I will never be able to work again"), which contributed to his suicidal ideation.

Thus, the case formulation suggested that working on Paul's appraisals of the trauma, updating the worst moments of the trauma memory, identification and discrimination of triggers of reexperiencing symptoms, and reversing his maintaining behaviors would be helpful in reducing both PTSD and depression symptoms. The therapist checked during therapy whether Paul's depression and suicidal ideation changed in parallel with his PTSD symptoms so that additional interventions could be considered if necessary.

Treatment

Paul attended 11 therapy sessions lasting between 60 and 90 min.

Work on Appraisals

Some of Paul's appraisals concerned *interpretations of his symptoms* (e.g., "I will never get better," "I will never be able to work again"). These were addressed with the following interventions in Session 1: *Normalization of symptoms* (e.g., "Nightmares are a sign that the trauma memory is being triggered. Working together on the trauma memory will help to process it and put it in the past, which will help to reduce nightmares"), *information about the nature of trauma memories* (e.g., "Trauma memories often feel like they are happening now and give you the sense that there is immediate danger. For example, one of your trauma memories is seeing the body bag. This makes you think of your son and gives you the sense that he is in danger. This feeling comes from the trauma memory"), and the introduction of *reclaiming your life assignments*. Examples of the assignments Paul completed over the course of therapy included: (a) building up exercise and by the end of treatment, running in a charity race; (b) watching football with his son; (c) inviting an old friend over to his house; (e) attending a computing course; (e) seeing an advisor about job options; and (f) volunteering in a charity shop. These activities helped reduce Paul's conviction in his appraisals of not recovering and raised his hope that he would be able to lead a less restricted life and eventually be able to work again.

"I am a failure." As Paul's belief that he was a failure stemmed from a moment during the trauma when he could not understand what the teenager was trying to say, the *updating trauma memories* procedure was used. In Session 2, Paul went through the event in imaginal reliving and identified two relevant hot spots that corresponded to his intrusive memories, namely, the moment when the teenager died and the moment he saw the body bag, which made him think of his son.

To identify updating information for the first hot spot, the therapist and Paul wrote a narrative and reviewed carefully what had happened (Session 3). The therapist used guided discovery to help Paul realize that not understanding what the teenager had said was probably due to the teenager's injuries and fading consciousness rather than his own incompetence. Paul wrote down what he knew about the teenager's injuries and what he had done to help him. Considering what he had written carefully, he realized that he had followed the protocol. However, some doubts remained. The therapist discussed with Paul how best to test his concern that he may not have followed the protocol. They decided to ask for an expert opinion. The therapist arranged for Paul to have a discussion with an experienced paramedic in Session 4. The expert agreed that Paul had done everything that was possible and that the injuries had been too severe to save the teenager's life.

Paul then updated the memory of this hot spot with a summary of his conclusions from the discussion with the therapist and the expert feedback (Session 4). The therapist guided Paul to visualize the moment when he could not understand the teenager and had felt incompetent. While holding this moment in mind, Paul reminded himself that the teenager was fading in and out of consciousness and was not speaking properly. He also reminded himself that the expert had confirmed that Paul had done everything possible. Paul also included the updating information in his trauma narrative so that he could refer back to the updating information when he found himself ruminating about the event.

"The teenager's family will permanently suffer and never again feel close to their son." To reduce the distress linked to Paul's appraisal of the family's suffering and loss, the therapist used imagery (Session 5). She first had Paul describe qualities he would associate with the teenager, having had a few brief, important moments with him. Paul said that the teenager represented strength and positivity despite his suffering after being stabbed. When asked what he thought could represent strength and positivity today, Paul thought of a ray of sunshine and how the sun generally makes people smile. He then imagined the teenager's family being touched with rays of sunshine, connecting them to qualities they loved about their son. Paul brought this imagery to mind when the trauma memory and thoughts about the family's loss were triggered.

"Something terrible will happen to my son or my wife." Paul's belief that his family were at risk was contrasted with the alternative hypothesis that his strong memory of the trauma, especially the intrusive images of the body bag, was giving him the impression that his son was in danger. The updating trauma memories procedure was used to update this hot spot. Paul realized that when he had seen the body bag, it had felt as if his son was inside. Updating this moment in memory in Session 3 with the information that his son was alive felt "like a surprise and relief."

The therapist also guided Paul to consider that his safety behaviors contributed to his sense of threat. Paul conducted a series of behavioral experiments that involved dropping his safety behaviors and hypervigilance. For example, he experimented with letting his son go to school and come home on his own without telephoning him on one day of the week. He predicted that it was 90 % likely that his son would have an accident or be attacked and not make it home. This never happened and Paul then experimented with increasing the number of days his son went to school on his own. With the help of his therapist and these experiments, he learned that the actual likelihood of his son having an accident was no more likely now than before the trauma and that the likelihood was extremely low. At home, he experimented with focusing on danger and checking that his wife and son were still breathing several times an evening and contrasting that to an evening when he focused his attention on assignments for his computer class. He discovered that when he focused on danger and checking for safety, he felt more frightened and worried than when he focused on his tasks for his class. He concluded that focusing on danger made him feel as though danger was imminent and that checking on his wife and son kept him focused on thoughts of accidents, illness, and death.

Memory Work to Reduce Reexperiencing

As described above, imaginal reliving and writing a narrative, together with detailed discussions with the therapist and an expert, helped Paul identify hot spots and helped him understand that he had done everything possible to help the teenager. Updating Paul's hot spots led to a significant reduction in his intrusive memories and nightmares.

In sessions 5 and 6, Paul explored with his therapist possible triggers of his intrusive memories. Through systematic observation and attention to sensory similarities between possible triggers and the trauma, he spotted a range of triggers that he had not noticed before. Examples included: objects the same color as the body bag, ambulance sirens, blood, and seeing his son asleep. He practiced discriminating these from the stimuli he encountered in the trauma by focusing on differences in both the stimuli and context, both during the session (e.g., listening to recordings of sirens, objects of the same color) and at home (e.g., looking at his son in bed).

After Paul had made good progress with the stimulus discrimination training, he went to the site where the stabbing had taken place with the therapist (Session 8). They focused on the differences between "Then" and "Now." When an ambulance drove by, Paul focused on that no one was hurt at present and the ambulance was driving past. He felt very relieved, as he had felt apprehensive about the site visit and had felt as if he would again find a dying child there. Paul remembered an important detail about the event. He remembered holding the teenager's hand, and the teenager briefly squeezing his hand. This made him realize that the teenager had acknowledged his efforts to help him and was unlikely to have experienced his efforts as incompetent. He felt a sense of relief. After the site visit, Paul felt that he could now look back at the event, rather than reexperience it.

Work on Maintaining Behaviors and Cognitive Strategies

To address Paul's *rumination*, the therapist guided Paul to distinguish between having a memory of the event and ruminating about it. They discussed the advantages and disadvantages of ruminating. Paul concluded that it had not helped and had made him feel even worse. He decided that the best time to think about what he should have done during the assault was in the therapy sessions and to ruminate less at home. He discussed triggers of rumination and found that during the day, a common trigger was sitting at home alone doing nothing, and at night, lying in bed when he woke up. He agreed that when he found himself ruminating, he would remind himself that this style of thinking was unhelpful. During the day, he would do one of his reclaiming your life assignments instead.

As discussed above, Paul's *hypervigilance, safety behaviors, and avoidance* were addressed by considering the hypothesis that Paul's trauma memory made him feel his family was in danger and with a series of behavioral experiments, both in the session and as homework. Hypervigilance was replaced with stimulus discrimination, focusing his attention on differences between the current situation and the trauma.

Paul experimented with having cannabis-free days to see if this helped his sleep. He found it difficult to fall asleep in the short term, but after 2 weeks of cannabis-free days and further therapy sessions, his sleep had improved. Paul also discovered that he felt more energetic on days when he did not use cannabis and had fewer intrusive memories. He concluded that cannabis actually did not help him feel less worried.

Outcome

At the end of treatment, Paul no longer suffered from PTSD or depression. He no longer had suicidal thoughts. He occasionally still felt sad when he thought about the tragic death. His relationship with his son had improved. He slept 7 h per night. He had resumed contact with some former work colleagues and was applying for work. At follow-up 1 year later, he had maintained his treatment gains and was working as a paramedic again.

9.3 Special Challenges

9.3.1 Comorbidity

Many patients with PTSD have comorbid conditions that need to be addressed in treatment.

Depression that is secondary to PTSD will usually be successfully reduced with treating PTSD. However, in some cases, depression may become so severe that it needs immediate attention (i.e., suicide risk) before PTSD treatment can commence. In some trauma survivors (especially after multiple trauma), depression may dominate the clinical picture to the extent that it makes a treatment focus on the trauma impossible and warrants treatment first. Depressive symptoms most likely to interfere with PTSD treatment are severe suicidal ideation, extreme lack of energy, social withdrawal, inactivity, and poor concentration. As in cognitive therapy for depression, the first goal in treatment will be to lift the patient's mood sufficiently so that cognitive therapy can commence, for example, with behavioral activation or antidepressant medication.

Anxiety disorders such as agoraphobia, obsessive-compulsive disorder, generalized anxiety disorder, or social anxiety disorder may be preexisting conditions or develop as a complication of PTSD. The therapist needs to determine whether the comorbid anxiety disorder needs treatment in its own right. If this is the case, the case formulation and treatment plan will need to integrate the treatment of both the PTSD and the other anxiety disorders. It is not always easy to determine in the initial assessment whether patterns of avoidance are part of the patient's PTSD or part of another anxiety disorder. An important question is "What is the worst thing that could happen if you … (encounter the feared situation, do not take special precautions)?" In PTSD, the patient's concern would usually be another trauma ("I will be attacked again," "I will die in another accident"). Other concerns suggest other anxiety disorders, for example, panic disorder ("I will have a heart attack," "I will faint") or social phobia ("I will make a fool of myself," "People will think I am weird"). It is also often difficult to determine initially whether or not a panic attack or strong anxiety response in a certain situation constitutes a reexperiencing symptom (as patients are usually not aware of the subtle sensory triggers of reexperiencing). In these cases, an ongoing assessment of the need for separate work on the other anxiety disorder is needed as treatment progresses.

In most cases with comorbid anxiety disorders, treatment starts with the CT-PTSD program. An important exception are patients with panic disorder who believe that a catastrophe will happen if they become very anxious or put their body under stress, for example, believing that they will have a heart attack, they will faint, or they will go crazy. These misinterpretations will often need to be addressed *before* working on the trauma memory as these patients are unlikely to engage in treatment or may drop out if their concerns are not addressed.

Many patients with PTSD use alcohol, cannabis, or other substances to numb their feelings or distract themselves from trauma memories. This may include heavy smoking or even consumption of caffeinated beverages in large quantities. Substance misuse is not a contraindication for treatment. Treatment of the PTSD will help patients to reduce their substance use. The therapist will need to incorporate the substance use as a maintaining behavior in the case formulation and address it together with the other maintaining factors in the overall treatment plan. However, if physical substance dependence has developed (i.e., the patient has withdrawal symptoms, tolerance, and acquiring and consuming the substances takes up much of the patient's life), withdrawal is usually necessary before the patient can benefit from the treatment described here. If in doubt, a useful strategy is to explain to patients with very high substance use that the treatment will only work if they are not intoxicated and do not have a hangover in the session, so that they can process fully what is being discussed and benefit from the treatment. The therapist will need to educate patients about the negative effects of the substance on their symptoms (e.g., alcohol may help the patient get to sleep but will lead to more awakenings at night and feeling irritable and emotional the next day; cannabis may make the patient feel more unreal or more paranoid; smoking leads to brief relief and then increased anxiety; caffeine can lead to irritability, poor sleep, and concentration). The therapist should then ask whether patients would be willing to try to reduce their substance consumption before treatment commences. Many patients will agree to give it a try if they have the prospect of receiving help for their PTSD. These patients often find that the reduction in substance use in itself has a positive effect on their PTSD symptoms. If the patient does not feel able to reduce the substance consumption, treatment will need to target the dependence first.

9.3.2 Dissociation

Patients with PTSD differ in the extent to which they dissociate when trauma memories are triggered. Some feel unreal, feel numb, or have "out-of-body" experiences but remain aware of their current environment. Therapeutic interventions for this milder form of dissociation include normalization of the experience as a common response to trauma (the therapist may want to link dissociation to freezing in animals who face predators) and work on interpretations of the experience such as

"I am going crazy," "I live in a different reality to other people," or "The real me died and I am an alien/ghost now." It can also be helpful to guide patients who had "out-of-body" experiences during imaginal reliving to return to their body and perceive the event from the perspective of their own eyes.

Other patients may lose awareness of current reality completely and feel and behave as if the trauma were happening again. This severe form of dissociation can involve significant risk to self and others and needs to be assessed carefully. Adaptations of the treatment procedures include a strong emphasis on stimulus discrimination from the outset of therapy and the use of grounding objects or strategies that help them stay aware of the present (e.g., touching a small toy or pebble from a beach, using room perfume, consuming a sour sweet or a strong mint, or listening to music when memories are triggered). The therapist explains that strong emotional reactions linked to the trauma can occur without any images of the event itself (e.g., strong urge to leave a situation, strong anger) and guides the patient to become increasingly aware that these are signs that trauma memories are being triggered. The work on trauma memory elaboration is done in a graded way that allows the patient to remain aware of the present safe environment. For example, the therapist and patient may write a narrative in small steps in combination with stimulus control strategies, taking many breaks to remind the patient of their present safe situation. Precautions that minimize risk to self and others are agreed if indicated, for example, talking to family members about how to spot dissociation and how to bring the patient's attention back to the present. For some patients, for example, survivors of prolonged childhood sexual abuse, training in emotion regulation strategies before the trauma memory work commences can be helpful (Cloitre et al. 2010).

9.3.3 Multiple Trauma

Many patients with PTSD have experienced more than one trauma but not all traumas are necessarily linked to their current PTSD. In order to determine which traumas need to be addressed in therapy, the therapist and patient discuss which traumas still bother them, for example, are represented in reexperiencing symptoms or are linked to personal meanings that trouble the patient at present. The discussion also involves a first assessment of problematic meanings that link several traumas. For example, Laura who was raped and physically assaulted on several occasions concluded "People can spot that I am an easy target." Patient and therapist discuss which trauma to start with. This would usually be either a trauma that the patient currently finds the most distressing or a trauma when an important problematic meaning originated. A narrative with a time line of the different events can be helpful in this discussion. The therapist also notes whether elements from other traumas come up when the patient relives the identified trauma, as these may have influenced its personal meanings. Once the hot spots from the identified trauma have been updated, the therapist checks whether this decreases the reexperiencing of other traumas that carry related meanings. The remaining traumas that are still distressing or relevant for problematic appraisals are then addressed in turn. Dissociation may be pronounced and will need to be addressed with the methods described above.

Work on reclaiming and rebuilding the patient's life is especially important after multiple trauma since these patients may lead very restricted lives and may need much support from the therapist with problem solving about how to best build up a social network, reengage in the job market, etc. Work on maintaining behaviors is also especially important as patients may show extreme forms of these behaviors, for example, chronic hypervigilance and complete social withdrawal. For patients with long-standing multiple traumas, additional work on self-esteem may be helpful (e.g., keeping a log of things they did well or positive feedback from others).

9.3.4 Physical Problems

The injuries contracted in the traumatic event may lead to ongoing health problems that significantly affect the patient's life. Chronic pain is common. Sometimes the traumatic event leads to a permanent loss of function, for example, difficulty walking, inability to have children, or blindness. Patients often need help in adjusting to these physical problems and the impact they have on their lives. This may require additional treatment strategies such as pain management or using coping strategies similar to those for coping with chronic illness.

For other patients, the physical injuries may have compromised their appearance, which may have negative effects on their job or social life. They may need support in learning to adapt to these changes. It is also not uncommon for patients to perceive a loss of attractiveness or a disfigurement that is greater than the objective change. For these patients, video feedback is helpful as it helps patients update the image of how they believe they appear to others (which is influenced by the trauma memory) with a more accurate image. Patients watch themselves in a short video recording, with the instruction to watch themselves objectively as if they were another person they do not know. For example, a patient who believed that his facial scars were repulsive saw bright red scars when he visualized how he would appear to others. His face was filmed with different red objects in the background. Comparing his face with the objects made him realize that the scars did not look red any longer and were much less visible than he had imagined. Surveys are helpful in testing patients' beliefs about what other people think about their appearance. For example, the patient agreed with the therapist for some other people to watch the video recording and answer a series of questions about his appearance, starting with neutral questions and ending with direct questions about the patient's concern: "Did you notice anything about this person's appearance?" "Did you notice anything about this person's face?" "Did you notice that he had scars?" "What did you think about the scars?" "Did you think he looked repulsive?" The therapist fed back the responses in the following week, and the patient was relieved to find that no one thought he looked repulsive and most people had not even noticed the scars.

Other health problems that existed before the traumatic event may influence the course of treatment. For example, patients with some medical conditions, such as poorly controlled diabetes, may find it hard to concentrate for long periods of time and require shorter sessions or sessions with frequent breaks. Patients with chronic heart conditions may require a graded approach in recalling the trauma and visiting the site.

9.4   Evaluations of Cognitive Therapy for PTSD

The efficacy of CT-PTSD has been evaluated in several randomized trials in adults (Ehlers et al. 2003, 2005, 2014, in prep) and children (Smith et al. 2007). Table 9.1 gives an overview of key results. A series of randomized controlled trials found that

Table 9.1 Evaluations of cognitive therapy for PTSD

	Patient sample	% Dropouts	Intent-to-treat size for PTSD symptoms (PDS)[a]	Intent-to-treat % patients in full remission[b]	% Patients with symptom deterioration (PDS)
Randomized controlled trials					
Ehlers et al. (2003)	Adults, acute PTSD following road traffic accidents	0	2.46	78.6	0
Ehlers et al. (2005)	Adults, chronic PTSD, wide range of traumas	0	2.82	71.4	0
Ehlers et al. (2014)	Adults, chronic PTSD, wide range of traumas	3.2	2.53	77.4	0
Smith et al. (2007)	Children, wide range of traumas	0	3.43	92.0	0
Open trials, consecutive samples					
Ehlers et al. (2005)	Adults, chronic PTSD, wide range of traumas	5.0	2.81	85.0	0
Gillespie et al. (2002)	Adults, PTSD following Omagh bombing		2.47		0
Brewin et al. (2010) (subsample treated with CT-PTSD)	Adults, PTSD following London bombings	0	2.29	82.1	0

(continued)

Table 9.1 (continued)

	Patient sample	% Dropouts	Intent-to-treat size for PTSD symptoms (PDS)[a]	Intent-to-treat % patients in full remission[b]	% Patients with symptom deterioration (PDS)
Effectiveness studies					
Duffy et al. (2007)	Adults, chronic PTSD, wide range of traumas, multiple traumas common	20.0	1.25	63.0	1.8
Ehlers et al. (2013)	Adults, chronic PTSD, wide range of traumas, multiple traumas common	13.9	1.39	57.3	1.2

N/A not assessed, *PDS* Posttraumatic Diagnostic Scale, *BDI* Beck Depression Inventory
[a]Cohen's *d*, pooled standard deviation
[b]Patient recovered from PTSD according to diagnostic assessment or clinically significant change on PDS (within 2 standard deviations of nonclinical population)

CT-PTSD is highly acceptable to patients (as indicated by very low dropout rates and high patient satisfaction scores). It led to very large improvements in PTSD symptoms (intent-to-treat effect sizes of around 2.5), disability, depression, anxiety, and quality of life. Over 70 % of patients fully recovered from PTSD. Outreach trials treating consecutive samples of survivors of the Omagh and London bombings replicated these results (Brewin et al. 2010; Gillespie et al. 2002). It was noteworthy that the percentage of patients whose symptoms deteriorated with treatment was close to zero and smaller than in patients waiting for treatment (Ehlers et al. 2014). This suggests that CT-PTSD is a safe and efficacious treatment.

Two further studies (Duffy et al. 2007; Ehlers et al. 2013) implemented CT-PTSD in routine clinical services. The samples treated in these studies included a very wide range of patients including those with complicating factors such as serious social problems, living currently in danger, very severe depression, borderline personality disorder, or multiple traumatic events and losses. Therapists included trainees as well as experienced therapists. Outcomes remained very good, with large intent-to-treat effect sizes of 1.25 and higher for PTSD symptoms. Around 60 % of the patients who started therapy remitted from PTSD. Dropout rates were somewhat higher than in the trials of CT-PTSD, but rates were still below the average for trials of trauma-focused cognitive behavior therapy of 23 % (Bisson et al. 2013). Hardly any patients experienced symptom deterioration.

Does CT-PTSD work by changing problematic meanings of the trauma? Kleim et al. (2013) analyzed the time course of changes in symptoms and appraisals. As predicted from the treatment model, changes in appraisals predicted subsequent symptom change, but not vice versa.

Ehlers et al. (2013) investigated whether patient characteristics influence treatment response. Encouragingly, very few did. Only social problems and having reexperiencing symptoms from multiple traumas were associated with a somewhat less favorable response. This was because treatment was less trauma focused, that is, patients and therapists spent more time discussing other problems, such as housing and financial problems, and spent less time working on the patient's trauma memories and their meanings. It remains to be tested whether an extension of the treatment duration (the mean was 10 sessions) would have led to better outcomes in these cases. Higher dropout rates were associated with patients' social problems and inexperienced therapists. This suggests that attention to skills that help engage patients in trauma-focused work is needed in therapist training.

Overall, the evaluations showed encouraging results and support CT-PTSD as an evidenced-based treatment.

Acknowledgments The development and evaluation of the treatment program described in this chapter was funded by the Wellcome Trust (grant 069777). We gratefully acknowledge the contributions of David M. Clark, Ann Hackmann, Melanie Fennell, Freda McManus, and Nick Grey. We are grateful to Edna Foa for her collaboration and advice.

References

Bisson, J. I., Roberts, N. P., Andrew, M., Cooper, R., & Lewis, C. (2013). Psychological therapies for chronic post-traumatic stress disorder (PTSD) in adults. *The Cochrane Library.* doi:10.1002/14651858.CD003388.pub4.

Bourne, C., Frasqilho, F., Roth, A. D., & Holmes, E. A. (2010). Is it mere distraction? Peritraumatic verbal tasks can increase analogue flashbacks, but reduce voluntary memory performance. *Journal of Behavior Therapy and Experimental Psychiatry, 41,* 316–324.

Brewin, C. R. (2014). Episodic memory, perceptual memory, and their interaction: Foundations for a theory of posttraumatic stress disorder. *Psychological Bulletin, 140,* 69–97. doi:10.1037/a0033722.

Brewin, C. R., Fuchkan, N., Huntley, Z., Robertson, M., Scragg, P., & Ehlers, A. (2010). Outreach and screening following the 2005 London bombings: Usage and outcomes. *Psychological Medicine, 40,* 2049–2057. doi:10.1017/S0033291710000206.

Cloitre, M., Stovall-McClough, K. C., Nooner, K., Zorbas, P., Cherry, S., & Petkova, E. (2010). Treatment for PTSD related to childhood abuse: A randomized controlled trial. *American Journal of Psychiatry, 167,* 915–924.

Duffy, M., Gillespie, K., & Clark, D. M. (2007). Post-traumatic stress disorder in the context of terrorism and other civil conflict in Northern Ireland: randomised controlled trial. *British Medical Journal, 334,* 1147–1150. doi:10.1136/bmj.39021.846852.BE.

Duffy, M., Bolton, D., Gillespie, K., Ehlers, A., & Clark, D. M. (2013). A community study of the psychological effects of the Omagh car bomb on adults. *PLoS One, 8*(9), e76618. doi:10.1371/journal.pone.0076618.

Dunmore, E., Clark, D. M., & Ehlers, A. (2001). A prospective study of the role of cognitive factors in persistent posttraumatic stress disorder after physical or sexual assault. *Behaviour Research and Therapy, 39,* 1063–1084.

Ehlers, A. (2015). Intrusive reexperiencing in posttraumatic stress disorder: Memory processes and their implications for therapy. In D. Berntsen, & L. A. Watson (Eds.), *Clinical perspectives on autobiographical memory* (pp. 109–132). Cambridge: Cambridge University Press.

Ehlers, A., & Clark, D. M. (2000). A cognitive model of posttraumatic stress disorder. *Behaviour Research and Therapy, 38*, 319–345.

Ehlers, A., Mayou, R. A., & Bryant, B. (1998). Psychological predictors of chronic posttraumatic stress disorder after motor vehicle accidents. *Journal of Abnormal Psychology, 107*, 508–519.

Ehlers, A., Clark, D. M., Hackmann, A., McManus, F., Fennell, M., & Mayou, R. (2003). A randomized controlled trial of cognitive therapy, a self-help booklet, and repeated assessments as early interventions for posttraumatic stress disorder. *Archives of General Psychiatry, 60*, 1024–1032.

Ehlers, A., Hackmann, A., & Michael, T. (2004). Intrusive re-experiencing in post-traumatic stress disorder: Phenomenology, theory, and therapy. *Memory, 12*, 403–415.

Ehlers, A., Clark, D. M., Hackmann, A., McManus, F., & Fennell, M. (2005). Cognitive therapy for post-traumatic stress disorder: Development and evaluation. *Behaviour Research and Therapy, 43*, 413–431.

Ehlers, A., Ehring, T., & Kleim, B. (2012). Information processing in posttraumatic stress disorder. In J. G. Beck & D. M. Sloan (Eds.), *The oxford handbook of traumatic disorders* (pp. 191–218). New York: Oxford University Press.

Ehlers, A., Grey, N., Wild, J., Stott, R., Liness, S., & Clark, D. M. (2013). Implementation of cognitive therapy in routine clinical care: Effectiveness and moderators of outcome in a consecutive sample. *Behaviour Research and Therapy, 51*, 742–752. doi:10.1016/j.brat.2013.08.006.

Ehlers, A., Hackmann, A., Grey, N., Wild, J., Liness, S., & Clark, D. M. (2014). A randomized controlled trial of 7-day intensive and standard weekly cognitive therapy for PTSD and emotion-focused supportive therapy. *American Journal of Psychiatry, 171*, 294–304. doi:10.1176/appi.ajp.2013.13040552.

Ehlers, A., Wild, J., Stott, R., Warnock-Parkes, E., Grey, N., & Clark, D. M. (in prep). *Brief self-study assisted cognitive therapy for PTSD: a randomized clinical trial.*

Ehring, T., Ehlers, A., & Glucksman, E. (2008). Do cognitive models help in predicting the severity of posttraumatic stress disorder, phobia and depression after motor vehicle accidents? A prospective longitudinal study. *Journal of Consulting and Clinical Psychology, 76*, 219–230.

Evans, C., Ehlers, A., Mezey, G., & Clark, D. M. (2007). Intrusive memories and ruminations related to violent crime among young offenders: Phenomenological characteristics. *Journal of Traumatic Stress, 20*, 183–196.

Foa, E. B., & Rothbaum, B. O. (1998). *Treating the trauma of rape. Cognitive-behavior therapy for PTSD.* New York: Guilford.

Foa, E. B., Ehlers, A., Clark, D. M., Tolin, D., & Orsillo, S. (1999). The Post-traumatic Cognitions Inventory (PTCI). Development and validation. *Psychological Assessment, 11*, 303–314.

Gillespie, K., Duffy, M., Hackmann, A., & Clark, D. M. (2002). Community based cognitive therapy in the treatment of post-traumatic stress disorder following the Omagh bomb. *Behaviour Research and Therapy, 40*, 345–357.

Halligan, S. L., Michael, T., Clark, D. M., & Ehlers, A. (2003). Posttraumatic stress disorder following assault: The role of cognitive processing, trauma memory, and appraisals. *Journal of Consulting and Clinical Psychology, 71*, 419–431.

Jelinek, L., Randjbar, S., Seifert, D., Kellner, M., & Moritz, S. (2009). The organization of autobiographical and nonautobiographical memory in posttraumatic stress disorder (PTSD). *Journal of Abnormal Psychology, 118*, 288–298.

Kleim, B., Wallott, F., & Ehlers, A. (2008). Are trauma memories disjointed from other autobiographical memories in PTSD? An experimental investigation. *Behavioural and Cognitive Psychotherapy, 36*, 221–234.

Kleim, B., Ehlers, A., & Glucksman, E. (2012a). Investigating cognitive pathways to psychopathology: Predicting depression and posttraumatic stress disorder from early responses after assault. *Psychological Trauma: Theory, Research, Practice, and Policy, 4*, 527–537. doi:10.1037/a0027006.

Kleim, B., Ehring, T., & Ehlers, A. (2012b). Perceptual processing advantages for trauma-related visual cues in posttraumatic stress disorder. *Psychological Medicine, 42*, 173–181. doi:10.1017/S0033291711001048.

Kleim, B., Grey, N., Hackmann, A., Nussbeck, F., Wild, J., & Ehlers, A. (2013). Cognitive change predicts symptom reduction with cognitive therapy for posttraumatic stress disorder. *Journal of Consulting and Clinical Psychology, 81*, 383–393. doi:10.1037/a0031290.

Michael, T., Ehlers, A., Halligan, S., & Clark, D. M. (2005). Unwanted memories of assault: What intrusion characteristics predict PTSD? *Behaviour Research and Therapy, 43*, 613–628.

Resick, P. A., & Schnicke, M. K. (1993). *Cognitive processing therapy for rape victims.* Newbury Park: Sage.

Rothbaum, B. O., Foa, E. B., Riggs, D. S., Murdock, T., & Walsh, W. (1992). A prospective examination of post-traumatic stress disorder in rape victims. *Journal of Traumatic Stress, 5*, 455–475.

Smith, P., Yule, W., Perrin, S., Tranah, T., Dalgleish, T., & Clark, D. M. (2007). Cognitive-behavioral therapy for PTSD in children and adolescents: A preliminary randomized controlled trial. *Journal of the American Academy of Child and Adolescent Psychiatry, 46*, 1051–1061.

Sündermann, O., Hauschildt, M., & Ehlers, A. (2013). Perceptual processing during trauma, priming and the development of intrusive memories. *Journal of Behavior Therapy and Experimental Psychiatry, 44*, 213–220. doi:10.1016/j.jbtep.2012.10.001.

Cognitive Processing Therapy

10

Tara E. Galovski, Jennifer Schuster Wachen,
Kathleen M. Chard, Candice M. Monson,
and Patricia A. Resick

Cognitive processing therapy (CPT) is an evidence-based, cognitive-behavioral treatment designed specifically to treat posttraumatic stress disorder (PTSD) and comorbid symptoms. This chapter will first review the theoretical underpinnings of the intervention and then provide more detail about the actual protocol including a clinical case description. We then will review several special considerations and challenges in administering the protocol to specific groups of trauma survivors and finally end with an overview of the published randomized controlled clinical trials demonstrating the efficacy of the therapy.

10.1 Theoretical Underpinnings

The theoretical basis of CPT is cognitive theory, one of the most prominent theories explaining the onset and maintenance of PTSD. A predominant notion underlying cognitive theory of PTSD is that PTSD is a disorder of non-recovery from a

T.E. Galovski, PhD (✉)
Department of Psychological Sciences, Center for Trauma Recovery,
University of Missouri – St. Louis, St. Louis, MO, USA

J.S. Wachen, PhD
Women's Health Sciences Division, National Center for PTSD,
VA Boston Healthcare System, Boston University School of Medicine, Boston, MA, USA

K.M. Chard, PhD
Department of Psychiatry and Behavioral Neuroscience, Cincinnati VA Medical Center,
University of Cincinnati, Cincinnati, OH, USA

C.M. Monson, PhD
Department of Psychology, Ryerson University, Toronto, ON, Canada

P.A. Resick, PhD
Department of Psychiatry and Behavioral Neuroscience,
Duke University Medical Center, Durham, NC, USA

© Springer International Publishing Switzerland 2015
U. Schnyder, M. Cloitre (eds.), *Evidence Based Treatments for Trauma-Related Psychological Disorders: A Practical Guide for Clinicians*,
DOI 10.1007/978-3-319-07109-1_10

traumatic event (Resick et al. 2008b). Thus, PTSD is not a condition with a prodromal phase or one in which early signs and symptoms are observed. Rather, in the majority of cases, the widest variety and most severe symptoms of PTSD are experienced in the early days and weeks after exposure to the traumatic event has ended. With time, the majority of individuals who have been exposed to a traumatic event(s) will experience an abatement of PTSD symptoms, or a natural recovery from the trauma. In a substantial minority of cases, individuals will continue to experience symptoms consistent with a diagnosis of PTSD. In other words, for this minority of all trauma survivors, natural recovery from the trauma has been impeded.

According to cognitive trauma theory of PTSD, avoidance of thinking about the traumatic event, as well as problematic appraisals of the traumatic event when memories are faced, contributes to this non-recovery. More specifically, individuals who do not recover are believed to try to assimilate the traumatic event into previously held core beliefs that are comprised of positive or negative beliefs about the self, others, and the world. Assimilation serves as an attempt to construe the traumatic event in a way that makes it fit, or to be consistent, with these preexisting beliefs. A common example of assimilation in those with PTSD is just-world thinking, or the belief that good things happen to good people and bad things happen to bad people. In the case of traumatic events (i.e., bad things), the individual assumes that he/she did something bad that may have led to the event or that the event is punishment for something he/she may have done in the past. An example of this type of thinking by a sexual assault survivor: "If I just hadn't been drunk that night (i.e., bad behavior), then I wouldn't have been assaulted (i.e., bad consequence)." Another common type of assimilative thinking is hindsight bias, or evaluating the event based on information that is only known after the fact (Fischhoff 1975). We will see an example of hindsight bias later in our clinical case description. At its essence, assimilation is an effort to exert predictability and control over the traumatic event after the fact that paradoxically leaves the traumatized individual with unprocessed traumatic material that is perpetually reexperienced.

Another tenant of cognitive trauma theory is that problematic historical appraisals about traumatic events (i.e., assimilation) lead to, or seemingly confirm, overgeneralized maladaptive schemas and core beliefs about the self, others, and the world after traumatization. In other words, individuals over-accommodate their beliefs based on the traumatic experience. Over-accommodation involves the modification of existing schemas based on appraisals about the trauma, but these modifications in schemas are too severe and overgeneralized. A common example of over-accommodation is when a traumatized individual comes to believe, based on his/her appraisals of his/her trauma, that the world is a completely unsafe and unpredictable place when he/she previously believed that the world was relatively benign or at least that bad things would not happen to him/her. Alternatively, traumatized individuals may have preexisting negative schemas, usually a result of a history of prior traumatization or other negative life events, that others cannot be trusted or that they have no control over bad things happening to them. In these cases, traumatic experiences are construed as proof for the preexisting negative schemas. Borrowing from earlier work by McCann and Pearlman (1990), cognitive trauma theory identifies beliefs related to the self and others that are often over-accommodated and contribute to non-recovery. These beliefs are related to safety, trust, power/control, esteem, and intimacy. A strength of cognitive trauma theory of PTSD is that it accounts for varying preexisting beliefs in each area that may have been positive or negative based on the client's prior trauma history. In CPT, assimilated and over-accommodated beliefs are labeled "stuck points," describing thinking that interferes with natural recovery thereby keeping people "stuck" in PTSD. Stuck points are targeted in therapy.

According to cognitive trauma theory, clients must allow themselves to experience the natural emotions associated with the event that are typically avoided in the case of PTSD. Natural emotions are emotions that are considered to be hardwired and emanate directly from the traumatic event (perhaps sadness of loss of loved one during trauma, fear of the danger associated with the trauma, etc.). Natural emotions that have been suppressed or avoided contribute to ongoing PTSD symptoms. According to cognitive trauma theory, natural emotions do not perpetuate themselves and thereby, contrary to behavioral theories of PTSD (Foa and Kozak 1986), do not require systematic exposure to achieve habituation to them. The client is encouraged to approach and feel these natural emotions, which have a self-limiting course once they are allowed to be experienced.

In contrast, maladaptive misappraisals about the trauma in retrospect (i.e., assimilation), as well as current-day cognitions that have been disrupted (i.e., over-accommodation), are postulated to result in manufactured emotions. Manufactured emotions are the product of conscious appraisals about why the trauma occurred and the implications of those appraisals on here-and-now cognitions. In the case of a natural disaster survivor who believed that the outcomes of the disaster occurred because he/she or others did not do enough to protect himself/herself and his/her family (self or other blame), he/she is likely to feel ongoing guilt and/or anger and be distrustful of himself/herself or others. In this way, trauma-related appraisals are manufacturing ongoing negative emotions that will be maintained as long as he/she continues to think in this manner. The key to recovery with regard to manufactured emotions is to foster accommodation of the information about the traumatic event. In other words, clients are encouraged to change their minds enough to account for the event in a realistic manner without changing their minds too much resulting in overgeneralized and maladaptive beliefs.

10.2 Clinical Description of CPT

CPT has historically been administered over 12 sessions in individual, group, or combined formats. The administration of CPT can be most briefly explained in terms of phases of treatment. During the pretreatment phase (Phase 1), the clinician will assess the presence of PTSD as well as consider the host of usual treatment priorities (suicidality, homicidality) and the presence of potentially interfering comorbid conditions such as current mania, psychosis, and substance dependence. Special challenges to treatment will be discussed later in this chapter. The next phase (Phase 2; sessions 1–3) consists of education regarding PTSD and the role of thoughts and emotions in accordance with cognitive theory described above. Phase 3 (sessions 4–5) consists of processing the actual traumatic event and allowing the client to engage with the trauma memory. The goals are the discovery of stuck points preventing the client's recovery and the expression of natural affect associated with the trauma memory. In Phase 4 of treatment (sessions 6 and 7), the clinician uses Socratic questions to begin to aid the client in challenging stuck points. This process is complemented by clinical tools (a series of worksheets) that aid the client in implementing formal challenging of stuck points between sessions at home. Phase 5 (sessions 8–12) often marks the transition to a more specific focus on over-accommodated stuck points with individual sessions dedicated to the trauma themes of safety, trust, power and control, esteem, and intimacy. Phase 5 also includes "facing the future" and focuses on relapse prevention, specifically targeting stuck points that might interfere with the maintenance of therapeutic gains. The following provides an overview of a recent case in our clinic of a young woman treated for PTSD secondary to a home invasion. Although, with this client's permission, this case depiction is based on true events, details have been altered to protect the identity of the client and those involved in the traumatic event.

Molly is a young woman who appeared in our clinic seeking assistance for distress she was experiencing following exposure to a traumatic event. She had recently moved to town to begin graduate training at a nearby university. She reported that she was trying to start a new life for herself and leave the past behind but, after a couple of months, realized that her distress actually seemed to be getting worse. We began the assessment process, typically a 2-h interview in which we take the time to hear the client's story, conduct a thorough clinical interview, and assess any psychopathology. Molly described a difficult childhood history in which she was raised primarily by her grandfather, who was physically and emotionally abusive to her and her siblings. During the interview, Molly demonstrated pride at her life accomplishments, getting herself out of a very bad neighborhood (while some of her siblings succumbed to drug addiction, engaged in criminal activity, and suffered from other types of psychopathology) and eventually graduating from the police academy and taking a job on the force in a major city on the East coast. She served as a police officer for 4 years with excellent reviews and even an early recommendation for promotion.

Approximately 3 years into her job as a police officer, she left work one night and headed over to visit an old friend (Jack) who was in town visiting his grandmother and mother. When she arrived, Molly was delighted that Jack's sister, Beth, had also come into town with her three kids to visit their uncle. The grandmother, mother, Beth, and kids went to bed and eventually Jack walked Molly to her car. At the curb, two hooded gunmen approached and demanded money. Molly and Jack did not have anything of value, so the gunmen forced them back into the home. They woke Jack's mother, the grandmother, and Beth. The tension escalated and eventually Molly made the decision to physically charge at the gunman. Multiple shots were fired with Molly taking five bullets directly in the chest and upper body, Jack getting shot multiple times, and Beth being fatally wounded. During the interview, Molly sobbed, repeating over and over that if only she had not made her move, this would not have happened and Beth would be alive. Molly met full criteria for PTSD and major depression. The event had occurred 2 years ago.

We began a course of CPT. During session 1, the results of Molly's diagnostic assessment were discussed with an emphasis on explaining the disorder of PTSD. In general, the goals of session 1 include gaining a thorough understanding of PTSD and why we believe (from a cognitive theory perspective) that some people develop the disorder. Our job in therapy was described as taking Molly's trauma memory and "airing it out," looking for places where interpretations about the actual event may not be entirely accurate (assimilation) and places where one might have drastically (and inaccurately) altered worldviews (over-accommodation). These inaccurate beliefs likely played a role in keeping Molly "stuck" in the recovery process. So we labeled such inaccurate beliefs as "stuck points." Throughout the assessment and into session 1, the therapist offered the example of a possible trauma-related stuck point that she had heard Molly repeat several times, "If I had not attacked the gunman, Beth would be alive today." In other words, Molly believed that Beth's death had been her fault. The role of emotion was also discussed in session 1, and Molly was clearly able to assert that she avoided memories of this event and any feelings associated with the memory whenever possible, even to the extent of cutting off old relationships and moving out of town. Molly agreed that it would be helpful to spend some time thinking about the beliefs around why that night happened and the influence of those events on her current beliefs by writing an impact statement (CPT assignment 1) for session 2.

Through the course of reading her impact statement and expanding on the information therein, we accumulated more examples of assimilated stuck points and present-focused stuck points (over-accommodated beliefs). Molly blamed herself for nearly every aspect of the events that unfolded during the home invasion. Specifically, stuck points such as, "I should have given the gunmen the keys to my car and they never would have gone in the house," "I should have fought them outside the house and never let them in," "I should have gone to the back of the house with them and they would have left," and "I never should have attacked them." We also identified a number of over-accommodated stuck points demonstrating substantial shifts in the way Molly viewed herself, others, and the world since the traumatic event. "I am a failure," "I am incompetent," "The world is a dangerous place and I am unsafe in it," "I cannot trust myself or my abilities," and "I am not the person I thought I was." We collected and recorded these on Molly's stuck point log and talked through the relationship between these types of thoughts and the significant distress that they were causing her. She agreed to continue this process outside of session by recording events, thoughts, and feelings on ABC sheets (a worksheet used in CPT to aid clients in identifying thoughts that might lead to emotion as well as help the client to understand the relationship between thoughts and emotions) for session 3.

The use of Socratic dialogue to challenge stuck points is termed the "cornerstone of CPT practice" in the training workshops and manual. Session 3 most typically begins the start of this Socratic process by gently challenging the stuck points that most likely lie at the heart of PTSD. Although the extent of the challenging can differ across clients in session 3 (depending on how tightly they are holding onto the beliefs, defensiveness, emotional arousal, etc.), Molly responded very well to this process from the start despite significant distress and the firmly held conviction that she was at fault. She made significant advances on several assimilated stuck points during this session. The following discourse is an example of a section of this dialogue, starting about a third of the way into the session.

Therapist: Tell me more about how this all started on that night. You mentioned that you should have given them your car keys at the very beginning and they wouldn't have killed Beth…

Molly (sobbing): Yes, if I had given them my car keys, they would have taken off. Better my car than Beth.

Therapist: Tell me about that moment when the gunmen came up to you and Jack. What were the choices and decisions that you were making at that moment?

Molly: Well, I did not want Jack to get hurt. I figured these were just punks that were trying to get some quick cash. I did not want to give them my car keys because my own weapon and uniform was in my gear bag on the seat.

Therapist: Oh, so it sounds like you were worried about them getting another weapon and where that would go? What about the car? Were you worried about that getting stolen?

Molly (kind of laughs): No, the car was a piece of junk. But I didn't know if their guns were real or loaded. It was so dark. I did know that my gun was very real with very real bullets. I was also worried about them seeing my uniform.

Therapist: Why is that?

Molly: They didn't know I was a cop, but if they found out, they might feel like they'd gone too far and couldn't risk getting caught. At this point, they hadn't even asked for my car keys, they'd just asked for cash. And neither of us had any on us.

Therapist: So, if we think back to what you've been telling yourself, the stuck point, "I should have given them the car keys and they wouldn't have shot Beth," it almost sounds as if the choice were between your car and Beth? But when we think it through a little more, would you say that was accurate? Was Beth even in the story at this point?

Molly (after a long pause): No, I was more worried about protecting Jack, making sure these guys didn't get hold of my gun and not letting them know I was an officer and freaking them out even more. You know, I never even considered that they actually never even asked for my car keys. I just remember being so focused on making sure they didn't get my gun…

Therapist: So, given the information you had at the time and not having any idea at all about the eventual outcome, what do you think about not giving the gunman your car keys?

Molly: I think at the time, keeping the perps away from my car was the priority. That changed quickly.

Therapist: Ok – How about we do this? How about if you take some time between now and the next session and write out in detail exactly what happened that night? I wonder if, by going slowly through some more of this event, we may find other places that are keeping you stuck. (Therapist then assigns trauma narrative for session 4).

Sessions 4 and 5 allowed the client the opportunity to really engage with the trauma memory. Molly wrote out her whole trauma narrative in significant detail and was able to express natural affect throughout both sessions. Socratic questions continued in both sessions around assimilated stuck points. Molly tightly held onto the idea that she could have prevented Beth's death and that her actions and decisions throughout the night caused the shooting. Specifically, two big stuck points included "I should never have let them in the house." and "I should never have attacked the gunman." The former stuck point was fairly easily challenged as Molly recalled that Jack had panicked and let the gunmen into the house before she could intervene. She had actually said that they did not know who lived in the house. Molly recalled considering at the time trying to fight or run for help, but after Jack let the gunmen in, she was more concerned that she would be leaving all the inhabitants of the house helpless and would infuriate the gunmen further by escaping. At the time, she felt the best plan was to get them what they wanted and get them out of there as quickly and calmly as possible. In other words, she was thinking like the trained officer that she was.

The big stuck point, "If I had not attacked the gunman, the shooting would not have started and Beth would be alive" remained. At session 5, the Socratic questions around this stuck point (following the reading of the second trauma narrative) transpired as such:

Therapist: Let's take a minute and think more about the stuck point that your action caused Beth's death. From what I'm understanding about your story, the gunmen became more and more agitated as time went on. They had tried to force Beth into the basement and Jack's mom had become extremely upset, screaming, "don't go down there, Beth." Where were you at this point?

Molly: They had me on my knees with my hands over my head facing a wall. When they told Beth to go down to the basement, I shouted for Beth to come to me and she ran over to me. I'll never forget her eyes. It was like she wanted me to do something about all this. I stood up and told the men I would go down to the basement.

Therapist: Why did you do that?

Molly: Because I thought that they were going to rape Beth and I knew she would scream and further exacerbate the situation. I thought I could survive being raped and would be able to handle it. But they wouldn't agree to it and then decided everyone had to go to the basement. Things got quickly out of control. I was terrified that the sleeping kids would wake up and come down with all the screaming and shouting. I knew that these guys had no plan and were getting agitated and crazy. The whole time, I had been thinking I needed to get my gun, but I could not figure out a way to get out of the house.

Therapist: So it sounds like things were quickly spiraling out of control.

Molly: Yes – before I had thought they were just looking to rob us and get out, but they were acting crazy and they hadn't really gotten anything of value. I knew that if we went down to the basement, no one was coming up out of there. There was no other reason to bring everyone down there.

Therapist: That sounds like an important piece of the puzzle. Things were rapidly changing, giving you the impression that going down to the basement was not going to have a good outcome? When you think back now, do you still think that going down there would have been terrible?

Molly (thinks about this): Yes, I do.

Therapist: So, in weighing your options in that moment, was there a choice?

Molly: I think the choices at the time were to go down and probably be killed, or fight. There was no reasoning with them. I should've fought sooner?

Therapist: Why didn't you? What was different sooner?

Molly: A few minutes earlier I had thought Beth was going to be targeted, and I tried to prevent that by offering to take her place. But they said no. This was the first time in the whole ordeal that it seemed like they were going to lose it and we were all going down. I remember thinking if I was going to die anyway, I was going to give the rest of them a fighting chance by taking one of them down with me.

Therapist: And so you tried to save everyone's life by literally throwing yourself in harm's way?…(long pause) See, it's almost as if you are now, in hindsight, assuming that no action would have had a better outcome. But it sounds like there is very little in your story to suggest these guys were going to suddenly decide to leave? (silence as Molly thinks about this for a couple of minutes). Is it possible that, as bad as the outcome was and I understand how very awful it was, it could have been even worse if you had not defended everyone? (Molly is nodding and sobbing. We sit with this for awhile.)… Who caused Beth's death?

Molly: Those men.

Therapist: Yes, I agree… It sounds like you did absolutely everything humanly possible to <u>prevent</u> Beth's and others' deaths.

We continue this conversation a little while longer and weave the next practice assignment (the challenging questions worksheet) into challenging this big stuck point. At session 5, the therapist introduces the first of the worksheets designed to help the client formally challenge stuck points on his/her own between sessions. Molly agrees to continue this work at home as well as to practice challenging other stuck points from her log. Molly returns to session 6 and has struggled a bit with the worksheets. We review them in session and figure out the pieces that troubled her. Her affect is much brighter and she reports that she has done a lot of thinking about the event and honestly feels as if a weight has been lifted off her shoulders. Her PTSD symptoms have substantially decreased as assessed by our self-report measure. We introduce the next of the worksheets designed to help the client identify overall patterns of thought in which she tends to engage.

When Molly returned to session 7, her belief that it was her fault had significantly decreased. She reported feeling quite a bit of sadness and spending time thinking about Beth and her children who now have to go through life without their mom. The sadness was hard but felt a lot different than the awful guilt she had been carrying. The focus of therapy shifted to some of the more present-focused (over-accommodated) stuck points including, "I don't trust myself," "I am powerless/incompetent," and "There is danger everywhere." The last five sessions of CPT specifically focus on five types of beliefs that are typically disrupted following the experience of a traumatic event, including safety, trust, power/control, esteem, and intimacy. We used the final worksheet (the challenging belief worksheet) to challenge stuck points in each of these areas. At one point prior to session 10, Molly traveled home for Jack's wedding. She saw everyone who had been present during the crime and felt enormous guilt. She returned to therapy thinking again as if she had somehow caused Beth's death by doing something wrong or not doing enough. Using the full worksheet and relying on Socratic questions, this old stuck point was fairly easily challenged. At this point in the therapy, Molly took the reins of challenging and thinking through stuck points with the therapist acting as a consultant. By the end of session 12, Molly no longer had PTSD or major depression. Almost a year later, she has begun a new career, remains PTSD free, and has recaptured her life.

10.3   Special Challenges

We are frequently asked how long a therapist should work with a client prior to starting CPT. The answer changes depending on a number of variables. If this is a new client, CPT can start right away after an initial assessment definitively determining a diagnosis of PTSD. If the therapist has been working with the client for a long time using more supportive or unstructured therapy, it may be necessary to discuss how CPT will look different in terms of the structure of the session and the homework expectations than what was previously being done in therapy. We often find that delaying the start of trauma treatment causes the client's avoidance to increase and reduces the likelihood that he/she will stay committed to the protocol. In fact, we commonly see that the therapist's avoidance or belief that the client "cannot tolerate" CPT is more often the reason for the delay of treatment than the client's desire to hold off.

Because the efficacy of CPT was tested with women who described complex trauma histories as well as a variety of comorbid psychological disorders, most clients can complete the treatment protocol as designed. For example, in clinical and research settings, we have implemented the protocol with individuals who were recently traumatized (days) and those who were 70 years posttrauma. In addition, the protocol has been utilized with those who are sub-threshold for PTSD diagnosis as well as those individuals who meet the full criteria for PTSD. Finally, we have successfully implemented the full protocol [CPT or CPT-cognitive only (which is CPT with the written trauma narrative component of the therapy removed)] with individuals who have been additionally diagnosed with many Axis I and all Axis II disorders (Chard, et al. 2011; Kaysen, et al. 2014; Walter et al. 2012). Most typically, in our research trials, individuals can have a diagnosis of bipolar disorder or schizophrenia; however, we first stabilize any manic or psychotic symptoms prior to commencing the trauma-focused work. To our knowledge, CPT has not been tested with individuals diagnosed with dementia.

There are a few situations in which delaying the start of trauma-focused work, such as CPT, may be warranted (such as stabilizing a client physically or psychologically). Ensuring that the individual is not a danger to self or others and in personal danger due to a current abusive relationship is an important consideration before beginning any kind of therapy. If danger is a concern, then safety planning needs to be prioritized before CPT is considered. Conversely, we have successfully treated individuals who are likely to face trauma in their near future with CPT, e.g., military service members, police, and firefighters. The likelihood of experiencing trauma in the future is a universal risk, so the possibility of future violence or trauma exposure should not be a reason to delay trauma treatment but should be an area where additional stuck points can be identified and challenged. Additional areas of physical safety that may delay treatment include those individuals with an eating disorder that places them at a severe health risk or those engaging in potentially lethal self-injurious behaviors. In both of these cases, attempts to stabilize the client should be made prior to starting CPT.

Another factor that may delay the start of CPT treatment is the client's psychological functioning. For example, if depression is so severe that the client is rarely attending sessions, if dissociation is so significant that he/she cannot sit through most of a therapy hour, or if severe panic attacks are preventing discussion of the trauma even in remote detail, then other therapeutic interventions may need to precede CPT (e.g., coping skill building, panic control treatment (See Chap. 17 and Part IV "comorbidities"). With respect to concurrent substance use disorders, we have commonly implemented the CPT protocol with those who are abusing substances with great success, but typically not in an outpatient setting if they are substance dependent and requiring detoxification (Kaysen et al. 2014). However, once someone has stabilized after detoxification, the individual is typically able to engage in CPT. Both research studies and clinical effectiveness trials have found that symptoms of depression, anxiety, substance use, anger, and guilt all decrease after CPT and individuals maintain these gains at treatment follow-up. Finally, if an individual has an unmedicated psychotic disorder or unmedicated bipolar disorder, it will likely be necessary to stabilize the individual on a medication regimen prior to starting CPT.

Several studies have shown that individuals with comorbid personality disorders (including borderline personality disorder; BPD) do very well in CPT. Although their initial PTSD score may start higher than individuals without a comorbid personality disorder, participants with BPD features (Clarke et al. 2008) and with full BPD (Walter et al. 2012) show equivalent gains in therapy as compared to those without personality disorders. The challenge for many therapists working with clients who have a personality disorder and PTSD is keeping the treatment on track with the protocol and not getting derailed by unrelated issues. We have found that clients often have developed maladaptive cognitions and coping strategies to manage their reactions to the trauma. These beliefs and behavioral patterns most likely served a functional purpose at some point in the person's life and eventually became dogmatic schemas about the world. The client then began to view all experiences through these schemas, ignoring or distorting information that challenges these beliefs. Our goal is to remain trauma-focused and provide the client with additional skills for specifically challenging trauma-related cognitions in an effort to reduce posttraumatic distress.

Modifications of the protocol are most often not recommended. That being said, our studies have shown that specific modifications may occasionally be necessary to achieve optimal outcomes (Galovski et al. 2012; Resick et al. 2008b). For example, we have used the protocol with individuals who have minimal formal education (4th grade) and those with an IQ around 75. However, in several of these cases, we have had to simplify the protocol. In addition, with the number of returning veterans with a history of traumatic brain injury (TBI), many clients with PTSD are also coping with post concussive symptoms that resulted from their injury. Clinical data supports the use of CPT or CPT-C in their current formats with a majority of these clients, but if the client is struggling to comprehend the purpose of the assignment, the worksheets have been simplified for different levels of understanding (Chard et al. 2011). For example, we have created versions of the worksheets that can be used throughout the treatment instead of moving on to the more advanced sheet. Bass et al. (2013) completed a randomized controlled trial of group CPT-C (cognitive-only version without accounts) in the Democratic Republic of Congo, in which the clients were illiterate and had no paper and the therapist had only a few years of education beyond elementary school. The worksheets and concepts had to be simplified so that the clients could memorize them. Results are discussed below.

In summary, therapists should not assume that CPT cannot be implemented with clients who have extensive trauma histories or be daunted by comorbid disorders accompanying PTSD. The decision the clinician must make in collaboration with the client is whether the comorbid disorder is so severe that it will preclude the client's participation in PTSD treatment. For the most part, however, the treatment of PTSD will improve the comorbid symptoms and may even eliminate the necessity of further treatment for those symptoms. Thus, decisions on when to start CPT, and with whom, should be made on a case-by-case basis in collaboration with the client.

10.4   Empirical Support

There is a large body of literature supporting the efficacy and effectiveness of CPT in diverse populations. The first randomized controlled clinical trial (RCT) compared CPT, prolonged exposure (PE), and a wait list (WL) control group in a sample of 171 female rape survivors (Resick et al. 2002). Results showed that both the CPT and PE groups demonstrated significant reductions in PTSD and depressive symptoms between pretreatment and posttreatment compared to the WL condition. There were very few differences between the two active treatments with the exception of significantly more improvement on guilt (Resick, et al. 2002), health-related concerns (Galovski et al. 2009), hopelessness (Gallagher and Resick 2012), and suicidal ideation (Gradus et al. 2013) reported by the participants who received CPT. These improvements were sustained at the 3-month and 9-month follow-up points. A subsequent long-term follow-up assessment of these participants (Resick et al. 2012) revealed no significant change in PTSD symptoms 5–10 years following original study participation, indicating that treatment gains were maintained over an extended period of time.

In an effort to more fully understand the possible individual contributions of the theorized active ingredients in the full CPT protocol, a dismantling study of CPT (Resick et al. 2008a) next compared the full protocol to a cognitive-only version (CPT-C) that does not include the written account and a written account-only (WA) condition. One hundred and fifty adult women with histories of physical and/or sexual assault were randomized into one of the three conditions. Participants in all three conditions showed significant improvements in PTSD and depressive symptoms during treatment and at the 6-month follow-up. Although the initial hypotheses predicted that the complete CPT protocol would be superior to both the CPT-C and WA conditions, in fact, when examining PTSD symptoms over the course of treatment, the CPT-C group had significantly lower scores than the WA condition during treatment, while the CPT condition did not differ significantly from CPT-C or WA. This finding suggests that cognitive therapy is a viable option in the treatment of PTSD. Although the WA component of the CPT protocol is important for some individuals to facilitate the experiencing of previously avoided trauma-related emotions, CPT-C may be an effective alternative for individuals who have a tendency to dissociate, are reluctant to undergo focused retelling of the event, or have a limited number of sessions to attend treatment (Resick et al. 2008a, b).

CPT also is shown to be effective in veteran populations. Monson and colleagues (2006) conducted the first RCT with a veteran sample and found that veterans receiving CPT demonstrated significant improvements in PTSD symptoms compared to treatment as usual through 1-month follow-up. Improvements in co-occurring symptoms including depression, anxiety, affect functioning, guilt distress, and social adjustment also were found. Forbes and colleagues (2012) examined the effectiveness of CPT compared to treatment as usual in three veterans' treatment clinics across Australia. Results showed significantly greater improvements in PTSD and secondary outcomes including anxiety and depression for the CPT group. In the first RCT examining CPT in a sample of veterans with military sexual trauma, CPT was compared to present-centered therapy (PCT), an active control group (Suris et al. 2013). Results revealed that both treatment groups showed significant improvement through 6-month follow-up in PTSD and depression, although veterans who received CPT showed significantly greater reductions in self-reported PTSD symptom severity at the posttreatment assessment compared to those who received PCT. No differences were observed between the two treatments on clinician-measured PTSD as assessed by the CAPS.

Chard (2005) developed an adaptation of CPT (CPT-SA) for survivors of sexual assault consisting of 17 weeks of group and individual therapy specifically designed to address issues salient to abuse survivors, such as attachment, communication, sexual intimacy, and social adjustment. In an RCT of this treatment, 71 women were randomized to CPT or a minimal attention (MA) wait list control group. The CPT group showed significant improvements from pretreatment to posttreatment compared to the MA group on PTSD, depression, and dissociation. PTSD symptomatology continued to improve from posttreatment to the 3-month follow-up and remained stable through 1-year follow-up.

Recent research has demonstrated effective ways in which CPT may be adapted to increase efficiency and accessibility of the treatment to a wide variety of populations. Galovski and colleagues flexibly administered a variable-length protocol of CPT (modified cognitive processing therapy; MCPT) in which the number of sessions is determined by client progress toward a predetermined good end-state functioning (Galovski et al. 2012). Results of an RCT in a sample of 100 male and female interpersonal trauma survivors found that MCPT demonstrated greater improvement on PTSD and depression, as well as secondary outcomes such as guilt, quality of life, and social functioning, compared to a minimal contact control group. Moreover, 58 % of participants receiving MCPT reached good end-state in fewer than 12 sessions, while only 8 % reached session 12 and 34 % required 12–18 sessions. Gains were maintained at the 3-month follow-up. These results suggest that the CPT protocol may be shortened for early responders, while adding additional sessions may improve outcomes for those previously deemed nonresponders after the standard 12-session protocol.

Another adaptation to CPT includes telehealth technology to deliver treatment. Morland and colleagues (2014) conducted an RCT in a sample of 125 male combat veterans in Hawaii comparing group CPT delivered via telehealth to in-person treatment. Results found that both groups had significant reductions in PTSD symptoms following treatment and maintained through 6-month follow-up. There were no significant between-group differences in clinical or process outcome variables. These findings support the feasibility and effectiveness of using telehealth technology to deliver CPT, which would greatly extend the reach of CPT and improve access to care for those with geographic limitations.

In the most unique adaptation of CPT to date, Bass and colleagues (2013) conducted a controlled trial with female sexual assault survivors in the Democratic Republic of Congo. Sixteen villages were randomly assigned to provide CPT-C (157 women) or individual support (248 women). CPT-C was delivered in a group format following an initial individual session. Results showed that participants in the CPT-C groups had significantly greater improvements in PTSD, depression, and anxiety symptoms than those in the individual support group, with effects maintained at 6-month follow-up. These findings demonstrate that CPT can be effectively implemented in diverse and challenging settings.

References

Bass, J. K., Annan, J., McIvor-Murray, S., Kaysen, D., Griffiths, S., Cetinoglu, T., Wachter, K., Murray, L., & Bolton, P. A. (2013). Controlled trial of psychotherapy for Congolese survivors of sexual violence. *New England Journal of Medicine, 368*(23), 2182–2191.

Chard, K. M. (2005). An evaluation of cognitive processing therapy for the treatment of posttraumatic stress disorder related to childhood sexual abuse. *Journal of Consulting and Clinical Psychology, 73*(5), 965–971.

Chard, K. M., Schumm, J. A., McIlvain, S. M., Bailey, G. W., & Parkinson, R. (2011). Exploring the efficacy of a residential treatment program incorporating cognitive processing therapy-cognitive for veterans with PTSD and traumatic brain injury. *Journal of Traumatic Stress, 24*(3), 347–351. doi:10.1002/jts.20644.

Clarke, S. B., Rizvi, S. L., & Resick, P. A. (2008). Borderline personality characteristics and treatment outcome in cognitive-behavioral treatments for PTSD in female rape victims. *Behavior Therapy, 39*(1), 72–78. doi:10.1016/j.beth.2007.05.002.

Fischhoff, B. (1975). Hindsight is not equal to foresight: The effect of outcome knowledge on judgment under uncertainty. *Journal of Experimental Psychology: Human Perception and Performance, 1*(3), 288–299. doi:10.1037/1076-898X.11.2.124.

Foa, E. B., & Kozak, M. J. (1986). Emotional processing of fear: Exposure to corrective information. *Psychological Bulletin, 99*(1), 20–35. doi:10.1037//0033-2909.99.1.20.

Forbes, D., Lloyd, D., Nixon, R. D. V., Elliot, P., Varker, T., Perry, D., Bryant, R. A., & Creamer, M. (2012). A multisite randomized controlled effectiveness trial of cognitive processing therapy for military-related posttraumatic stress disorder. *Journal of Anxiety Disorders, 26*(3), 442–452.

Gallagher, M. W., & Resick, P. A. (2012). Mechanisms of change in cognitive processing therapy and prolonged exposure therapy for PTSD: Preliminary evidence for the differential effects of hopelessness and habituation. *Cognitive Therapy and Research, 36*(6), 750–755. doi:10.1007/s10608-011-9423-6.

Galovski, T. E., Monson, C., Bruce, S. E., & Resick, P. A. (2009). Does cognitive-behavioral therapy for PTSD improve perceived health and sleep impairment? *Journal of Traumatic Stress, 22*(3), 197–204. doi:10.1002/jts.20418.

Galovski, T. E., Blain, L. M., Mott, J. M., Elwood, L., & Houle, T. (2012). Manualized therapy for PTSD: Flexing the structure of cognitive processing therapy. *Journal of Consulting and Clinical Psychology, 80*(6), 968–981.

Gradus, J. L., Suvak, M. K., Wisco, B. E., Marx, B. P., & Resick, P. A. (2013). Treatment of posttraumatic stress disorder reduces suicidal ideation. *Depression and Anxiety, 30*(10), 1046–1053. doi:10.1002/da.22117.

Kaysen, D., Schumm, J., Pedersen, E., Seim, R. W., Bedard-Gilligan, M., & Chard, K. (2014). Cognitive processing therapy for veterans with comorbid PTSD and alcohol use disorders. *Addictive Behaviors, 39*, 420–427. doi:10.1016/j.addbeh.2013.08.016.

McCann, I. L., & Pearlman, L. A. (1990). *Psychological trauma and the adult survivor: Theory, therapy, and transformation.* Philadelphia: Brunner/Mazel.

Monson, C. M., Schnurr, P. P., Resick, P. A., Friedman, M. J., Young-Xu, Y., & Stevens, S. P. (2006). Cognitive processing therapy for veterans with military-related posttraumatic stress disorder. *Journal of Consulting and Clinical Psychology, 74*(5), 898–907.

Morland, L. A., Mackintosh, M. A., Greene, C., Rosen, C. S., Chard, K. M., Resick, P. A., & Frueh, B. C. (2014). Cognitive processing therapy for posttraumatic stress disorder delivered to rural veterans via telemental health: A randomized noninferiority clinical trial. *Journal of Clinical Psychiatry, 75*(5), 470–476.

Resick, P. A., Nishith, P., Weaver, T. L., Astin, M. C., & Feuer, C. A. (2002). A comparison of cognitive-processing therapy with prolonged exposure and a waiting condition for the treatment of chronic posttraumatic stress disorder in female rape victims. *Journal of Consulting and Clinical Psychology, 70*(4), 867–879.

Resick, P. A., Galovski, T. E., Uhlmansick, M. O., Scher, C. D., Clum, G. A., & Young-Xu, Y. (2008a). A randomized clinical trial to dismantle components of cognitive processing therapy for posttraumatic stress disorder in female victims of interpersonal violence. *Journal of Consulting and Clinical Psychology, 76*(2), 243–258.

Resick, P. A., Monson, C. M., & Chard, K. M. (2008b). *Cognitive processing therapy: Veteran/military manual.* Washington, DC: Veterans Administration.

Resick, P. A., Williams, L. F., Suvak, M. K., Monson, C. M., & Gradus, J. L. (2012). Long-term outcomes of cognitive-behavioral treatments for posttraumatic stress disorder among female rape survivors. *Journal of Consulting and Clinical Psychology, 80*(2), 201–210.

Suris, A., Link-Malcolm, J., Chard, K., Ahn, C., & North, C. (2013). A randomized clinical trial of cognitive processing therapy for veterans with PTSD related to military sexual trauma. *Journal of Traumatic Stress, 26*(1), 28–37.

Walter, K. H., Bolte, T. A., Owens, G. P., & Chard, K. M. (2012). The impact of personality disorders on treatment outcome for Veterans in a posttraumatic stress disorder residential treatment program. *Cognitive Therapy Research, 36*(5), 576–584.

38. ... ...
39. ... ...

EMDR Therapy for Trauma-Related Disorders

11

Francine Shapiro and Deany Laliotis

Eye movement desensitization and reprocessing (EMDR) therapy is an integrative eight-phase approach that emphasizes the role of physiologically stored memory networks and the brain's information processing system in the treatment of pathology. It is guided by the Adaptive Information Processing (AIP) model, which conceptualizes mental health problems, excluding those caused by organic deficits (e.g., genetic, toxicity, injury), to be the result of inadequately processed memories of adverse life experiences. According to this view, presenting symptoms result from memories of disturbing experiences that have been dysfunctionally stored, encoded with the original emotions, beliefs, and physical sensations (Shapiro 2001, 2012a, 2014). Since the model's development in the early 1990s, a substantial body of research has confirmed the primacy of such disturbing life events for a wide range of psychological and somatic symptomatology (e.g., Mol et al. 2005; Felitti et al. 1998).

11.1 The Adaptive Information Processing (AIP) Model

More generally, the AIP model explains the development of personality and pathology, and predicts successful clinical outcomes, while guiding EMDR therapy case conceptualization and procedures. Pivotal to the model is the widely recognized fact that the brain's information processing system is designed to make sense of current

F. Shapiro, PhD (✉)
Mental Research Institute,
Palo Alto, CA, USA
e-mail: fshapiro@mcn.org

D. Laliotis, LICSW
EMDR Institute,
Watsonville, CA, USA

© Springer International Publishing Switzerland 2015
U. Schnyder, M. Cloitre (eds.), *Evidence Based Treatments for Trauma-Related Psychological Disorders: A Practical Guide for Clinicians*,
DOI 10.1007/978-3-319-07109-1_11

situations by linking the experience with related extant memory networks. For example, the experience of falling off a bicycle will link with networks containing memories of other accidents and the general category of being physically hurt. Or a conflict with a friend will be integrated with memories pertaining to interpersonal relationships. Also pivotal is the recognition that another fundamental purpose of the information processing system is to alleviate emotional distress via a return to homeostasis. In most circumstances, disturbing experiences will be resolved automatically by linking with networks containing mitigating or qualifying information, such as "these things have occurred before" or "I have already successfully dealt with this kind of thing and moved past it." Whether through the passage of time, thinking about it, or dreaming about it, the information processing system may be said, metaphorically, to "metabolize" or "digest" the experience. What is useful is stored in the appropriate memory networks and serve as a functional guide for future perception, reactions, and behavior; what is useless is discarded. In short, processed memories are the foundation of good mental health.

According to the AIP model, an adverse life experience is sometimes so disturbing that it overwhelms the information processing system. When this happens, the memory becomes "stuck," frozen in time, and incapable of making the appropriate associations with other memory networks of adaptively stored life experiences. These disturbing events are neurophysiologically maintained in memory together with the negative affect, sensations, and beliefs engendered by the original event. According to some memory researchers, the failure to process a traumatic event involves the lack of integration of episodic memory into the semantic memory system (see Stickgold 2002). Inadequately processed memories of disturbing events are easily triggered by both internal and external stimuli, resulting in a variety of clinical symptoms that may include inappropriate emotions, beliefs, and behaviors. The flashbacks, nightmares, and intrusive thoughts of PTSD are the most striking examples. However, as predicted by the AIP model, highly disturbing adverse life experiences that do not qualify as "Criterion A trauma" can also be dysfunctionally stored and provide the foundation for a wide range of pathologies such as negative affective, cognitive, and somatic responses. In fact, general adverse life experiences have been found to generate even more PTSD symptoms than major traumatic events (Mol et al. 2005).

When unresolved, these disturbing experiences shape the individual's perception of the present, resulting in a vicious cycle of dysfunction. As indicated previously, an important aspect of unprocessed memories is their inclusion of the emotions and physical sensations that occurred at the time of the critical event. For example, when a child undergoes a traumatic experience whose memory remains unprocessed, the associated reactions of helplessness, perceived danger, and lack of control, which are not uncommon in childhood, persist into adulthood. Since perceptions of current situations are automatically linked with associated memory networks, these unprocessed affective and cognitive responses emerge, coloring the perceptions of the present, as current stimuli trigger the stored associations. In short, the past becomes present. These experiences are stored in turn, expanding the negative memory network and reinforcing a negative sense of self, others, and life circumstances.

According to the AIP model, self-characterizations such as "I am an unworthy person" are not the cause of present clinical problems, but rather symptomatic of unprocessed earlier life experiences, along with their emotional concomitants. Dysfunctional emotions, thoughts, and behavioral responses are viewed as manifestations of these unprocessed memories. This tenet is integral to EMDR treatment and contrary to therapies that view negative beliefs or dysfunctional behaviors as the basis of pathology and the restructuring of beliefs or manipulation of behavior as agents of therapeutic change.

Research has validated EMDR therapy as an effective trauma treatment across the life span and joins trauma-focused cognitive behavioral therapy as the only two psychotherapies recommended in the World Health Organization (2013) practice guidelines for the treatment of PTSD in children, adolescents, and adults. These two forms of therapy share certain characteristics, but also differ in significant ways. As noted in the World Health Organization (2013) practice guidelines: "[EMDR] therapy is based on the idea that negative thoughts, feelings and behaviours are the result of unprocessed memories. The treatment involves standardized procedures that include focusing simultaneously on (a) spontaneous associations of traumatic images, thoughts, emotions and bodily sensations and (b) bilateral stimulation that is most commonly in the form of repeated eye movements. Like CBT with a trauma focus, EMDR therapy aims to reduce subjective distress and strengthen adaptive cognitions related to the traumatic event. Unlike CBT with a trauma focus, EMDR does not involve (a) detailed descriptions of the event, (b) direct challenging of beliefs, (c) extended exposure, or (d) homework" (p.1).

While CBT utilizes behavioral, narrative, or cognitive tasks as agents of change, therapeutic change with EMDR therapy (as guided by the AIP model) is viewed as a by-product of processing produced by spontaneously generated internal associations that are elicited during the bilateral stimulation. As illustrated in the treatment section, the therapist instructs the client to access the memory by concentrating on certain specific components and then, guided by the therapist, to engage in simultaneous sets of eye movements while noticing whatever comes to mind. At the end of each set, the client is asked to briefly respond to the question, "What do you get now?" The client may report new thoughts, insights, emotions, body sensations, or entirely new memories. In contrast to CBT, the client may only attend directly to the initially targeted incident for a few moments in a given session. Rather, the client's response at the end of each set of eye movements is assessed to ensure that processing is occurring. Depending on the client's response, the clinician guides his or her next focus of attention according to standardized procedures to ensure that the entire memory network is addressed.

As seen in the EMDR session transcripts below, therapy progresses rapidly, as each set of bilateral stimuli brings with it greater client awareness and changes in the emotions, sensations, and memories associated with the critical event. According to the AIP model, the underlying basis for these changes is the establishment of links between the initially unprocessed experience and other, related memory networks. This has been posited to cause the disturbing episodic memory to become integrated within semantic networks (Stickgold 2002). Thus, as a result of successful EMDR therapy treatment, the memory is no longer isolated, but fully assimilated within a comprehensive set of adaptive networks of previous experiences. The original disturbing memory of the event, with all of its negative affects and cognitions, is resolved through an accelerated learning experience and stored with appropriate affect, serving as a foundation of resilience. This is posited to occur by means of a shift in brain states induced by the procedures that support the associational process and a prolonged orienting response (Stickgold 2002) elicited by the repeated bilateral stimulation. This brain state is thought to be similar to that occurring during rapid eye movement (REM) sleep, in which sleep-dependent processing of episodic memories has been shown to specifically facilitate (1) the development of insight into and understanding of the memories, (2) reduction or elimination of associated negative affect, and (3) the memories' integration into existing semantic networks, all of which contribute to their resolution.

It is further posited that EMDR therapy results in memory reconsolidation (Solomon and Shapiro 2008; Shapiro 2014), in which the original memory is transformed and stored in an altered form. As illustrated in the treatment section, this distinguishes EMDR therapy from trauma-focused cognitive behavioral therapies (TF-CBT) that rely on habituation and extinction, which appear to create a new memory during the therapeutic process, while leaving the original one intact. Significantly, research has indicated that the lengthy exposures used in TF-CBT cause extinction, while short exposures such as those of EMDR therapy cause memory reconsolidation (Suzuki et al. 2004). As described by Craske et al. (2006), "… recent work on extinction and reinstatement … suggests that extinction does not eliminate or replace previous associations, but rather results in new learning that competes with the old information" (p. 6). The distinction between extinction and reconsolidation has important clinical implications. As discussed in the research section below, memory reconsolidation may be responsible for a variety of EMDR treatment effects (e.g., elimination of phantom limb pain) not found with extinction-based therapies.

11.2 Treatment Overview

EMDR therapy is an eight-phase treatment approach that addresses the adverse life experiences assumed to be the basis of a wide range of pathologies with the exception of those caused by organic deficit (Shapiro 2001). The number of sessions and the length of the various phases depend upon the complexity of the case. For instance, single-trauma PTSD may be successfully treated within three sessions (e.g., Wilson et al. 1995, 1997). In such cases, the history-taking and preparation phases may take place during the first session, and the assessment and reprocessing phases (desensitization, installation, body scan) could be inaugurated during the second session and completed on the third. The closure phase returns the client to equilibrium and ends each session, while the reevaluation phase begins each session subsequent to reprocessing. For those with complex PTSD, the history-taking and preparation phases may span more sessions to ensure a comprehensive assessment of the case and that the client has sufficient affect stability to commence processing. Likewise, reprocessing will entail additional sessions to adequately treat the multiple traumas. Table 11.1 provides an overview of the goals and procedures used in the various phases.

An overall objective of EMDR therapy is to restore good mental health by helping clients reprocess memories of adverse life experiences, which results in spontaneous shifts of emotion, cognition, physical sensations, and behaviors. As demonstrated in the treatment section, standardized procedures are used to access

Table 11.1 Overview of eight-phase EMDR therapy treatment

Phase	Purpose	Procedures
History taking	Obtain background information. Identify suitability for EMDR treatment	Standard history taking questionnaires and diagnostic psychometrics
	Identify processing targets from events in client's life according to standardized three-pronged protocol	Review of selection criteria
		Questions and techniques (e.g., Floatback, Affect Scan) to identify (1) past events that have laid the groundwork for the pathology, (2) current triggers, and (3) future needs
Preparation	Prepare clients for EMDR processing of targets	Education regarding the symptom picture
		Metaphors and techniques that foster stabilization and a sense of personal control (e.g., safe place)
Assessment	Access the target for EMDR processing by stimulating primary aspects of the memory	Elicit the image, negative belief currently held, desired positive belief, current emotion, and physical sensation and baseline measures
Desensitization	Process experiences toward an adaptive resolution (no distress)	Standardized protocols incorporating eye movements (taps, or tones) that allow the spontaneous emergence of insights, emotions, physical sensations, and other memories
Installation	Increase connections to positive cognitive networks	Enhance the validity of the desired positive belief and fully integrate within the memory network
Body scan	Complete processing of any residual disturbance associated with the target	Concentration on and processing of any residual physical sensations
Closure	Ensure client stability at the completion of an EMDR therapy session and between sessions	Use of self-control techniques if needed
		Briefing regarding expectations and behavioral reports between sessions
Reassessment	Ensure maintenance of therapeutic outcomes and stability of client	Evaluation of treatment effects
		Evaluation of integration within larger social system

Reprinted from Shapiro (2012b)

the dysfunctionally stored memories while simultaneously facilitating the information processing system by fostering the internally generated associations that arise in consciousness during sequential sets of bilateral dual attention stimulation (visual, auditory, or tactile). This stimulation is applied by asking the client to follow a light or the clinician's finger back and forth in horizontal sweeping movements while tracking their internal responses. After about 30 s, the clinician stops the bilateral stimulation and asks the client to briefly report on what they are experiencing, insuring that processing is taking place.

Rather than maintaining the sustained attention on the original incident that characterizes exposure-based therapies, or attempting to reinterpret the experience, the EMDR client is generally encouraged to "let whatever happens, happen" and simply notice what arises in consciousness. The goal is to stimulate the inherent information processing system of the brain and, with as little clinical intrusion as possible, allow it to spontaneously make the appropriate connections. The associations constitute an accelerated learning process that generally evolves to an adaptive psychological resolution. It is believed that this approach maximizes the needed associations between the targeted memory and related extant neural networks, thereby fostering optimal therapeutic outcomes that include a new positive assessment of the event, appropriate affective response, functional behaviors, and generalization of the treatment effects to other life contexts. Two detailed case descriptions illustrate the clinical procedures and outcomes.

11.2.1 Single Trauma

Jennifer, a 31-year-old married woman with a 15-month-old toddler, underwent a traumatic experience while delivering her second child, Jake, 6 months earlier. Jennifer had told the doctors that she could actually feel what they were doing in preparation for the C-section and needed more anesthesia. However, the anesthesiologist denied that Jennifer could feel anything given the medication dose he had administered and made a unilateral decision to proceed with the C-section despite her protests. As she was cut open, Jennifer screamed from the intensity of the pain. It was only then that the doctors stopped, administered more medication, and waited until she was sufficiently anesthetized to proceed. She also described how disoriented she felt in the recovery room from the effects of the amount of anesthesia she was ultimately given.

The history-taking phase of EMDR therapy during the first appointment revealed that Jennifer was happily married, with no previous trauma history, and a stable childhood. However, her clinical complaints were textbook symptoms of PTSD: nightmares of the event, flashbacks, avoidance of reminders of the event, hyperstartle response, hypervigilance, irritability, difficulty concentrating, and sleep disturbance. She ruminated about the event often, wondering how things could have gone so wrong in the delivery room despite her best efforts to communicate. She was upset that her doctors had ignored her feedback and that her husband, who was there at the time, had failed to intervene on her behalf. She reported having difficulty bonding with Jake, since being with him brought on feelings of anxiety and fear. She also reported being short-tempered and irritated with her husband since the birth.

During the preparation phase, Jennifer was given a brief overview of trauma and the AIP model. She was then taught a safe place, one of the EMDR therapy self-control techniques (Shapiro 2001, 2012a) to ensure that she was able to achieve a state of calm both during and between sessions. In this technique, the client is asked to identify a real or imagined place of safety or calm and concentrate on deepening the experience until it is fully developed. The client is then asked to think of a mild irritant, focus on it for a few moments and then shift back to their safe place. This technique is often taught with short, slow sets of bilateral stimulation, both to facilitate a deepening of the experience and to introduce the client to the stimulation itself. The goal of this technique is to assess the client's ability to effectively shift states on demand as well as increase access to positive affective states. The client is encouraged to apply this technique on their own as a tool to manage stress responses.

Based on multiple factors, including readiness and motivation for treatment, no previous trauma history, mastery of the affect regulation skill, and the need to restore a level of functioning that would allow her to bond with Jake, it was decided to commence with EMDR reprocessing during the next meeting. At the beginning of that session, Jennifer was further prepared for processing by reminding her that she was in complete control and that if she needed to take a break, she had only to raise her hand as a signal. During processing, she was asked to "let whatever happens, happen." A standard EMDR therapy metaphor was used to support her ability to do this, as she was asked to imagine that she was on a train and that whatever emerged in consciousness was simply the scenery passing by.

In the assessment phase, the components of Jennifer's childbirth memory were identified. Additionally, she is asked to choose a positive cognition she would prefer to have at the end of treatment:

Image (representing the worst part of the experience in the present): "Seeing myself strapped down on the hospital bed screaming."
Negative cognition: "I am powerless."
Positive cognition: "I have power now in my life."
Validity of positive cognition (VoC) on a scale of 1–7, with 1 being completely false, 7 being completely true: 2
Emotions (currently experienced): Anger, fear, sadness
SUD (subjective units of distress scale) from 0 no disturbance to 10 highest: 10
Body sensations (experienced in the present)—tension in her throat, jaw, stomachache

The desensitization phase is initiated by asking the client to bring to consciousness the image, the negative belief, and the body sensations. Jennifer held in mind the image in the delivery room; the word, "I am powerless"; and the negative feelings in her throat, jaw, and stomach. She was instructed to maintain a dual awareness, noticing whatever might emerge internally as she followed the sets of eye movement and to indicate with her stop signal if she needed a break. She then began to follow the therapist's hand for a set of approximately 24–36 bilateral repetitions of eye movements. The length of each set is customized to the client's needs by observing nonverbal responses.

At the end of each set of stimuli, the therapist asks, "What are you noticing now?" The clinician is looking for indicators of change in the client's experience, making sure that processing is taking place. These range from changes in the initial memory (e.g., less emotional distress, unclear visuals, a change in reference point) to associations to other similar experiences. For example, if Jennifer or a close relative had previous negative experiences in childbirth, those associations would likely emerge. Other associations might involve experiences of powerlessness having nothing to do with childbirth per se. Depending on the response, the clinician may offer emotional support to the client by reminding them they are safe in the present or simply instructing them to "go with that (association or experience)" during the subsequent set of stimuli. At various times during the session, according to structured protocols, clients are asked to attend to various elements or to focus attention back on the original target to ensure that the entire memory has been fully processed.

Below is the transcript of Jennifer's EMDR reprocessing session, which encompasses phases four through six (desensitization, installation, and body scan). While every reprocessing session is structured to include phases three through seven, not all reprocessing is completed within the time frame of a single clinical session. In this case, the processing was completed in this one session. After each set of bilateral stimulation (BLS), Jennifer reports her associational experience:

Jennifer: *"I'm just seeing myself in the room frozen."*
Therapist: *"Ok, go with that…"*
Jennifer: *"Now, I'm hearing myself screaming. I'm not saying anything in particular, just screaming. My throat is hurting more now."*
Therapist: *"Ok, just notice that you're not actually there as you continue."*
Jennifer: *"I can't see what's going on behind the curtain…now I'm really scared because no one is listening to me and I don't know what they're going to do!"*
Therapist: *"You're doing fine, you're doing fine…just continue to notice what is happening now, keeping in mind that it's just a memory."*
Jennifer: *Now I'm hearing the anesthesiologist tell me that it's impossible for me to be feeling any sensations…oh, my god, now I can feel them cutting into me!"*
Therapist: *"Okay, just hang in there, remember that the worst is over and that you're okay now."*
Jennifer: *"Oh my god, I don't know if I can bear this again…I can't stand it! It feels like I'm going to die!"*
Therapist (during the BLS): *"I know this is hard. Notice that you're here and that you're safe and that nothing is actually happening to you. You're in complete control of this situation."*
Jennifer (during the BLS): *"Okay, okay!!! (hyperventilating). This is so awful! When is it going to end???"* (Long set of BLS to get through emotional response until intensity shifts).

Therapist: *"Just remember that it DID end and that it will end again, once and for all. You're doing great."*

Jennifer: *"Okay, okay."* (Minutes later): *"The pain in my abdomen is lessening now."*

Therapist: *"That's great. Stay with that."*

Jennifer: *"Now I'm seeing my husband's face. He looks shocked his face is white. He's not moving."*

Therapist: *"Okay, just notice that and whatever sensations you might still be having."*

Jennifer: *"Oh my god, I'm realizing that he* (husband) *was frozen with shock and that it was happening to him, too! I'm a little calmer now."*

Therapist: *"Good. Stay with it. You're doing fine."*

Jennifer: *"I'm getting now that he was being traumatized, too. No wonder he couldn't do anything to help me! It wasn't because he was weak or that he didn't get what was going on."*

Therapist: *"That's right. Stay with that. Notice how that feels in your body..."*

Jennifer: *"I feel soooo much better knowing that! My body is really calming down now."*

Therapist: *"Good. Let's give your body plenty of time to process through all the leftover sensations..."* (Longer set to make sure all residual body sensation was being processed).

Therapist: *"So, how are you doing?"*

Jennifer: *"Much better. It feels like it's over."*

Therapist: *"Good. Stay with that."*

Jennifer: *"It really feels done...my body feels that way, too."*

Therapist: *"Okay, great. So, let's go back to the memory of what actually happened. What are you noticing now?"*

Jennifer: *"I'm still upset that it happened, but it seems more distant than when we started."*

Therapist: *"Okay, go with that."*

Jennifer: *"Now I'm feeling really woozy. (Long pause) I guess I'm in the recovery room now."*

Therapist: *"Okay, go with that."*

Jennifer: *"Now I'm getting a really bad headache; I feel disoriented. I guess this is the anesthesia."*

Therapist: *"Sounds like it. Just keep going. You're doing fine."*

Jennifer: *"Okay, I'm starting to feel better now."*

Therapist: *"Good. Stay with it. We're almost done."*

Jennifer: *"Okay, good. The headache is gone, and my head is clearing up. I can even see more clearly than I could just a minute ago."*

Therapist: *"That's great. Just stay with it a little bit longer to make sure it's all cleared out."*

Jennifer: *"It feels pretty good now."*

Therapist: *"Okay. So, let's go back to the memory as a whole. What are you noticing now?"*

Jennifer: *"I can't believe that the doctor didn't listen to me! I'm so angry! How could he do that?"*

Therapist: *"Good question. Go with that."*

Jennifer: *"I just can't believe it. I can't believe that this actually happened to me. I'm so relieved that nothing happened to Jake and that he is okay."*

Therapist: *"That's right. Just notice that."*

Jennifer: *"I guess there's a happy ending to this nightmare after all, isn't there?"*

Therapist: *"Yes, there is. Notice that. Notice how THAT feels in your body."*

Jennifer: *"I feel calm. It's over."*

Therapist: *"Yes, it IS over. So, when you think of the memory now, on a scale of 0–10, where 0 is no disturbance and 10 is the highest disturbance you can imagine, how does it feel to you now?"*

Jennifer: *"It's about a 1.* (Pauses with disbelief) *Wow!"*

Therapist: *"Okay. So, notice what's left in your body right now..."*

Jennifer: *"I had a shadow of pain in my abdomen. Now it's completely gone."*

Therapist: *"That's great."*

The reprocessing indicates the comprehensive changes in cognitive, emotional, and somatic domains, including insight regarding her husband's reactions, a recognition that event is in the past, and an elimination of disturbing physical sensation. In the installation phase, the previously identified desired positive belief about the self, or a preferred one that may have emerged, is processed along with the neutralized memory. This enhances the self-affirming evaluation in the context of the memory and strengthens the affective connection to the client's adaptive memory networks.

Therapist: *"When you think of the memory of giving birth to Jake, do the words, 'I have power in my life now,' still fit? Or, is there another statement that fits even better?"*

Client: *"Yes, that still fits."*

Therapist: *"On a scale of 1–7, where 1 feels completely false and 7 is completely true, how true do the words, 'I have power now in my life,' FEEL to you now?"*

Client: *"They're a 7."*

Therapist: *"Good! Bring to mind the memory and the words, 'I have power now in my life.' Hold them together and follow my fingers."* (Therapist inaugurates a set of eye movements.)

During the body scan phase, Jennifer was asked to hold the positive belief and memory of the delivery room in her mind as she scanned her body to identify any residual negative sensations. She reported that her body felt, "Clear and relaxed."

During the closure phase at the end of the session, Jennifer was told that additional associations might emerge during the week as processing continued and was asked to briefly jot down any disturbance in a log (e.g., indicating image/thought/affect). She was also reminded to use her self-control technique if needed.

At the next session, during the reevaluation phase the memory is reaccessed to evaluate whether further processing is needed. The clinical symptoms are evaluated, and the client is asked to report any changes that have occurred since the last session. This indicated that Jennifer's symptoms were resolved. In the subsequent session, Jennifer reported that she was sleeping well again and was no longer preoccupied with the events of the delivery nor hypervigilant or hyperaroused about potential danger and uncertainty. There had been no more flashbacks, nightmares, or avoidance of stimuli that reminded her of the incident. When asked about the relationship problems she had had with Jake and her husband, she reported that they were now resolved. For example, she was no longer experiencing anxiety or fear or reminded of the delivery when she was interacting with Jake. Further, the irritation she had felt with her husband over various random events had completely vanished. Instead, she actually had a long talk with him about her experience of his role (which she had not disclosed to him before) and how that had shifted as a by-product of the reprocessing. When she considered the thought of having another baby, she remarked, "If we decide to have more children, that will be our choice. This experience has nothing to do with what we decide for ourselves and our family." She confirmed in a telephone follow-up that she felt "like herself" again.

Although unnecessary with Jennifer because of the comprehensive generalization of treatment effects, additional procedures used to complete the three-pronged protocol involve the processing of current triggers and imaginal templates for positive future actions. These will be described in the next case.

11.2.2 Developmental Trauma

Developmental trauma refers to the category of early life experiences that are formative, pervasive, and have a significant negative impact on self and psyche. As illustrated in this case, the eight phases of EMDR therapy and standardized three-pronged approach involve a thorough evaluation of the comprehensive clinical picture, client preparation, and the processing of (a) past events that set the foundation for pathology, (b) current situations that trigger disturbance, and (c) skills needed to address future challenges.

Carla is a 30-year-old woman, twice divorced, who came for EMDR therapy to deal with anxiety and depression due to her off-again, on-again relationship with Joe, her current boyfriend of 5 years, who often ignored her needs. She had struggled during this time to do "whatever it takes" to make the relationship work. After two failed marriages, she believed that this was her last chance to have a family of her own.

Carla grew up as the youngest of four children, with three older brothers. Her parents both worked full-time, leaving her at home with her grandfather who lived with them until he died when she was 6 years old, devastating her. Subsequently, she spent a great deal of time at home alone with the family dogs. Even when others were home, she experienced an overwhelming sense of loneliness. She gave up asking; she gave up wanting. She would dress herself in the mornings to get herself to school, often forced to wear the same clothes day after day to the point where the school called to see if her family needed financial assistance. Her mother never took an active interest in parenting her. When she paid attention to Carla, it was to scold her or blame her for her unhappiness. Her father was passive and detached. Her brothers bullied her or ignored her altogether.

From an AIP-informed perspective, Carla's symptoms of anxiety, depression, low self-esteem, and poor relationship skills stem from her unprocessed memories of neglect and abuse as well as early loss of a primary attachment figure. It was clear that she was an unwanted pregnancy and that her mother resented having to care for her. So, when her boyfriend ignored her, it triggered the childhood feeling that she is not good enough to warrant his attention, causing her to shut down emotionally rather than considering that there may be something wrong with the situation or with him. Reacting the same way in the present as she did when she was a child, feeling not good enough, and powerless to do anything about it, she again gives up asking, gives up wanting.

In the history-taking phase of EMDR therapy, the clinician evaluates the clinical picture looking for connections between the client's current problems and past experiences triggering those difficulties. Using the floatback technique, the clinician uses a recent experience such as the one where Carla finds herself feeling alone and unimportant while at home with Joe. She is then asked to bring that experience fully to mind, noticing the image, thoughts, feelings, and sensations that emerge and to allow her mind to "float back" to earlier, similar experiences in her life. Carla's floatback revealed several stored experiences in her memory network: scenes of being alone in her marriages; her grandfather's death; being pinched by her brother at the family dinner table with no one responding to her protests; seeing herself alone with her family dogs; and being 8 years old and scolded by her mother for going to the neighbor's house on a dark, rainy afternoon when no one was home and she was scared. While these associations are not by the usual definition "traumatic," in and of themselves, Carla had numerous early, adverse life experiences that were pervasive and cumulatively had a lasting negative effect on her sense of self and relationships with others. These experiences are processed during EMDR therapy by systematically targeting memories that represent each cluster of similar events (being ignored, bullied, etc.). Successful processing of one memory often results in a generalization of treatment effects to other memories within the cluster of associated experiences.

It is important in the early phases of EMDR therapy to assess the client's desired outcomes and readiness to address the presenting problems. Many clients enter psychotherapy for symptom reduction but with little understanding of the larger emotional landscape that lies beneath. Creating a sense of safety and a climate of collaboration to bring about a mutual understanding of the problem(s) is critical. Carla understood that her early childhood experiences contributed to her low self-esteem and her relationship difficulties. However, she was less clear about the degree of neglect she had endured and its profound impact on her. Part of the effect of those experiences was to cause her to shut down and act as if everything was all right when it was not. Eventually she learned to compartmentalize her feelings and her needs to the point where she had difficulty accessing her true emotional experience. Understanding these developmental deficits in the early phases of treatment helps to establish the treatment frame and identify the memories that should be targeted. For example, Carla's proclivity to abandon her needs and defer to the desires of others at her personal expense was best addressed by targeting the childhood memory of getting in trouble for going to the neighbor's house during a storm. That experience embodied the sense that she was not worthwhile and that bad things will happen when you try to get your needs met. When that memory and pertinent associations were successfully reprocessed, Carla felt like she could have a say in her own life, no longer shutting down and reacting passively to a challenging situation in the present.

During the preparation phase the clinician evaluates the client's readiness and affect regulation skills. As a memory-focused approach that relies on addressing disturbing experiences, it is important in EMDR therapy to establish that the client can: (a) access a critical memory and tolerate the resulting experience for a period of time, (b) maintain a dual focus of attention between the past and present, (c) shift from one emotional state to another, and (d) access memory networks of adaptive experiences. A variety of self-control and resource development techniques (e.g., safe place) can be used, differing as a function of the client's level of debilitation. In addition, as with many clients with developmental trauma, it was important to help Carla access her full emotional response since she was so accustomed to suppressing her feelings. Although earlier experiences are generally targeted first in EMDR therapy, a current situation was used since its immediacy enabled her to feel the intensity of her emotional reaction to being ignored. As indicated below in a transcript excerpt of the desensitization phase, a variety of childhood experiences emerged during the first processing session, using a recent disagreement with Joe as the target memory. After each set of eye movements, Carla reported to the therapist the associations that emerged:

Carla: I'm a kid sitting on the couch while everyone is running around and I'm just sitting there.

Carla: I remember being in school and the school calling to ask if we had enough money to buy clothing. At that point, they could afford to buy me clothing, but I wore the same thing every day...and sometimes I would dress myself and I would wear something crazy...my grandfather had died and he was the one who really took care of me...

Carla: I was in the playground and I was playing, and a bee stung my finger and it really hurt, and I didn't do anything about it. I didn't scream, I just didn't do anything. I knew at the time, I was thinking, "Why aren't you screaming?" I just shoved it down, it didn't hurt.

Carla: I see myself with my mother criticizing me as she always did. I wasn't pretty enough, I wasn't smart enough...that I was doing it all wrong."

After multiple sets of negative associations, the clinician may use a cognitive interweave, which is a statement or a question designed to elicit the adaptive information that is unavailable to the client in the moment. Guided by the AIP model, the clinician is minimally intrusive, eliciting just enough information to jump-start spontaneous processing:

Therapist: So, if this were a girlfriend telling you these things, what would you say to her, knowing her as well as you do?
Carla: I would say to her that she is good enough, that it was her mother who had problems!
Therapist: That's right. Go with that."
Carla: I can see that my Mom used to do that to everyone. She was just not a happy woman.

After further processing of the target event, adaptive information continues to automatically link in:

Carla: I just saw myself bouncing around, wondering, "Who is good for me?" I saw quick flashes throughout my life asking my parents who's good for me asking friends going to fortune tellers, psychics, and not listening to me. That's why I don't trust my intuition because I've always looked outside for whoever else is the expert other than me. I also have a knack for picking the wrong guy. It's like the bee sting: I feel it, but I don't do a thing!

The resultant insight about the bee sting and its correlation to how she responds when in relationships is a revelatory moment as she realizes that her response is a childhood adaptation to being neglected, not "how she is as a person."

Therapist: That's right. Focus on that.
Carla: Wow, that was cool! I went through this journey in my mind imagining some-one [herself] strong, independent, successful, with self-esteem, not arrogant. I just felt like that for a little bit. And I imagined feeling that way going back to my house and talking to Joe. I tried that for a while and I felt like just saying what I needed to say. It was about what I was feeling, not about what he was feeling and that felt really good!

Carla's positive image of seeing herself as strong is an association that is sponta-neously accessed from her adaptively stored memory network, a typical by-product of processing as the negative arousal diminishes.

Therapist: That's really great. So, just notice that.
Carla: And now I'm remembering times as a little girl when I did have these feel-ings of self-worth and now I feel like they were squashed, but I feel like I have rekindled that feeling a little bit.
Therapist: Yes, it's like reconnecting to that younger self that really did feel good about herself and bringing her forward.
Carla: I feel like it's a miracle!

Therapist: Let's go back to thinking about what actually happened that night on the couch with Joe. What are you noticing now?

Carla: Oh my god, hang on! It's weird because it feels like there are shifting gears going on in my head. I feel this physical reaction. I know what I need to tell him and I'm nervous because of it. So, I actually feel it now. That's wild!

Therapist: Great. Are you okay with that?

Carla: Yes! And this is the anxiety I feel whenever I have to give a presentation at work, and it's probably all that bottled up stuff!

Therapist: Yes. It's all that bottled up stuff. Focus on that.

Carla: I just feel exhilarated! I think that's the right word. I haven't felt this before.

Therapist: Going back to the other night at home with Joe, on a scale of 0–10, how much does it bother you?

Carla: 1 or 2, but, actually it's a 0 because I feel worth it!

At the following session, Carla reported that her mood had improved and she felt better about herself as a person. She was discouraged about her relationship with Joe, but that seemed "ecologically" appropriate. That is, there were no outward signs of change in his behavior toward her, and she continued to struggle in her ability to speak up for herself in the moment. She described that, instead of feeling numb and shut down, she felt anxious and insecure because she knew that what she had to say would be likely to generate conflict between them and that he might leave her. While discussing her reluctance to speak up for herself, other memories in need of processing were revealed. As is often the case when treating developmental trauma, resolving one type of experience brings up that which is beneath. In this case, processing her reaction of numbness when she is unattended to reveals the underlying anxiety of needing care and attention and being anxious about having to ask for it, anticipating the negative reactions she would get in response. Consequently, it is necessary to carefully monitor the clients' progress via an ongoing evaluation of current symptoms, identifying the remaining difficulties in the present, processing both the current triggers and the past experiences that are driving them, and helping them integrate the changes into their larger social system. Attention should be paid to the comprehensive clinical picture. In Carla's case, this included resolving the presentation anxiety she had revealed during processing. Her treatment continued over a 6-month period bringing her to a robust feeling of self-confidence and mental health.

The interplay between the past, present, and future is the cornerstone of the three-pronged protocol of EMDR therapy and insures that the clinician is targeting the relevant past experiences connected to the client's difficulties in the present. Additionally, the absence of distress and the associated distortions about self and others do not necessarily translate into a functioning set of responses to meet future demands, especially when the client has incurred significant developmental deficits. For clients with developmental trauma, it is likely that the clinician will need to help them learn appropriate relational skills so they can respond adaptively in the future, which is the third prong of the three-pronged protocol of the past, present, and future. For instance, Carla was taught assertiveness skills through interactive role-play, during this phase. These were later developed into templates for future actions by imagining herself asserting her needs to Joe appropriately. This takes place in the reprocessing phases of EMDR therapy as a future template, generating new neural networks of adaptive responses to challenge situations. Seeing no positive response from him, she eventually ended the relationship and began dating candidates more suitable to her newfound sense of self-worth.

11.3 Clinical Challenges

As with every psychotherapeutic approach, EMDR therapy must factor into effective treatment plans a variety of clinical challenges. While it is beyond the scope of this chapter to review all of the cautions and strategies articulated in comprehensive treatment guides for these specialty populations, some specific observations will be made regarding EMDR treatment.

11.3.1 Children

The standard three-pronged EMDR therapy protocol has been made developmentally appropriate for children by the incorporation of simplified language and the potential use of art and play strategies. Children tend to be enormously resilient and responsive to EMDR therapy. However, there are inherent challenges in the treatment of this population since the presenting problem is often defined by a third party and the clinician's primary sources of information are family members, who may play a role in the child's symptoms. For example, a child whose parents have divorced may experience severe anxiety about leaving the house, refusing to go to school or play with friends out of fear that the remaining parent will not be home when they return. Thus, it may be necessary to treat both child and parent by reprocessing the experiences associated with the disruption of the family (Shapiro et al. 2007). In the absence of this dual treatment, the continuing emotional pain of the parent may exacerbate the problem by enhancing and reinforcing the child's negative emotions. For children with pervasive developmental trauma, resource development techniques are crucial, along with specific protocols to assist extremely debilitated children, which include memory processing in the presence of a supportive caregiver (Wesselmann et al. 2012).

Children with language and communication deficits can benefit greatly from the use of EMDR therapy since it does not require the creation of a narrative or a verbalized story. Clinicians can use a wide range of strategies to assist these children in processing their experiences of trauma and adversity in EMDR therapy through play, drawings, art, and the use of figures and symbols from sand tray therapy (Gómez 2012). All strategies are geared to the child's level of cognitive and emotional development and their communication capacities. Without words, children may be invited to use art or music to express what they are experiencing as processing takes place.

11.3.2 Complex PTSD

A broad range of presenting complaints are rooted in trauma during the developmental years. Client history can reveal problems stemming from single episodic instances of adverse childhood events to those suffering from pervasive experiences of abuse and neglect that are more debilitating and complex. Clearly, it is important to evaluate each client's ability to effectively manage arousal states, which may be compromised due to traumatic experiences in early life. However, while this is a legitimate concern for any therapist treating complex developmental trauma, it is also important not to underestimate the client's capacities based on history alone. The challenge is to evaluate the client's actual skills through clinical observations and client self-reports. Careful attention must be paid to forging a supportive therapeutic relationship and stabilizing the client sufficiently to undertake memory processing, as this in turn will reduce emotional turmoil. Depending on the level of client debilitation, preparation ranges from the use of individual EMDR therapy techniques that can be implemented in one or more sessions to integration of these strategies within a more structured stabilization program (e.g., Cloitre et al. 2006).

EMDR therapy utilizes self-control and resource development techniques to enhance access to memories of positive experiences (e.g., feeling confidence, mastery, hope) or skills that the client has in other areas of life (see Shapiro 2001, 2012a). These are taught to foster the client's ability to self-monitor and change emotional states both during and between sessions. While these strategies can be introduced at any point during the treatment according to need, they are often applied in the preparation phase in order to stabilize the client or optimize the capacity to manage stressful situations until the memories informing their maladaptive reactions can be processed. So, for example, the client with a long history of medical trauma is likely to need a specific self-soothing strategy such as a safe place visualization to help manage the stress response to an upcoming medical procedure. While the usual cautions prevail (e.g., confirming the client's ability to use social supports and change states), the fact that EMDR therapy does not demand detailed descriptions of the event or homework assignments means that preparation time can be adjusted accordingly. Since all treatment takes place in-session with the regulating presence of the therapist, clients' readiness to commence processing can generally be determined by observing their level of arousal and capacity to manage and change emotional states when asked to bring up a distressing memory. This is particularly important since the diagnosis of complex PTSD usually assumes the presence of dissociative processes, as well as a pervasive belief that one is defective. The clinical challenge when processing traumatic memory networks in EMDR therapy is to manage the arousal states and potential peritraumatic dissociation by tracking the client's ongoing ability to maintain simultaneous awareness of past and present conditions, particularly during intense emotional responses. Since research has indicated that a single memory can generally be completely processed within three EMDR sessions (see research section), stability can also be enhanced through the use of extended or consecutive-day sessions to allow a rapid resolution of a highly disturbing targeted trauma, particularly in the early stages of therapy.

11.3.3 Addictions

A common conception of clinicians treating addictions is that clients must abstain from all of their prohibited substances before trauma treatment can commence. However, using the evaluation criteria discussed in the previous section, it has been reported that introducing targeted EMDR trauma reprocessing early on, before full abstinence is demonstrated, can reduce the client's emotional distress while increasing motivation and the capacity to respond to the treatment demands (Brown et al. 2011). Clients struggling with addiction often experience significant ambivalence and denial about the severity of their disorder, despite the fact that by the time they seek help, they have suffered major adverse consequences as a direct result of their destructive behaviors. As negative as these consequences can be, their addiction has also been a "solution" to otherwise unmanageable negative emotional states. Thus, clients experience both positive and negative effects from their substance abuse or other addictive/compulsive behaviors. For example, a woman suffering from an eating disorder may report it to be highly pleasurable for her to binge on sugary foods because she feels she is giving herself a "treat," which in turn results in a state of euphoria that can be as rewarding as a drug. This behavior also serves as an escape from the feelings of emotional pain and deprivation rooted in her childhood traumatic experiences. The avoidance of the underlying distress, coupled with euphoria, makes sugar consumption enormously compelling and difficult to resist, especially when she is guaranteed to feel good every time she binges. The Adverse Childhood Experience study (Felitti et al. 1998) demonstrated a strong correlation between early adverse life experiences and later health problems, including addictive behaviors, which are maladaptive strategies for coping with the negative effects of these experiences. Therefore, processing the memories that are fueling the addiction is a high priority, as is uncoupling the appropriate need for positive affective states (to feel lovable, in control, confident) from the destructive addictive behaviors with which positive states have been inappropriately linked. Therefore, in addition to using the standardized EMDR three-pronged trauma processing protocol, the therapist should specifically target the urges and positive states associated with the addictive substance or activity while helping the client develop alternative healthier means of accessing the desired positive states to prevent a relapse.

11.3.4 Military Personnel

Combat veterans' exposure to trauma is rarely a single event, and hence the need for self-regulation skills is critical to effective treatment. They may also feel that the pain they are experiencing from the wartime experiences is an important way to honor the dead. This challenge can be dealt with by assuring them they will not forget and that EMDR therapy research indicates that processing the trauma memories actually results in greater positive recall of the deceased (Sprang 2001). Additionally, their need to maintain control over their circumstances is paramount, as they have often endured many situations where a loss of control resulted in serious consequences. Specific preparation time may be required with the combat veteran to allow the clinician and client to clearly establish the "rules of engagement" for the therapy to allow access to the difficult and sometimes unspeakable experiences of horror. The kinds of experiences that haunt veterans can include events in which they participated that resulted in one or more people being killed. Military personnel who observed or participated in acts that violated their personal values experience "moral injury" (Nash et al. 2013). While all acts of moral injury are hauntingly painful when they involve people being killed, it can be particularly challenging when these people are unarmed civilians such as women and children as an unintended consequence of military operations. Such distressing memories can haunt the veteran until treated. EMDR therapy is effective in treating shame, guilt, and other wounds of moral injury along with other aspects of combat trauma. However, shame over their involvement makes it challenging to address, especially because they will invariably be concerned about how the therapist will perceive them. In addition to demonstrating an open and nonjudgmental therapeutic stance, the clinician can assure veterans that with EMDR therapy, it is unnecessary for them to provide detailed descriptions of the event(s) for effective processing to occur.

Veterans are also challenged by their difficulty in distinguishing between real and perceived threats to their safety as they continue to suffer from the hyperarousal and hypervigilance that kept them alive in combat conditions. In these cases, it is often necessary to first address the intrusive symptoms (such as sleep-disrupting nightmares) that make it difficult to meet the demands of daily living. The nightmare image and accompanying affect can be directly targeted and processed, which generally results in an adaptive resolution of the dream and subsequent cessation of the nightmare. Additionally, those veterans suffering from phantom limb pain or medically unexplained physical complaints can often be relieved of these symptoms by directly targeting the traumatic event and the physical sensations associated with the somatic complaint (Russell and Figley 2012; Silver et al. 2008).

Another challenge in working with combat veterans is treating "anniversary reactions," where the client becomes acutely symptomatic leading up to an anniversary of a significant event. While such reactions are not unique to this population, it is almost a universal phenomenon in this group to "remember" significant events where people close to them died. This is compounded by the repeated admonition that soldiers "do not leave anyone behind." While facing the demands of their military service, veterans are frequently faced with lingering issues regarding the loss of friends either in combat operations or suicide afterwards. Anniversary dates involving grieving over the death of a battle buddy are further complicated by survivor's guilt, a sense of personal responsibility that a friend died while the veteran lived. The impact of such losses is amplified whenever there is a death of another comrade with whom they served. It is vital that the clinicians recognize this phenomenon and prioritize the events for treatment. These intense, emotional reactions can be averted if the event(s) associated with these losses can be reprocessed with EMDR therapy prior to the anniversary date itself. Further, since the emotional responses associated with anniversary dates may not be accompanied by visual cues, unexplained spikes in emotional lability should be traced back with EMDR memory retrieval techniques such as the affect scan to identify the needed targets. In addition, it is important to help the veteran identify another way to acknowledge the event by means of the future template such as honoring those who have died by writing a letter to them or volunteering at a soup kitchen.

11.4 Research

Over 20 randomized controlled trials (RCT) have demonstrated the effectiveness of EMDR therapy with a wide range of trauma populations, and it is designated an empirically supported PTSD treatment (e.g., World Health Organization 2013). Research has demonstrated that 84–100 % of single-trauma victims no longer have PTSD after the equivalent of three 90-min sessions (Marcus et al. 2004; Rothbaum 1997; Wilson et al. 1997). However, the appropriate dose of treatment varies with both the number of traumatic events and age of onset. For instance, in a study funded by Kaiser Permanente (Marcus et al. 2004), a mean of six 50-min sessions resulted in the remission of PTSD diagnoses in 100 % of single-trauma survivors, but only 77 % of multiple-trauma survivors. Similarly, after 12 sessions, 78 % of multiple-traumatized Vietnam veterans no longer had PTSD (Carlson et al. 1998), while earlier studies using only two sessions or treating only one memory produced only limited effects (Silver et al. 2008). An RCT comparing eight sessions of EMDR therapy and 8 weeks of fluoxetine (van der Kolk et al. 2007) recommended lengthier EMDR treatment for adults with childhood trauma. At a 6-month follow-up, 91.7 % of those EMDR participants in the adult-onset group had lost their PTSD diagnosis, as compared to 88.9 % of those in the child-onset group. However, asymptomatic end-state functioning was achieved by 75 % of EMDR participants with adult-onset trauma, compared to only 33.3 % with childhood trauma (and no participants in the fluoxetine group). These findings underscore the value of more extensive targeting and reprocessing for adults with child-onset complex PTSD in order to sufficiently address the comprehensive clinical picture, due to the pervasive nature of early experiences as well as the time needed for them to develop a healthier sense of self (see Shapiro 2001; Wesselmann et al. 2012).

A recent meta-analysis (Lee and Cuijpers 2013) examined the 26 RCT that compared the eye movement component of EMDR therapy to an exposure condition while participants concentrated on a disturbing memory. Pre/post differences demonstrated significantly greater declines in the eye movement condition on standardized outcome measures, negative emotions and imagery vividness. These findings indicate that the eye movements used in EMDR therapy contribute to the positive treatment effects and the processing of emotional memories. Three dominant hypotheses regarding the mechanism of action underlying the eye movements that have received research support (Schubert et al. 2011) are that they (a) tax working memory, (b) elicit an orienting response causing parasympathetic activation, and (c) link into the same processes that occur during rapid eye movement sleep. The various documented memory effects (e.g., emotional de-arousal, increased recognition of true information, episodic retrieval) suggest that the three mechanisms appear to come into play at different times in the therapy process. Therefore, clinicians may observe a rapid decrease in emotional disturbance, reduction in the vividness of the trauma image, emergence of associated memories, and increased insight along with the spontaneous emergence of positive emotions and beliefs.

All but one out of ten RCT have reported that EMDR therapy is equivalent or superior on some measures to exposure-based CBT, with five demonstrating more rapid treatment effects (for review, see Shapiro 2014). Therefore, the fact that EMDR, unlike CBT, requires no homework, detailed descriptions of the event, or extended exposures suggests that different neurophysiological memory processes are responsible for the therapeutic outcomes of the two approaches. As previously noted, research has indicated that the extended exposures used in TF-CBT result in extinction, creating a new memory and leaving the original memory intact, while short exposures, as used in EMDR therapy, result in reconsolidation (Suzuki et al. 2004), in which the original memory is stored in altered form. This difference has important clinical implications, as reconsolidation may explain certain treatment outcomes that occur for EMDR but not for exposure-based therapies. For instance, a recent open trial (van den Berg and van den Gaag 2012) reported that six sessions of EMDR trauma processing with psychotic patients resolved PTSD in 77 % of the patients and had "a positive effect on auditory verbal hallucinations, delusions, anxiety symptoms, depression symptoms, and self-esteem" (p. 664). The majority of patients initially suffering from auditory hallucinations were free of them by the end of treatment. The researchers noted that, in contrast, CBT treatments with this population result in a continuation of auditory hallucinations, although with less distress.

Other research has found that EMDR therapy processing of the trauma memory causes a substantial reduction or complete elimination of phantom limb pain (e.g., de Roos et al. 2010). The explanation for why no such observation has been reported for CBT may lie in the fact that the memory changes produced by EMDR entail reconsolidation, rather than extinction. As discussed previously, clinical problems, according to the AIP model, have their basis in the physiologically stored perceptions (images, thoughts, beliefs, emotions, sensations, smells, etc.) of the critical event, which remain encoded in the unprocessed memory. It follows that if the dysfunctionally stored memory is successfully processed and reconsolidated, the physical sensations will no longer be present. This conclusion was further supported in a study by Ricci et al. (2006) with a group of child molesters who had themselves been sexually assaulted in childhood. They found that EMDR therapy processing of the perpetrators' trauma memories resulted in both increased empathy for their victims and a substantial decrease in deviant arousal, as measured by penile plethysmography. This outcome was maintained at 1-year follow-up. Such results are predicted by the AIP (Shapiro 2001, 2012a) model guiding EMDR therapy. As illustrated in the previous clinical transcripts, the trauma memory is transmuted during EMDR therapy to an adaptive resolution, along with spontaneous changes in affective, cognitive, and somatic domains. It is posited that the transformation of the original distressing episodic memory through integration and reconsolidation eliminates the overt symptoms, which would otherwise persist if the original memory remains intact.

As indicated previously, research has supported the AIP tenet that adverse life experiences not rising to the level of full-blown trauma are also a major source of PTSD symptoms (Mol et al. 2005). Therefore, a thorough evaluation of such experiences should be conducted with clients who present with symptoms such as depression, emotional volatility, hypervigilance, and anxiety (Shapiro 2014). Research has demonstrated the successful treatment of such experiences within three EMDR therapy sessions. For instance, Wilson et al. (1997) reported that equivalent effects were found in a mixed sample when comparing those with and those without full PTSD diagnoses, with an 84 % remission for those who met full criteria at pretest.

Since EMDR therapy does not involve homework or the need to describe the traumatic memory in detail, it has been reported to be particularly beneficial for patients in physical rehabilitative services (e.g., Arabia et al. 2011). In addition to the rapid decline in depression and trauma symptoms, a significant change in trait anxiety was observed. It was posited that EMDR therapy would be particularly amenable for patients debilitated by cardiac conditions, since the eye movements have been correlated with physiological calming due to parasympathetic activation (e.g., Schubert et al. 2011). RCT have demonstrated that subjective distress significantly declines during the initial EMDR therapy sessions, in contrast to increases in exposure-based therapy (e.g., Rogers et al. 1999).

Research has also indicated that EMDR therapy is effective for both acute and chronic PTSD subsequent to both natural and manmade disasters (e.g., Jarero and Uribe 2012; Silver et al. 2005). Field teams of therapists have successfully treated victims with consecutive-day sessions and with a single extended session of 90–120 min. EMDR therapy group protocols have also been effective for both adults and children (e.g., Fernandez et al. 2004). Research has indicated the need of efficient and effective treatment for such populations worldwide.

References

Arabia, E., Manca, M. L., & Solomon, R. M. (2011). EMDR for survivors of life-threatening cardiac events: Results of a pilot study. *Journal of EMDR Practice and Research, 5*, 2–13.

Brown, S. H., Stowasser, J. E., & Shapiro, F. (2011). Eye movement desensitization and reprocessing (EMDR): Mental health-substance use. In D. B. Cooper (Ed.), *Intervention in mental health-substance use* (pp. 165–193). Oxford: Radcliffe.

Carlson, J., Chemtob, C. M., Rusnak, K., Hedlund, N. L., & Muraoka, M. Y. (1998). Eye movement desensitization and reprocessing (EMDR): Treatment for combat-related post-traumatic stress disorder. *Journal of Traumatic Stress, 11*, 3–24.

Cloitre, M., Cohen, L. R., & Koenen, K. C. (2006). *Treating survivors of childhood abuse: Psychotherapy for the interrupted life*. New York: Guilford Press.

Craske, M., Herman, D., & Vansteenwegen, D. (Eds.). (2006). *Fear and learning: From basic processes to clinical implications*. Washington, DC: APA Press.

de Roos, C., Veenstra, A., de Jongh, A., den Hollander-Gijsman, M., van der Wee, N., Zitman, F., & van Rood, Y. R. (2010). Treatment of chronic phantom limb pain (PLP) using a trauma-focused psychological approach. *Pain Research and Management, 15*, 65–71.

Felitti, V. J., Anda, R. F., Nordenberg, D., Williamson, D. F., Spitz, A. M., Edwards, V., Koss, M. P., & Marks, J. S. (1998). Relationship of childhood abuse and household dysfunction to many of the leading causes of death in adults: The adverse childhood experiences (ACE) study. *American Journal of Preventive Medicine, 14*, 245–258.

Fernandez, I., Gallinari, E., & Lorenzetti, A. (2004). A school- based EMDR intervention for children who witnessed the Pirelli building airplane crash in Milan, Italy. *Journal of Brief Therapy, 2*, 129–136.

Gómez, A. M. (2012). *EMDR therapy and adjunct approaches with children: Complex trauma, attachment and dissociation.* New York: Springer.

Jarero, I., & Uribe, S. (2012). The EMDR protocol for recent critical incidents: Follow-up report of an application in a human massacre situation. *Journal of EMDR Practice and Research, 6*, 50–61.

Lee, C. W., & Cuijpers, P. (2013). A meta-analysis of the contribution of eye movements in processing emotional memories. *Journal of Behavior Therapy and Experimental Psychiatry, 44*, 231–239.

Marcus, S., Marquis, P., & Sakai, C. (2004). Three- and 6-month follow-up of EMDR treatment of PTSD in an HMO setting. *International Journal of Stress Management, 11*, 195–208.

Mol, S. S. L., Arntz, A., Metsemakers, J. F. M., Dinant, G., Vilters-Van Montfort, P. A. P., & Knottnerus, A. (2005). Symptoms of post-traumatic stress disorder after non-traumatic events: Evidence from an open population study. *British Journal of Psychiatry, 186*, 494–499.

Nash, W. P., et al. (2013). Psychometric evaluation of the moral injury events scale. *Military Medicine, 178*, 646–652.

Ricci, R. J., Clayton, C. A., & Shapiro, F. (2006). Some effects of EMDR treatment with previously abused child molesters: Theoretical reviews and preliminary findings. *Journal of Forensic Psychiatry and Psychology, 17*, 538–562.

Rogers, S., Silver, S. M., Goss, J., Obenchain, J., Willis, A., & Whitney, R. L. (1999). A single session, group study of exposure and eye movement desensitization and reprocessing in treating posttraumatic stress disorder among Vietnam War veterans: Preliminary data. *Journal of Anxiety Disorders, 13*, 119–130.

Rothbaum, B. O. (1997). A controlled study of eye movement desensitization and reprocessing in the treatment of post-traumatic stress disordered sexual assault victims. *Bulletin of the Menninger Clinic, 61*, 317–334.

Russell, M. C., & Figley, C. R. (2012). *Treating traumatic stress injuries in military personnel: An EMDR practitioner's guide.* New York: Routledge.

Schubert, S. J., Lee, C. W., & Drummond, P. D. (2011). The efficacy and psychophysiological correlates of dual-attention tasks in eye movement desensitization and reprocessing (EMDR). *Journal of Anxiety Disorders, 25*, 1–11.

Shapiro, F. (2001). *Eye movement desensitization and reprocessing: Basic principles, protocols, and procedures* (2nd ed.). New York: Guilford Press.

Shapiro, F. (2012a). *Getting past your past.* New York: Rodale.

Shapiro, F. (2012b). *EMDR therapy training manual.* Watsonville: EMDR Institute.

Shapiro, F. (2014). The role of eye movement desensitization & reprocessing (EMDR) therapy in medicine: Addressing the psychological and physical symptoms stemming from adverse life experiences. *The Permanente Journal, 18*, 71–77.

Shapiro, F., Kaslow, F., & Maxfield, L. (Eds.). (2007). *Handbook of EMDR and family therapy processes.* Hoboken: Wiley.

Silver, S. M., Rogers, S., Knipe, J., & Colelli, G. (2005). EMDR therapy following the 9/11 terrorist attacks: A community-based intervention project in New York City. *International Journal of Stress Management, 12*, 29–42.

Silver, S. M., Rogers, S., & Russell, M. C. (2008). Eye movement desensitization and reprocessing (EMDR) in the treatment of war veterans. *Journal of Clinical Psychology: In Session, 64*, 947–957.

Solomon, R. M., & Shapiro, F. (2008). EMDR and the adaptive information processing model: Potential mechanisms of change. *Journal of EMDR Practice and Research, 2*, 315–325.

Sprang, G. (2001). The use of eye movement desensitization and reprocessing (EMDR) in the treatment of traumatic stress and complicated mourning: Psychological and behavioral outcomes. *Research on Social Work Practice, 11*, 300–320.

Stickgold, R. (2002). EMDR: A putative neurobiological mechanism of action. *Journal of Clinical Psychology, 58*, 61–75.

Suzuki, A., Josselyn, S. A., Frankland, P. W., Masushige, S., Silva, A. J., & Kida, S. (2004). Memory reconsolidation and extinction have distinct temporal and biochemical signatures. *Journal of Neuroscience, 24*, 4787–4795.

Wesselmann, D., Davidson, M., Armstrong, S., Schweitzer, C., Bruckner, D., & Potter, A. E. (2012). EMDR as a treatment for improving attachment status in adults and children. *European Review of Applied Psychology, 62*, 223–230.

Wilson, S., Becker, L. A., & Tinker, R. H. (1995). Eye movement desensitization and reprocessing (EMDR): Treatment for psychologically traumatized individuals. *Journal of Consulting and Clinical Psychology, 63*, 928–937.

Wilson, S., Becker, L. A., & Tinker, R. H. (1997). Fifteen-month follow-up of eye movement desensitization and reprocessing (EMDR) treatment of post-traumatic stress disorder and psychological trauma. *Journal of Consulting and Clinical Psychology, 65*, 1047–1056.

World Health Organization. (2013). *Guidelines for the management of conditions that are specifically related to stress.* Geneva: WHO.

van den Berg, D. P. G., & van den Gaag, M. (2012). Treating trauma in psychosis with EMDR: A pilot study. *Journal of Behavior Therapy and Experimental Psychiatry, 43*, 664–671.

van der Kolk, B., Spinazzola, J., Blaustein, M., Hopper, J., Hopper, E., Korn, D., & Simpson, W. (2007). A randomized clinical trial of EMDR, fluoxetine and pill placebo in the treatment of PTSD: Treatment effects and long-term maintenance. *Journal of Clinical Psychiatry, 68*, 37–46.

Narrative Exposure Therapy (NET): Reorganizing Memories of Traumatic Stress, Fear, and Violence

12

Thomas Elbert, Maggie Schauer, and Frank Neuner

this is my story, I am

12.1 The Theoretical Basis of NET: Trauma-Related Disorders Are Disorders of Memory

The question "Who are we and how did we become what we are?" has remained one of the oldest questions of mankind. We can ask this question in a somewhat different manner: what shapes us as individuals and what are our cultural memories? Evolution has equipped us with various forms of memory, however, only to handle the future not the past. To imagine future scenarios, our mind can reshuffle the memory traces of experiences in playing and replaying past and future scenarios. Memory thus means remodeling the mind and body in order to adapt to a future that is to be expected on the basis of past experience. With any ability to adapt, however, one runs the risk of becoming inept. For example, it may not be adaptive for stored carbohydrates to be converted into blood sugar for a soldier who, at a family picnic, spends the entire evening hiding under a pickup truck because the fireworks remind him of the battles that he fought in Afghanistan. While earlier psychological models of PTSD had characterized such symptoms primarily as a disorder of anxiety, a radical change occurred at the turn of the century, with trauma-related symptoms coming to be understood as

T. Elbert (✉)
Department of Psychology, Clinical Psychology and Behavioural Neuroscience,
University of Konstanz, Konstanz, Germany
e-mail: Thomas.Elbert@Uni-Konstanz.de

M. Schauer
Department of Psychology, Clinical Psychology and Centre for Psychotraumatology,
University of Konstanz, Konstanz, Germany
e-mail: Maggie.Schauer@Uni-Konstanz.de

F. Neuner
Department of Psychology, Clinical Psychology and Psychotherapy,
University of Bielefeld, Bielefeld, Germany
e-mail: Frank.Neuner@Uni-Bielefeld.de

© Springer International Publishing Switzerland 2015
U. Schnyder, M. Cloitre (eds.), *Evidence Based Treatments for Trauma-Related Psychological Disorders: A Practical Guide for Clinicians*,
DOI 10.1007/978-3-319-07109-1_12

a disorder of memory (Ehlers and Clark 2000; Brewin and Holmes 2003). Memories are formed from emotionally arousing experiences, that is, those with strong positive or negative valence, activating either approach or avoidance responses. And they then develop their own intrinsic dynamics, not only driven by the original experiences themselves but also by the memories thereof, thus remodeling cognition, emotion, and behavior to the extent that clinical symptoms may arise. From episodic threats to social exclusion to the continuous wear and tear associated with living in adverse situations, stressors not only cause a set of responses but also modify the body's defensive systems. In other words, we argue that a disordered memory representation lies at the core of posttraumatic stress disorder (PTSD) and that, for a therapeutic intervention to be successful, it must initiate a process of self-regulation. This self-regulation of memory paves the way for a reorganization of the individual, a development that continues well after treatment and eventually results in healing.

We will therefore, in this chapter, first present the specific structure of traumatic memories before we present the logic of NET and then detail its procedure. Finally, we will present a case as an example.

12.1.1 The Structure of Traumatic Memories

During a traumatic event, mainly sensory and perceptual information (e.g., the sound of gunshots, the smell of blood) is stored in memory. The mind and body become extremely aroused (rapid heartbeat, sweating, trembling) and are braced for actions such as hiding, fighting, or escape. The sensory elements, together with the related cognitive emotional and physiological responses, then form associations in memory related to the traumatic experiences. We refer to the storage of this information as *hot memory* (Metcalfe and Jacobs 1996; Elbert and Schauer 2002; it has also been termed situationally accessible memory, or sensory perceptual representation; see Brewin et al. 2010; Schauer et al. 2011; Neuner et al. 2008a). For a new type of experience, this hot memory is connected to the contextual information, the *cold memory* (which has been referred to also as verbally accessible memory or contextual representation): the individual will remember the event within its context, that is, where and when it has happened. Repeatedly experiencing similar types of events fosters a generalization of their memory representation. Therefore, evolution has prearranged the organization of memory such that sensory and emotional experiences are stored in brain circuits separate from those relevant for contextual information. Following principles of associative learning, any important experience is stored in an interconnected neural network, which, for repeated adversities, may establish a "trauma network" (Fig. 12.1). This trauma network encompasses sensory, cognitive, and physiological representations and includes the emotional response related to the experience (hot memory). In PTSD, the hot memories have lost their association to the contextual cold memory system (Fig. 12.1). Environmental stimuli (e.g., a smell or noise) and internal cues (e.g., a thought) can still activate the trauma structure. The ignition of just a few elements in the network may be sufficient for activating the whole structure. The survivor will experience this as intrusive recollection or even a "flashback," that is, the perception that one is back in the traumatic situation with its sound of bullets, smell of fire, feeling of fear, defensive response propositions, and thoughts (Fig. 12.1).

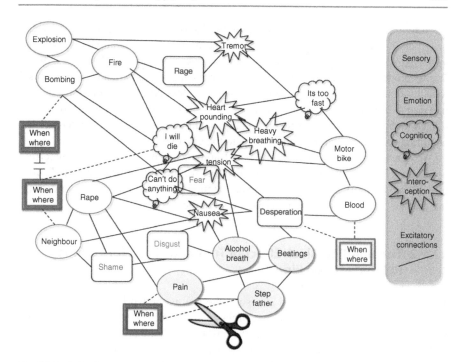

Fig. 12.1 A fear/trauma network is composed of mutually excitatory connections. It results from multiple fearful experiences: the representation of a single event may well connect to the particular context, the "when" and "where" it happened. If, however, an additional stressful experience cues an already existing network of traumatic hot memories, the connection to the cold memory is lost, while sensory, cognitive, emotional, and physiological representations interconnect with increasingly mutual excitatory power. Cold, contextual memories, that is, codes of the "where" and "when," however, are not consistently co-activated as the brain's architecture does not support the simultaneous activation of two different places (coded by "place cells" in the hippocampus) (Elbert et al. 2006). Thus the fear/trauma network becomes disconnected (symbolized by the scissors) from time and place, and the fear generalizes, giving rise to feelings of impending threat. Narrative Exposure Therapy is thought to reverse this process by reconnecting hot and cold memories while segregating the memory traces of the different events (Figure modified from Schauer and Elbert 2010)

Since the activation of the trauma network serves as a frightening and painful recollection, many PTSD patients learn to avoid cues that act as reminders of the traumatic event. They attempt not to think or talk about any part represented in the trauma network and to stay away from persons and places that remind them of the frightening event. In contrast to their prominent hot trauma memories, survivors who suffer from PTSD have difficulties with autobiographical cold context; that is, they are unable to orient the fear associated with the events appropriately in time and space or to clearly structure these traumatic events in chronological order (Schauer et al. 2011). Such challenges, in conjunction with the avoidance of activating the trauma structure, make it difficult for PTSD patients to narrate their traumatic experiences (Neuner et al. 2008a). It is likely that these mechanisms of traumatic memories are not restricted to PTSD. Individuals suffering from other anxiety disorders, depression, or eating disorders frequently also report repeated vivid intrusive recollections abounding in highly distressful content but lacking cold memory contextual elements (Brewin et al. 2010).

Note that the network connects to response dispositions (= emotions), which can be either an alarm response involving fight and flight or a dissociative response (up to the extent of fainting, i.e., playing dead; Schauer and Elbert 2010). Thus, dissociative amnesia or "shutdown" can occur, replacing intrusions and hyperarousal with dissociation and passive avoidance. Both response types are evolutionarily prepared, and a patient may show either one, depending on the cues that activate the related memory. Narrative Exposure Therapy is thought to reverse these detrimental conditions by strengthening connections to the context.

We conclude that repeated exposure to traumatic events results in the distortion of not merely the content of events but also the overarching organization and structure of both memory storage and retrieval; the more seriously threatening or damaging the survived experiences, the greater degree the disorganization.

12.1.2 The Building Block Effect of Traumatic Load for Trauma-Related Mental Illness

With cumulative adversities and stressors, the trauma network becomes enlarged, ultimately leading to forms of trauma-related suffering (Fig. 12.1): survivors are unable to contextualize cues, and thus the past becomes the present. The writer and Holocaust survivor Primo Levo describes such experiences in his work *The Truce:* "...I am sitting... in a peaceful relaxed environment, apparently without tension or affliction; yet I feel a deep and subtle anguish, the definite sensation of an impending threat. And in fact ..slowly and brutally.. everything collapses, and disintegrates around me, the scenery, the walls, the people, while the anguish becomes more intense and more precise. I am alone in the centre of a grey and turbid nothing, and I know what this thing means, and I also know that I have always known it: *I am in the Lager* (death camp).., *and nothing is true outside the Lager. All the rest was a brief pause, a deception of the senses, a dream.*"

All symptoms of traumatic stress (PTSD) and depression have repeatedly been shown to correlate in their severity with the cumulative exposure to traumatic stress (Mollica et al. 1998; Neuner et al. 2004a; Kolassa and Elbert 2007; Kolassa et al. 2015, Chap. 4). More recently it has become obvious that childhood adversity is the other major dimension in predicting trauma-related mental illness (Catani et al. 2009b,c, 2010; Neuner et al. 2006; Nandi et al. 2014).

12.2 The Rationale and Logic of NET

Given the structure of traumatic memory representations, the goal of an etiologically oriented trauma therapy must be to reconnect hot and cold memory, focusing on the most arousing experiences. Therefore, in NET, the client, with the assistance of the therapist, constructs a chronological narrative of her/his life story with a focus on the traumatic experiences. Within a predefined number, usually about 4–12, of 90 min sessions, the fragmented reports of the traumatic experiences will be transformed into a coherent narrative. Empathic understanding, active listening, congruency, and unconditional positive regard are key components of the therapist's behavior and attitude. For traumatic stress experiences the therapist explores sensory information, resulting cognitions, affective and physiological responding in detail and probes for respective observations. The patient is encouraged to relive these experiences while narrating, without losing the connection to the "here and now." Using permanent reminders that the feelings and physiological responses result from activation of (hot) *memories*, the therapist links these mnemonic representations to episodic facts, that is, time and place (cold memory). The imagined exposure to the traumatic past is not terminated until the related affection, especially the fear presented by the patient, demonstrably decreases. In this way, the therapist is supportive yet directive in eliciting the narrative in order to recover the implicit information of the trauma in its entirety. For survivors of domestic or organized violence, the testimony can be recorded and used for documentary purposes.

After an assessment of the individual's mental health status, a *psychoeducational introduction* is presented to the survivor, focusing on the explanation of his or her disturbance and symptoms, and, if appropriate a statement about the universality of human rights, followed by an outline of the treatment rationale tuned to the cognitive capacity of the survivor (age, formal education, etc.).

Narrative Exposure Therapy then starts with a biographical overview of the life span. Figure 12.2 schematically indicates the goal of the therapist: to determine arousal peaks across the life span. Lifetime periods and important biographical events of the survivor are symbolized in a ritual called *the lifeline*. The *lifeline* exercise consists of placing positive and negative life events, symbolized by flowers and stones, along a "line" (e.g., rope) in chronological order. With the guidance of the therapist, the patient places the symbols next to the line while classifying them only briefly – just a label will do. The purpose of the *lifeline* is the reconstruction of subjectively significant life events in their chronological order. An initial, cursory overview of the times and locations in which events occurred within the overarching context of the individual's life, it serves as introduction to the logic of the therapeutic process. The therapist asks questions concerning the "when" and "where" an event took place, that is, focuses on cold memory and moves on before hot memory contents become strongly activated. The therapist attends to the body language of the patient. When the patient shows any signs of emotional arousal or begins to recall pictures or other sensations, the therapist reminds the patient that a detailed processing and narration of the event will be constructed later, beginning in the next session. The lifeline exercise should be concluded within one session. Otherwise an avoidance conspiracy between client and therapist may delay the essential healing agent, that is, the imagined exposure of the traumatic experience.

In the next session, the narration starts with essential background information and then the earliest arousing events in life and continues sequentially over time. A pre-trauma period may be used as the time during which a foundation for the therapeutic core process is laid and a good rapport between therapist and patient is established. In this phase, for example, the telling of emotional, warm, or exciting moments in the patient's early life offers themselves as a training ground for emotional processing and communication between the patient and therapist.

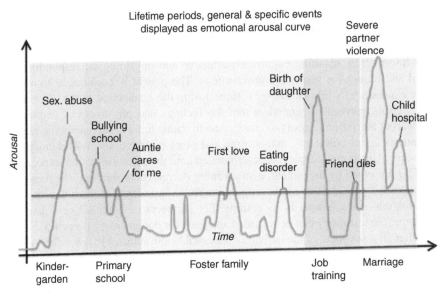

Fig. 12.2 Emotional arousal varies greatly across the life span. The lifeline exercise marks the arousal peaks above a threshold with a symbol, negative valence with a stone and positive valence with a flower, and assigns them to a place (e.g., "hometown") and a time, ideally a specific event (like "the night before my 12th birthday") or at least a general event ("when my uncle visited us"). A life period (when I went to school, college; when I was working in New York) can always be assigned (for more details, see Schauer et al. 2011; Schauer and Ruf-Leuschner 2014)

During the narrative procedure, the survivor continues recounting his/her life story in chronological order. Wherever a "stone" (traumatic incident) occurs, the event is relived in a moment-by-moment reprocessing of the sensory, cognitive, emotional, and bodily details of the traumatic scenes, ensuring the interweaving of hot and cold memory elements, meaning-making, and integration. During the telling of the events, the therapist structures the topics and helps to clarify ambiguous descriptions. The therapist assumes an empathic and accepting role. Inconsistencies in the patient's report are gently pointed out and often resolved by raising in-depth awareness about recurring bodily sensations or thoughts. The patient is encouraged to describe the traumatic events with sensory details and to reveal the perceptions, cognitions, and emotions that had been experienced at that time. During or after the session, the therapist either writes down a version of the patient's narration or drafts brief notes next to the *lifeline* that has been sketched or photographed.

In the subsequent sessions, the autobiography is briefly repeated, now emphasizing the cold memories of the event. The patient may add details that may have been missed and that he/she feels are important. Then subsequent emotionally arousing peaks (the next stones and flowers) are processed, that is, additional traumatic experiences are added to the narration. The procedure is repeated in subsequent sessions until a final version of the patient's life span and complete biographical highlights are created.

There are several options for the closing session. The *lifeline* may be completed and used as review of the patient's life. In cases where the narration has been fully recorded in written form, the document may be read aloud to the patient. The patient, the translator, if present, and the therapist sign the lifeline and/or written narration. A copy of the signed document is handed to the patient. With the agreement or upon request of the patient, another copy may be passed on to lawyers or (in anonymized form) to human rights organizations as documentation of these events. In addition, rituals can be used to ease the mourning and grief. Lastly, the patient may be counseled how to go on with life and is potentially offered further, but now future-oriented sessions (such as adjusting to a new role for a refugee or coping with relationships for a battered woman).

12.3 NET Step by Step

The following procedure follows the treatment manual by Schauer et al. (2011).

12.3.1 Session 1: Diagnosis and Psychoeducation

Prior to the diagnostic assessment for trauma-related disorders, we recommend an extensive checklist of family violence and other traumatic stressors encompassing the entire life span. For adversities during childhood, we recommend the MACE (*Ma*ltreatment and *A*buse *C*hronology of *E*xposure) and for organized violence the vivo checklist (for both see Schauer et al. 2011; German version of the MACE in Isele et al. 2014). The checklists provide the therapist with an indication of the traumatic history of the patient and suggest which events might and should appear on the *lifeline*.

For survivors of trauma it is vital that they learn to conceptualize and understand their condition. Moreover, they need an explanation about the motivation of the therapist and her/his ability to listen to the worst stories ("I am here to assist people who have experienced extremely stressful conditions such as war (rape, forced migration, torture, massacre, natural disaster) and to document the human rights violations that have taken place. …. We hope to use what we learn from you to improve the way survivors of extreme stress are supported and respected in the future…").

If the person suffers from symptoms of trauma-related illness, it is advisable to proceed with psychoeducation immediately following the diagnosis. It is important to explain to the patient that alarm and/or dissociative responses are part of the defense repertoire of all humans and that trauma symptoms result when extreme and harmful events have been repeatedly experienced. Explain that memories of the trauma are intrusive memories, which may be triggered by single sensory cues, or internal states, in the mind and body. Provide information that these intrusions are perceived as a current threat, keeping the survivor in a state of vigilance as long as the trauma remains unresolved. The intrusive pictures, sounds, and smells, together with the feelings they elicit, require conscious processing before they can be assigned to the past. This will occur during the course of therapy. The therapeutic procedure is outlined to the patient as an offer. At times, some patients believe that they are an "ill-fated creation of God" or "cursed" and are unworthy of treatment. The reasoning that documentation of human rights violations alone justifies the joint effort involved in therapy is often helpful in these cases. Others found joy in the violence they committed and were proud of the team spirit in gangs or armed groups. There are several reasons that a survivor might feel ashamed or guilty or believe that the therapist will not like what they hear about certain details of the individual's life. As the therapist, it is important to assure the individual that they have the professional skill to support testifying and that their main job is to provide a beneficial experience, regardless of the details, controversial or otherwise.

12.3.2 Session 2: The Lifeline Exercise

The *lifeline* in NET displays the emotional highlights of the individual's life in a ritualized and symbolic way. Hereby the survivor places objects that symbolise major events along a rope or string that symbolizes the continuous flow of biographical time (Fig. 12.3). Flowers designate happy major events and the good times in life, for example, for positive, empowering occurrences; moments of achievement; important relationships; experiences of bliss and acceptance. In this way, flowers can serve as resources. Stones symbolize fearful ordeals, especially

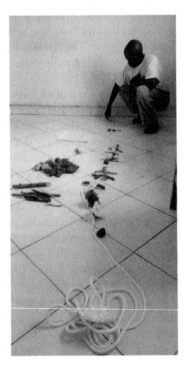

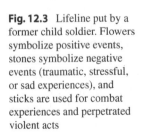

Fig. 12.3 Lifeline put by a former child soldier. Flowers symbolize positive events, stones symbolize negative events (traumatic, stressful, or sad experiences), and sticks are used for combat experiences and perpetrated violent acts

traumatizing experiences such as life-threatening events or anything that triggers an alarm response or evokes a dissociative response, like abuse, rape, assault, injury or harm, captivity, natural disasters, accidents, etc. Survivors usually also place stones for difficult moments in life, such as times of hardship (divorce, dismissal, sickness). While further symbols may complicate the exercise – flowers – stones carry a clear message and give structure. Nevertheless, additional symbols may meet the needs for special cases: For very sad experiences that cause continuous grief, like the death of a loved one, a candle can be placed and lit. Criminal offenders or perpetrators committing violent acts may not necessarily be of negative valence, and thus a stone may not be an appropriate symbol, neither would a flower be adequate for victory after a massacre. A more neutral symbol may thus be introduced for these cases: we use a small stick to symbolize participation in any form of aggression or violence, including combat (Elbert et al 2012; Hermenau et al. 2013; Crombach and Elbert 2014). It is good to offer a variety of differently sized, colored, and shaped stones and flowers, so as to give choices for the representation of events.

When the rope/string is put on the floor, the therapist encourages the individual to start placing the symbols along the line. The therapist guides the patient to name and mark important events and turns in life, following a chronological order. For each arousing event, the questions "when?" "where?" and "what?" should be answered with only a few words, without going into the details (e.g., "in secondary school, living in my hometown, I was raped by my neighbor," "a few months ago, living here in this town, a car hit me," "during the birth of my first child named 'Jonnie,'" "at the hospital, I was forced to undergo a Cesarean section," etc.). The therapist affixes a name to each symbol and notes the where and when. Clear brief naming of the symbol and appropriating it a title is important to build confidence in approaching the hot memories. However, it is crucial to not go any deeper at this point, as the lifeline exercise is not the designated time to begin confronting the content of the event. During this stage of the lifeline procedure, the therapist guides the individual in staying on the *cold memory* side (questions focus on facts, names, dates, etc., rather than on emotions, sensations, physiology, etc.). The lifeline exercise is only an *overview* of important life events – a "roadmap." In this regard, it is helpful to settle and cool down after each symbol placement, especially stones, before placing the next event. The focus remains on the "when?" – naming the lifetime period – and "where?" not on the "what?" Otherwise, feelings "pile up" toward the end of the lifeline and emotions get mixed up and confused. In this way, the *lifeline* tool in *Narrative Exposure Therapy* is a useful first step toward discussing the traumatic material (Schauer and Ruf-Leuschner 2014; Schauer et al. 2014).

The *lifeline* was first introduced in trauma therapy with children: KIDNET (Schauer et al. 2004; Onyut et al. 2005) and continues to be utilized as such (Schaal et al. 2009; Catani et al. 2009a; Ruf et al. 2010; Ertl et al. 2012; Hermenau et al. 2012; Crombach and Elbert 2014). Later, the classic *lifeline* method was adopted in NET for different groups of adult survivors of multiple and complex trauma (Bichescu et al. 2007; Neuner et al. 2008b, 2010; Schaal et al. 2009; Halvorsen and Stenmark 2010; Hensel-Dittmann et al. 2011; Pabst et al. 2012, 2014; Stenmark et al. 2013), sometimes as a paper-and-pencil version, in which the patient marks the biographical highlights along the timeline on a piece of paper (Dōmen et al. 2012; Ejiri et al. 2012; Zang et al. 2013). There is clear evidence for the effectiveness of Narrative Exposure Therapy (NET) with the *lifeline* being included in the treatment plan. However, treatment success has also been confirmed for Narrative Exposure Therapy *without* the *lifeline* module (Neuner et al. 2004b; Schauer et al. 2006; Hijazi 2012) and also, alternatively, with the *lifeline* module at the end of the therapy (Zang et al. 2014). Conversely, clinical efficacy of the lifeline as a stand-alone procedure in the treatment of traumatized individuals has not been demonstrated and would not be predicted on the basis of the theoretical assumptions presented at the beginning of this chapter.

12.3.3 Session 3: The Narration

The narration begins during the third session, starting at the very beginning of life. The chronology of the narration should address the most arousing events of the patient. The family background should not be neglected: how the patient grew up, what the relationship to his parents was, and what other attachment figures and bonds played a role during the early stages of development ("When are you born and where? Who was bringing you up? Which people were your family? What did they tell you about your first years of life, before your own memory sets in? Any pictures, documents?"). Depending on the resources in terms of the amount of sessions, discussion of the pre-trauma period should remain limited, so as not to avoid narrating the more difficult material later on. Usually time is allocated to work through the first traumatic experience during the same double session (90–120 min) that the narration is initiated. Full expression of the fearful and defensive responding is desirable now during the imagined exposure, allowing for the individual to subsequently experience the reduction in arousal that occurs while narrating the period that followed the most threatening "hot spot."

The contextual information must first be clearly recollected, and then the event is reported in detail, and, finally, it is put into the past from its present perspective:

- *WHEN? Time and setting*: Establish *when* the incident took place. Lifetime period? Season of the year? Time of day?
- *WHERE? Location and activity*: Establish as precisely as possible *where* the incident took place. Where was the person at that time? Begin asking for sensory details of the scenery, the house, the road, etc.
- *WHAT? Begin the narration, when the arousal begins to rise.* Only then, the therapist shifts to *slow motion*. It may take some courage for both the client and the therapist to deliberately slow down and recall in detail what happened. The therapist supports the processing of the material by allowing the emotional responses to run their course. *Hot memory* (the associated elements of the fear/ trauma structure) is activated involving the following sequence: *sensation* (what did you see, hear, smell… body position…), *cognition* (what did you think?), *emotion* (what did you feel? Note that a therapist will not be able to understand

the feelings of a client, as long as the respective thoughts are not known), *physiological responses* (heartbeat, sweating, cold hands, etc.), and *meaning* content (Fig. 12.1). The therapist helps to put the hot memory into words and connect them to autobiographical flow, that is, fit them into the narrative. Basically, the therapist keeps pushing on until the experience, especially the emotions, have been put into words and the client starts to feel relief. Stopping anytime before that point is detrimental. The therapist has reached the goal, when a good movie could be made from the client's descriptions. For the therapist, it is a good idea to let this little film play in one's mind, although only as if moving together, shoulder by shoulder with the survivor through the scene.

- *NOW!* Let the patient contrast the past and present feelings together with the current bodily sensations: Individual: "At the time of the disaster, I felt horrified, now as I look back, I am getting sad." Therapist: "I can see you are sighing." "Your eyes are tearing up now." "Can you feel the fear in your body now? Where do you feel it?" This will allow the individual to develop better sensorial awareness. There is no need for hesitation when attempting to label the patient's affective responses: a patient will inform the therapist immediately if the feelings have been labeled incorrectly. Once the fear has been put into words, the client realizes that there is no current danger and that the source of arousal is the memory of a threat rather than an instant threat itself. Consequently, the arousal will decrease.

- After the arousal has noticeably reduced, be sure to bring the narrative to a close for this session. Even if time in the session is running out, it is of utmost importance to establish a clear ending to the traumatic event that has been worked on. The way to bring this closure is by transitioning to the time that occurred immediately following the event. To do this, the therapist wants to have the client verbalize in at least a few sentences what happened in the time period following the incident. In case it seems difficult to let go of the emotions of the imagined exposure, a question helpful for moving forward can be to ask how the survivor subsequently managed to live through the aftermath of this event (the hours, days, weeks, and months afterward). This strategy assists in transitioning from stress and discomfort of the hot memory toward session closure by aligning with the directionality of the NET lifeline to which the individual is already accustomed. It is important to clarify the time period following the traumatic event in order to enable the patient to integrate the incident into the greater life story. During "exposure," arousal and negative emotions are escalating. During "closure," arousal is decreasing, and the therapist supports this calming down process. Always be clear about the direction in which you are headed.

- *BOND!* The therapist attends to the healing of social pain. The warm, empathic, and nonjudgmental attitude of the therapist while processing the events allows for the healing of attachment wounds. This undertaking invites the establishment of corrective relationship experiences by revisiting old social pain situations in the presence and with the support of a therapeutic relationship.

Hence, the arc of tension within a session begins with storytelling prior to the trauma, proceeds to the details constituting the trauma itself, and then extends to the period occurring shortly after the traumatic event concludes. This allows for the trauma to be contextually situated and for the patient to orient the time and space, as well as the emotional and meaning context, of the event. Before drawing the session to a close, the therapist will ascertain through observation and questioning as to whether the patient's arousal level has subsided and that the individual once again has their bearings in the present reality.

12.3.4 Session 4 and Subsequent Sessions: Completing the Narration

In the subsequent session, the narrative elaborated in the previous session will be summarized, and the narration of subsequent life and traumatic events is continued. The number of sessions (usually 10–12) required depends on the setting and the severity of PTSD. In complex cases, e.g., in patients with borderline personality disorder, a greater number of sessions may be required (see the case presentation). However, a limit to the number of exposure sessions should be set early on so to circumvent avoidance or delaying of the narration of the worst events.

12.3.5 Cognitive Restructuring and the Days After

At the end of a session, patients often begin to reflect on the meaning content. A more formal *cognitive restructuring* process may be supported by explicitly pointing out the following:

- *New insights about the meaning of the event* for the patient's life. Patients may realize how the everyday emotions and unhealthy behavioral patterns (such as general anxiety, mistrust, rage, outbursts of anger) have their origins in the traumatic experience.
- The detailed narration leads to a *more thorough understanding of a person's behavior during the event*. This might help to modify feelings of guilt and shame.
- The recognition of interrelated life patterns and incidents, allowing integration.

Much of the beneficial process of increased awareness of what has happened takes place between sessions. When the therapist and patient meet again, the therapist should be open to positively receiving any thoughts and considerations the patient might have had since they last met.

12.3.6 Final Session of the NET Module

During the final session the events constituting the individual's life are reviewed as a contextualized and integrated narration. The patient might look at the narrative with a sense of distance (it's a sad but true story), or she/he might look at the document as a tool for peace building or educational purposes (awareness raising). Laying out the complete *lifeline* at the end of the NET treatment – this time including all the formerly inaccessible memories – enables the person to oversee the biographical work done and to perceive the "Gestalt" of the course of life. After the completion of the NET, patients are less preoccupied with their past and now focused on how to find their way back to life and how to construct a livable, productive future.

12.3.7 Follow-Up Period

Ideal times for evaluation are at 4–6 months and 1 year posttreatment. Over time, one can anticipate symptom remission to a degree at which PTSD is no longer diagnosable. NET initiates a healing process that requires months, if not longer, to fully unfold (see case presentation and Fig. 12.4).

12.3.8 Overview of the Therapeutic Elements of NET

Several elements of NET have been identified as contributing to its efficacy that the clinician may wish to keep in mind (c.f. Schauer et al. 2011). They are summarized below.

1. Active chronological reconstruction of the autobiographical/episodic memory
2. Extended exposure to the "hot spots" and full activation of the fear memory in order to modify the emotional network (i.e., learning to separate the traumatic memory from the conditioned emotional response and understanding triggers as cues, which are just temporarily associated) through detailed narration and imagination of the traumatic event
3. Meaningful linkage and integration of physiological, sensory, cognitive, and emotional responses to one's time, space, and life context (i.e., comprehension of the original context of acquisition and the reemergence of the conditioned responses in later life)
4. Cognitive reevaluation of behavior and patterns (i.e., cognitive distortions, automatic thoughts, beliefs, responses) as well as reinterpretation of the meaning content through reprocessing of negative, fearful, and traumatic events – completion and closure
5. Revisiting of positive life experiences for (mental) support and to adjust basic assumptions
6. Regaining of one's dignity through satisfaction of the need for acknowledgement through the explicit human rights orientation of "testifying"

Case Report

This case indicates that Narrative Exposure (NET) can be helpful also for individuals with complex PTSD which frequently include serious comorbid disorders, such as depression or borderline personality disorder (Pabst et al. 2012, 2014). While just a few sessions may be sufficient for survivors with limited exposure to traumatic stressors, such as survivors of natural disasters, more sessions are needed for those with complex trauma-related disorders.

When Sue S. sought treatment at our outpatient clinic, she was 33 years old. She had been referred with PTSD, recurrent major depression, and borderline personality disorder. Her symptoms were being managed with medication including SSRI and benzodiazepines. Medication was stable for more than 3 months. She had been unemployed for many years and was receiving support through social welfare. She had to be admitted to inpatient care frequently (several acute admissions per year). She had received repeated in- and outpatient treatment by experts for borderline personality disorder (largely DBT-based, but also cognitive interventions). Due to her severely compromised functionality, she was placed in an assisted living unit and assigned a state guardian and a social worker.

The previous therapist indicated that while Sue stated a desire to detail her traumatic experiences, she would not yet be stable enough to do so. The therapist recommended further stabilization prior to trauma-focused therapy. Self-injurious behavior, such as forearm cutting with a razor blade, anorexic, self-induced starvation, bulimic binging with gastrointestinal purging, and suicidal acts, were cited as reasons that no exposure therapy had been previously offered to the client. In addition, Sue was severely dissociative with spells of vasovagal shutdown syncope (Schauer and Elbert 2010), for example, during therapeutic group settings.

Procedure

After a detailed diagnosis that included a checklist of traumatic events and also childhood adversities (the MACE [*M*altreatment and *A*buse *C*hronology of *E*xposure] as listed in Schauer et al. 2011), psychoeducation prepared Sue for treatment with NET. Informed consent was obtained, and a pretreatment evaluation was conducted by an independent assessor, confirming a borderline personality disorder diagnosis, DSM-IV PTSD diagnostic criteria, and manageable suicidal ideation. There was no current substance abuse. At the beginning of treatment, Sue had been staying in an inpatient ward at the center for psychiatry for already 3 weeks. She had been admitted to emergency inpatient treatment due to her unstable conditions. The last documented serious suicide attempt was about one and a half years ago, and the interview revealed that Sue chronically suffered from suicidal ideations up to the current examination. At treatment beginning with Narrative Exposure Therapy, she still showed self-injurious behavior (in particular: cutting the skin of her arms and legs with sharp objects and anorectic eating patterns). Sue showed severe symptoms of dissociation with spells of fainting. After the sixth session she was released from the psychiatric ward and completed the treatment in an ambulatory setting.

Treatment

Treatment was delivered in 15, 90-min individual sessions conducted weekly over a 5-month period. Session 2 was devoted to the *lifeline* exercise (as described above). The *lifeline* was a new experience for Sue, initially piquing both interest and insecurity. Once settled into the process, she became fully engaged in the exercise but had obvious difficulties chronologically recalling and labeling biographical events. The therapist emphasized respective lifetime periods and explained that it would be sufficient in the first step to place the events of the most frequently intruding aversive memories (symbolized as stones) within their corresponding time periods. The therapist also reminded the patient to include any highlights (flowers) that could be recalled and suggested candles be used to symbolize losses and grief.

In session 3, the narration commenced and proceeded in chronological order throughout the subsequent 15 double sessions. Sue disclosed her most emotionally charged experiences, both positive and negative, beginning from her earliest memories. Along the way working through the periods of childhood and adolescence, Narrative Exposure was facilitated (different instances of childhood sexual abuse, being sold in child pornography and experiencing severe violence and social interpersonal victimization). Whenever dissociative detachment from reality or first signs of *tonic* or *flaccid immobility* occurred, the therapist grounded Sue using sensational and perceptional contrasting of the "here and now" (dual awareness) as well as motoric countermaneuvers. Active muscle tension appears the frontline treatment of reflex syncope, inducing significant blood pressure increase to avoid shutdown. Motor activation (using, e.g., applied muscle tension, leg crossing, external pressure to the lower extremities) helped Sue staying conscious with good enough circulatory function while working on her trauma material. In this way, the therapist responded to prodromal fainting symptoms by engaging in context-contrasting grounding activities to counteract the incipient syncope. Keeping a good contrast between the imagined trauma reality and the reality in the therapy room is an anti-dissociative strategy facilitated through continuous shifting of attention between the presence and the exposed scene by recalling reality and sensory stimulation during the exposure session, for example, tactile stimulation, presentation of positive fragrances like lemon or tasting samples like peppermint oil or chili gum, switching on bright light, allowing to notice the body position, letting describe the room, touch textures or feel the cold of an ice pack, leading attention to auditory stimuli (further practical examples to counter dissociation are presented in Schauer and Elbert 2010, p. 121).

Working through the biography from session to session, the complete testimony was transcribed by the therapist and read to the survivor, providing a full reprocessing without dissociation and adding more details to the traumatic scenes and their meaning contents, that is, most importantly, allowing integration by examining the intertwining of events and emotional contexts. Since Narrative Exposure Therapy aims at targeting all of the traumatic events (–types), a one-time narrating of the events and the active participation and engagement in the reexperiencing through rereading and complementing of the text often is enough. But some of Sue's experiences of sexual violence in prostitution were so horrific that a second extensive in sensu exposure in slow motion was needed to allow habituation and to complete a comprehensive narrative of the scene. After this, the therapy process proceeded chronologically along the lifeline heading toward the next symbol.

Whenever the patient seemed amnestic for an entire time period, the therapist carefully helped Sue explore the different contexts and spatial environments, that is, locations, rooms, and typical scenes (Example: "In which street did you live when you where 14 years old? How did the apartment/school/sports club look like? Let's walk through the rooms. What do you see? Let us open the doors. Which furniture is there? How does it smell? How do you feel in the environment?…"). In vivo exploration of these worlds of the past allows activation of the associative network elements (trauma/fear structure). Subsequently, in conjunction with an onset of physiological arousal, impressions and images appeared in Sue's mind. Once prompted to describe thoughts, feelings, and perceptions associated with these newly intruding images, typically the full trauma material evolved from disconnected "snapshots" into a fluid motion scene. The therapist in NET accompanied the patient step-by-step through the experience and assisted in verbalizing the accompanying emotions of the events in great detail. In this autobiographical context, Sue managed to retrieve memories of traumatic and sadistic abuse scenes that had taken place, and she was able to confront the material. She could reprocess the incidents and as well revisit the "flowers" (positive moments, successes, loving relationships, resources, etc.) of the different lifetime periods. Whenever we came to "candles" in the lifeline, she recounted how it was for her and what it meant to lose her dear grandmother and a beloved pet in childhood. All of these experiences were included in the autobiographical testimony of her life.

In the last session, Sue felt competent in delineating her *lifeline* once again. This time it was a much faster exercise; stones and flowers were quickly named and marked on small notes next to the symbols – divisions between major lifetime periods were also indicated. In addition, she added sticks as symbols for her delinquent acts. In a small ritual, the therapists handed a picture of the final *lifeline* and the transcription of the biography to a very proud survivor. In honor of her hopes for the future, Sue memorialized her accomplishments of the courageous recounting of the trauma with flowers, which she took home as a symbol of her hopes for the future.

Instruments

In addition to a complete pre- and follow-up diagnosis of an independent assessor from a different clinic, the following clinician-rated measures were incorporated to track the course of symptoms: PSSI (interview version of the posttraumatic diagnostic scale – PDS) for PTSD symptoms, the HSCL (Hopkins Symptom Checklist) for depressive and anxiety symptoms, the BSL (borderline symptom checklist), and the DES (Dissociative Experiences Scale) for dissociative symptoms.

Assessments were conducted pretreatment and across subsequent 3-month periods (as indicated in Fig. 12.4). The patient did not receive any monetary compensation.

Results and Discussion

The change in symptom scores from pretreatment to posttreatment and an extended follow-up period are illustrated in Fig. 12.4. A marked decline in response to treatment was observed for all measures. By 3 months posttreatment, the self-injurious behavior had completely ceased, and the eating behavior normalized. By 6 months, PTSD symptoms, including dissociative symptoms, largely subsided, and the borderline score indicated a substantial reduction in symptoms. The quality of life began to increase when Sue started to plan her future. To realize her goals, she utilized social assistance, allowing for her to find her own apartment and a job. After 3 years, an independent assessor confirmed that she no longer met criteria for any mental disorder, including borderline personality disorder or PTSD. Sue wrote to her NET therapist: "I am finally in my own flat, and things have worked out. I am doing quite well and like my job. I can go out shopping and meet my friends for coffee. I don't cling to people so much anymore. And the best part: I haven't fainted since and have never cut myself after I said goodbye to you. I am so glad that there are no more admissions to those psychiatric wards. Yes, I really enjoy my autonomous life. Although, sometimes I miss all the people that have helped me so much over the years. But, you know, it was their job. Now I found some real friends who hopefully like me for who I am!"

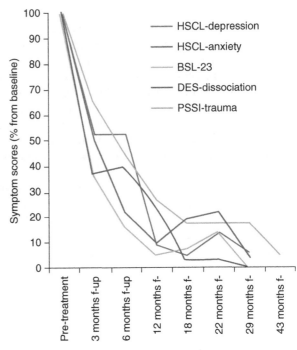

Fig. 12.4 Change in symptom scores (in %, baseline =100 %) during the follow-up period of survivor Sue S (*HSCL* Hopkins Symptom Checklist. *BSL* borderline symptom list, *PSSI* posttraumatic diagnostic scale – PDS – in interview form)

12.4 NET as an Evidence-Based Treatment

Results from more than a dozen treatment trials in adults and children have demonstrated the power of using NET in reducing the suffering of interpersonal or organized violence, as well as other disasters, for survivors. These stressors frequently produce detrimental effects in combination with childhood abuse and neglect, issues directly addressed in NET. By the very nature of NET, it is constructed to counter the impact of multiple and complex traumatic stress experiences that have occurred across an entire lifetime. NET provides a proven treatment option to complex trauma survivors (Pabst et al. 2012, 2014) and survivors of repeated torture as evidenced by large effect sizes (Hensel-Dittmann et al. 2011; Neuner et al. 2010). The most pronounced improvements are observed at follow-up, suggesting a sustained change in psychopathological symptoms, physical health, functioning, and quality of life. NET has effectively been applied in situations that remain volatile and insecure, such as in continuous trauma settings. It effectively reduces PTSD symptoms in the individual while bearing witness to the atrocities endured. A number of reviews identified NET as an evidence-based treatment, especially for survivors of violence (Robjant and Fazel 2010; Crumlish and O'Rourke 2010; McPherson 2012; Nickerson et al. 2011). A number of studies showing the effectiveness of NET have been independently conducted (Zang et al. 2013, 2014; Hijazi 2012; Gwozdziewycz and Mehl-Madrona 2013; Ejiri et al. 2012; Dōmen et al. 2012; Hijazi 2012; Hijazi et al. 2014), and thus, the NET procedure has been taken up in a variety of countries (e.g., Zech and Vandenbussche 2010; Jongedijk 2012, 2014). Manuals have appeared in print in Dutch, English, French, Italian, Japanese, Korean and Slovak.

An interesting strength for the evidence of NET is the validation of its effectiveness by means of markers from neurophysiology and molecular biology. Successful psychotherapeutic interventions reorganize memory and, with it, modify the architecture of the brain. Imaging of corresponding changes may indeed be possible, even on a macroscopic level: in a controlled trial, NET was compared to treatment as usual of traumatized asylum seekers (Schauer et al. 2006). The success was not only demonstrated in symptom scores but also in parameters of magnetic brain activity. During the 6-month follow-up, oscillatory neural activity in the NET group, but not in the control group, became more similar to that of healthy controls. Moreover, using magnetic source imaging of the brain, Adenauer et al. (2011) observed that NET causes an increase of activity associated with cortical top-down regulation of attention toward aversive pictures. The increase of attention allocation to potential threat cues obviously allowed treated patients to reappraise the actual danger of the current situation, thereby reducing PTSD symptoms.

PTSD is a well-documented risk factor for various somatic diseases, including chronic pain, cancer, cardiovascular, respiratory, gastrointestinal, and autoimmune diseases (Boscarino 2004; Kolassa et al. 2015). The poor physical health found in individuals with PTSD seems moderated by altered immune functions and inflammatory processes (Pace and Heim 2011). The study of Neuner et al. (2008b) indicated that NET reduced the frequencies of cough, diarrhea, and fever. Morath et al. (2014a) showed that symptom improvements were mirrored in an increase in the originally reduced proportion of regulatory T cells in the NET group at the 1-year follow-up. These cells are critical for maintaining balance in the immune system, regulating the immune response, and preventing autoimmune diseases. Moreover, NET is able to reverse in individuals with PTSD the increased levels of damaged DNA back to a normal level (Morath et al. 2014b). These findings may have implications for physical health, in particular for carcinogenesis. The reversibility of pathophysiological processes in individuals with PTSD via psychotherapy indicates that there is a therapeutic window not only to revert the psychological burden of the disease PTSD but also to reduce the long-term, and potentially lethal, somatic effects of this mental disorder. However, it should also be noted that other immune parameters (like the proportion of naïve T lymphocytes) have not changed and thus might render these patients more susceptible to infectious diseases across extended periods even after the completion of successful treatment.

Two decisive strengths of NET include its very low dropout rate and its high potential for dissemination, including to counselors in low-income countries and war and crisis regions (Catani et al. 2009a; Neuner et al. 2008b; Ertl et al. 2011; Jacob et al. 2014; Schauer and Schauer 2010). Stenmark et al. (2013) showed that with NET, in the case of central Norway, refugees as well as asylum seekers can be successfully treated for PTSD and depression in the general psychiatric health care system.

12.5 Challenges

Some survivors of childhood abuse, continuous trauma or personality disorders are utterly unable to retrieve reliable memories of their past. This often results from severe dissociative responding when attempting to retrieve autobiographical memories (Schauer and Elbert 2010). Laying the *lifeline* at the opening of the NET procedure therefore takes place without requiring completeness. It is worth the effort to attempt to structure the autobiography at the beginning of treatment, even when voluntary retrieving of hot memories is a serious challenge. The laying of the *lifeline* should be concluded within one session of up to 120 min, regardless of level of completion. Narration must begin in the following session for the following reasons: delaying the exposure may strengthen the avoidance and reject a patient who finally is prepared to talk about the worst drama. Alternatively, it is possible to start with the narration immediately and have the *lifeline* exercise only at the very end of the treatment (Zang et al. 2014).

Like any other imagined exposure procedure, dissociation as well as avoidance of either the client or the therapist, or both, may be a topic to be aware of. Furthermore, social (self-conscious) emotions such as shame, experiences of social pain, or feelings of guilt may cause a challenge for the narrative work. Particularly shame, with its confusion of mind, downward cast eyes and lowered head, but most of all its, silence and speechlessness may create a formidable challenge to any story telling. Pathological shame-proneness is ultimately the fear of being rejected and socially excluded because deep inside it feels impossible to meet the (moral) requirements of the community. A client thus hides everything deep inside as showing it will cause others to dislike and reject the individual. NET is then like a behavioral experiment: as a client reveals portions of the true inner self, she/he will expect rejection. The therapists respond with the opposite, showing true and honest compassion – that is, sets an inclusive social signal. At times, socially traumatized (e.g., raped) individuals may be so sensitive that they will suspect that the therapist may not be honest. Thus, shame caused by social threat cannot be treated by either exposure or compassion alone, but only by the combination of both. Attempts to cure shame with self-compassion will not work; individuals need to feel included by others not by themselves. Obviously, relief from shame requires knowledge of cultural values by the therapist.

If a patient is acutely intoxicated, abuses drugs, suffers from a severe, current eating disorder, or demonstrates an acute psychotic crisis, the facilitation of narrative exposure is neither possible nor advisable. Trials that start NET during detox are underway and case studies seem promising.

Ideally, a patient may have regularly eaten prior to a treatment session, and water is offered during the session. A therapist may routinely ask about nutrition.

Serious complications, such as an uncertain asylum status of refugees in the host country or living in a conflict zone with continuous traumatic stress conditions, do not necessarily undermine positive treatment outcomes. Even under unsafe conditions, survivors can benefit from narrative exposure treatment owing to the symptom remission and enhanced functionality. Repeated exposure to traumatic stressors, however, may negatively impact the longer-term outcome success.

Conclusion

The healing attributed to NET extends well beyond the alleviating of core PTSD symptoms. Empathic listening creates a unique and secure venue in which survivors can provide testimony and bear witness to human rights violations, contribute to collective memories via their individual narrative, and reap and confirm the benefits of autobiographical storytelling. These additional assets cumulate and pave the way to not only an honorable tribute to a survivor's experience but also the restoration of their dignity.

On a personal level, successful NET treatment can lead to quite practical changes and developments in an individual's life. While scientifically sound documentation of these changes remains a challenge, the informal evidence abounds: Former trauma inpatients go on to successfully complete job training. Go shopping in a crowded mall without panicking or fainting. Begin wearing skirts and earrings after decades of avoiding attention by hiding under bulky clothes. Meet friends at a public café after years of isolation. Establish a romantic relationship. Or even simply apply lotion to their body without feelings of disgust. Survivors may be able to experience moments of sudden joy again. Take a leisurely stroll out in nature. Or as one survivor put it in her own words: "... *It already helps to tell myself that the scary and unpleasant feelings probably have nothing to do with the current moment and perception. Already to explore the dates and time, when things happened gives me support and – finally – a feeling of identity! Even bad experiences, as long as you can locate them can give you the feeling of "this is my story, I am." Without that, every day is a gauntlet – and when a day gets worse, you have NOTHING to hold against it. If you have a past, this defuses immensely and it is a huge relief. Also to describe things reduces the bad feelings often truly enormous... And I keep on working through my own story...*"

Acknowledgment We greatly appreciate the editing and comments on earlier versions of this chapter by Danie Meyer-Parlapanis and the editors of this book.

References

Adenauer, H., Catani, C., Gola, H., Keil, J., Ruf, M., Schauer, M., & Neuner, F. (2011). Narrative exposure therapy for PTSD increases top-down processing of aversive stimuli – Evidence from a randomized controlled treatment trial. *BMC Neuroscience, 12*(1), 127. doi:10.1186/1471-2202-12-127.

Bichescu, D., Neuner, F., Schauer, M., & Elbert, T. (2007). Narrative exposure therapy for political imprisonment-related chronic posttraumatic stress disorder and depression. *Behaviour Research and Therapy, 45*, 2212–2220.

Boscarino, J. (2004). Posttraumatic stress disorder and physical illness: Results from clinical and epidemiologic studies. *Annals of the New York Academy of Sciences, 1032*, 141–153.

Brewin, C. R., and Holmes, E. A. (2003). Psychological theories of posttraumatic stress disorder. *Clinical Psychology Review, 23*(3), 339–376.

Brewin, C. R., Gregory, J. D., Lipton, M., & Burgess, N. (2010). Intrusive images in psychological disorders: Characteristics, neural mechanisms, and treatment implications. *Psychological Review, 117*(1), 210–232. doi:10.1037/a0018113.

Brewin, C. R., & Holmes, E. A. (2003). Psychological theories of posttraumatic stress disorder. *Clinical psychology review*, 23(3), 339–376.

Catani, C., Kohiladevy, M., Ruf, M., Schauer, E., Elbert, T., & Neuner, F. (2009a). Treating children traumatized by war and tsunami: A comparison between exposure therapy and meditation-relaxation in north-east Sri Lanka. *BMC Psychiatry, 9*, 22. doi:10.1186/1471-244X-9-22.

Catani, C., Schauer, E., Elbert, T., Missmahl, I., Bette, J. P., & Neuner, F. (2009b). War trauma, child labor, and family violence: Life adversities and PTSD in a sample of school children in Kabul. *Journal of Traumatic Stress, 22*(3), 163–171. doi:10.1002/jts.20415.

Catani, C., Adenauer, H., Keil, J., Aichinger, H., & Neuner, F. (2009c). Pattern of cortical activation during processing of aversive stimuli in traumatized survivors of war and torture. *European Archives of Psychiatry and Clinical Neuroscience, 259*(6), 340–351. doi:10.1007/s00406-009-0006-4.

Catani, C., Gewirtz, A. H., Wieling, E., Schauer, E., Elbert, T., & Neuner, F. (2010). Tsunami, war, and cumulative risk in the lives of Sri Lankan schoolchildren. *Child Development, 81*(4), 1176–1191. doi:10.1111/j.1467-8624.2010.01461.x.

Crombach, A., & Elbert, T. (2014). Controlling offensive behavior using Narrative Exposure Therapy: A RCT of former street children. *Clinical Psychological Science*, http://dx.doi.org/10.1177/2167702614534239.

Crumlish, N., & O'Rourke, K. (2010). A systematic review of treatments for post-traumatic stress disorder among refugees and asylum-seekers. *Journal of Nervous and Mental Disease, 198*(4), 237–251.

Dōmen, I., Ejiri, M., & Mori, S. (2012). Narrative Exposure Therapy for the treatment of Complex PTSD: An examination of the effect and adaptation. *The Japanese Journal of Psychotherapy, 13*(1), 67–74.

Ehlers, A., & Clark, D. M. (2000). A cognitive model of posttraumatic stress disorder. *Behaviour Research and Therapy, 38*(4), 319–345.

Ejiri, M., Dōmen, I., & Mori, S. (2012). A trial study for introducing Narrative Exposure Therapy into psychiatric practice: An examination of the effect and adaption. *The Japanese Journal of Psychotherapy, 13*(1), 59–65.

Elbert, T., & Schauer, M. (2002). Burnt into memory. *Nature, 419*(6910), 883. doi:10.1038/419883a.

Elbert, T., Rockstroh, B., Kolassa, I.-T., Schauer, M., & Neuner, F. (2006). The influence of organized violence and terror on brain and mind: A co-constructive perspective. In P. B. Baltes, P. A. Reuter-Lorenz, & F. Rösler (Eds.), *Lifespan development and the brain* (pp. 326–349). Cambridge: Cambridge University Press.

Elbert, T., Hermenau, K., Hecker, T., Weierstall, R., & Schauer, M. (2012). FORNET: Behandlung von traumatisierten und nicht-traumaisierten Gewalttätern mittels Narrativer Expositionstherapie. In J. Endrass, A. Rossegger & B. Borchard (Hrsg.), *Interventionen bei Gewalt- und Sexualstraftätern. Risk-Management, Methoden und Konzepte der forensischen Therapie* (S. 255–276). Berlin: MWV Medizinisch-Wissenschaftliche Verlagsgesellschaft.

Ertl, V., Pfeiffer, A., Schauer, E., Elbert, T., & Neuner, F. (2012). Community-implemented trauma therapy for former child soldiers in Northern Uganda: a randomized controlled trial. *JAMA, 306*(5), 503–512.

Gwozdziewycz, N., & Mehl-Madrona, L. (2013). Meta-analysis of the use of narrative exposure therapy for the effects of trauma among refugee populations. *The Permanente Journal, 17*(1), 70.

Halvorsen, J. O., & Stenmark, H. (2010). Narrative exposure therapy for posttraumatic stress disorder in tortured refugees: A preliminary uncontrolled trial. *Scandinavian Journal of Psychology, 51*, 495–502.

Hensel-Dittmann, D., Schauer, M., Ruf, M., Catani, C., Odenwald, M., Elbert, T., & Neuner, F. (2011). Treatment of victims of war and torture: A randomized controlled comparison of Narrative Exposure Therapy and Stress Inoculation Training. *Psychotherapy and Psychosomatics, 80*, 345–352.

Hermenau, K., Hecker, T., Ruf, M., Schauer, E., Elbert, T., & Schauer, M. (2012). Childhood adversity, mental ill-health and aggressive behavior in an African orphanage: Changes in response to trauma-focused therapy and the implementation of a new instructional system. *Child and Adolescent Psychiatry and Mental Health, 5*, 29.

Hermenau, K., Hecker, T., Schaal, S., Mädl, A., & Elbert, T. (2013). Narrative Exposure Therapy for Forensic Offender Rehabilitation – a randomized controlled trial with ex-combatants in the eastern DRC. *Journal of Aggression, Maltreatment & Trauma, 22*(8), 916–934.

Hijazi, A. M. (2012). *Narrative exposure therapy to treat traumatic stress in middle eastern refugees: A clinical trial.* Wayne State University. http://digitalcommons.wayne.edu/oa_dissertations/543

Hijazi, A. M., Lumley, M. A., Ziadni, M. S., Haddad, L., Rapport, L. J., & Arnetz, B. B. (2014). Brief narrative exposure therapy for posttraumatic stress in Iraqi refugees: A preliminary randomized clinical trial. *Journal of Traumatic Stress, 27,* 314–322.

Isele, D., Teicher, M., Ruf-Leuschner, M., Elbert, T., Kolassa, I. T., Schury, K., & Schauer, M. (2014). KERF – ein Instrument zur umfassenden Ermittlung belastender Kindheitserfahrungen. *Zeitschrift für Klinische Psychologie, 43*(2), 1–10.

Jacob, N., Neuner, F., Mädl, A., Schaal, S., & Elbert, T. (2014). Dissemination of psychotherapy for trauma-spectrum disorders in resource-poor countries: a randomized controlled trial in Rwanda. *Psychotherapy & Psychosomatics, 83*(6), 354–363.

Jongedijk, R. A. (2012). Hoofdstuk (chapter) 34. Narratieve Exposure Therapie. In E. Vermetten, R. J. Kleber, & O. van der Hart (red). *Handboek Posttraumatische stress stoornissen* (pp. 551–564). Utrecht: De Tijdstroom.

Jongedijk, R. A. (2014). *Levensverhalen en psychotrauma. Narratieve Exposure Therapie in theorie en praktijk* [Life stories and psychotrauma. Narrative exposure therapy in theory and practice]. Amsterdam: Uitgeverij Boom (Boom Publishers).

Kolassa, I.-T., & Elbert, T. (2007). Structural and functional neuroplasticity in relation to traumatic stress. *Current Directions in Psychological Science, 16*(6), 321–325. doi:10.1111/j.1467-8721.2007.00529.x.

Kolassa, I.-T., Illek, S., Wilker, S., Karabatsiakis, A., & Elbert, T. (2015). Neurobiological findings in post-traumatic stress disorder. In U. Schnyder & M. Cloitre (Eds.), *Evidence based treatments for trauma-related psychological disorders* (chap. 4). Cham: Springer.

McPherson, J. (2012). Does narrative exposure therapy reduce PTSD in survivors of mass violence? *Research on Social Work Practice, 22*(1), 29–42.

Metcalfe, J., & Jacobs, W. (1996). A "hot-system/cool-system" view of memory under stress. *PTSD Research Quarterly, 1996*(7), 1–3.

Mollica, R. F., McInnes, K., Poole, C., & Tor, S. (1998). Dose-effect relationships of trauma to symptoms of depression and post- traumatic stress disorder among Cambodian survivors of mass violence. *The British Journal of Psychiatry, 173*(6), 482–488.

Morath, J., Moreno-Villanueva, M., Hamumi, G., Kolassa, S., Ruf, M., Schauer, M., Bürkle, A., Elbert, T., & Kolassa, I. T. (2014a). Effects of psychotherapy on DNA strand break accumulation originating from traumatic stress. *Psychotherapy & Psychosomatics, 83*(5), 289–297.

Morath, J., Gola, H., Sommershof, A., Hamuni, G., Kolassa, S., Catani, C., Adenauer, H., Ruf-Leuschner, M., Schauer, M., Elbert, T., Groettrup, M., & Kolassa, I.-T. (2014b). The effect of trauma-focused therapy on the altered T cell distribution in individuals with PTSD. Evidence from a randomized controlled trial. *Journal of Psychiatric Research.* doi:10.1016/j.jpsychires.2014.03.016.

Nandi, C., Crombach, A., Bambonye, M., Elbert, T. & Weierstall, R., (2014). Predictors of posttraumatic stress and appetitive aggression in active soldiers and former combatants. (submitted for publication).

Neuner, F., Schauer, M., Karunakara, U., Klaschik, C., Robert, C., & Elbert, T. (2004a). Psychological trauma and evidence for enhanced vulnerability for PTSD through previous trauma in West Nile refugees. *BMC Psychiatry, 4*(1), 34.

Neuner, F., Schauer, M., Klaschik, C., Karunakara, U., & Elbert, T. (2004b). A comparison of narrative exposure therapy, supportive counseling, and psychoeducation for treating posttraumatic stress disorder in an African refugee settlement. *Journal of Consulting and Clinical Psychology, 72*(4), 579–587.

Neuner, F., Schauer, E., Catani, C., Ruf, M., & Elbert, T. (2006). Post-Tsunami stress: A study of posttraumatic stress disorder in children living in three severely affected regions in Sri Lanka. *Journal of Traumatic Stress, 19,* 339–347.

Neuner, F., Catani, C., Ruf, M., Schauer, E., Schauer, M., & Elbert, T. (2008a). Narrative exposure therapy for the treatment of traumatized children and adolescents (KidNET): From neurocognitive theory to field intervention. *Child and Adolescent Psychiatric Clinics of North America, 17*(3), 641–664.

Neuner, F., Onyut, P. L., Ertl, V., Odenwald, M., Schauer, E., & Elbert, T. (2008b). Treatment of posttraumatic stress disorder by trained lay counselors in an African refugee settlement: A randomized controlled trial. *Journal of Consulting Psychology, 76*, 686–694.

Neuner, F., Kurreck, S., Ruf, M., Odenwald, M., Elbert, T., & Schauer, M. (2010). Can asylum-seekers with posttraumatic stress disorder be successfully treated? A randomized controlled pilot study. *Cognitive Behaviour Therapy, 39*(2), 81–91.

Nickerson, A., Bryant, R. A., Silove, D., & Steel, Z. (2011). A critical review of psychological treatments of posttraumatic stress disorder in refugees. *Clinical Psychology Review, 31*(3), 399–417.

Onyut, L. P., Neuner, F., Schauer, E., Ertl, V., Odenwald, M., Schauer, M., & Elbert, T. (2005). Narrative Exposure Therapy as a treatment for child war survivors with posttraumatic stress disorder: Two case reports and a pilot study in an African refugee settlement. *BMC Psychiatry, 5*, 7.

Pabst, A., Schauer, M., Bernhardt, K., Ruf, M., Goder, R., Rosentraeger, R., Elbert, T., Aldenhoff, J., & Seeck-Hirschner, M. (2012). Treatment of patients with borderline personality disorder (BPD) and comorbid posttraumatic stress disorder (PTSD) using narrative exposure therapy (NET): a feasibility study. *Psychotherapy and Psychosomatics, 81*, 61–63.

Pabst, A., Schauer, M., Bernhardt K., Ruf, M., Goder, R., Elbert, T., Rosentraeger, R., Robjant, K., Aldenhoff, J., & Seeck-Hirschner, M. (2014). Evaluation of Narrative Exposure Therapy (NET) for borderline personality disorder with comorbid posttraumatic stress disorder. *Clinical Neuropsychiatry, 11*(4), 108–117.

Pace, T. W. W., & Heim, C. M. (2011). A short review on the psychoneuroimmunology of post-traumatic stress disorder: From risk factors to medical comorbidities. *Brain, Behavior, and Immunity, 25*, 6–13.

Robjant, K., & Fazel, M. (2010). The emerging evidence for narrative exposure therapy: A review. *Clinical Psychology Review, 30*(8), 1030–1039.

Ruf, M., Schauer, M., Neuner, F., Catani, C., Schauer, E., & Elbert, T. (2010). Narrative exposure therapy for 7- to 16-year-olds: A randomized controlled trial with traumatized refugee children. *Journal of Traumatic Stress, 23*(4), 437–445.

Schaal, S., Elbert, T., & Neuner, F. (2009). Narrative exposure therapy versus interpersonal psychotherapy: A pilot randomized controlled trial with Rwandan genocide orphans. *Psychotherapy and Psychosomatic, 78*(5), 298–306.

Schauer, M., & Elbert, T. (2010). Dissociation following traumatic stress: Etiology and treatment. *Journal of Psychology, 218*(2), 109–127.

Schauer, M., & Ruf-Leuschner, M. (2014). Die *Lifeline* – Zugang zur Narrativen Exposition (NET) in der Traumatherapie. *Psychotherapeut, 59*, 226–238.

Schauer, M., & Schauer, E. (2010). Trauma-focused public mental-health interventions: A paradigm shift in humanitarian assistance and aid work. In E. Matz (Ed.), *Trauma rehabilitation after war and conflict* (pp. 361–430). New York: Springer.

Schauer, E., Neuner, F., Elbert, T., Ertl, V., Onyut, P. L., Odenwald, M., & Schauer, M. (2004). Narrative exposure therapy in children – A case study in a Somali refugee. *Intervention, 2*(1), 18–32.

Schauer, M., Elbert, T., Gotthardt, S., Rockstroh, B., Odenwald, M., & Neuner, F. (2006). Wiedererfahrung durch Psychotherapie modifiziert Geist und Gehirn. *Verhaltenstherapie, 16*, 96–103.

Schauer, M., Neuner, F., & Elbert, T. (2011). *Narrative exposure therapy: A short-term treatment for traumatic stress disorders.* Cambridge, MA: Hogrefe-Verlag.

Schauer, M., Ruf-Leuschner, M., & Landolt, M. (2014). Dem Leben Gestalt geben: Die *Lifeline* in der Traumatherapie von Kindern und Jugendlichen (im Druck). In K. Priebe & A. Dyer (Eds.), *Metaphern und Symbole in der Traumatherapie*. Göttingen: Hogrefe.

Stenmark, H., Catani, C., Neuner, F., Elbert, T., & Holen, A. (2013). Treating PTSD in refugees and asylum seekers within the general health care system. A randomized controlled multicenter study. *Behaviour Research and Therapy, 51*, 641–647.

Zang, Y., Hunt, N., & Cox, T. (2013). A randomized controlled pilot study: The effectiveness of narrative exposure therapy with adult survivors of the Sichuan earthquake. *BMC Psychiatry, 13*, 41.

Zang, Y., Hunt, N., & Cox, T. (2014). Adapting Narrative Exposure Therapy for Chinese earthquake survivors: A pilot randomised controlled feasibility study. *BMC Psychiatry, 14*, 262.

Zech, E., & Vandenbussche F. (2010). La thérapie par exposition à la narration de Schauer, Neuner et Elbert: Manuel de traitement de l'état de stress post-traumatique après la guerre, la torture et la terreur. Presses universitaires de Louvain.

Brief Eclectic Psychotherapy for PTSD

13

Berthold P.R. Gersons, Marie-Louise Meewisse, and Mirjam J. Nijdam

13.1 Introduction

Brief eclectic psychotherapy for PTSD (BEPP), developed during the 1980s and 1990s of the last century, has proven to be as effective as other trauma-focused treatments (Gersons et al. 2000; Lindauer et al. 2005; Bradley et al. 2005; NICE 2005; Bisson et al. 2013; Schnyder et al. 2011). What makes BEPP special is that it is a comprehensive treatment especially developed for PTSD in which effective elements from various psychotherapy schools have been integrated into a logical sequence. In contrast to other trauma-focused treatments, BEPP focuses on the expression of strong emotions like sorrow and anger which stem from the traumatic event and on learning from the way the event has changed someone's life. Some trauma-focused treatments

B.P.R. Gersons (✉)
Department of Psychiatry, Academic Medical Center, University of Amsterdam, Amsterdam, The Netherlands

Arq Psychotrauma Expert Group,
Nienoord 5, Diemen 1112 XE, The Netherlands
e-mail: b.p.gersons@arq.org

M.-L. Meewisse
Center for Personality Disorders and Psychological Trauma,
GGZ Noord-Holland Noord (institute for mental health),
Bevelandseweg 3, Heerhugowaard, 1703 AZ , The Netherlands
e-mail: m.meewisse@ggz-nhn.nl

M.J. Nijdam
Center for Psychological Trauma, Academic Medical Center, University of Amsterdam,
Meibergdreef 5, Amsterdam, 1105 AZ, The Netherlands
e-mail: m.j.nijdam@amc.uva.nl

© Springer International Publishing Switzerland 2015
U. Schnyder, M. Cloitre (eds.), *Evidence Based Treatments for Trauma-Related Psychological Disorders: A Practical Guide for Clinicians*,
DOI 10.1007/978-3-319-07109-1_13

disregard that the losses of trauma bring forth a lasting change and therefore seem to give the message that the patient will be the same as before the trauma, whereas the message in BEPP is that one becomes "sadder and wiser" and finds a new equilibrium with the surrounding world. BEPP is structured and delivered in 16 sessions.[1]

This chapter starts with the theoretical underpinnings of BEPP, followed by a description of the protocol which is illustrated with a case description and special challenges. The next part is devoted to the scientific evidence of BEPP treatment. This chapter ends with conclusions and practical suggestions.

13.2 Theoretical Underpinnings of BEPP

Acceptance of emotions, understanding the meaning of feelings, and facing the often horrific reality of the traumatic event(s) and its consequences are the three central themes of brief eclectic psychotherapy for PTSD (BEPP).

13.2.1 Acceptance of Emotions

A patient with PTSD is still struggling with strong emotions that originate from the trauma and its aftermath. When treating PTSD with BEPP, it is crucial to focus on tolerating and accepting emotions caused by the trauma.

> A man of 43 tells about a terrible incident when he was 10 years old. His sister of 3 fell in the milking machine and was chopped into pieces. He had always felt guilty about the loss of his little sister because he was older and therefore thinks he should have prevented her death. During imaginal exposure, he held the small red dress of his sister on his lap, and he could let go all the sorrow and grief and feel relieved.

Originally, BEPP was based on the neoanalytic work of Mardi Horowitz (1986). Psychoanalysts like Horowitz (1976) and Davanloo (1987) tried to shorten psychoanalytic treatment in order to adapt it for specific brief disordered states that resulted from negative life events (Erikson 1968). For the person involved, these states cause insecurity about himself or herself leading to anxious and/or negative mood reactions. When the environment of the person subsequently enforces the feeling of insecurity by a lack of understanding or care for this person, the disordered state could spiral down toward a more chronic condition. This justified development of interventions to stop worsening the condition and to find a way back up. Names of such interventions were *crisis intervention* and *short-term dynamic psychotherapy.*

To know at which point an intervention was necessary, one needed to understand how healthy processing of negative life events differed from pathological processing. Mardi Horowitz has been a pioneer in the study of traumatic stress. In his book *Stress Response Syndromes* (Horowitz 1976), he showed a model for steps in healthy and pathological processing (see Fig. 13.1).

---

[1] The BEPP protocol can be requested from the authors and through the BEPP website www.traumatreatment.eu. The protocol is available in Dutch, English, German, Lithuanian, and Georgian and will be also translated in Rumanian, Italian, and Polish.

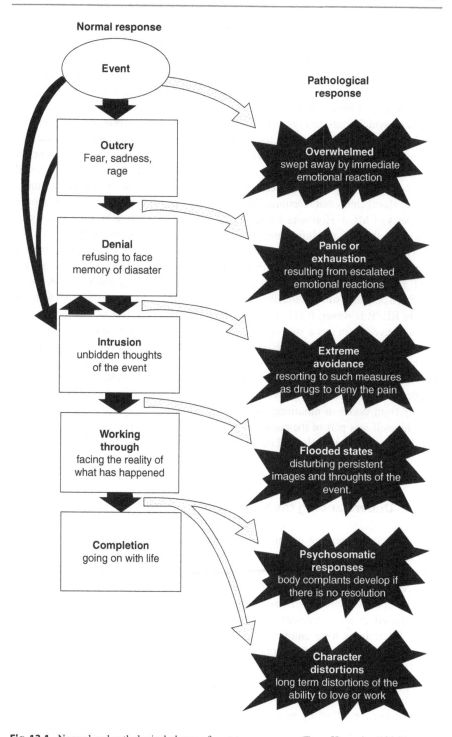

Fig. 13.1 Normal and pathological phases of poststress response (From Horowitz (1986))

As in the work of Lindemann (see later), the loss of a loved person and following mourning was seen as analogous to processing a traumatic event. The normal process starts with an *outcry* of emotions like fear, sadness, and rage. This is followed by *denial*, refusing to face the memory of the disaster which subsequently leads to *intrusions*. Horowitz hypothesized a dynamic alternation between intrusions and avoidance (Gersons 1989). The next step is *working through*, facing the reality of what happened which ends in *completion*, going on with life. In principle, a person is capable of processing a loss of a loved one without professional mental healthcare.

On the right side of the figure, pathological responses are summarized in hierarchical order. It is interesting to carefully study the wording used by Horowitz. It starts with *overwhelmed* directly after the event. He then described *panic or exhaustion* "resulting from escalated emotional reactions." The ability to tolerate extreme emotions is the key hypothesis of Mardi Horowitz for healthy processing of trauma. When emotions are suppressed, this will result in panic and exhaustion that disturbs the daily life of a person. This is in accordance with psychoanalytic theory stating that feeling and accepting emotions is essential for coping with negative events. This is the central hypothesis in BEPP. In learning theory, the central hypothesis is that PTSD is a conditioned response in which a person is still irrationally fearful for recurrence of a traumatic event from the past. In BEPP, however, it is hypothesized that the irrational fear of repetition of the traumatic event is in fact a subconscious anxiety for the suppressed intense emotions. This is in line with the model of Horowitz in which panic and exhaustion are explained as results from escalated emotional reactions. In earlier days, Erich Lindemann (1944) described the diversity of grief reactions after a huge fire in a night club in which 500 people died. His observations were not limited to the consultation room but came directly from stories of mourning families, friends, and colleagues in the Boston area as he himself was part of the community. Besides a healthy process of mourning, he also described more pathological routes. Like Horowitz, he also showed that denial and suppression of emotions are the driving force of unhealthy patterns.

13.2.2 Understanding the Meaning of Emotions

Tolerating and accepting extreme emotions is the key toward a healthy outcome after negative life events. When no energy is taken up for suppression and avoidance anymore, the dysfunctional high level of arousal will diminish which helps to relax. Unnecessary scanning for danger that results from high levels of arousal will subsequently stop. Acceptance of strong emotions like grief and anger helps to understand the effect of the traumatic experiences on one's life and the meaning of life itself. Tolerating strong emotions will help to feel self-compassion for what one went through and also self-acceptance as someone who survived and wants to go on with life. Remembering the traumatic event and just feeling powerless will not lead to improvement; however, contact with underlying emotions of healthy anger because of the terrible experiences will activate the patient to feel in control of one's personal territory. Feeling anger is also very valuable because it helps to accept one's own reaction toward evil. When someone expresses anger in a controlled manner, it helps to prevent the acting out of aggression because the idea of being powerless vanishes. Subsequently, others will no longer be pushed away. Commonly, it also helps patients to get in touch with underlying emotions of sorrow as this promotes attachment to others.

Notwithstanding the negative consequences of avoiding emotions after trauma, patients with PTSD have had their reasons to do so. When people become highly emotionally aroused, they need others for their psychological support. Intense emotions in themselves become a danger when they lead to distancing from important others and to abandonment. Research findings emphasize the role of past and current attachment relationships in trauma-related psychopathology. Parental neglect for instance is a risk factor for enduring psychopathology after a traumatic event in adulthood (Meewisse et al. 2011), and the most important predictor for PTSD is a lack of perceived social support after trauma (for review, see Ozer et al. 2003; Brewin et al. 2000). When one has experienced a life-threatening event and there is no one to share this horrific threatening experience with, the danger continues and one will feel terribly lonesome.

Patient: "I am haunted by my son's accident. I have a loving relationship with my wife, but I am afraid to lose her when I reveal the details of what is troubling me as she will learn that I am a monster as part of it was my fault."

Patient: "I cannot allow myself to think about what has happened as it is pointless and painfully repelling. I'd better forget it all because when I open up about the sexual acts my father did, others will be disgusted by me and it will drive my family apart."

Intense emotions become overwhelming when they are perceived as a threat for the self and the relationships with others.

13.2.3 Facing the Often Horrific Reality of the Trauma

Rebuilding one's life after trauma implies that one faces reality and stops denying the current circumstances even if this means risking rejection or abandonment. After a crisis, people frequently reevaluate their relationships with others. Some people are valued much more than before because of their unexpected support; others who have been disappointing are set at a distance.

Lindemann (1944) also paid attention to the context of loss of a loved one. This is not only a personal emotional process but also a process in which one has to deal with the reaction of others like family or community members. For instance, someone's children will miss their deceased brother and sister or react to the loss of the other parent. When a loved one has died, the daily life and routines have changed. Positions and responsibilities of family members shift, and unexpected financial problems can arise due to loss of income. The method of crisis intervention was based on Lindemann's paper (1944). Crisis intervention combines working through the emotions and uses problem solving until a new equilibrium has been found and established.

In BEPP, the first part of the treatment is devoted to the expression of emotions which helps to diminish the symptoms of PTSD. The second part which is called "the domain of meaning" is focused on the awareness and realization of fundamental change in daily life.

After imaginal exposure, patients often use words like "it is as if I wake up and see the world again, but differently." Ulman and Brothers (1988) and also Wilson et al. (2001) have pointed to the importance of loss of trust in the world and changes in the view on oneself after traumatic events. Without severe traumatic events, one experiences a constant safety of the surrounding world. One can trust others and institutions like the government, employers, doctors, and police. Traumatic experiences like floods, earthquakes, traffic accidents, and especially interpersonal events like murder, rape, and assaults dissolve trust in others and in the world. Subsequently, a person will blame himself or herself for the tragedy he or she has experienced and for not having been prepared enough to avoid the horror. In trauma-focused treatments like EMDR and CBT, this self-blame is targeted by cognitive restructuring to let people realize that the self-blame is irrational. In BEPP, these feelings are more often accepted as such while their origin is explored. Memories of similar feelings in childhood might surface which can help patients understand why they cling to such interpretations. Going back to childhood is not a prerequisite in BEPP; however, it is often helpful to understand that expectations about others, the world, and oneself originate from critical experiences in childhood. Ulman and Brothers (1988) described how traumatic events can destroy feelings and fantasies of invulnerability and how this may lead to a shattered self. Self-blame, which is frequently felt, is often a shield for feelings of anger caused by failure and deception about oneself. When the pain of the loss of illusions is felt and understood in the second part of BEPP, it helps to redefine oneself as vulnerable and resilient at the same time. It also helps to adopt a realistic view on the world, one that is not totally safe, nor completely dangerous. This helps a person to be aware of future negative life experiences and also motivates to enjoy the gift of life more. Posttraumatic growth is seen as a very valuable opportunity in BEPP to learn from trauma and to overcome the sadness.

From crisis theory we know that a period of uncertainty follows an unknown or unexpected incident or situation. This will result in stress and in loss of control. People suffering from PTSD excessively try to keep control over everything around them because they expect danger to strike again. In BEPP, we therefore start the treatment with psychoeducation to start restoring the feeling of being in control. By explaining the symptoms of PTSD as resulting from the traumatic experiences, people start to understand they are not "mad" and that the symptoms have a function in the face of real danger.

In developing BEPP, we have discovered that solely talking about the traumatic incident and emotions resulting from the experience will help to better understand what happened to the patient. However, this will not lead to a decrease in PTSD symptoms.

Patient: "I have told over a hundred times how I was robbed, but that did not help me."

Involuntary vivid reexperiencing symptoms which spontaneously arise or are evoked in response to triggers need more specific intervening. Theories about memory systems (Brewin 2014) help to give some explanation of these special memories. It is remarkable how patients with PTSD easily forget ordinary things like groceries, while specific details of an assault vividly stay present in memory. It seems that a traumatized person is not able to forget the details of the traumatic incident because information about danger is extremely important for survival.

In BEPP, imaginal exposure is applied as the method by which the traumatic memories are treated and changed to become a memory of a past event instead of an overly significant one for the present. After a brief relaxation exercise, imaginal exposure is started. The therapist helps the patient to return to the traumatic events with eyes closed for a detailed and vivid mode. This results in feeling tense and frightened. Just bringing a person back to such a nasty memory is not helpful. In BEPP, we therefore focus on feelings of sorrow about what happened. Commonly, patients start to cry intensely or show 'silent' grief. When they open their eyes after exposure, they feel sad and tired but relieved that they felt the pain and that they accepted to feel this as it led to self-compassion. We discovered that it is necessary to go back in such vivid details to discharge the emotions. In 4–6 exposure sessions, we follow the chronological course of the event in great detail until all moments with an affective load have been addressed. The result is that patients may still feel sad about what has happened, but that it is not so overwhelming anymore. This outcome is similar to other trauma-focused treatments like CBT and EMDR. The method of exposure however is different in these three treatment modalities for PTSD. In all three, the patient has to go back to the worst images of the event. In CBT, the result of the exposure is explained by the extinction of fear by repetitive confrontation with the trauma memories. In EMDR also a repetitive confrontation is used directly followed by a visual or audible distraction. Therapists report that such forms of exposure are also often accompanied by crying or sadness, but it is not considered to be the essential ingredient like it is hypothesized in BEPP.

13.3 BEPP Protocol

The BEPP protocol consists of 16 weekly sessions of 45 min each. The sessions are structured in the following order (Gersons and Olff 2005):

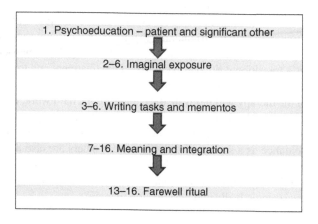

The overlapping numbers indicate that the separate elements of the therapy may both be the focus in a single session. In practice, the number of sessions needed for the different modules can vary dependent on the complexity of the case and the experience of the therapist.

13.3.1 First Session: Psychoeducation

Psychoeducation is a powerful tool to help patients understand the relationship between the traumatic event(s) and their symptoms of PTSD. Symptoms of PTSD are explained as a psychological and physiological state which is functional when danger looms but is dysfunctional and exhausting when there is no threat anymore. For instance, to avoid walking on the grass because one fears mines under the surface, like in Afghanistan, is not functional in most other countries. Most symptoms are beyond control and triggered by conscious and unconscious associations related to past traumatic experiences. One is hyperalert, agitated, and easily startled and has difficulty sleeping and concentrating on the daily routines, because one cannot relax and does not feel safe due to experiencing ongoing danger. By explaining the symptoms of PTSD as resulting from the traumatic experiences, people start to understand that they are not crazy and that the symptoms have had their function in the face of real danger. Avoidance of triggers of the trauma helps to briefly suppress emotions but is counterproductive in the long run. When a traumatized person wants to process the trauma, it is necessary and very helpful to feel, accept, and understand the strong emotions. Being overwhelmed by remembrances of the traumatic event and the feeling as if this is going to happen again creates the feeling of being powerless and in desperate need of control. Psychoeducation helps to regain some feeling of control. The next step in this first, or sometimes second, session is to explain the rationale of the BEPP treatment. The imaginal exposure, the letter writing, and the use of memorabilia are explained as tools to return to the terrible experiences in a vivid way in order to feel and accept the intense emotions and connect them to the trauma. It concerns emotions like sorrow, grief, anger, hate, shame, disgust, and horror. After this phase, which is emotionally heavy, the meaning-making part will start. The patient learns that the world is not as safe as we want it to be and that we are not invulnerable. It will take time and effort to start trusting others again. Also the farewell ritual will be explained as the last confrontation with the frightening memories of the trauma and one's suffering from the experiences for closure, followed by celebrating the comeback to normal life. In fact, it is a transitional ritual as well, to end the treatment and to go on without the therapist from this point on. Prediction of the difficult processes involved in the various parts of the therapy will motivate the patient for the hard work, especially during imaginal exposure. As dropout is a significant problem during trauma treatment (Bisson et al. 2013; Schnyder 2005; Bradley et al. 2005), therapists explicitly draw attention to avoidance as a serious pitfall. Significant others are also asked to attend this first session of psychoeducation, as they usually play a supportive role in keeping patients motivated. Appointments are made in collaboration with the patient on how to act when they struggle badly and wish to stop therapy.

13.3.2 Sessions 2–6: Imaginal Exposure

The following five sessions aim to accept and express emotions to process the trauma using several interventions: imaginal exposure, mementos of the trauma, and letter writing. During imaginal exposure, patients recount their trauma in the first person and present tense while they have their eyes shut. This is preceded by a brief muscle and breathing relaxation to facilitate focus and concentration. In every session, a part of the trauma narrative is recounted in chronological order. The therapist helps patients to experience and label feelings by focusing on sensory information. What is happening, and what do patients see, hear, feel, and think? Those moments with a high emotional load are specifically explored during imaginal exposure. These so-named hotspots can be recognized by a change in intonation of the patient's voice, body language, lack of detail due to speeding up the story, a change of subject, or suddenly opening the eyes. The responsibility of the therapist is to locate the hotspot, reflect on the feelings of the patient, and, if necessary, slow down the pace of the exposure when encountering such a moment.

During exposure, arousal has to be at an optimal level for the patient to be able to process the trauma emotionally and make sense of one's reactions.

When arousal is too low, for instance in the case of dissociation, no change will occur in information processing, as emotions are lacking. To help patients get in touch with their feelings, therapists prompt for sensory information. Following these prompts, they focus on physical awareness of emotions to make the bridge to the feelings.

Patient: (in a calm voice) "He just grabs my bag and walks away."
Therapist: "Stop for a second and rewind a bit. Look at him; watch his face when he grabs your bag. What do you see?"
Patient: "His face has no emotional expression. His eyes are dead."
Therapist: "You seem to shiver. What do you feel now?"
Patient: "I am so afraid."
Therapist: "What scares you so much about his appearance?"
Patient: "It is like I am nothing to him. One wrong move and he will shoot me."

When arousal is too high, information processing stops also because it blocks the possibility to think logically. In this case, the therapist helps the patient to label the current feelings as this will downregulate the arousal. Following a reflection on the patient's feelings, the therapist prompts a new perspective in order to let the feeling emerge in a controlled way. In the case of repression of sorrow, this could be worked out during a session in the following way:

Patient: "My heart is beating. He tries to suffocate me and I am powerless. I am afraid to die" (silently crying).
Therapist: "You almost died? You were so scared. It is really upsetting to realize what you went through, isn't it?"

In the case of repression of aggression, it could be done like this:

Patient: "I am 12 years old and I am held down by this man. I cannot move. It leaves me no choice but to let him do what he wants" (patient shivers).
Therapist: "He is so much stronger than you are. You shiver by what he does to you. You despise him, am I right? (pause)."

The usual course in BEPP is that the perspective turns from fear, as was experienced during the actual traumatic event, to feelings of sorrow in the present. This is accomplished by looking back from the present how awful it has been. The result is that the trauma is experienced as an event that happened in the past, which is crucially different from flashbacks that lack context and feel as if the traumatic event happens in the here and now. During exposure, patients usually remember details of the trauma that were forgotten and that shed a new perspective on the event.

In BEPP, the focus is on the meaning of the trauma for the sense of self and the view on others. Since it is not aimed at habituation of fear or decrease of arousal as such, exposure is not prolonged. The first half of the session is spent on imaginal exposure, while the second half of the session is spent to elaborate on issues that patients become aware of during exposure.

After imaginal exposure, patients feel sad and tired but also relieved as they start to understand their anguish. It feels awful to remember how helpless one has been during the traumatic event, but at the same time it helps to realize that there was no choice but to act during the trauma as they did. This is essential to modify one's perspective on guilt and self-blame. Feelings of sadness arise as patients experience the loss of cherished beliefs, particularly, the illusion of safety and of a sense of self as master of one's own experiences.

Recounting a personal trauma narrative can be retraumatizing when it leads to rejection and distancing in the therapeutic relationship, as arousal levels are high and subsequently attachment needs increase. In therapy, patients often start recounting little bits of a horrifying experience. Usually patients attend carefully to how a therapist reacts to hearing the story. The interpretation of the reaction of the therapist may affirm the meaning of the trauma. For instance, seeing an aversive reaction on the therapists face when recounting a sexual trauma could confirm the patients' idea that they themselves are disgusting as a person. On the other hand, an assertive reaction of the therapist that this traumatic event is horrible may be interpreted as a sign that the trauma is too cruel and scary for others to hear, which leaves the patient alone once again. In BEPP, therapists use their own emotions as a guideline to understand internal states of patients. The therapist's own emotions are also used to encourage patients by normalizing their fears, such as in the following example:

Therapist: "I get goose bumps now that you tell me. I am touched; you are so brave to tell me as it has been so awful for you."

When therapists show compassion about what happened, patients will start crying commonly. The task of the therapist is to stay present and available, since this moment could become a breakthrough. Crying leads to relief when there is someone who cares. It opens a window to a new perspective on attachment to others: from rejection and abandonment to compassion and a willingness to be close. Consolation and support was not available at the time one needed it the most, and this is a first experience that someone is able and willing to stand next to the person, without taking over control. A result is that the trauma loses its intensity.

13.3.3 Mementos and Letter Writing

Another way to work on acceptance and expression of emotions to process the trauma is by the use of mementos and letter writing. Mementos with a specific meaning in the context of trauma like statements, newspaper articles, pictures, or clothes that the person wore at the time are frequently kept by survivors for years, although these usually are stored far from sight. Taking such an item to therapy opens a tangible perspective to the trauma and its sequelae and helps to relive it. The patient is invited to elaborate on the meaning of the item while they watch or hold the memento closely.

Patient: "After the assault I took this bag along for a while as I wanted to overcome the horror. I stopped doing it as I was so ashamed of these tiny bloodstains. Probably they aren't even visible to others, but it felt so degrading that all of this had happened to me. Like I am a beast of prey and I do not count. I still feel like that, and as such it pisses me off every time someone takes me for granted."

It is desirable to further explore the meaning regarding intense emotions that spring from imaginal exposure or discussion of mementos. Therefore, therapists prompt the patient to start writing a letter. In this letter, which is addressed to a particular person or institute, patients express their repressed feelings of anger or grief. This homework assignment is performed in the form of an uncensored letter, which will never be sent. Expression of the meaning of the trauma in written words promotes acceptance of emotions and confronts the person with the reality and the consequences of the trauma. As such, letter writing will bring about self-compassion and activates patients to act and stand up for themselves. Yet, painting or drawing is a good alternative to writing if the patient expresses himself or herself better in that way.

In the case of repressed anger, the letter is written to someone who is held responsible for the trauma, such as the perpetrator. However, it is worth to note that patients with PTSD frequently experience the biggest shock by the way they are treated by people whom they expected support from in the aftermath, like family, friends, colleagues, employers, police, government, or bystanders. Therefore, letters are usually addressed to others who did not show any interest in what patients went through.

In the case of repressed grief, the letter is written to the person they lost due to the traumatic event.

Patient writing: "Dear Jon, my chest aches every time I see your empty chair at the table. I still set the table for you and imagine you are here with me. I feel so guilty to go on with life; it is as if it doesn't mean anything to me that you are gone...."

13.3.4 Sessions 7–15: Meaning and Integration

The first part of the treatment in which we work on the catharsis and acceptance of the strong emotions has the effect that PTSD symptoms diminish substantially. Subsequently, patients become at ease and regain energy to work on the important second part named "the domain of meaning." Traumatic events not only bring about feelings of fear and horror but also challenge trust in others, in oneself, in institutions, and sometimes in society as a whole. Subsequently, people have to redefine themselves, others, and society. There is often no place anymore for a naïve trust in the world, in honesty, and in high morale. Contrary to this loss, often these topics become much more fundamental and important than before. This is what we call learning from traumatic experiences, to give the traumatic experiences meaning by looking at the consequences and by integrating a changed view of oneself and the world. This is often referred to as posttraumatic growth. Often patients relate their traumatic experiences to significant events in their childhood that resemble aspects of the trauma or on how one coped with the horror. This part also focuses on the realization of change in daily life. Current real-life issues regarding social functioning, work, and the way patients relate to others are addressed. Moreover, patients are encouraged to investigate fundamental issues regarding their core beliefs, coping style, and subsequent choices in life and make changes accordingly.

13.3.5 Session 16: Farewell

In the last session, a review of the therapy is performed to consolidate its effectiveness with a relapse prevention plan. To mark the end of therapy and specifically the difficult period in the life of patients, a farewell ritual is advised. During this ritual, patients and their loved ones explicitly dwell on the traumatic event and its aftermath one more time. Patients mourn by what they have lost and share what they have learned from it. The ritual is worked out in a way that does justice to the meaning of the trauma. The therapist encourages the patient and their partner to work out the plans together as it is time for the therapist to withdraw from the patient's life and for others to step in. During the ritual, patients usually burn their mementos of the trauma and letters they have written during the therapy. Regularly, they write a speech to read out loud to their loved ones during a special dinner. The ritual also marks the end of the therapy and the therapeutic relationship, and as such it is a transition to show significant others that they feel better and are no longer preoccupied by the past. They are ready for the future.

Case Description

Mr. B is a 45-year-old police officer and veteran. He is married and has five children and is known as someone who can be relied upon. He had experienced many critical incidents during work with which he had been able to cope. However, since he had been involved in a raid as the officer in charge in order to detain illegal refugees 5 years ago, he started to have intrusions and nightmares. He felt emotionally unstable, restless, and continuously on guard which affected both his social life and work. During a clinical assessment, PTSD was diagnosed and brief eclectic psychotherapy for PTSD (BEPP) was indicated.

Psychoeducation

Mr. B and his wife both attended the first session on psychoeducation. Mr. B recognized the feeling of being constantly alert while the actual danger had passed. He felt preoccupied by the trauma and said it stood in his way to focus on his five children. He also felt guilty about letting down his subordinates due to his loss of energy. Mr. B said that one of the reasons he had avoided speaking about the traumatic incident was that he did not want others to worry about him or be a burden. His wife had experienced an unsafe childhood herself and also recognized the symptoms of PTSD. She struggled with issues from the past herself and had been in therapy unsuccessfully several times. She was supportive toward Mr. B, and she was pleasantly surprised to hear that this therapy had predefined steps for specific goals as it was much different than the unstructured way of therapy she had been in. Mr. B stated that he was looking forward to treatment even though he heard the therapist say that it would have an emotional impact. He wanted to get over his issues as soon as possible to be able to be more supportive to his family and colleagues.

Imaginal Exposure

In the following session, imaginal exposure was performed after a brief relaxation and breathing exercise. As Mr. B just hurried from work to be in time, the exercise helped him to shift his attention from rush hour to being in the here and now. During imaginal exposure, Mr. B remembered how reluctant he was to go and raid homes in order to bust illegal refugees. He did what he had to do and coordinated his team to enter a suspicious apartment. The moment they entered it, one man fled away to the balcony. Mr. B went outside and saw this man holding on to a railing 6 floors high.

Mr. B: There is a glass window between me and this man. I see him hanging there, and I am worried that his hands will slip and that he will fall. I am afraid to scare him, but I need to act due to the urgency of the situation.
Therapist: Look at the man's face, what do you see?
Mr. B: He looks me in the eye. I see the panic in his face, but also some sort of decisiveness when he looks down. I see him open his hands deliberately and let go.

Therapist: What do you feel now that he lets go?

Mr. B: My energy floods away. I am nailed to the ground. I see him hitting the balconies below like a ragdoll. I am completely powerless.

Therapist: I see you are touched now you are telling me this.

Mr. B: I know he won't survive (crying while holding his face in his hands). It was so unnecessary.

Following imaginal exposure, Mr. B felt sad. He felt relieved also, because he became aware that the man made the decision to let go. He felt less responsible as he now remembered that his hands did not slip. In the next session, imaginal exposure continued where it was stopped last time. Mr. B recounted that he ran down the stairs, even though he knew that it was a hopeless situation. His fear was confirmed when he saw the man lying as a sack of bones in a pit caused by the speed of his fall. He had no hope that medical aid could be of any use. This man would die any minute. His final job was to protect bystanders from the sight of the scene. When citizens of the neighborhood came closer, they turned their anger toward him and his colleagues. After imaginal exposure, Mr. B said that the anger of the crowd had hit him hard as he already felt guilty and ashamed of what had happened. Mr. B continued to talk that he detested this part of his job in which he had to chase people who were not criminals but just sought asylum. It felt as if he haunted people, some of whom were really scared due to war experiences in their land of origin. He had been in charge of the operation. However, due to the new government policies, they had to act increasingly forceful and refugees had become very frightened of the police.

Mementos and Letter Writing

Upon request of the therapist, he brought a memento to the next session. It was a newspaper report on the death of the man, and it stated that it was caused by the police who were racists. It felt so unfair and it raged him to be seen as a racist. He himself was happily married to a dark-skinned woman. Moreover, after the incident the locals had put up banners on the spot stating that the police were scum. Mr. B said that the worst thing about it was that he felt completely unprotected by his superiors. They did not set things straight in the media or pull down the banners as the spot was seen as a memorial place. Ever since, he had felt unsafe in the streets in his job uniform as he felt the anger of the citizens. As a homework assignment, Mr. B wrote an angry letter to his superiors whom he held responsible for the situation. The situation reminded him of his time in the army in former Yugoslavia where he had been powerless to stand up for his safety and rights. Mr. B and the therapist jointly decided to park this important subject to the later phase of meaning making in therapy. He also wrote a letter to a minister whom he held responsible for the policies regarding refugees. These letters helped him to express his anger. He wrote a third letter to the mother of the man who deceased.

He expressed his condolences and regret. He had never intended for this to happen. The three letters helped him to describe his ideology clearly. He had joined the force in order to stand next to those in need and to help to create a safer world for everyone, and he mourned that things had turned out otherwise. Bit by bit Mr. B felt relief of what was bothering him.

Midterm Evaluation

During a brief evaluation at session 7, Mr. B said that he started to sleep much better and felt much more at ease. His mind was less preoccupied by the event, and it was time for the next phase of therapy of meaning and integration of the trauma in his life.

Meaning and Integration

The following several sessions were spent on his peace mission during the war in former Yugoslavia as it had been a meaningful period in his life. He had felt powerless in several situations at the time and learned that it was better not to rely on those who are in charge. It had changed his view on authorities that claimed to offer safety but instead were pretty ignorant and inconsiderate to the well-being of their subordinates. Repeatedly, his force was not allowed to act when they got robbed by persons who had put up a roadblock. They were an army which one could disregard and humiliate without any consequences. The situation at the time had motivated him to work hard and get in a responsible position where he would be in charge. It had felt bitter to be in a similar situation in his current work as he had decided at the time never to be part of an operation in which he had no control and had to be submissive to others again.

Just an hour before the start, session 10 was canceled. His wife called that Mr. B was sleeping because he had worked a double shift. Since it was the second time that Mr. B canceled a session because he felt obliged to help out others, the therapist put this topic on the agenda of the next session.

Mr. B said that he always considered where he was needed the most as he felt competent and responsible to help out. His priorities were set in this way. However, in his function as officer in charge and as a father of five children, this meant that he hardly had any time left to relax. On the other hand, it helped him to focus on others when he was not feeling well. While he reflected on the last 5 years, he noticed that he had been increasingly busy with the well-being of others while at the same time he felt less and less like he did a meaningful job. He wanted to change his behavior that seemed to serve as a defense against awareness of his disturbed self-image as an incompetent person. He now realized that the gratitude he received after helping out others was his way to counterbalance his self-image and instead feel competent. However, his pattern of solving everything for others had frustrated him and has led to exhaustion in the past 5 years. In the following weeks, Mr. B stopped taking over responsibilities of others. A positive side effect was that he was better able to listen to others; he did not get agitated as much anymore as he did not need to keep everything under control. The urge to jump in as soon as someone mentioned a problem disappeared, as he learned that others were able to take responsibility also. It changed his view on his kids from helpless to reliable persons, when he saw that they took over some of the duties at home he had been doing for years. He now no longer felt guilty when he did not help out everyone, as he started to rely on others to be competent to do the job themselves.

Farewell Ritual

The therapy came to an end, and as a farewell ritual Mr. B and his wife visited the site of the incident. They went up to the floor of the apartment where he had seen the refugee fall down 5 years ago. His heart pumped while he told his wife exactly what happened that day, but it felt good also to share this life-changing event with her. During the dinner that followed, which they had planned just for the two of them, he told his wife about his plan to apply for a job within the police force in which he could work on rebuilding the lives of hardened criminals.

Six-Month Follow-Up

At the follow-up session half a year later, Mr. B said he was feeling fine. He did not suffer from PTSD symptoms anymore. He felt at ease even though his life continued to be hectic and demanding. He had changed his job, and his wife had decided to seek psychotherapy herself. She was hopeful for the future, now that she had seen the positive effect on her husband.

13.4 Special Challenges

Commonly, therapists face special challenges in BEPP of which several are described below.

13.4.1 Choice of Trauma for Imaginal Exposure

Often patients report multiple traumata. It is not necessary and even logical to address every single trauma with imaginal exposure. The content or theme of reexperiencing symptoms and the memory that is currently most upsetting is leading for choosing the right traumatic experience. The patient himself or herself often helps to choose which experience has been the most upsetting and also which aspect has caused the ongoing fear. When one or sometimes two traumatic experiences have been focused on in the exposure, the irrational fear disappears. The impact and meaning of the various other traumatic events will be addressed extensively in the domain of meaning phase.

13.4.2 Understanding the Rationale Is Vital

Patients with PTSD have difficulties concentrating, and treatment seems less beneficial among those with poorer pretreatment performance on verbal memory measures (Nijdam 2013). As such, it seems wise to deliver psychoeducation on PTSD and the rationale of the treatment repeatedly and in several modalities, spoken, written, and visual. During imaginal exposure, it is essential that patients understand the purpose of reliving the traumatic experience. The therapist checks whether patients have understood the rationale of why it is necessary to tolerate and accept intense emotions related to the trauma. When patients continue to avoid intense emotions during imaginal exposure, it is necessary to explain again that repression of intense emotions is the driving force for their fear in the present. The therapist opens the conversation to explore why the patient keeps avoiding. In the worst case, patient and therapist mutually decide to stop therapy when the timing appears to be wrong in this moment of the patient's life.

13.4.3 Avoidance of Writing

Patients may avoid the homework assignment of writing an angry letter to someone they hold responsible for the trauma or to someone who let them down in the aftermath. It is necessary to trace and understand the reason of the avoidance. Fear of becoming overwhelmed with anger and subsequently is act of being completely irresponsible are examples of a reason to avoid writing. Awareness of this fear can help patients to start writing. When patients think they will harm themselves or others when they get in touch with their anger, in-session writing is helpful to let them feel safe and experience that expressing anger relieves tension. Another reason to avoid writing can be strong feelings of guilt and self-blame instead of anger toward others. Those feelings are also important to face and to discuss in the treatment. One may write the angry letter as if they are an advocate that defends the self. It is written to the part of the self that criticizes the self and keeps oneself small and down.

Patient writing: "To the blamer in me, Stop calling me names. I know I ran away while Sarah was in trouble. If I could turn back time and had the information I have now, I would have done things differently. At the time it seemed best to get off and look for help. I feel terrible that Sarah is gone. I miss her daily. It hurts me and depresses me that you keep pointing at me like I am to blame. It is unfair that you call me selfish. It holds me down and it scares me to get near to others as it gives me the impression that I am a danger to everyone. I do care for others, and I have always been that way. Do not bother me anymore as it affects me and everyone I love."

Sometimes patients like to first write a letter in which they can express feelings of grief about people who died and were loved. Also writing can be helpful in reporting all events in a timeline with all the connected details.

13.4.4 Therapist Skills

BEPP requires specific skills of the psychotherapist. The attitude of the therapist in the beginning of the treatment is like a teacher, followed by the attitude of a listener who visualizes the events the patient went through and feels sympathy for him or her. It is also vital to offer hope and determination that one can overcome the horror and trust in the treatment. This is essential especially when the therapy is intense and difficult for the patient. The confrontation with the gruesome details of traumata is intense in BEPP treatment, and feelings of powerless and hopelessness of the patient may be transferred to the therapist. In the phase of meaning, the therapist becomes someone who understands, explains, and interprets in a mutual process with the patient. The therapist and patient will reflect and find new understandings and solutions. At the end, the therapist should show trust in the patient and end the treatment. Since patients usually are very positive about the therapeutic relationship, it may be hard for the therapist to lose this gratifying contact. The person who suffered from PTSD explicitly stops being a patient and will go on in life with more experience, trust, and capacity to cope with difficulties in the future. The richness of these processes makes BEPP a valued treatment for people who appreciate depth and contextualization in the processing of traumatic events. Furthermore, the interpersonal processes and social context of trauma processing are explicitly addressed during the treatment by involvement of the partner during the different phases of BEPP.

13.5   BEPP Research

13.5.1 BEPP in the Police Force

Since BEPP was originally developed for police officers, its efficacy has first been investigated in this population. In a randomized controlled trial, 42 police officers were included, and results showed a significant difference on clinician-assessed PTSD after treatment in favor of BEPP compared to wait list (Gersons et al. 2000). PTSD symptoms further diminished during the follow-up period of 3 months of this study. BEPP yielded large treatment effects (Cohen's d 1.30) on PTSD and had significant effects on return to work, clinician-rated agoraphobia, and several indices of self-reported symptoms, in comparison with wait list. No patients prematurely dropped out of treatment.

After its efficacy had been established, BEPP became the first-line treatment for police officers with PTSD who were referred to the Police Outpatient Clinic of the Psychotrauma Diagnosis Center, the Dutch center for trauma-related mental health problems for police officers. Analysis of the charts collected during the 16 years of existence of this center showed that 96 % of the policemen and policewomen who received BEPP lost their diagnosis of PTSD (Smit et al. 2013). This study thus confirmed that BEPP is a highly efficacious treatment for the police population. Sixty percent of the police officers reported some residual symptoms after their treatment. The most frequently endorsed residual symptom was difficulty concentrating, present in 16.4 % of the police officers after treatment.

13.5.2 BEPP in General Outpatient Populations

As BEPP was increasingly applied in the general population of patients who had developed PTSD as a result of various other traumatic events, a second randomized controlled trial was conducted in which 24 patients from a general outpatient clinic participated. Lindauer et al. (2005) investigated them before and after treatment and found a significant difference between BEPP and wait list on clinician-assessed PTSD diagnosis and symptoms with large treatment effects for BEPP (Cohen's d 1.62). Five patients dropped out before or during treatment. Besides diminished PTSD symptoms, BEPP also led to significant improvement in self-reported general anxiety symptoms. In this study, no differences were found between BEPP and wait list on self-reported depressive symptoms, sick leave, or relationship problems.

An independent research group in Zurich, Switzerland, took the initiative to conduct a randomized controlled trial that compared BEPP to a minimal attention intervention in 30 outpatients with PTSD. Besides a replication of the effects of BEPP on clinician-assessed PTSD, this study also found that treatment effects were stable after a follow-up of 6 months (Schnyder et al. 2011). Treatment effects were large sized (Cohen's d 1.5). In this trial, significant differences were found between the groups on self-reported depressive and general anxiety symptoms and posttraumatic growth. The authors attributed the increased posttraumatic growth to a strong focus on meaning making and integration during the second phase of BEPP treatment.

The largest randomized controlled trial to date compared BEPP to another active trauma-focused psychotherapy, Eye Movement Desensitization and Reprocessing therapy (EMDR), in 140 outpatients. Both interventions were administered as in clinical practice, allowing for the number of sessions to vary depending on recovery. Patients received an average of 14.7 BEPP sessions of 45–60 min or an average of 6.5 EMDR sessions of 90 min in the trial. BEPP and EMDR were found to be equally effective in reducing PTSD symptom severity, but the speed of change was different in these treatments (Nijdam et al. 2012). EMDR led to a significantly faster decrease in self-reported PTSD symptoms than BEPP, also when we corrected for the difference in session duration in the analyses. Dropout rates were similar for both treatments (around 30 %). Since a considerable number of BEPP treatments were conducted by psychiatrists in their clinical training, BEPP proved to be effective even when therapists had little treatment experience or trauma expertise. Both treatments yielded large effects for both self-reported PTSD (Cohen's d 1.55 for BEPP) and clinician-rated PTSD (Cohen's d 1.95 for BEPP), indicating that the majority of the patients benefitted from these treatments. The PTSD diagnosis remained present for 14 % of BEPP patients posttreatment. Large improvement effect sizes were found for self-reported depressive and general anxiety symptoms, and the treatments also had positive effects on comorbid major depressive disorder and anxiety disorders other than PTSD. Over the course of BEPP and EMDR, significant improvements were also found on measures of memory and executive functioning (Nijdam 2013).

A small pilot study assessed the impact of attending to hotspots on BEPP treatment outcome. In this pilot, hotspots in imaginal exposure sessions were coded in 10 successful and 10 unsuccessful BEPP treatments according to a manual. We found that the number of hotspots did not differ between the successful and unsuccessful BEPP treatments, but hotspots were more frequently addressed by the therapist in successful treatments, as compared to unsuccessful ones (Nijdam et al. 2013). Furthermore, more characteristics of hotspots, such as an audible change in affect, were present in successful treatments than in unsuccessful ones. Although we cannot draw causal inferences from this study, we concluded that it seems important for successful BEPP therapy to repeatedly address the most difficult moments of the trauma memory and to observe characteristics of hotspots during imaginal exposure. This may not only be important in BEPP but also in other trauma-focused psychotherapies.

13.5.3 Neurobiological Research

Lindauer and colleagues assessed various neurobiological parameters before and after BEPP treatment as part of their randomized trial (2005) and in a related study. Twenty-four civilian patients with PTSD, 15 police officers with PTSD, and 15 trauma-exposed healthy control participants were asked to listen to personalized scripts that were neutral, stressful, or trauma-related in nature. Lindauer et al. (2004, 2006) assessed their heart rate, blood pressure, and subjective anxiety ratings during the scripts. Both civilians and police officers with PTSD proved to have significantly higher heart rate responses when listening to the trauma script, as compared to healthy controls. Normalized heart rate responses in reaction to the trauma scripts were seen in those civilians with PTSD who were treated with BEPP, while patients on wait list showed no difference. The civilian patients also underwent trauma script-driven PET scans before and after BEPP to investigate functional alterations in the brain. Lindauer et al. (2008) found significant alterations after BEPP in several PTSD-related frontal and temporal brain areas. It seems that the higher cortical regions, responsible for conscious thinking about a situation and making a thorough judgment, regain more control over the limbic system (known to be responsible for a fast response in case of danger). In another open trial with civilian PTSD patients, various neuroendocrine parameters were assessed in plasma before and after BEPP treatment. Successful BEPP treatment led to an increase in the levels of the anti-stress hormone cortisol (Olff et al. 2007). Cortisol functions to inhibit the stress response via a negative feedback loop to the brain. It also regulates bodily functions and is therefore very important for a good regulation of stress over a longer period of time.

13.6 Conclusion

Brief eclectic psychotherapy for PTSD offers a trusted effective treatment protocol. Since the effect sizes of PE/CBT, EMDR, and BEPP are equal, other factors are important to indicate which specific treatment to offer to patients. The principle of stepped care in mental health may be helpful. When a person had a stable life but got PTSD after a single event, one of the short trauma-focused treatments should be offered. When the effect of the traumatic events is more severe and complex and when a person needs or wants to learn from it, BEPP offers more than the other trauma-focused treatments. A more severe clinical picture and more comorbidity may ask for a stay at a day clinic where BEPP can be combined with group treatment.

References

Bisson, J., Roberts, N.P., Andrew, M., Cooper, R., & Lewis, C. (2013). Psychological therapies for chronic post-traumatic stress disorder (PTSD) in adults. *Cochrane Database Systematic Reviews, 12*:CD003388.

Bradley, R., Greene, J., Russ, E., & Westen, D. (2005). A multidimensional meta-analysis of psychotherapy for PTSD. *The American Journal of Psychiatry, 162*(2), 214–227.

Brewin, C. R. (2014). Episodic memory, perceptual memory, and their interaction: Foundations for a theory of Posttraumatic Stress Disorder. *Psychological Bulletin, 140*(1), 69–97.

Brewin, C. R., Andrews, B., & Valentine, J. D. (2000). Meta-analysis of risk factors for posttraumatic stress disorder in trauma-exposed adults. *Journal of Consulting and Clinical Psychology, 68*, 748–766.

Davanloo, H. (1987). *Short-term dynamic psychotherapy: Basic principles and techniques.* New York/London: Spectrum Publ.

Erikson, E. H. (1968). *Identity: Youth and crisis.* New York: Norton.

Gersons, B. P. R. (1989). Patterns of posttraumatic stress disorder among police officers following shooting incidents; The two-dimensional model and some treatment implications. *Journal of Traumatic Stress, 2*(3), 247–257.

Gersons, B. P. R., Carlier, I. V. E., Lamberts, R. D., & van der Kolk, B. (2000). A randomized clinical trial of brief eclectic psychotherapy in police officers with posttraumatic stress disorder. *Journal of Traumatic Stress, 13*(2), 333–347.

Gersons, B.P.R., & Olff, M. (2005) *Behandelingsstrategieën bij posttraumatische stress stoornissen,* Bohn Stafleu van Loghum.

Horowitz, M. J. (1976). *Stress response syndromes.* Northvale: Jason Aronson.

Horowitz, M. J. (1986). *Stress response syndromes* (2nd revised ed.). Northvale: Jason Aronson.

Lindauer, R. J. L., Booij, J., Habraken, J. B., Uylings, H. B., Olff, M., Carlier, I. V., den Heeten, G. J., van Eck-Smit, B. L., & Gersons, B. P. R. (2004). Cerebral blood flow changes during script-driven imagery in police officers with posttraumatic stress disorder. *Biological Psychiatry, 56*(5), 356–363.

Lindauer, R. J. L., Gersons, B. P. R., van Meijel, E. P. M., Blom, K., Carlier, I. V. E., Vrijlandt, I., & Olff, M. (2005). Effects of Brief Eclectic Psychotherapy in patients with posttraumatic stress disorder: Randomized clinical trial. *Journal of Traumatic Stress, 18*, 205–212.

Lindauer, R. T., van Meijel, E. P., Jalink, M., Olff, M., Carlier, I. V., & Gersons, B. P. (2006). Heart rate responsivity to script-driven imagery in posttraumatic stress disorder: Specificity of response and effects of psychotherapy. *Psychosomatic Medicine, 68*(1), 33–40.

Lindauer, R. J., Booij, J., Habraken, J. B., van Meijel, E. P., Uylings, H. B., Olff, M., Carlier, I. V., den Heeten, G. J., van Eck-Smit, B. L., & Gersons, B. P. (2008). Effects of psychotherapy on regional cerebral blood flow during trauma imagery in patients with post-traumatic stress disorder: A randomized clinical trial. *Psychological Medicine, 38*(4), 543–554.

Lindemann, E. (1944). Symptomatology and management of acute grief. *American Journal of Psychiatry, 101*, 141–148.

Meewisse, M. L., Olff, M., Kleber, R., Kitchiner, N. J., & Gersons, B. P. R. (2011). The course of mental health disorders after a disaster: Predictors and comorbidity. *Journal of Traumatic Stress, 24*(4), 405–413.

National Institute for Clinical Excellence. (2005). *The Management of PTSD in primary and secondary care*. London: NICE.

Nijdam, M. J. (2013). *Memory traces of trauma: Neurocognitive aspects of and therapeutic approaches for posttraumatic stress disorder*. The Netherlands: BOXpress, 's Hertogenbosch.

Nijdam, M. J., Gersons, B. P. R., Reitsma, J. B., de Jongh, A., & Olff, M. (2012). Brief eclectic psychotherapy versus eye movement desensitization and reprocessing therapy in the treatment of posttraumatic stress disorder: Randomized controlled. *British Journal of Psychiatry, 200*, 224–231.

Nijdam, M. J., Baas, M. A., Olff, M., & Gersons, B. P. (2013). Hotspots in trauma memories and their relationship to successful trauma-focused psychotherapy: A pilot study. *Journal of Traumatic Stress, 26*(1), 38–44.

Olff, M., de Vries, G. J., Guzelcan, Y., Assies, J., & Gersons, B. P. (2007). Changes in cortisol and DHEA plasma levels after psychotherapy for PTSD. *Psychoneuroendocrinology, 32*(6), 619–626.

Ozer, E. J., Best, S. R., Lipsey, T. L., & Weiss, D. S. (2003). Predictors of posttraumatic stress disorder and symptoms in adults: A meta-analysis. *Psychological Bulletin, 129*(1), 52–73.

Schnyder, U. (2005). Why new psychotherapies for posttraumatic stress disorder? *Psychotherapy and Psychosomatics, 74*, 199–201.

Schnyder, U., Müller, J., Maercker, J., & Wittmann, L. (2011). Brief eclectic psychotherapy for PTSD: A randomized controlled trial. *Journal of Clinical Psychiatry, 72*(4), 564–566.

Smit, A. S., Gersons, B. P. R., van Buschbach, S., den Dekker, M., Mouthaan, J., & Olff, M. (2013). *PTSD in the police – A better view; 16 years police outpatient department, 1000 clients,* [PTSS bij de politie – een beter beeld; 16 jaar politiepoli, 1000 gebruikers]. Politieacademie, (in Dutch).

Ulman, R. B., & Brothers, D. (1988). *The shattered self: A psychoanalytic study of trauma*. Hillsdale: The Analytic Press.

Wilson, J. P., Friedman, M. J., & Lindy, J. D. (2001). A holistic, organismic approach to healing trauma and PTSD. In J. P. Wilson, M. J. Friedman, & J. D. Lindy (Eds.), *Treating psychological trauma and PTSD* (pp. 28–58). New York/London: Guilford Press.

STAIR Narrative Therapy

14

Marylene Cloitre and Janet A. Schmidt

Anold soldier who is now a successful professional contemplates his time as a prisoner of war (POW) during the Vietnam conflict. He describes himself as young fearless pilot, a master of himself and of his machine. Captured and beaten, he realized that his arms were broken in several places so badly he could not lift a finger. Fellow captive squadron mates took turns spooning food so he could eat. They did this for several weeks. He would not have survived without their aid. The experience transformed his understanding of himself and others. He says, "In the sky, alone, I believed I was invincible but I realized we are all individually nothing. We cannot live without each other, plain and simple."

14.1 Introduction

Skills Training in Affective and Interpersonal Regulation (STAIR) Narrative Therapy is an evidence-based psychosocial treatment that provides a combination of traditional PTSD trauma-focused work (Narrative Therapy) with skills training that addresses a wide range of problems in day-to-day functioning that emerge from difficulties in emotion and relationship management (Cloitre et al. 2006). There are

M. Cloitre (✉)
Division of Dissemination and Training, National Center for PTSD,
Menlo Park, CA, USA

Department of Psychiatry and Child and Adolescent Psychiatry,
New York University Langone Medical Center, New York, NY, USA
e-mail: marylene.cloitre@nyumc.org

J.A. Schmidt, PhD
Division of Dissemination and Training, National Center for PTSD, Menlo Park, CA, USA

© Springer International Publishing Switzerland 2015
U. Schnyder, M. Cloitre (eds.), *Evidence Based Treatments for Trauma-Related Psychological Disorders: A Practical Guide for Clinicians*,
DOI 10.1007/978-3-319-07109-1_14

many therapies that are effective in reducing PTSD symptoms, and the most effective of these include the review and reappraisal of traumatic memories (National Research Council 2014). However, even when PTSD symptoms resolve, functional impairment frequently remains (Westphal et al. 2011). The primary goal of STAIR Narrative Therapy is to improve functioning by reducing PTSD as well as by improving or rehabilitating emotion regulation and interpersonal skills.

Traumatic events diminish social and emotional resources for managing day-to-day life. Post-event, emotions typically become raw or get shut down, relationships can become conflict-ridden, hostilities and misunderstanding develop, and social networks by dint of the trauma (e.g., natural disasters, wars) become frayed or fall apart (e.g., Norris and Kaniasty 1996; North et al. 2002; Shalev et al. 2004). While many people recover their equilibrium, others – in addition to developing PTSD – seem to lose the ability to rely on friends, family, and community as part of the recovery process, and old coping strategies for managing distress do not seem equal to the task. STAIR was developed to rehabilitate or strengthen important emotion management and social skills that are adversely affected by traumatic events. STAIR was initially created for individuals with childhood trauma, who, as a result of repeated and chronic traumatization (e.g., sexual or physical abuse), did not appear to have developed strong emotion management and social skills. However, years of clinical practice indicated that, even among those confronting trauma for the first time in adulthood, such experiences, particularly those that are sustained (e.g., civil wars and conflicts), wear down emotion regulation and social engagement capacities. Paradoxically, of course, emotional regulation and social engagement are resources that facilitate trauma recovery and more generally are critical for effective living. Thus, the purpose of STAIR interventions are to provide strategies for recouping from psychological and social resource losses which are integral to the trauma experience but without which one does not fully recover (Hobfoll 2002). In its philosophy, structure, and interventions, STAIR Narrative Therapy emphasizes the maintenance of a balance between attending to past events via recollection of traumatic events while responding effectively to the demands of the present by strengthening important emotion management and social skills.

This chapter will provide a review of the rationale for the development of the treatment, a summary of the treatment protocol illustrated with a case example, potential challenges in the implementation of the treatment, and a summary of the research on STAIR Narrative Therapy.

14.2 Theoretical Underpinnings

14.2.1 The Role of Emotion Regulation and Relational Capacities as Contributors to Good Functioning

STAIR Narrative Therapy was initially developed in response to the observed needs of patients who had PTSD but who had also experienced significant childhood adversity such as sexual abuse, physical abuse, emotional abuse, and neglect.

PTSD was frequently a presenting complaint, and symptoms could relate to childhood trauma, adulthood trauma, or both. However, patients more often described difficulties with managing social and intimate relationships and with a broad array of problems related to emotions: difficulties with mood, emotional lability, distrust of their emotions, inability to use emotions for effective decision making, and sometimes entire lack of awareness of emotions. Analyses of baseline assessment measures of approximately 100 consecutive patients with histories of childhood abuse seen at our New York City clinic revealed that predictors of functional impairment were consistent with patient complaints. While PTSD symptoms represented about 50 % of the identified contribution to impairment, the remaining 50 % derived from emotion regulation problems and difficulties in managing relationships including problems with assertiveness, sociability, and intimacy (Cloitre et al. 2005).

This symptom profile is consistent with what might be expected when viewed from the perspective of developmental theory and with the results of prospective developmental studies regarding the effects of maltreatment. There are several studies that have identified that childhood sexual, physical, and emotional abuse are predictive of PTSD in the childhood and adolescent years (Copeland et al. 2007; Fergusson et al. 1996; Saigh et al. 1999; Seedat et al. 2004). However, abuse is also associated with disruption of critical developmental goals, which are called in the developmental literature "socio-emotional competencies." In ideal circumstances, adult caregivers guide the development of emotional awareness, emotion regulation, and expression through a variety of means including verbal labeling (e.g., statements of "you look sad" matching child's face or mood), behavioral strategies (soothing with tone of voice), direct instruction (have a glass of water, you will feel better), and role modeling (parental self-management). The development of emotion regulation competencies is predictive of good functioning, which in the childhood years is measured by outcomes such as good school performance, being perceived in a positive way by peers and teachers and having friends (see Shipman and Zeman 2001). These emotional competencies emerge from the context of the relationship between the child and caregiver, such that the caregiver serves as the "external" emotion regulator. This function shifts from the caregiver to the child over the course of development as the child learns and internalizes these competencies. As this developmental shift occurs, the caregiver provides encouragement and praise, which reinforces the child's sense of competence and worth. During times of stress or in unfamiliar circumstances, the caregiver provides additional emotion regulation support or skills training to facilitate recovery from stress or success in meeting the challenges of the unfamiliar. These interpersonal dynamics create expectations of support, positive regard, and safety when in the presence of the caregiver.

However, these important socializing experiences are disturbed in caretaking environments marked by sexual, emotional, or physical abuse. A child who is whipped and then told "that did not hurt" is receiving a verbal label that is dyssynchronous with her/his internal experience. Soothing parental behaviors, if present, are mixed with painful physical, emotional, or sexual experiences. Effective role modeling of parental self-management is clearly compromised by abusive behaviors toward the child. Indeed, cross-sectional and prospective studies of mistreated children indicate that such interaction has adverse effects on emotion regulation and social engagement. Children with histories of maltreatment show diminished emotional self-awareness, difficulty modulating excitement in emotionally arousing situations, and difficulty recovering from episodes of upset (Shields et al. 1994; Shipman et al. 2000, 2005). Such children are more likely to isolate themselves or withdraw under conflictual circumstances (Sroufe et al. 1983), expect little help under stressful circumstances, and tend to interpret the ambiguous or even supportive efforts of others as hostile (Suess et al. 1992). Longitudinal studies have found that compared to nonmaltreated children, those who have experienced abuse have more difficulty managing their emotions adaptively throughout childhood (see Shipman and Zeman 2001).

Similarly as adults, victims of childhood abuse and neglect show difficulties in emotion regulation, especially in the context of interpersonal relationships. Several studies have demonstrated that compared with women who have suffered first-time traumas as adults (e.g., rape, physical assault), childhood abuse victims have more difficulty managing anger, hostility, anxiety, and depression (Browne and Finkelhor 1986; Meewisse et al. 2011) and report more problems in interpersonal functioning in work, home, and social domains (Cloitre et al. 2008; Zlotnick et al. 1996). Adults who have experienced childhood abuse report less satisfaction in intimate relationships, lower perceptions of social support, and lower expectations of help from others which has been found to adversely affect functioning (Cloitre et al. 2008; Schumm et al. 2006).

The documented presence of these compromised essential life skills and their impact on adult functioning provided the impetus for the development of STAIR Narrative Therapy. The introduction of STAIR partnered with an exposure-based intervention (Narrative Therapy) was intended to acknowledge the presence of these difficulties and to provide habilitative or rehabilitative interventions to improve social and emotional competencies.

The potential value of the STAIR component may also be as a resiliency building intervention that reduces risk for future episodes of PTSD upon exposure to additional stressful life events. Over the past decade, data from both retrospective and prospective studies indicate that low perceptions of social support either before or after a traumatic event are a risk factor for the development of PTSD and conversely the presence of social support can be protective against its development (see Charuvastra and Cloitre 2008). Similarly, emotion regulation difficulties have been identified as a mediator of PTSD, with suggestions that emotion regulation problems contribute to the development and maintenance of PTSD among childhood abuse survivors (Arias 2004; Stevens et al. 2013). Thus, the introduction of interventions concerning emotion regulation and social and interpersonal functioning contributes not only to improve functioning but also may strengthen important personal characteristics that protect against or reduce risk of future episodes of PTSD.

14.2.2 Social Bonds and Emotion Regulation More Broadly Considered

Recent studies indicate that many kinds of trauma, not only childhood trauma, adversely affect interpersonal and emotion regulation capacities (Hobfoll 2002) and that, regardless of the nature of the trauma, the loss of these resources contributes to functional impairment (e.g., Malta et al. 2009). Moreover, problems in social and emotion regulation management appear to contribute to the development and maintenance of PTSD (e.g., Zoellner et al. 1999) and conversely effective emotion regulation and social resources are protective against risk for PTSD (Coifman and Bonanno 2007; Papa and Bonanno 2008).

Social bonds across the entire lifespan serve to support, soothe, and facilitate recovery of those who are traumatized. As noted in children, the ideal caregiver or parent acts as an "external regulator" when the child becomes emotionally overwhelmed by challenges or stressors, providing soothing, support, and direction. Similarly, in adulthood and through the lifespan, important others (partners) or even collectives of people or communities such as firefighters, Red Cross, therapists, church members, and coworkers act as "external regulators" to an individual or group of individuals who are overwhelmed in the face of trauma. Words of comfort by leaders and friends and offers of a safe environment are soothing; support in terms of clothing, food, and completion of important tasks; and help provide practical resources and direction in the steps required for recovery (see Hobfoll 2002; Johns et al. 2012; Stevens et al. 2013).

The implications for treatment are that rehabilitation of social and emotional competencies can be considered for trauma survivors of all kinds. At the first year anniversary of the 9/11 attacks on the World Trade Center, we assessed individuals with 9/11-related PTSD symptoms regarding predictors of PTSD symptom severity to determine whether, controlling for early life trauma, functional impairment would be predicted by social and emotion regulation disturbances. Results were similar to our previous study a decade earlier with childhood abuse survivors. Negative social perceptions, relationship status (single/divorced/widowed), and emotion regulation problems were significant contributors to functional impairment and together created more burden to effective functioning than PTSD symptoms (Malta et al. 2009). A benchmark trial of STAIR Narrative Therapy for individuals with PTSD symptoms related to 9/11 resulted in statistically and clinically significant reductions in PTSD, emotion regulation difficulties interpersonal problems, and low social support. The results suggest the feasibility and utility of the treatment for trauma survivors of various kinds.

14.3 Description of the Protocol

STAIR Narrative Therapy is a 16-session treatment in which the first module STAIR (sessions 1–8) focuses on the development of emotion regulation and social/interpersonal skills. The Narrative Therapy (NT) module (sessions 9–16) introduces the narration of traumatic experiences, but there is continued attention to skills training in every session relevant to the day-to-day problems the patient is experiencing. During the STAIR module, a key intervention is the identification of trauma-related interpersonal expectations about relationships and about social interactions more generally. Typically, these interpersonal schemas once had an adaptive function but currently in changing circumstances (post-trauma) may be compromising social functioning and the development of healthy relationships. During STAIR, alternative more adaptive schemas are considered and experientially explored. The success of these alternative schemas often relies on improvement in emotion regulation skills and on a shift in the feelings experienced as generated by the alternative schemas.

The narrative work in the second module is based on a modified version of prolonged exposure (PE) in which the client organizes a narrative or story of the traumatic events experienced with a beginning, middle, and end. Traumatic memories from across the lifespan are identified, and a hierarchy of the memories is organized according to the distress they elicit. As in PE, the first memory selected is one which elicits distress but which feels manageable. In addition, the memory is selected according to the relevance it has to the patient's symptoms and current difficulties. The selection of additional memories is made in a similar fashion by the patient in collaboration with the therapist. The number of memories reviewed typically ranges from 3 to 6 traumas, with patients working with a single memory from one to three sessions, until emotional distress related to the memory is substantially reduced. Often, similar meaning or affective themes emerge across the different memories (e.g., shame, guilt). These are explicitly identified and represented in the treatment as "core" schemas.

The narration of each memory is told with attention to perceptual-sensory detail and to the emotions elicited at the time. After the narrative is completed, therapist and client identify the interpersonal schema or schemas embedded in the narrative. The identified interpersonal schema is reviewed for its adaptive function in the past environment. Often the schema, or a similar version of it, has been identified in the STAIR module, but the schema identified in the narrative work tends to be more precise and "emotionally real" than its earlier version. The trauma schema is then contrasted with a new alternative schema which has typically been proposed and tested during the STAIR module.

The comparison of the old and new schemas is conducted in a way that provides validation of both old and new expectations, respecting the old trauma-generated schemas but allowing room for the development of alternative interpersonal expectations in a new social context. The concept of multiple schemas is based on the notion of multiple "working models of relating" proposed by Bowlby (1988), which suggests that different social contexts and different relationships are associated with different expectations, feelings, and actions. The larger goal is for the client to develop greater flexibility in their thoughts, feelings, and actions, to function in more adaptive ways as they transition out of traumatic contexts. Table 14.1 provides a summary of the topics for 16 sessions of STAIR Narrative Therapy.

Table 14.1 Session-by-session overview

Module 1
Session 1: Introduction to treatment. Treatment overview and goals; introduction to focused breathing; building the therapeutic alliance
Session 2: Emotional awareness. Psychoeducation and identification of impact of childhood abuse on emotion regulation; importance of recognizing feelings; exploration and guidance in feeling identification; practice of self-monitoring
Session 3: Emotion regulation. Focus on connections among feelings, thoughts, and behaviors; identification of strengths and weaknesses in emotion regulation; tailoring and practicing emotion coping skills; identification of pleasurable activities
Session 4: Emotionally engaged living. Acceptance of feelings/distress tolerance; assessment of pros and cons of tolerating distress; awareness of positive feelings as a guide to goal identification
Session 5: Understanding relationship patterns. Introduction of interpersonal schemas and relationship between feelings and interpersonal goals; guided use of Interpersonal Schemas Worksheet
Session 6: Changing relationship patterns. Therapist introduces the use of role-plays to practice relevant interpersonal situations with alternative behaviors; generation of alternative schema
Session 7: Agency in relationships. Psychoeducation on assertiveness; discussion of alternative schemas and behavioral responses; role-plays requiring assertiveness; review and expansion of alternative schemas
Session 8: Flexibility in relationships. Focus on flexibility in interpersonal relationships; continued role-playing on interpersonal situations requiring flexibility using client material; discussion of transition from phase I to phase II of treatment
Module 2
Session 9: Motivating and planning for memory work. Rationale for narrative work and creation of traumatic memory hierarchy
Session 10: Introduction to exposure. Review rationale for narrative work; practice with neutral memory; conduct and tape record first narrative; therapist and client listen together and explore emotions and beliefs about the self and others revealed in the narrative; therapist reinforces patient's learnings and behavior changes
Session 11: Deepening exploration of memories and contrasting with the present. Emotional check in; review analysis of last memory; conduct narrative (same or new memory); review and revise narrative-based interpersonal schemas; practice role-plays relevant to new schemas, review trauma in context of present life
Session 12–15: Exploration of other affective themes. Continue selection of memories; explore affective themes other than fear, such as shame, grief, and loss; identify and revise schemas related to shame and loss.
Session 16: Closure. Summary of patients gains in skills and changes in self/other schemas; discussion of future goals and challenges as well as relapse risks

Case Description

In the following section, we use the case example of Virginia to put STAIR Narrative Therapy into clinical context and highlight specific key points in the therapy process.

Virginia, a 50-year-old divorced African American woman who worked as a hospital maintenance manager, came into treatment after being referred by her primary care physician whom she had been seeing for years and with whom she had a trusting relationship. A routine HIV test had come back positive. The news had shocked Virginia and had led to her revealing to her physician that she had been raped a year earlier but had told no one about it and had "put the event in a closet and closed the door." She also disclosed she has been repeatedly sexually assaulted by her stepfather as a child, something she had never told anyone else. While relieved to share this history, after the HIV diagnosis, Virginia began experiencing nightmares about the abuse, the rape, and being sucked into a deep dark dirty pit that suffocated her. Virginia understood that being HIV positive was not the "death sentence" it once was but that her health required that she adhere to the medication regime in a strict fashion. Despite this knowledge, Virginia and her doctor noticed that she was missing quite a lot of her doses. Her nightmares were worsening, and she was becoming angry with herself and getting into arguments with her coworkers. She had told no one about her HIV status. Upon her doctor's recommendation, she decided to visit a therapist so that she could better manage her moods, deal with her HIV diagnosis, and be able to function at her job.

At the end of her evaluation visit with the therapist, Virginia was surprised to find out that she had PTSD. Both the rape and the HIV diagnosis were traumatic events for her. And indeed, she had nightmares about the assault and about the moment she was told she was HIV positive. Most importantly, it became clear that going to the clinic and taking the medications were traumatic reminders not only of her HIV status but the assault that lead to it. Her avoidance was understandable but life-threatening. However, given an explanation for behavior that had otherwise seemed counterintuitive, Virginia felt supported and understood by the therapist and agreed to try treatment.

14.3.1 History and Symptoms/Commitment to the Treatment (Session 1)

In the first session, the therapist took time to review more about Virginia's relationships and early life. Typical of many patients who are referred for STAIR Narrative Therapy, Virginia suffered betrayals by both her primary caretakers: her stepfather abused her from age 5–11 with the knowledge of her mother. Virginia married at age 19 to a man fifteen years older and who had been married previously and had two teenage children. While they remained married for over 10 years, repeated infidelities by her husband and his drinking and financial difficulties within the family finally resulted in their divorce. The therapist and Virginia concluded that she had not had many people to confide in or to trust. Based on these experiences, there was little reason for Virginia to believe that she could disclose a difficult truth and expect a supportive or concerned response. The therapist used direct language to confirm that the doctor had told her about Virginia's HIV status and expressed her sympathies about the status as a difficult situation. The therapist also mentioned she had worked with other HIV-positive individuals and was informed about medications and their actions. She also told Virginia she would follow up with the physician as needed with newer medications with which she might not be as familiar. They agreed that one practical goal of the therapy would be to help Virginia manage the emotional reactions she was having to the HIV diagnosis, resolve her PTSD and depression, and identify barriers that were keeping her from managing her medications better.

14.3.2 Identifying and Expressing Feelings (Sessions 2–4)

Virginia's first task was to focus on her emotions so that she could become more aware of the sources of distress and introduce coping strategies to manage them better. A simple tracking form was introduced to identify emotions, triggers, thoughts, and actions. Specifically, the therapist asked Virginia to track the feelings and thoughts she had when she was taking her medications. The tracking form was also used to identify situations that gave her peace and pleasure, in order to recognize and engage in them in a purposeful and planned way when they might be used to change a mood or protect her from the dark moods she could feel coming on some days. Before this work began, however, the therapist asked Virginia to review how emotions were handled in her family when she was growing up.

Virginia's home life had been one in which emotions had no place, children were to be seen and not heard. As far as her mother was concerned, feelings were to be happy ones or otherwise swept under the rug. Virginia had the sense her mother did not really like her or have any genuine interest in her well-being. During this session, Virginia spontaneously disclosed about some aspects of her abuse, an unusual action for her. Virginia described that her stepfather would come into her bedroom at night and put his hand over her mouth. He told her to be quiet and tell no one and everything would be alright. At other times, he told her she was "bad" and that problems in the house were her fault. The therapist did not dwell on the details of the trauma but rather focused on explicitly acknowledging the disclosure ("I am so sorry to hear that happened to you") with compassion and neither going into details nor moving too quickly away from the disclosure. The therapist did explore the impact of those experiences on her expectations and reactions in intimate relationships in the present, stating "No wonder you feel like you are suffocating when you get physically close to someone."

Virginia wrote down her feelings and thoughts to the experience of taking her first set of pills of the day. She logged fear (I have HIV, and am sick and going to die), nausea (I am stuffing poison into my body), disgust (I am a bad person), and shame (I deserve this). The therapist broke down these reactions into the three channels of experiencing (feeling, thoughts, and behaviors) and for each one explored coping strategies that would be a good fit for Virginia to act as an "antidote" to the negative experience.

In reviewing the tracking sheets, it became clear that the medications had become a traumatic stimulus, a reminder to Virginia of her HIV status, which elicited fear as well as a reminder of what she believed about herself, that she was a bad and shameful person. The therapist proposed reframing the medications as an ally in her goal toward health rather than as an enemy. Virginia was willing and the therapist proceeded to provide an intervention for each of the channels of emotional experience identified.

Therapist: OK, let's start with your fear reaction to the pill. Let's take out one. How about the blue and white ones?

Virginia: Here they are.

Therapist: Now it is true that you have HIV, but it is also true that these pills will get you and keep you healthy. These pills will improve your white blood cell count, the important healthy cells of your body. Do you want to try a statement about these pills while looking at them?

Virginia: OK. This is crazy, talking to a pill, but here goes: "Pill, every time I take you, I take a step towards health."

Therapist: Excellent! Repeat that and really look at the pill. Add any elaborations you might like that come to mind about what you hope for in managing your HIV and about a positive future for yourself.

Virginia: "Pill, every time I take you, I take a step towards health. I imagine you in my body lighting up the way, fighting my enemies."

Therapist: How about your nausea? Can you take the pills with something tasty? Think about the soothing tea you like. Take them together…

Virginia used this exercise effectively. The above exchange focuses on changing beliefs but along with certain visual and gustatory associations that were involved in taking the medications. The therapist also explored positive associations of the pills to other sensory modalities (e.g., the blue and white colors of the pills like blue sky and clouds on a beautiful day).

The exercise in revising cognitions, emotions/sensations, and actions (taking the pills) engaged Virginia's curiosity in linking sensations with names of feelings and with the idea that feelings could be helpful rather than to be ignored and avoided. The therapist introduced the STAIR "feelings wheel" to help Virginia learn to identify and label more feelings.

Virginia was initially amazed at the number of feelings on the wheel and used them to complete the feelings monitoring form typically using at least three feeling words for every situation. New coping strategies were introduced that were targeted for each channel that was feasible and acceptable to Virginia. These included daily focused breathing to reduce anxiety (feelings) and difficulty concentrating (cognition). Behavioral strategies included knitting for her step-grandchildren, which she found a soothing activity and which also had the function of getting her more socially engaged with her stepchildren with whom she had maintained a good relationship. The therapist proposed that she attend an HIV support group (at a different hospital) but Virginia turned this down because she did not want to take the risk of being recognized by someone in her community.

She reported that she could see the happiness in the grandchildren's eyes as they looked at her, crawled on her lap, and hugged her. She wrote down these experiences in her feelings monitoring form, allowing herself the pleasure of acknowledging their affection (emotional awareness). As part of her therapy, she made a commitment to call, e-mail, or visit the grandchildren at least once a week (behavior change). In addition, she countered thoughts that she was a bad, shameful person and focused on a mantra for herself "I am a good person and worthy of love" (cognitive change). Her daughter was pleased that her mother and children were spending more time together and this improved the relationship with her daughter. As she was making progress with her family, Virginia realized that she could possibly do better in her relationships at work as well.

14.3.3 Interpersonal Schemas (Sessions 5–8)

Sessions 5–8 have several goals one of which is the identification of interpersonal schemas from childhood and recognition of how the client is being currently influenced by expectations and feelings from the past. Interpersonal schemas are the emotionally charged "templates" created by early life experiences that continue to unconsciously influence the client's life in the present. Another goal is the generation of new schemas based on adult understandings of the self and others gained from treatment. The following vignette describes how Virginia's therapist accomplishes these goals.

Guided by the interpersonal schemas worksheet, the therapist and Virginia considered a specific recent interpersonal interaction that had been distressing. Virginia and a male coworker had an argument about how to conduct an inventory check. Together they considered what happened ("I blew up, yelled at him, and then left the room"), how Virginia felt ("I am out of control; I should not have screamed; no one really wants to listen to me; I am ashamed of myself"), and how she expected her colleague to act ("He should respect my 25 years of experience but he doesn't"). The therapist asked how the interaction ended: Virginia admitted she was more stressed about the increase in tension and felt ashamed about her behavior. Virginia and her therapist considered the situation in light of her childhood abuse. Virginia had learned to believe "no one listens to her," so in order to achieve her goals, she would hold back on her thoughts and feelings, until they exploded. The resulting consequence was actually the thing she feared and was trying to prevent. She had been minimizing her effectiveness on the job and the respect of her coworkers by screaming. Virginia's therapist asked her to consider what she might do differently, a step toward beginning to change core beliefs about the self *and others*.

14.3.4 Role-Playing (Sessions 5–8)

An important therapist skill in STAIR Narrative Therapy is the ability to engage patients in role-playing with the primary objective of developing and testing alternatives to old childhood schemas. Role-playing commonly encountered relationship dynamics (assertiveness, control, flexibility) creates opportunities to practice new behaviors in a safe environment, explore how they feel, and revise as needed. The therapist acts as regulator of the patient's emotions, pulling for the contextually salient emotions, helping the patient sustain or reduce emotional intensity as needed, and helping the patient identify alternative emotions (e.g., joy, or sadness, instead of guilt, or shame) through the use of collaborative exploration.

At the next session, Virginia's therapist asked about how her problem with her coworker and completion of the inventory process was going. Virginia said that her colleague had avoided her during the week and she was handling the inventory on her own. She was angry but felt unable to ask for help. The therapist suggested roleplaying the situation as a way to practice some alternatives in a safe environment. Before the role-play, the therapist normalized Virginia's anger in light of the stress of her diagnosis and all that it had churned up. The therapist also suggested that Virginia have a bit more compassion for herself under these circumstances. While the behavior was rude and not particularly effective, it was also not necessary for Virginia to feel so shamed by it. Virginia had difficulty accepting that her behavior was not a product of her being a bad person but rather a situation in which a good person engaged in some bad behavior. While Virginia agreed she should apologize, she could not find a way to do it without feeling like she was groveling and humiliating herself as she believed she would be exposing her essential "badness." The therapist then modeled a statement of apology in tones of mutual respect for both the apologizer and the one being apologized to and asked Virginia to "try it out." Once Virginia had practiced the statement, the therapist and Virginia practiced an exchange in which the therapist infused some humor.

Therapist: Let's start by you playing yourself and I will be your colleague Jim. My part is easy, I don't have to say anything, I just walk right by you because I am really mad at you! Imagine steam coming out of my ears and a really sulky face.

Virginia (Starting role-play): Hey Jim, can you stop for a minute, I would like to talk to you about the inventory.

Therapist: No thanks, just send me an e-mail, I don't want to get my head chewed off again.

Virginia: Yes, I know I was having a bad day and took it out on you. That inventory project has me really on edge. If you can pitch in, it will be easier for everyone, but especially me.

Therapist: You have a lot of bad days, if you were more relaxed, people around here would help out more. But sure…

The therapist used a bit of humor ("I just walk on by") to reinforce that the role-play was not "real." The therapist's affective approach and responses, particularly expressions of curiosity and playfulness can shape the meaning of these experiences to the patient. Playfulness and humor are incompatible with feelings of fear, and their presence in skills practice such as role-plays conveys the idea that the patient can explore or "try on for size" feelings and attitude that approximate and finally represent a skilled presentation of the message that the patient wishes to give. Playfulness also recognizes that there is both a pretend and real aspect to role-playing. In the pretend aspect, the emotional experience is not as intense because the context does not elicit it (e.g., "I am just pretending to be angry at you, but you are not really Jim"), while the real aspect pulls for a more genuinely felt emotion (e.g., "If I really imagine you are my coworker, it is scary to feel this much anger sitting here in your office"). While this brand of humor will not work with every patient, the goal is to give the individual an authentic emotional experience in which they feel positive self-efficacy in the context of safety and acceptance provided by the therapist.

14.3.5 Narrative Therapy (Sessions 9–16)

The interventions in the first module of treatment focus on improving quality of life and functional capacity, stressing emotion regulation. In addition, the experience with the therapist in the titration of emotions during role-play and discussion of emotionally daily-life matters reinforces confidence in the working relationship. Building on these gains, the second module of treatment (sessions 9–16) focuses on the working through of the traumatic past.

Emotional awareness and engagement in feelings associated with the trauma are elicited through explicit verbalization and description of the memories and associated feelings. The telling of these feelings and memories are organized within the structure of a narrative with a beginning, middle, and end. The use of autobiographical narration and its inherent structure help support, reinforce, and consolidate important self-regulatory activities. In the telling of a narrative, the patient (1) learns to regulate the flow of emotion as the narrator of the story; (2) experiences directed, contained, and goal-oriented emotional expression through the presence of an explicitly defined narrative structure; and (3) strengthens metacognitive functioning and self-awareness as the patient is both in the story as its subject and also removed from the story as its narrator.

All narratives are tape-recorded. After the first tape recording, the patient and therapist listen to the tape together and engage in an analysis that explores the meaning of the event as experienced at the time as well as a revision of its meaning through the incorporation of new information gleaned from the therapy work. These reappraisals often involve the recognition that the chronic fear experienced in the present belongs to an event in the past which can no longer harm the person, that the chronic shame or guilt experienced about the event is misplaced, and that the loss intrinsic to the experience (of a person, a sense of worth, a capacity to relate to others) can be purposefully reworked and transformed in the present. The second and all future recordings include both the narrative and the meaning analysis. The patient listens to the taped narrative at home, ideally on a daily basis. The purpose of this "homework" is to facilitate extinction of fear and other negative emotions associated with memory and to reinforce a revision of the trauma memory that includes the alternative, more adaptive interpretations of the event.

In this phase of work, the therapist moves from coach and teacher to listener, witness, and sometimes cocreator of the new meaning of the trauma. Despite some change in role, we reiterate the centrality of the positive relationship of the therapist to the patient. Evidence from the psychotherapy process literature indicates that in the treatment of many disorders, emotional arousal is a substantial contributor to positive change but only in the presence of a strong therapeutic alliance (reviewed in Whelton 2004). Process research of this module-based treatment suggests that a positive therapeutic alliance can be forged from effective work in skills development in the initial module of treatment and that this in turn contributes to the effective use of emotion regulation skills during the memory processing. Specifically, we found that the therapeutic alliance established early in treatment reliably predicted emotion regulation capacity during the memory processing phase of the treatment which in turn predicted good outcome at posttreatment as measured by reduction of PTSD symptoms (Cloitre et al. 2004). The vignette below illustrates how Virginia and her therapist approach reorganizing her past trauma into an integrated life story.

At this point, Virginia and her therapist felt she had made progress in managing her suppressive/explosive anger. Virginia had also been having success in taking her medications regularly, and her viral load was decreasing and white cell count was improving. She was beginning to feel a sense of self-efficacy managing her illness. However, she was still troubled by nightmares and flashbacks of her rape. Because Virginia liked and trusted her therapist, she was anxious but willing to begin the process of identifying memories of incest abuse. Virginia chose to work on the traumatic memory from the time she was eleven of telling her mother that her father had fondled her and being slapped and belittled in response. Recording the session, the therapist prompted Virginia to imagine the situation was occurring in the present. What was she sensing, feeling, and thinking during the episode?

Therapist: You just told me your mother didn't believe you…can you remember what she said and how she acted? Describe what you are seeing and how you are feeling.

Virginia: She screams, "you little liar….you are making that up! How could you say something so dirty? Shut up, shut up, shut up!!" She backs out of the room and closes the door.

Therapist: I know this is difficult to share…you are doing a great job……what did you do then?

Virginia: I ran and hid in my closet. It felt safe, dark, and warm. I never wanted to see my mother or dad again. I decided I would never talk about it ever again either.

After this emotionally charged experience, the therapist and Virginia explored the meaning of this experience. It came as no surprise to either of them that schemas of shame, worthlessness, and anger were apparent. A central schema that emerged from the narrative was "If I tell about bad things happening to me, I will be blamed and rejected by others." The schema arose from the reaction she received from her mother about the abuse and guided her interactions with not only her mother but in all of her relationships. The schema-guided behavior (hiding information) kept her safe in relationship to her mother. But the application of the schema was overgeneralized to other relationships which was not necessary or helpful. Virginia noted that her strong feelings about how her HIV status would be interpreted by others were based on the above schema. The therapist provided an alternative schema during module 1 ("If I tell about bad things that happen to me, I will be helped and accepted"). During the treatment, Virginia had positive experiences with her therapist that provided evidence supporting the alternative schema. The therapist also pointed out that her physician knew much of the "bad" that had happened to her but had positive regard and deep concern for her, providing more support for the alternative schema.

In addition, through the collaboration of her therapist and physician, Virginia had begun participating in a confidential peer program in which she was mentored by a woman who was also HIV positive. The peer helped her in finding practical ways to manage her medication regime better and accompanied Virginia on her visits to the clinic for her HIV checkup. These visits were often distressing experiences where Virginia would lose track of her medication summary sheets. The peer would help keep all relevant medical information organized, provide emotional support, and practice STAIR skills with Virginia including positive self-statements and focused breathing in the waiting room. The peer mentoring gave Virginia a way to meet other people, "good" people who were HIV positive and who also liked and respected her, regardless of her HIV status.

Virginia's relationships at work improved in part because she was less angry and developed assertiveness skills that increased her confidence. She began to sing in the church choir, a commitment which took her out of the house and brought new friends. Virginia's therapist summarized these positive changes in emotional regulation and interpersonal skills as well as the development of new, more accurate schemas. They discussed her future goals and what might continue to be challenging. During the course of treatment, Virginia had created a notebook with all of her therapy worksheets. She decided on the last day to create a "top ten" list of positive actions, thoughts, and activities which she later put on her smartphone in case of relapse. She and her therapist reviewed the list, highlighting which activities could be done alone when her slowly growing social support network was unavailable. While still concerned that her first response to any emotionally ambiguous situation would be shame and anger, Virginia felt she had some new skills which enabled her to step back and consider alternatives. Finally, she agreed to touch base with her therapist if needed.

14.4 Challenges to Implementing STAIR Narrative Therapy

As noted in the introduction, STAIR Narrative Therapy was originally developed for PTSD patients suffering from complex trauma. Given the variety and intensity of their experiences, this population of client may offer special challenges to the STAIR Narrative Therapy therapist. Common to these challenges is *the degree and extent of client fears (emotional component)* and intense *preference for avoidance (behavioral response)*. In order to achieve emotional regulation, a targeted outcome of treatment, therapists must be prepared to deal with patients' fears. Experienced clinicians have identified five specific fears that can impede therapeutic progress in the use of STAIR Narrative Therapy (Jackson et al. 2009).

First is fear of feelings themselves. Some patients may come into treatment wanting to get rid of their emotions, as feelings have only caused them distress and conflict. They may carry beliefs that having feelings is a weakness and that not having feelings at all is the only way they can be successful. Second is fear of being exposed to the feelings of others, in life and in the therapy room. Patients may not have the skills to respond to emotional expression in others which reinforces their feelings of inadequacy. Third is the fear that the recognition of any feeling will result in its exacerbated expression (becoming out of control). Consistent with an "all or nothing" view of emotions, many STAIR Narrative Therapy patients fear once they either recognize their own feelings or are exposed to those of others, their reactions will be explosive. The fourth fear is of experiencing positive feelings. Patients who have experienced complex trauma may believe that feeling positive emotions or being happy is invalidating of their trauma. Trauma survivors often develop extraordinarily negative views about themselves and their competence and worth as humans which impact their right to experience pleasure. The fifth and final fear is fear of a changed or changing self-identity.

In regard to the first three fears, STAIR Narrative Therapy is organized explicitly so that exposure to emotions occurs in a graded fashion and is supported by the introduction of emotion management skills. Exposure to emotions in the context of daily life is typically less frightening and threatening than exposure to emotions as they relate to traumatic events. Moreover, demonstrated success in managing feelings in day-to-day transactions creates a sense of competence and self-efficacy. Both the actual skills and the sense of self-efficacy can be recruited for the narrative work which can be emotionally more challenging.

Fear of positive emotions or pleasurable experiences can similarly be managed through graded exposure, providing "evidence" counter to beliefs that bad things happen when positive emotions are experienced. Rejection of positive experiences because they are inconsistent with identity as a "bad" person is more challenging and may be understood as related to a sense of being undeserving as well. This is related to the final fear of a changing and unknown self. Individuals who hold on to their old identity of the "traumatized self" sometimes note they are comfortable in this "self." The idea of a changing self may provoke the feeling that "the devil that I know is better than the devil that I don't." In addition, patients may replay past self-other relational patterns in current interpersonal interactions because previous schemas were adaptive to survival in traumatic environments and were to some degree of successful (Cloitre et al. 2002; van der Kolk 1996).

The dislocated or changing sense of self can be frightening to the trauma-identified patient. Graded success experiences associated with the proposed alternative more adaptive schemas can support the transition. In addition, validation of the "old self" and respect for its origins in a traumatic past can be maintained through reference to the idea of "working models of relating." The analogy of the development of an "autobiography" can help create a sense of coherence in a changing sense of self, and it is frequently and repeatedly used in the treatment to organize the experience of change. Memories that have been reviewed represent different chapters in the patient's life and several of these chapters may be thematically related as the story of the "traumatized self." The therapist should point out that the patient has successfully created meaning and coherence to the past traumatic events and that the patient can now similarly create and be the author of the chapters that remain to be written regarding their current life and future plans. Lastly, of course, insight is easier than behavioral change, and the therapist should convey to the patient that insight about the need to change and the benefit of changing may come more quickly than the actual change itself. Expression of compassion and support for the patient in his or her struggles and acknowledgment that recovery from trauma is a lifelong journey will set more realistic expectations. The short-term nature of the treatment requires the acknowledgment that the process of recovery will continue after the therapy ends. Practical plans, such as guidelines for continued use of skills, and an invitation to making return visits or "booster" sessions as needed may be proposed as part of the termination work.

14.5 Research

The efficacy of STAIR Narrative Therapy has been evaluated in four studies with adults: two studies of adult survivors of childhood trauma (Cloitre et al. 2002, 2010), one study of survivors of mass violence (9/11) (Levitt et al. 2007), and a fourth study of a sample of inpatients dually diagnosed with PTSD and schizoaffective disorders (Trappler and Newville 2007). Results support the utility of STAIR Narrative Therapy for PTSD reduction and improvements in emotional and social functioning. An additional two studies have been completed with adolescents, one an open trial for youth in inpatient settings and the other a comparison study of group STAIR for adolescent girls in a school-based setting. Both studies found significant improvement in coping skills and reduction in symptoms. These studies are discussed in greater depth in Chap. 20.

The first randomized controlled trial with adult participants compared STAIR Narrative Therapy to a wait-list control (Cloitre et al. 2002b). Relative to those in the control condition, STAIR Narrative Therapy intervention participants demonstrated significant improvements in PTSD symptoms, affect regulation, interpersonal problems, perceived social support, and overall functioning in family, work, and social domains. Gains were maintained at 3- and 9-month follow-up periods. Moreover, strength of therapeutic alliance and improvement in negative mood regulation established during the STAIR component predicted participants' responses to the narrative component as measured by decrease in PTSD symptoms during this work (Cloitre et al. 2004). Thus, the therapeutic relationship and skills work appear to contribute to effective use of the narrative work.

More recently, Cloitre and colleagues (2010) conducted a component study of STAIR Narrative Therapy to assess the relative contributions of the STAIR and the Narrative Therapy components as compared to their standard sequenced combination. This randomized controlled study of 104 women with PTSD related to childhood trauma had three treatment conditions, the standard treatment (i.e., STAIR Narrative Therapy), and then test conditions in which one of the modules was eliminated and replaced with a nonspecific active treatment, supportive counseling (SC) (i.e., STAIR/SC and SC/Narrative Therapy). This design allowed control of number of sessions, treatment duration, and therapist contact across the three conditions. Results indicated that participants who received STAIR Narrative Therapy were more likely to achieve sustained and full remission of PTSD in comparison to the two control conditions. In addition, participants in the STAIR Narrative Therapy intervention group evidenced greater improvements in emotion regulation, perceptions of social support, as well as reduction in interpersonal problems than participants in the two control conditions. Of note, the benefits of STAIR Narrative Therapy emerged primarily at the 3- and 6-month follow-up assessments. We speculate that the continuing improvements following treatment may have resulted from the use of skills in effectively managing day-to-day life stressors with greater skill and confidence over time, including previous situations that might have "triggered" reexperiencing symptoms. Success in managing stressful situations may have reinforced the message of the exposure work that the traumatic past was truly in the past.

A third investigation evaluated a flexible application of STAIR Narrative Therapy in the treatment of survivors of the 9/11 World Trade Center terrorist attack (Levitt et al. 2007). Clinicians were allowed to skip or repeat protocol sessions based on their relevance to the patients' symptom presentation and end treatment prior to completing the entire protocol if satisfactory improvement had occurred. Therapists could also incorporate non-protocol sessions in order to address a current life stressor or crisis that warranted clinical attention. Length of treatment varied between 12 and 25 sessions. Therapists' experience ranged from no to extensive prior training in cognitive behavioral therapy intervention. The results of this benchmark trial were compared to the 2002 RCT study results. Significant improvements were obtained in PTSD, depression, and interpersonal problems in the flexible application, and the effect sizes were equivalent to those obtained in the 2002 RCT. In addition, coping strategies were measured and found to significantly change: use of alcohol and drugs to cope significantly decreased, while use of social support to cope significantly increased. STAIR Narrative Therapy proved to be effective in reducing distress when delivered in a flexible manner, suggesting a potential for tailored treatments that may be applicable to a wide range of trauma populations and clinical settings.

The implementation of only the STAIR module as a group-based intervention has been shown to be efficacious for men and women who were diagnosed with PTSD and comorbid schizoaffective disorders and whose PTSD was derived from a variety of stressors. Trappler and Newville (2007) examined the efficacy of STAIR group treatment (n=24) compared to a treatment as usual (TAU) (n=24) on an inpatient unit. Patients who received the STAIR group showed significant improvement on measures of PTSD and psychotic symptoms, as well as improvements in affect and emotional expression and management.

Lastly, fMRI evaluation of women with PTSD related to childhood (n=21) who completed STAIR Narrative Therapy found that treatment response was associated with reduced amygdala activation but increased recruitment of the ventral medial prefrontal cortex (vmPFC) suggesting that posttreatment symptom changes were associated with greater emotion regulation of fear responses (Brown et al. 2011).

To summarize, STAIR Narrative Therapy is an efficacious treatment intervention for PTSD as well as for trauma-related social and emotional impairments. The STAIR module alone has been used in a group format and shown to be effective among individuals with PTSD and comorbid psychotic spectrum disorders. STAIR Narrative Therapy, in its entirety, is effective for both men and women, and for those who have experienced prolonged and chronic trauma as well as those with single incident traumas. It has also been shown to be effective when flexibly applied an attractive quality for clinicians.

References

Arias, I. (2004). Report from the CDC. The legacy of child maltreatment: Long-term health consequences for women. *Journal of Women's Health, 13*(5), 468–473.

Bowlby, J. (1988). *A secure base*. New York: Basic Books.

Brown, A. D., Root, J. C., Cloitre, M., Perez, D., Teuscher, O., Pan, H., & Stern, E. (2011, November). *Changes in fear reactivity in response to STAIR/NST: A preliminary analysis*. Paper presented at the Symposium at the Annual Conference International Society for Traumatic Stress Society, Baltimore.

Browne, A., & Finkelhor, D. (1986). Impact of child sexual abuse: A review of the research. *Psychological Bulletin, 99*(1), 66.

Charuvastra, A., & Cloitre, M. (2008). Social bonds and posttraumatic stress disorder. *Annual Review of Psychology, 59*, 301.

Cloitre, M., Cohen, L. R., & Scarvalone, P. (2002a). Understanding revictimization among childhood sexual abuse survivors: An interpersonal schema approach. *Journal of Cognitive Psychotherapy, 16*(1), 91–111.

Cloitre, M., Koenen, K. C., Cohen, L. R., & Han, H. (2002b). Skills training in affective and interpersonal regulation followed by exposure: A phase-based treatment for PTSD related to childhood abuse. *Journal of Consulting and Clinical Psychology, 70*(5), 1067–1074.

Cloitre, M., Chase Stovall-McClough, K., Miranda, R., & Chemtob, C. M. (2004). Therapeutic alliance, negative mood regulation, and treatment outcome in child abuse-related posttraumatic stress disorder. *Journal of Consulting and Clinical Psychology, 72*(3), 411.

Cloitre, M., Miranda, R., Stovall-McClough, K. C., & Han, H. (2005). Beyond PTSD: Emotion regulation and interpersonal problems as predictors of functional impairment in survivors of childhood abuse. *Behavior Therapy, 36*(2), 119–124.

Cloitre, M., Cohen, L. R., & Koenen, K. C. (2006). *Treating survivors of childhood abuse: Psychotherapy for the interrupted life*. New York: Guilford Press.

Cloitre, M., Stovall-McClough, K. C., Zorbas, P., & Charuvastra, A. (2008). Adult attachment, emotion regulation and expectations of support among treatment seeking adults with childhood maltreatment. *Journal of Traumatic Stress, 21*, 282–289.

Cloitre, M., Stovall-McClough, K. C., Nooner, K., Zorbas, P., Cherry, S., Jackson, C. L., & Petkova, E. (2010). Treatment for PTSD related to childhood abuse: A randomized controlled trial. *The American Journal of Psychiatry, 167*(8), 915–924. doi: 10.1176/appi.ajp.2010.09081247 [pii].

Coifman, K. G., & Bonanno, G. A. (2007). Emotion context sensitivity in adaptation and recovery. In A. M. Kring & D. M. Sloan (Eds.), *Emotion regulation and psychotherapy: A transdiagnostic approach to etiology and treatment*. New York: Guilford Press.

Copeland, W. E., Keller, G., Angold, A., & Costello, E. J. (2007). Traumatic events and posttraumatic stress in childhood. *Archives of General Psychiatry, 64*, 577–584.

Fergusson, D. M., Horwood, L. J., & Lynskey, M. T. (1996). Childhood sexual abuse and psychiatric disorder in young adulthood: II. Psychiatric outcomes of childhood sexual abuse. *Journal of the American Academy of Child and Adolescent Psychiatry, 35*, 1365–1374.

Gudino, O. G., Wies, R., Havens, J. G., Biggs, E. A., Diamond, U. N., Marr, M., Jackson, C. J., & Cloitre, M. (2014). Group trauma-informed treatment for adolescent psychiatry inpatients: A preliminary uncontrolled trial. *Journal of Traumatic Stress, 27*(4), 496–500.

Hobfoll, S. E. (2002). Social and psychological resources and adaptation. *Review of General Psychology, 6*(4), 307–324.

Jackson, C. L., Nissenson, K., & Cloitre, M. (2009). Treatment of complex PTSD. In R. Leahy & D. Sookman (Eds.), *New approaches to treatment-resistant anxiety disorders* (pp. 75–103). New York: Jason-Aronson.

Johns, L. E., Aiello, A. E., Cheng, C., Galea, S., Koenen, K. C., & Uddin, M. (2012). Neighborhood social cohesion and posttraumatic stress disorder in a community-based sample: Findings from the Detroit Neighborhood Health Study. *Social Psychiatry and Psychiatric Epidemiology, 47*(12), 1899–1906. doi:10.1007/s00127-012-0506-9.

Levitt, J. T., Malta, L. S., Martin, A., Davis, L., & Cloitre, M. (2007). The flexible application of a manualized treatment for PTSD symptoms and functional impairment related to the 9/11 World Trade Center attack. *Behaviour Research and Therapy, 45*(7), 1419–1433.

Malta, L. S., Levitt, J. T., Martin, A., Davis, L., & Cloitre, M. (2009). Correlates of functional impairment in treatment-seeking survivors of mass terrorism. *Behaviour Therapy, 40*(1), 39–49. doi:10.1016/j.beth.2007.12.007.

Meewisse, M. L., Olff, M., Kleber, R., Kitchiner, N. J., & Gersons, B. P. (2011). The course of mental health disorders after a disaster: Predictors and comorbidity. *Journal of Traumatic Stress, 24*(4), 405–413. doi:10.1002/jts.20663.

National Research Council. (2014). *Preventing psychological disorders in service members and their families: An assessment of programs*. Washington, DC: The National Academies Press.

Norris, F. H., & Kaniasty, K. (1996). Received and perceived social support in times of stress: A test of the social support deterioration deterrence model. *Journal of Personality and Social Psychology, 71*(3), 498–511.

North, C. S., Tivis, L., McMillen, J. C., Pfefferbaum, B., Cox, J., et al. (2002). Coping, functioning, and adjustment of rescue workers after the Oklahoma City bombing. *Journal of Traumatic Stress, 15*(3), 171–175.

Papa, A., & Bonanno, G. A. (2008). Smiling in the face of adversity: The interpersonal and intrapersonal functions of smiling. *Emotion, 8*(1), 1–12. doi:10.1037/1528-3542.8.1.1.

Saigh, P., Yasik, A., Sack, W., & Koplewicz, W. (1999). Child-adolescent post traumatic stress disorder: Prevalence, risk factors, and co-morbidity. In P. Saigh & J. D. Bremner (Eds.), *Posttraumatic stress disorder: A comprehensive text* (pp. 18–43). Boston: Allyn & Bacon.

Schumm, J. A., Briggs-Phillips, M., & Hobfoll, S. E. (2006). Cumulative interpersonal traumas and social support as risk and resiliency factors in predicting PTSD and depression among inner-city women. *Journal of Traumatic Stress, 19*(6), 825–836. doi:10.1002/jts.20159.

Seedat, S., Nyamai, C., Njenga, F., Vythilingum, B., & Stein, D. J. (2004). Trauma exposure and post-traumatic stress symptoms in urban African schools. Survey in Cape Town and Nairobi. *British Journal of Psychiatry, 184*, 169–175.

Shalev, A. R., Tuval-Mashiach, R., & Hadar, H. (2004). Posttraumatic stress disorder as a result of mass trauma. *Journal of Clinical Psychiatry, 65*(Suppl. 1), 4–10.

Shields, A. M., Cicchetti, D., & Ryan, R. M. (1994). The development of emotional and behavioral self-regulation and social competence among maltreated school-age children. *Development and Psychopathology, 6*(1), 57–75. doi:10.1017/s0954579400005885.

Shipman, K. L., & Zeman, J. (2001). Socialization of children's emotion regulation in mother-child dyads: A developmental psychopathology perspective. *Development and Psychopathology, 13*(2), 317–336.

Shipman, K., Zeman, J., Penza, S., & Champion, K. (2000). Emotion management skills in sexually maltreated and nonmaltreated girls: A developmental psychopathology perspective. *Development and Psychopathology, 12*(1), 47–62.

Shipman, K., Edwards, A., Brown, A., Swisher, L., & Jennings, E. (2005). Managing emotion in a maltreating context: A pilot study examining child neglect. *Child Abuse and Neglect, 29*(9), 1015–1029. doi:10.1016/j.chiabu.2005.01.006.

Sroufe, L. A., Fox, N. E., & Pancake, V. R. (1983). Attachment and dependency in developmental perspective. *Child Development, 54*, 1615–1627.

Stevens, N. R., Gerhart, J., Goldsmith, R. E., Heath, N. M., Chesney, S. A., & Hobfoll, S. E. (2013). Emotion regulation difficulties, low social support, and interpersonal violence mediate the link between childhood abuse and posttraumatic stress symptoms. *Behaviour Therapy, 44*(1), 152–161. doi:10.1016/j.beth.2012.09.003.

Suess, G. J., Grossmann, K. E., & Sroufe, L. A. (1992). Effects of infants attachment to mother and father on quality of adaptation in preschool: From dyadic to individual organization of self. *International Journal of Behavioral Development, 15*(43–65), 43.

Trappler, B., & Newville, H. (2007). Trauma healing via cognitive behavior therapy in chronically hospitalized patients. *Psychiatric Quarterly, 78*(4), 317–325. doi:10.1007/s11126-007-9049-8.

Van der Kolk, B. A. (1996). The complexity of adaptation to trauma: Self-regulation, stimulus discrimination, and characterological development. In B. A. van der Kolk, A. C. McFarlane, & L. Weisaeth (Eds.), *Traumatic stress: The effects of overwhelming experience on mind, body, and society*. New York: Guilford Press.

Westphal, M., Olfson, M., Gameroff, M. J., et al. (2011). Functional impairment in adults with past posttraumatic stress disorder: Findings from primary care. *Depression and Anxiety, 28*(8), 686–695.

Whelton, W. J. (2004). Emotional process in psychotherapy: Evidence across therapeutic modalities. *Clinical Psychology and Psychotherapy, 11*(58–71), 58.

Zlotnick, C., Zakriski, A. L., Shea, M. T., Costello, E., Begin, A., Pearlstein, T., & Simpson, E. (1996). The long-term sequelae of sexual abuse: Support for a complex posttraumatic stress disorder. *Journal of Traumatic Stress, 9*(2), 195–205.

Zoellner, L. A., Foa, E. B., & Brigidi, B. C. (1999). Interpersonal friction and PTSD in female victims of sexual and nonsexual assault. *Journal of Traumatic Stress, 12*, 689–700.

Complicated Grief Treatment (CGT) for Prolonged Grief Disorder

15

M. Katherine Shear

Sixty million people in the world die every year, leaving loved ones struggling to adjust. We expect to react strongly to the death of a loved one, but loss of a close relationship often creates havoc beyond what we expect. Close relationships anchor us, enrich our lives, and provide some of our greatest joys and deepest satisfactions. Dysregulated emotions and disruption of functioning occur when they die and the feelings are unfamiliar and disconcerting. People often wonder how they can ever accommodate to the new reality. Interestingly most people make this adjustment, often more quickly than they predict (Boerner et al. 2005; Wilson 2002). Grief is permanent after we lose someone very close, but symptoms usually decrease in frequency and intensity over time and we find ways to reenvision our own lives. However, people suffering from complicated grief (CG) (Shear et al. 2011) get lost in acute grief, unable to come to terms with the loss and unable to imagine purpose, meaning, or joy in life without their loved one.

The purpose of this chapter is to describe an efficacy-tested complicated grief treatment (CGT) for the syndrome in which acute grief is complicated and prolonged (Shear et al. 2005). Although there is not yet consensus on its name or on which criteria should be used to diagnose this grief-related syndrome, there is extensive data, reviewed in Chap. 6 of this book, to support its existence. Both DSM-5 and ICD-11 have proposed preliminary criteria. In the meantime, the 19-item Inventory of Complicated Grief (ICG) (Prigerson et al. 1995) is a simple screening tool with excellent psychometric properties that can be used to identify people suffering in this way. Participants in two clinical trials who scored over 30 on this scale and were

M.K. Shear, MD
Columbia University School of Social Work,
Columbia University College of Physicians and Surgeons,
1255 Amsterdam Avenue, New York, NY 10027, USA
e-mail: ks2394@columbia.edu

© Springer International Publishing Switzerland 2015
U. Schnyder, M. Cloitre (eds.), *Evidence Based Treatments for Trauma-Related Psychological Disorders: A Practical Guide for Clinicians*,
DOI 10.1007/978-3-319-07109-1_15

judged to have CG as their primary problem showed a significantly better response to CGT than to grief-focused interpersonal psychotherapy (IPT).

15.1 Theoretical Underpinnings

In order to explain the theoretical underpinnings of CGT, we need to clarify the way our group uses terminology. Bereavement is defined as the situation of having lost someone close (Stroebe et al. 2003). As such, bereavement meets the definitions of trauma that entail confrontation with death, though not all bereavement is considered to be a trauma in the DSM-5. The impact of bereavement is related to the importance of the person who is lost as well as the circumstances and consequences of the death. In general, loss of a child or a romantic partner is the most challenging. Violent, unexpected death is also especially difficult (Kristensen et al. 2010).

Grief, defined as the response to bereavement, contains thoughts, feelings, behaviors, and physiological changes. The pattern, frequency, and intensity of these symptoms vary and evolve over time. Grief, like the love that spawns it, is unique to each person and each relationship. Still, certain features of grief are universal, including yearning and sadness, frequent thoughts and memories of the lost person, and feelings of disbelief and of alienation from ongoing life. The usual response to a loss includes an initial acute grief period that can be intensely painful and disruptive and that is gradually transformed to a permanent integrated grief that is much less insistent, no longer dominating the mind (Shear and Shair 2005). Most people are able to regulate emotions and to experience brief periods of positive emotions during acute grief (Moskowitz et al. 2003), and this facilitates the assimilation of information about the death and transformation of acute to integrated grief.

CGT utilizes attachment theory (Bowlby 1980; Mikulincer and Shaver 2003), self-determination theory (Ryan and Deci 2000), concepts of self-compassion (Neff and Vonk 2009) and neurobiological research on memory (Reber 2013; Hassin et al. 2009), reward system functioning (Burkett and Young 2012), and emotion regulation (Min et al. 2013). The approach utilizes strategies and procedures modified from prolonged exposure for PTSD (PE) (Foa et al. 2005), motivational interviewing (MI) (Miller and Rollnick 2013), and interpersonal therapy (IPT) (Weissman et al. 2000). The dual treatment objectives are to resolve grief complications and facilitate a successful mourning process.

Attachment theory was first proposed by John Bowlby in the mid-twentieth century. Since then research data have been obtained that strongly support the premises of this theory. Humans as well as other species are biologically motivated to seek, form, and maintain close relationships with a small number of other people. The closest of these bonds is usually between parent and child and between romantic partners in adults. Yet virtually any relationship can meet the characteristics of attachment relationships, namely, that proximity to the significant other is rewarding and separation resisted and that the attachment figure provides a safe haven and secure base. Attachment security contributes to psychological and physiological regulatory processes, and the disruption of a secure attachment relationship typically leads to profound emotional and physiological dysregulation.

The third of Bowlby's famous trilogy provides a detailed discussion of the consequences of attachment loss. Bowlby defines mourning as "a fairly wide array of psychological processes set in train by the loss of a loved one irrespective of their outcome" (Bowlby 1980 p. 17) Successful mourning is the process by which a person adapts to loss. Typically, the mourner oscillates between confronting the painful reality and setting it aside such that information about the finality and consequences of the loss can be assimilated into the attachment working model. According to the CGT model, complicated grief is the condition that occurs when this assimilation is impeded by the presence of complicating thoughts, feelings, and behaviors.

Bowlby (1980) pointed to the importance of revising the internalized working model of the deceased person, essentially a form of working memory in which the mental representation of a loved one is used to devise goals and plans. Bowlby claimed that this revision is undertaken only slowly and with resistance. The usual process is one in which a bereaved person grapples with fully comprehending the finality and consequences of the loss by oscillating between attention to the reality and defensive exclusion. This oscillation produces bouts of intense emotional activation alternating with periods of respite. As a successful mourning process unfolds, the bereaved person comes to terms with the loss and regains a sense of relatedness, autonomy, and competence in his or her own life. The finality and consequences of the death are assimilated into long-term memory, a sense of self is restored, and the future holds the potential for happiness.

Self-determination theory provides another framework for understanding loss of a loved one. Bereavement is a life event that is usually ranked among the most stressful anyone can experience. One reason for this is that loss of a close attachment disrupts relatedness, autonomy, and competence, identified by Deci and Ryan (2000) as basic human needs. Our attachment relationships are an important source of our sense of relatedness defined as the sense of belonging and mattering to others. Attachment relationships provide a safe haven and secure base that facilitate autonomy and competence, and their loss can threaten these basic needs as well. From this perspective adjustment to loss is facilitated by reestablishing avenues for fulfilling basic needs.

Complicated grief is a form of prolonged acute grief in which this adaptive outcome does not occur. However, the problem is not grief itself which is seen as the manifestation of love after someone dies. Grief is permanent after a loved one dies, albeit usually transformed over time. However, with CG grief symptoms remain intense and interfere with the bereaved person's capacity to restore his or her own life. Complications, using the term in the medical sense of superimposed problems, alter grief and interrupt its natural course.

Grief complications take the form of maladaptive thoughts, feelings, or behaviors that block the natural progression of grief. Maladaptive thoughts include rumination over some issue related to the circumstances, consequences, or context of the death. Inordinate difficulty with emotion regulation can be a grief complication. Maladaptive behaviors include dysfunctional avoidance of painful reminders of the loss and/or futile proximity seeking to try to escape the painful reality. CGT targets acceptance of grief as a manifestation of love, resolution of complications, and facilitation of successful mourning.

Self-compassion, meaning kindness toward oneself, feelings of common humanity, and mindful balance of accepting negative emotions without overidentification (Neff and Vonk 2009), is important in facilitating successful mourning. The occurrence of any unwanted and highly emotionally activating experience challenges feelings of self-compassion. Loss of self-compassion may be one of the predisposing factors in complicated grief. Encouraging self-compassion is a core principle employed throughout CGT.

15.2 How to Do CGT

CGT is a 16-session weekly treatment initiated after a pretreatment assessment establishes that CG is present and the patient's most important problem. The treatment utilizes a set of key procedures that are employed in a structured sequence of four phases: getting started, core revisiting sequence, midcourse review, and closing sequence. Sessions begin by setting an agenda and reviewing the grief monitoring diary. Each session then addresses the goal of coming to terms with the loss followed by a focus on restoration of the potential for happiness in ongoing life. Sessions end with the therapist summarizing the session, obtaining feedback from the patient, and then discussing plans for the interval of time (usually one week) until the next scheduled session.

15.2.1 Pretreatment Assessment

CGT is designed to be used after completing an initial assessment in which complicated grief has been established as present and the most appropriate target for treatment. The existence of a condition in which acute grief symptoms are intense and prolonged is strongly supported in the literature. However, the current lack of consensus about how to identify such a syndrome can lead to some confusion. Our group opted to identify CG in a consistent manner until there are approved official criteria. Thus, all of our work, beginning in the late 1990s, has utilized the original 19-item ICG along with a semi-structured clinical interview. The 19-item ICG is a well-validated instrument that has been used throughout the world. Several other forms of this questionnaire exist, and this, again, can cause confusion, so we want to be clear about how we identify the individuals who have benefitted from CGT.

In CGT the therapist needs to have a basic understanding of the patient's history, including important relationships and autonomous functioning. It's a good idea to also complete a full psychiatric and medical evaluation to be sure that any associated problems are either addressed or monitored during the course of the treatment. Also, during the pretreatment assessment patients are provided with a general description of the treatment and its goals. They are given information that there are emotionally activating components to the treatment and that the success of the work will depend on their willingness to engage in these. The therapist also explains the importance of bringing the treatment into patients' ongoing lives.

15.2.2 Sessions 1–3: Getting Started

The first phase of CGT focuses on history taking, providing psychoeducation, and beginning grief monitoring diary, aspirational goals, and building support. The therapist uses these sessions to establish a companionship alliance. The therapist conveys warmth, acceptance, and recognition that grief is a universal experience. At the same time, the expertise and willingness to serve as a guide for the patient's grief journey are also apparent.

Introducing Marcy

Marcy is a 58-year-old woman who is neatly dressed. She sits in the waiting room filling out forms and crying. She enters the therapist's office, struggles to gain control, and says she is sorry to be so emotional – this is not at all like her. She is a mess since her beloved husband Daniel died 5 years ago and, no offense intended, she doesn't really see how anyone can help.

The therapist says there is no need to apologize for being emotional after a painful loss. Marcy seems to relax a little and thanks the therapist. Everyone else seems to think she is self-centered and pathetic, wallowing in her grief and not wanting to feel better. She wonders if this is true. She feels so lost like this is different from anything she ever dealt with and she doesn't know what to do.

Marcy's History

Marcy was the younger of two children, born in a tight-knit neighborhood close to where she currently lives. She describes her upbringing as difficult and lonely. Neither parent seemed very interested in her, and she often felt that she was just one more irritant in their sad lives. Her immigrant parents struggled to make ends meet, and her father was often irritable after long days at work. Her mother took in sewing and often seemed anxious and preoccupied during the day. In the evening, she focused on trying to pacify her husband, though she rarely succeeded. She remembers thinking that she was the one who caused her parents trouble and this made her scared and sad. She was close to her older brother, John, and they had a common group of friends. Marcy and John spent a lot of time together until he got to high school and started using drugs. After that they grew apart and were never close again. Now she is not sure where he is and has not talked to him since her father died more than 10 years ago. She met Daniel in college and always thought he reminded her of John. They got married a few years later. Marcy and Daniel were married for 35 years and had three children. They were unusually close. Their relationship was the envy of their friends.

Marcy's CG Symptoms

Marcy has not moved any of Daniel's things. His toothbrush is still in the bathroom. She can't bear to have anyone sit at his desk. She cannot bring herself to sell his pickup truck, though she doesn't know how to drive it. She avoids social occasions because she feels strangely incomplete when with other people and has painful feelings of sadness and shame. She avoids places where she is afraid she will miss Daniel too much – activities they enjoyed together, people they socialized with, and places where they spent time. Since his death, she has refused to go near the hospital where he died. She visits the cemetery infrequently because she can't bear to think of him lying in the cold ground. Marcy wishes she would have died with Daniel.

Her only comfort is in reveries in which she imagines being with Daniel and thinks about how beautiful her life was when he was alive. When not day dreaming, Marcy often ruminates, feeling angry and bitter about Daniel's death. She asks herself why they didn't do the surgery before it was too late. She still can't believe this nightmare really happened.

Marcy sometimes skips meals or forgets to take her cholesterol medicine, knowing this is not healthy. Even though she has lost her faith, her religious upbringing is all that keeps her from trying to take her own life. She and Daniel attended church regularly, but she lost faith in God after he died. What good is it to attend church if this is what you get? What kind of God would allow Daniel to die when people who are bad continue to live? She continues to work as an office manager for a medium-sized accounting firm but is having trouble concentrating. She no longer feels close to her children and describes herself as "just wandering around through life" thinking repeatedly, "why did he have to die? If only I had watched him more closely; if only I had convinced him to get to the doctor earlier; if only the doctors had treated him better....Why couldn't the doctors help him?"

Grief monitoring is introduced in session 1. The patient is asked to keep a record of grief levels during the treatment, rating grief intensity on a 1–10 scale. At the end of each day, they record the highest level of grief that day and the situation in which it occurred, the lowest level and the situation in which that occurred, and the average grief level. The therapist also introduces the idea of building support and encourages the patient to invite someone to session 3. The purpose of the joint session is to both get another perspective on the patient's situation and also to help a close friend or relative get some ideas about how they might help.

The restoration focus is introduced in session 2. The role of positive emotions is described along with self-compassion and self-determination needs for autonomy, competence, and relatedness. The therapist introduces the ideas of rewarding activities, aspirational goals, and rebuilding close relationships. The restoration-related component aims to help the patient access core values and interests and to use these in developing plans and goals. The patient also starts to build in simple activities that generate feelings of pleasure, interest, or satisfaction.

Marcy's Aspirational Goal

Toward the end of the second session, the therapist asked, "If I could wave a magic wand and your grief was at a manageable level, what would you want for yourself?" Marcy stared at the therapist, surprised, and said that all she wants is to feel like she used to when Daniel was alive. The therapist accepted this, gently reminding Marcy that of course they couldn't bring him back and that their job together was to help Marcy find some peace with this reality and a way to move forward in her life in a new way. If they succeeded in helping her somehow feel that she could deal with the painful reality, what would she want for herself? Marcy thought for a few minutes and then said, "OK I'll try – I always wanted to play the viola. My mother made me play the violin when I was a child because her cousin gave her one. I never liked it and another girl at school had a viola and it sounded so much better to me." Then she said that for some reason she had been thinking about this lately. She said Daniel always told her she should take viola lessons but she couldn't ever find the time. He wanted her to play in a quartet. She said, "It's so sad that I never did that when he was alive. I don't know how I would feel trying to do something like that." The therapist encouraged Marcy to keep thinking about the possibility of learning to play the viola.

Session 3 is usually held with a significant other. Its purpose is to reopen communication between the patient and a close friend or family member and foster support for the patient. Not infrequently, people with CG feel estranged from other people even though they have friends who want to help. However, eventually these friends start to feel helpless and become frustrated. The session gives the visitor the opportunity to express his or her affection for the patient, to air some of the frustration he/she has been feeling, and to share in supporting the treatment. The therapist learns about the visitor's relationship with the patient before the death and what it has been like since. Patients may be surprised to see how much the visitor cares.

Marcy Brings Her Daughter Jessica to Session 3

Marcy's 43-year-old daughter Jessica was eager to come and this surprised Marcy. She had thought that Jessica would be stressed by the invitation. Marcy hated feeling like she was a bother to her daughter. Jessica revealed that she had been feeling frustrated because her mother couldn't stop feeling sorry for herself and this was ruining everyone's life. Jessica said she had run out of things to try and had pretty much given up trying. She decided she had lost her mother along with her father and was now grieving them both. She longed to have her mother back but did not have much hope. Tearfully, she described her relationship with her mother as always very close. Marcy had always been the go-to person in the family when there was a problem and played the same role for her friends. But Jessica said that when her dad died, the mom she always knew disappeared too. It seemed like she was a shell of the person she used to be. Jessica thought it didn't have to be this way and did not see why her mother wasn't trying. Tears streamed down Marcy's face as she listened to this. She said she hated how she has been acting, but she felt so lost – like she didn't know how to try to cope with Daniel's death. They discussed Jessica's questions about CG and the plans for the treatment and discussed some possible ways Jessica might be able to support her mom in the treatment. As she left the session, Jessica hugged her mother and said, "I feel so relieved and more hopeful than any time since dad died."

15.2.3 Core Revisiting Sequence

Sessions 4–9 are core revisiting sessions that contain the heart of the treatment. The sessions are focused on revisiting the time of the death in order to reinvigorate a successful mourning process. They include situational revisiting and memories work. During this sequence the therapist works to help the patient resolve grief complications and focus on coming to terms with the reality of the loss. Each session also includes work on the three components of restoration-related work, including rewarding activities, aspirational goals, and building support.

Session 4 introduces the first imaginal revisiting exercise, and this is followed by a discussion of rewarding activities and aspirational goals. The session ends with a summary and feedback from the patient and a discussion of plans for the upcoming week. These include listening to a recording of the revisiting exercise daily. The therapist plans to talk with the patient by phone after the first time the patient listens to the tape.

The revisiting exercise is designed to confront the patient with the reality of the death. Patients are asked to close their eyes and to visualize the moment when they learned of the death. They tell the story of what happened from that point forward out loud to the therapist for 10 min. The therapist checks distress levels at regular intervals during the narrative and whenever it appears that emotionality increases. At the end of about 10 min, patients open their eyes, report distress levels, and spend the next 10 min reflecting on the exercise.

The imaginal revisiting exercise is repeated during 3–5 of the next 5 sessions. A new audio recording is made each time and patients are asked to listen to it during the week. With repetition the narrative usually becomes more detailed and distress levels decrease. Patients usually report that after telling and/or listening to this story a few times, they start to believe that their loved ones are "really gone." Before this, they knew it was true but somehow could not really believe it. A feeling of being lighter and more connected to the present is also common.

Marcy's Imaginal Revisiting Exercises

Marcy was very emotional during the first revisiting exercise. However, in repeatedly listening and doing the revisiting exercises, Marcy's memory of Daniel's death gradually became less acutely painful and less potent, and Marcy saw that she could tolerate the pain. She found that in listening to the tape, the reality of the death "really hit home – something about hearing myself tell that story." She was no longer afraid of loss of control. She began to reconsider whether it was reasonable to think his death could have been prevented and eventually came to believe that everyone tried his or her best. Maybe this was just Daniel's time to go. She also realized she had been struggling with an idea that he died without knowing how much she loved him. This continued to trouble her even though she thought it probably wasn't true. As Marcy told and listened to this story, she became freer to think about her relationship with her husband, and she could see clearly that there had never been a time when either of them questioned their love. She also realized that if Daniel had worried about anything at the end, it would have been about how she would manage. She began to think about how she could comfort and honor him by letting herself be happy now. She stopped thinking about the unfairness of Daniel's death and she began to realize that his untimely death did not mean that it was wrong for her to enjoy life without him. These changes in her thinking occurred with the revisiting exercises and the reflection periods but without much therapist input.

Situational revisiting is introduced in session 5. The patient is asked to identify situations – people, places, or things – that he/she is avoiding because they trigger painful reminders of the loss. The patient decides on an activity that entails confronting this situation. The therapist asks the patient to do this activity each day during the upcoming week and to record distress levels before, during, and after he/she does this activity. Usually, distress levels come down during the course of the week, and the patient's comfort level with the situation increases quite noticeably. The therapist then suggests they move to another situation, higher on the distress hierarchy. The process of planning and doing an activity that entails confrontation with this situation is repeated. Usually this process continues until the end of the treatment.

Marcy's Situational Avoidance

Marcy started situational revisiting by bringing in her favorite picture of Daniel. Marcy asked the therapist to hold her hand as she took the picture out of the envelope and the therapist agreed. Her distress spiked up to 100 as expected, but within a few minutes of looking at the picture, tears in her eyes, Marcy smiled. She began talking about the day this picture was taken and before long was laughing at the memory of Daniel's antics. Situational revisiting progressed to looking at more pictures at home and then to spending time with her children and grandchildren. Marcy realized that she wanted to tell her grandchildren stories about their grandfather and that she could do this when she was with them. She increased the frequency of her visits and they gradually became more and more fun for her and the children. She began to address other situations on her hierarchy with increased confidence each time, and each time, the situation quickly became easier. The most challenging was her visit to the hospital where Daniel died, but by the end of the treatment, she had begun to address this as well.

Work with memories and pictures begins in session 6 and continues for 5 sessions. The therapist asks the patient to use some of the interval time to write about positive memories such as the deceased person's most likeable characteristics, the most enjoyable times with the person, what this person added to the patient's life, and things the patient loved most about this person. The patient writes about positive memories after sessions 6, 7, and 8, and then after session 9 he/she is invited to think about the "not so positive" things about the person and their relationships. For example, they might write about their least favorite memories, what they liked least about their loved one, or what they wished might have been different.

15.2.4 Midcourse Review and Closing Sequence

Session 10 is devoted to a review of the treatment to date and to planning for the remaining sessions. The therapist reviews the CG model, discusses this with the patient, and considers what has changed and what still needs work. They discuss progress with situational revisiting, rebuilding support, and aspirational goals work. The therapist and patient work collaboratively to plan the last phase of treatment.

The last 6 sessions of CGT are used to complete and consolidate treatment gains and discuss thoughts and feelings about treatment termination. The loss component is focused on three goals: helping the patient make peace with the finality of the loss, understanding what the loss means to the patient, and fostering reconfiguration of his or her relationship with the deceased such that he/she feels an ongoing sense of connection in the context of accepting the reality of the loss and a separate sense of identity.

The primary loss-focused exercise in this sequence is the imaginal conversation with the deceased. This is usually done in session 11, but there is flexibility in the timing, based upon when the patient completes the imaginal revisiting sequence. The procedure for an imaginal conversation is to ask the patient to close his/her eyes and envision himself/herself with his/her deceased loved one shortly after the death. The patient talks to his/her loved one out loud and then takes the role of the deceased person and answers, also out loud. The patient is asked to imagine that the deceased person can hear and respond, even though of course they cannot. Patients are encouraged to ask or tell their loved ones anything they wish and then to take the other person's role and respond. Most people have some trepidation in doing this, but once they do, they find it a very powerful exercise.

Marcy's Imaginal Conversation

Marcy was hesitant at first but then agreed to do this exercise. She closed her eyes and told Daniel that it was so hard to watch him get so sick and die. She said she couldn't comprehend what was happening and thinks she was not as supportive of him as she should have been because she was focused too much on herself. "It wasn't about me. It must have been so much worse for you." She said that she loved him very much and she hoped he was OK. She is struggling to envision her life without him. She wasn't sure if he really knew how much she loved him. At the therapist suggestion, Marcy took Daniel's role and responded. Her voice changed as she said, "Please don't worry Marcy. I have always known you loved me. I am sorry to be gone but there was no way to change the course of my illness. I was glad you weren't there at the end because I know how hard that would have been for you. I still want more than anything for you to be happy. You know that's what I always wanted. ... I didn't want to die, but it was God's will and I am with God now and I am at peace."

The restoration component is focused on the goals of promoting rewarding activities in everyday life, envisioning an aspirational goal that feels like a true volitional choice that reflects a sense of personal authenticity, and rebuilding support. These activities continue in each session in the closing sequence.

Each of the closing sequence sessions addresses treatment termination. The therapist and patient reflect on the treatment together, highlighting progress in reorganizing the self-concept, making new goals and plans, and envisioning a future with the possibility of happiness. The therapist helps the patient identify his/her ongoing strengths and to see where vulnerabilities might lie as he/she thinks about plans for the future. Thoughts and feelings about ending treatment are elicited. The time allotted for termination discussions increases gradually from session 11 to 15. The termination discussion culminates in session 16 with a review of the CG model, personalizing the discussion and highlighting changes that have occurred during treatment.

Marcy's Last Session

Marcy's symptoms were markedly diminished at the end of the treatment. She still felt sad when she talked about Daniel or when she thought about him. She still felt occasional pangs of missing him immensely when she was out with friends. But she was going out regularly with her girlfriends and had several successful dinners with the old friends who were couples. One of them wanted to fix her up with a widower he knew, but she said she didn't know if she was ready for that yet. She told the therapist that dating was probably in her future. For now she wanted to concentrate on starting the viola and on working hard to repay the firm for their acceptance and understanding over the past 5 years. She said she owed them a lot. Marcy smiled as she shook hands with the therapist to say goodbye. "I am so grateful" she said, "You gave me my life back, and more. I feel stronger than I have ever felt. I am not quite sure how it happened, but it feels really good."

15.3 Challenges in Implementing CGT

Therapist comfort level in working with death and loss can be a challenge in implementing CGT. Confrontation with thoughts of death activates deeply rooted fears and triggers a response called "terror management" (Pyszczynski et al. 1999). Implicit terror management occurs when we suppress mortality salience, which makes us more rigid in our thinking, more concerned about being right, and more needy of bolstering our own self-esteem (Florian and Mikulincer 1998; Mikulincer et al. 2003). This can lead to rigid thinking and the need to be right, making it harder to learn new concepts and to work with patients. Clinicians need to monitor their own reactions and find effective ways to regulate their emotional response to death and loss.

CGT sessions are focused and relatively brief so much of the impact of the treatment derives from what the patient does between the sessions. Another challenge of the treatment is that therapists must convince avoidant patients and/or those with survivor guilt to engage with planned activities. Therapists may need to devise creative alternatives for people who are unwilling or unable to do interval work as planned. For example, if the patient resists the idea of doing grief monitoring, the therapist can start by getting him/her to just monitor the average grief levels, or just monitor the highest or lowest, or ask him/her to use fewer numbers or rate the levels as high, medium, or low instead of with numbers. The therapist might get him/her to monitor just 2 or 3 days of the week or only in the mornings.

Another common challenge is patient fear and resistance in doing revisiting exercises. Patients may try to postpone revisiting by being overly talkative or bringing up unrelated issues requiring the therapist to gently redirect the patient. Sometimes the patient does not want to close his or her eyes. The therapist can gently encourage the patient to try or agree to do the exercise with eyes open, looking down so the patient does not watch the therapist's reaction. The patient may tell a very abbreviated story. The therapist can simply let this happen, record the exercise as usual, and send the recording home with the patient. If the patient listens regularly, they will often tell a more extensive version of the story in the next session. Sometimes, patients refuse to do the exercise. In this case the therapist can try to approximate the experience by having the patient tell the story in a more narrative way or write the story. The imaginal revisiting exercise is an important component of the treatment; every effort should be made to do it as close to protocol as possible.

15.4   Our Complicated Grief Treatment Research

CGT was first pilot tested in a study of the 16-week protocol in the late 1990s (Shear et al. 2001). Eligible participants were at least 3 months post loss and scored in the CG range on the 19-item ICG. In addition, participants completed depression and anxiety ratings. Scores on the ICG decreased to less than half the baseline score. Depression and anxiety scores also decreased during the treatment to a level that was clinically and statistically significantly lower than at baseline. The large reduction in CG symptoms was about twice as great as we had previously observed for IPT in a study targeting bereavement-related depression.

We next obtained funding from the National Institute of Mental Health to conduct a randomized controlled trial comparing IPT to CGT, each administered over approximately 16 sessions (Shear et al. 2005). This study showed a statistically and clinically significant difference between the treatments. Completion rate was high for both treatments, and the response rate for CGT completers was twice that for IPT completers. Clinical characteristics and outcomes in African-American study participants showed no differences from Caucasians (Cruz et al. 2007). A paper reporting positive results of a randomized controlled trial comparing CGT to IPT among older adults has been accepted for publication. This second study was conducted in a different laboratory using different therapists and a population that was more than a decade older, on average, than in our first study.

Participants in our studies could take psychotropic medication providing they met criteria for being stable on that medication. Those with a comorbid mood or anxiety disorder were about twice as likely to be taking antidepressants as those without co-occurring disorders. A secondary analysis showed that antidepressant medication use was associated with much higher rates of treatment completion for CGT. This medication effect was not seen for IPT completion rates where completion rates were the same among those taking antidepressants as those not on antidepressants (Simon et al. 2008). Antidepressant medication increased response rates about 20 % points for both CGT and IPT. We concluded that antidepressant medication may augment the beneficial effects of CGT. An NIMH-funded study is currently underway to evaluate the efficacy of antidepressant medication when administered either with or without CG.

A pilot study of 16 individuals who met criteria for substance use disorder (7 alcohol, 4 cannabis, 3 cocaine, and 3 methadone) used an expanded 24-session form of CGT that included motivational interviewing and emotion coping and communication skills (Zuckoff et al. 2006). Outcome analyses showed a large, clinically significant reduction in ICG scores among both completers and the intent-to-treat group with large pre- and post-effect size. Percent days abstinent increased significantly for both groups with medium to large effect sizes pre- to posttreatment.

Secondary analyses of our randomized trial addressed comorbidity (Simon et al. 2007), suicidality (Szanto et al. 2006), daily life activities (Monk et al. 2006), sleep and dreams (Germain et al. 2005, 2006, 2013), and periloss dissociation (Bui et al. 2013). Most of the individuals we have treated in each of our studies meet criteria for a current DSM-IV Axis I mood and/or anxiety disorder. For example, in our first large study, participants were about evenly divided among groups having no comorbidity: 1, 2, and 3 or more comorbid disorders. Major depression and post-traumatic stress disorder were the most common comorbidities, each occurring in about half of the study participants.

Clinicians need to be aware of suicidality associated with CG. A majority of our CG patients had a wish to die following the death of their loved ones. This was about twice the rate which they had reported experiencing before their loved ones had passed away. A small proportion (less than ten percent) of these had actually made a suicide attempt. However, nearly a third had deliberately ignored their own health or safety because of not caring whether they lived or died, and slightly over a quarter thought they wanted to leave life or death to chance by being careless or reckless. Suicidal behavior was associated with CG after controlling for depression.

Sleep disturbance is not mentioned in the proposed diagnostic criteria for CG, yet sleep is often disrupted with this condition. CG participants in our study scored well above the cutoff for clinically significant sleep disturbance on the Pittsburgh Sleep Quality Index (PSQI). Another study showed that treatment response with CGT, but not IPT, was associated with a marked improvement in PSQI scores. Lastly, we examined dream reports in our study subjects and found that they differed from previously published normative dream data. Specifically, for our CG participants, dreams were overpopulated with familiar people but deficient in both positive and negative dream elements. Interestingly, this pattern also differed from previously reported dream patterns observed in both MDD (Barrett and Loeffler 1992) and PTSD (Esposito et al. 1999).

Daily life routines were also measurably different in our study participants compared to previously monitored healthy controls. Participants with CG were significantly more likely than controls to take an afternoon nap and to have an evening snack or drink. Correspondingly, they were more likely to skip meals and to stay inside all day. They were less likely to engage in work, housework, or to exercise. These changes suggest more escape-related behaviors and less social interaction, and this may contribute to maintenance and/or severity of CG symptoms.

Taken together our studies of complicated grief and its treatment provide a comprehensive picture of the clinical syndrome of CG presented by help-seeking individuals who met our criteria for CG and who signed consent for research participation. Notably, these participants have high rates of comorbidity and substantial functional impairment. We and others have documented high rates of suicidal thinking and behavior as well as marked sleep disturbance and disrupted daily activities. Most of our study participants had previously sought treatment with grief counselors or other mental health professionals without getting relief from their symptoms. We showed that these highly distressed and impaired individuals responded robustly to the brief targeted intervention described in this chapter. Study participants were often effusively grateful, telling us things like "you gave me my life back and more." In stark contrast, these individuals had only a minimal response to our comparison treatment, which was a high-quality treatment with strong efficacy data for depression. Our results provide clinicians with a clear picture of the clinical syndrome of complicated grief (aka prolonged grief disorder) and a simple, efficacious approach to treating these individuals.

References

Barrett, D., & Loeffler, M. (1992). Comparison of dream content of depressed vs nondepressed dreamers. *Psychological Reports, 70*(2), 403–406.

Boerner, K., Wortman, C. B., & Bonanno, G. A. (2005). Resilient or at risk? A 4-year study of older adults who initially showed high or low distress following conjugal loss. *Journals of Gerontology. Series B, Psychological Sciences and Social Sciences, 60*(2), P67–P73.

Bowlby, J. (1980). *Loss sadness and depression* (Attachment and loss, Vol. 3, p. 472). New York: Basic Books.

Bui, E., et al. (2013). Periloss dissociation, symptom severity, and treatment response in complicated grief. *Depression and Anxiety, 30*(2), 123–128.

Burkett, J. P., & Young, L. J. (2012). The behavioral, anatomical and pharmacological parallels between social attachment, love and addiction. *Psychopharmacology, 224*(1), 1–26.

Cruz, M., et al. (2007). Clinical presentation and treatment outcome of African Americans with complicated grief. *Psychiatric Services, 58*(5), 700–702.

Esposito, K., et al. (1999). Evaluation of dream content in combat-related PTSD. *Journal of Traumatic Stress, 12*(4), 681–687.

Florian, V., & Mikulincer, M. (1998). Symbolic immortality and the management of the terror of death: The moderating role of attachment style. *Journal of Personality and Social Psychology, 74*(3), 725–734.

Foa, E. B., et al. (2005). Randomized trial of prolonged exposure for posttraumatic stress disorder with and without cognitive restructuring: Outcome at academic and community clinics. *Journal of Consulting and Clinical Psychology, 73*(5), 953–964.

Germain, A., et al. (2005). Sleep quality in complicated grief. *Journal of Traumatic Stress, 18*(4), 343–346.

Germain, A., et al. (2006). Treating complicated grief: Effects on sleep quality. *Behavioral Sleep Medicine, 4*(3), 152–163.

Germain, A., et al. (2013). Dream content in complicated grief: A window into loss-related cognitive schemas. *Death Studies, 37*(3), 269–284.

Hassin, R. R., et al. (2009). Implicit working memory. *Consciousness and Cognition, 18*(3), 665–678.

Kristensen, P., Weisaeth, L., & Heir, T. (2010). Predictors of complicated grief after a natural disaster: A population study two years after the 2004 South-East Asian tsunami. *Death Studies, 34*(2), 137–150.

Mikulincer, M., & Shaver, P. R. (2003). The attachment behavioral system in adulthood: Activation, psychodynamics, and interpersonal processes. *Advances in Experimental Social Psychology, 35*, 53–152.

Mikulincer, M., Florian, V., & Hirschberger, G. (2003). The existential function of close relationships: Introducing death into the science of love. *Personality and Social Psychology Review, 7*(1), 20–40.

Miller, W. R., & Rollnick, S. (2013). *Motivational interviewing: Helping people change* (Applications of motivational interviewing 3rd ed., xii, 482 p). New York: Guilford Press.

Min, J. A., et al. (2013). Cognitive emotion regulation strategies contributing to resilience in patients with depression and/or anxiety disorders. *Comprehensive Psychiatry, 54*(8), 1190–1197.

Monk, T. H., Houck, P. R., & Shear, M. K. (2006). The daily life of complicated grief patients – What gets missed, what gets added? *Death Studies, 30*(1), 77–85.

Moskowitz, J. T., Folkman, S., & Acree, M. (2003). Do positive psychological states shed light on recovery from bereavement? Findings from a 3-year longitudinal study. *Death Studies, 27*(6), 471–500.

Neff, K. D., & Vonk, R. (2009). Self-compassion versus global self-esteem: Two different ways of relating to oneself. *Journal of Personality, 77*(1), 23–50.

Prigerson, H. G., et al. (1995). Inventory of complicated grief: A scale to measure maladaptive symptoms of loss. *Psychiatry Research, 59*(1–2), 65–79.

Pyszczynski, T., Greenberg, J., & Solomon, S. (1999). A dual-process model of defense against conscious and unconscious death-related thoughts: An extension of terror management theory. *Psychological Review, 106*(4), 835–845.

Reber, P. J. (2013). The neural basis of implicit learning and memory: A review of neuropsychological and neuroimaging research. *Neuropsychologia, 51*(10), 2026–2042.

Ryan, R. M., & Deci, E. L. (2000). Self-determination theory and the facilitation of intrinsic motivation, social development, and well-being. *American Psychologist, 55*(1), 68–78.

Shear, K., & Shair, H. (2005). Attachment, loss, and complicated grief. *Developmental Psychobiology, 47*(3), 253–267.

Shear, M. K., et al. (2001). Traumatic grief treatment: A pilot study. *The American Journal of Psychiatry, 158*(9), 1506–1508.

Shear, K., et al. (2005). Treatment of complicated grief: A randomized controlled trial. *Journal of American Medical Association, 293*(21), 2601–2608.

Shear, M. K., et al. (2011). Complicated grief and related bereavement issues for DSM-5. *Depression and Anxiety, 28*(2), 103–117.

Simon, N. M., et al. (2007). The prevalence and correlates of psychiatric comorbidity in individuals with complicated grief. *Comprehensive Psychiatry, 48*(5), 395–399.

Simon, N. M., et al. (2008). Impact of concurrent naturalistic pharmacotherapy on psychotherapy of complicated grief. *Psychiatry Research, 159*(1–2), 31–36.

Stroebe, M., Stroebe, W., & Schut, H. (2003). Bereavement research: Methodological issues and ethical concerns. *Palliative Medicine, 17*(3), 235–240.

Szanto, K., et al. (2006). Indirect self-destructive behavior and overt suicidality in patients with complicated grief. *The Journal of Clinical Psychiatry, 67*(2), 233–239.

Weissman, M. M., Markowitz, J. C., & Klerman, G. L. (2000). *Comprehensive guide to interpersonal psychotherapy* (Basic behavioral science, xii, 465 p). New York: Basic Books.

Wilson, T. D. (2002). *Strangers to ourselves: Discovering the adaptive unconscious*. Cambridge, MA: Harvard University Press.

Zuckoff, A., et al. (2006). Treating complicated grief and substance use disorders: A pilot study. *Journal of Substance Abuse Treatment, 30*(3), 205–211.

Trauma and Substance Abuse: A Clinician's Guide to Treatment

Lisa M. Najavits

Substance use disorder (SUD) frequently co-occurs with posttraumatic stress disorder (PTSD) and trauma symptoms broadly. This comorbidity is clinically important, with research showing that it signifies a more difficult course of recovery and greater impairment than either disorder alone (Ouimette and Read 2013). The presence of SUD also impacts how PTSD is addressed in treatment. The whole is not the sum of its parts—addressing PTSD/SUD is not simply about applying treatments for each, but requires conceptualization of how each disorder affects the other and how to engage in successful strategies to address each without worsening the other. It is like a seesaw that needs careful balancing to prevent tipping too far to one side.

Too often, either the SUD or the PTSD is not addressed by clinicians. Patients still frequently hear messages from earlier eras:

- "Get your substance use under control; only then can we address your PTSD."
- "You must go to Alcoholics Anonymous or other 12-step groups."
- "Your PTSD is the root issue—if we just address that, your substance use will decrease too."
- "If you don't stop using substances, I will not treat you."
- "Your substance use means you are avoiding your PTSD."
- "You need to hit bottom."

As will be explored in this chapter, these old messages are generally not helpful to PTSD/SUD patients and can impede recovery. Splits between PTSD and SUD

L.M. Najavits
Veterans Affairs Boston Healthcare System,
Boston, MA, USA

Department of Psychiatry, Boston University School of Medicine,
Boston, MA 02118, USA
e-mail: lisa.najavits@va.gov

© Springer International Publishing Switzerland 2015
U. Schnyder, M. Cloitre (eds.), *Evidence Based Treatments for Trauma-Related Psychological Disorders: A Practical Guide for Clinicians*,
DOI 10.1007/978-3-319-07109-1_16

treatment are well known, and most clinicians never receive formal training in both. Patients have often been left to try to integrate what our field has not. Although PTSD and SUD may be viewed separately, they are strongly intertwined in the day-to-day experience of patients' lives.

This chapter offers a brief summary of models for PTSD/SUD, key findings from outcome research, practice principles, and future directions.

16.1   Various Models

Recent years have seen the emergence of new therapies to address PTSD/SUD and research evaluating them. Table 16.1 provides a list of models that were either developed specifically for PTSD/SUD or studied in that population. In addition, for inclusion the model had to use a manual, was for treatment not prevention, and had to have at least one study addressing both PTSD and SUD outcomes, and a controlled or randomized controlled trial (RCT) had to provide outcomes for the experimental treatment. Thus, Substance Dependence PTSD Therapy (Triffleman 2000) was excluded. Due to space limits, it is not possible to describe each model nor list all research citations pertaining to them. One primary empirical citation is listed per model from which more information can be obtained; and if the model has a website, that is listed too. The number of studies listed is per Najavits and Hien (2013) plus a subsequent literature search.

Table 16.1   PTSD/SUD behavioral studies

Model and primary empirical citation	Number of outcome studies
Seeking Safety (SS) (Najavits and Hien 2013)	22
Trauma Recovery and Empowerment Model (TREM) (Fallot et al. 2011)	3
Helping Women Recover followed by *Beyond Trauma* (HWR/BT) (Covington et al. 2008)	2
Integrated CBT for PTSD and SUD (ICBT) (McGovern et al. 2009)	2
Prolonged Exposure plus *BRENDA SUD counseling* (PE/BRENDA) PE (Foa et al. 2013) BRENDA (Volpicelli et al. 2001)	1
Concurrent Prolonged Exposure (COPE)[a] (Mills et al. 2012)	1
Structured Writing Therapy for PTSD plus *manual-based SUD group therapy* (SWT) (van Dam et al. 2013)	1
Integrated Therapy (Sannibale et al. 2013)	1
Trauma Adaptive Recovery Group Education and Therapy (TARGET) (Frisman et al. 2008)	1
Creating Change (CC)[b]	1

[a]Prior version was Concurrent Treatment of PTSD and Cocaine Dependence (Brady et al. 2001)
[b]Prior version was Exposure Therapy-Revised (Najavits et al. 2005)

16.2 Major Findings

Several findings can be observed across the literature at this point, including some surprises. Even for clinicians who do not specialize in PTSD/SUD treatment, it is worth understanding the current state of the field. As it is said, every clinician has PTSD/SUD patients in their practice, whether they know it or not.

For details on the findings, see Najavits and Hien (2013), which is a comprehensive literature review on all outcome studies for PTSD/SUD. That review was written for clinicians as well as researchers and provides extensive descriptions of each study's methodology and results. Recent studies that emerged after that review are cited in Najavits (2013b); Hien et al. in press. Other reviews are available but are not comprehensive (e.g., Torchalla et al. 2012). Also more research is needed, given the methodology limitations of some studies (Najavits 2013b).

PTSD/SUD studies consistently show positive outcomes. In the 38 outcome studies conducted thus far, the pattern of results has consistently been positive. Improvements were found in PTSD, SUD, and other domains such as self-compassion, cognitions, coping skills, psychopathology, and functioning. Treatment satisfaction was strong in studies that addressed it. Early concerns that addressing PTSD in the context of SUD would worsen patients' state have not been borne out. But it is important to remember that all studies used new models specifically designed for PTSD/SUD or made major changes to classic PTSD therapies to make them tolerable and feasible for SUD samples.

All studies using a PTSD exposure (past-focused) approach combined it with a SUD coping skills (present-focused) approach—but none outperformed models that were present-focused alone. A major current discussion in the field is the relative merit of present- versus past-focused approaches to PTSD treatment. Broadly speaking, models that focus on exposure-based or other emotionally intense exploration of trauma memories are termed here *past-focused*. In contrast, *present-focused* models focus on coping skills and psychoeducation but do not explore trauma memories in detail (Najavits 2013a). Note that *trauma-focused* is often used to refer to exposure-based models. However, all present-focused PTSD models directly focus on trauma. The difference is how they approach it. Exposure-based models focus primarily on the past by exploring the intense trauma narrative and memories. Present-focused PTSD models explicitly omit detailed exploration of the past and instead offer psychoeducation and coping skills to help patients work on PTSD in the present (e.g., learn to identify and manage trauma symptoms; improve functioning; increase safety in their current actions, thinking, and behavior; and promote overall stabilization). Moreover, the term *non-trauma-focused treatment* for present-focused PTSD models is problematic; it is comparable to referring to women as "non-men" or children as "non-adults." Thus the terms *present- and past-focused* are used here.

The majority of PTSD/SUD studies thus far use present- rather than past-focused approaches. This is convergent with the widely endorsed stage-based approach to PTSD treatment in which present-focused stabilization occurs before moving into past-focused exposure (Cloitre et al. 2011; Herman 1992). This framework also helps explain why most of the PTSD literature has excluded SUD patients.

In recent years, there has been the healthy development of trying to evaluate whether past-focused approaches may be safely used with PTSD/SUD populations. Importantly, every study using a past-focused PTSD approach combined it with a present-focused SUD model. Concurrent Treatment of PTSD and Substance Use Disorders Using Prolonged Exposure (COPE; Mills et al. 2012) combines PTSD exposure therapy (Foa and Rothbaum 1998) with two CBT SUD models (Baker et al. 2003; Carroll 1998). The PE study (Foa et al. 2013) combined PE (Foa et al. 2007) with a motivational interviewing SUD model (Volpicelli et al. 2001). The Integrated Treatment Study (Sannibale et al. 2013) combined PTSD therapies (exposure and PTSD cognitive restructuring) with SUD treatment manuals from Project MATCH (Kadden et al. 1995) and Project COMBINE (Miller 2004). A study by van Dam et al. (2013) combined Structured Writing Therapy for PTSD (SWT; van Emmerik et al. 2008) with SUD group CBT (Emmelkamp and Vedel 2006). Creating Change uses a gentle approach to explore the past in relation to both PTSD and SUD, including preparation for the work, readiness evaluation, strong safety monitoring, and theme-based session topics (Najavits 2013a). In sum, no investigator has used any past-focused PTSD approach as-is with a SUD population.

Moreover, it is notable that all studies that included a past-focused component were delivered in individual modality rather than group and were almost always restricted to less complex samples than present-focused studies, in keeping with the PTSD-alone literature. "Less complex" means that patients were typically excluded if they had drug use disorders (rather than alcohol only), current domestic violence, homelessness, suicidality, violence, cognitive impairment, serious mental illness, and/or criminal justice involvement. In contrast, present-focused models were primarily group modality and accepted a much broader range of patients (Najavits and Hien 2013). (See below for more on this point.)

Many people believe that past-focused models are more powerful than present-focused models, perhaps because they are experienced as more emotionally intense. Yet all four RCTs that included past-focused PTSD treatment found null results (no difference) on either PTSD or SUD at the end of treatment compared to a control conditions that was present-focused only (Mills et al. 2012; Foa et al. 2013; Sannibale et al. 2013; van Dam et al. 2013) See Najavits 2013b for a summary. End of treatment is emphasized as that is the most rigorous time point for evaluating the impact of a model relative to a control. Both past- and present-focused models worked, but past-focused was not superior to present-focused, even on PTSD where it would be expected to if the "emotional intensity" hypothesis held. One explanation for the null results is that combining past-focused methods with present-focused diluted the past-focused work (Foa et al. 2013). Another explanation is that past-focused models may be too intense for patients who are struggling with SUD, which is consistent with the dropout problem Hoge et al. (2014), in various past-focused studies (e.g., (Foa et al. 2013; Mills et al. 2012; Brady et al. 2001)). See also the recent meta-analysis by Gerger et al. (2013), which found that the PTSD treatment models they reviewed, which were predominantly past-focused, worked best with simpler rather than more complex patients, when compared to nonspecific therapies such as supportive therapy and relaxation training. A study sample was identified as complex if 80 % met at least two of four clinical criteria: (a) duration of symptoms lasting more than 6 months; (b) presence of multiple problems (e.g., comorbid mental disorders, being in an ongoing violent relationship; being a refugee); (c) presence of a complex psychological traumatization, that is, childhood, multiple, or intentional trauma; and (d) the presence of a formal PTSD diagnosis per the DSM.

Overall, with PTSD/SUD patients, greater emotional intensity in sessions does not equal better outcomes. Both present- and past-focused models may be helpful to patients, based on readiness of the patient and clinician, training, setting, and other contextual factors. Such findings are consistent with psychotherapy research broadly, which shows that manual-based models perform equally well, including those developed for PTSD and those developed for SUD (Imel et al. 2008; Benish et al. 2007; Powers et al. 2010). The bottom line is that clinicians have a lot of choice in which models to use.

The most evidence-based model at this point is Seeking Safety (SS). SS has been very widely implemented in treatment programs for PTSD/SUD (as well as for either alone and for subthreshold patients). It has been the subject of the majority of PTSD/SUD studies, including 13 pilots, 3 controlled studies, and 7 RCTs (Najavits and Hien, 2013; Hien et al. in press). It is also the model with the most number of studies by independent investigators, which are less subject to positive bias (Chambless and Hollon 1998). SS has had consistently positive outcomes and is the only model thus far to outperform a control on both PTSD and SUD (Najavits and Hien 2013). However, some *partial-dose* SS studies were more mixed. Partial-dose studies used just 24–48 % of the model, including the largest study of SS, the National Institute on Drug Abuse Clinical Trials Network. SS is currently the only model for PTSD/SUD listed as having strong research support by professional entities, such as the International Society for Traumatic Stress Studies and Divisions 12 and 50 of the American Psychological Association.

Most studies addressed complex PTSD/SUD populations. It is heartening that the majority of PTSD/SUD studies addressed a broad range of patients: those with substance dependence rather than just substance abuse, those with drug disorders rather than just alcohol, and often including those with issues such as homelessness, domestic violence, suicidality, violence, serious and persistent mental illness, criminal justice involvement, unemployment, multiple prior treatment episodes, and low education. Inclusions and exclusions varied by study, but generally there were low to moderate exclusions in contrast to the relatively high exclusions in the PTSD-alone literature. Among PTSD/SUD studies, those with past-focused models had the most exclusions, in keeping with the PTSD-alone literature from which they derived. Exceptions, however, were Mills et al. (2012), Najavits and Johnson (2014), and Najavits et al. (2005), all of which had a broader range of patients.

Most studies used lower-cost formats for delivery of treatment models. The PTSD/SUD literature primarily uses group rather than individual therapy, open rather than closed groups, frontline clinicians who were native to the setting rather than brought in from the outside, and clinicians who were less highly trained (e.g., without advanced degrees). Such features are common in SUD treatment settings, which is where most of the studies were conducted. Here too, past-focused models differed overall, being conducted in individual modality and generally by highly trained clinicians brought in from the outside.

It appears easier to change PTSD than SUD. In the literature thus far, when there were differences between conditions, they were more often on PTSD or other mental health variables and less often on SUD. This may indicate that in PTSD/SUD patients, PTSD and mental health issues may be easier to treat than SUD. That remains a question for future research but does fit clinicians' perceptions (Back et al. 2009). This pattern also fits the current view of PTSD as amenable to time-limited treatment, whereas SUD (severe SUD in particular) is conceptualized as a chronic relapsing disorder needing ongoing care (Arria and McLellan 2012).

16.3   Recommendations for Practice

1. *Attend to both PTSD and SUD if the patient has both.* This may seem simple but all too often is not done in practice. There are many reasons for it, including lack of sufficient training on PTSD and/or SUD in professional degree programs. The disorders are also known to evoke strong emotional reactions in clinicians and, for SUD in particular, stigma and negative attitudes (Imhof 1991; Pearlman and Saakvitne 1995). Clinicians may shy away from addressing them, may feel incompetent to manage them, or may simply not notice them. Yet just as a patient with cancer and diabetes needs help with both, so too the patient with PTSD and SUD needs help with both. The treatment plan will depend on many factors. Some clinicians may be the primary treater for both; others may treat one or the other or refer out for both. But the "no wrong door" principle still applies: address both in some fashion if present.

2. *The first step in helping is accurate assessment.* Accurately identify both PTSD and SUD, along with other diagnoses and problems that may be present. Use validated instruments rather than homegrown instruments or ad hoc questions. There are at this point many assessments that are easy to obtain, including screening tools, diagnostic interviews, and self-report measures of problem areas. See (Najavits 2004; Ouimette and Read 2013; Read et al. 2002).

3. *The second step in helping is working together with the patient to explore treatment options.* Collaboration is crucial. Ultimatums often drive the patient away and reinforce distrust of professionals. "My way or the highway" approaches are sometimes used with SUD patients out of frustration or a misguided view that harsh confrontation or "hitting bottom" is needed to overcome SUD denial. Yet research shows that a supportive stance is best when working with SUD (Miller et al. 1993; Miller and Rollnick 1991) as well as PTSD. Offer the patient

as many treatment options as possible and empower patients to try out as many as possible before they choose which fit best for them. A helpful strategy is to encourage them to attend up to three sessions of various treatments. According to research, the therapeutic alliance is established by about the third session (Garfield and Bergin 1994). If the alliance is weak at that point, have the patient try other approaches. Pushing patients to stay in treatments they do not like is counterproductive and can drive patients away for good. To learn about treatment resources for PTSD and SUD, search online and find manuals that address PTSD/SUD.

4. *Be compassionate.* Listen closely and convey empathy. PTSD/SUD patients have typically lived lives of extraordinary pain. They are often highly sensitive and feel enormous self-hatred. They are used to being misunderstood by their own families, communities, and, unfortunately, sometimes by clinicians. If they perceive you as aloof or judgmental, they will be less likely to open up. They may drop out of treatment. A caring professional stance is the basis of good treatment. However, remember that true compassion does not mean letting go of standards, making excuses, tolerating unacceptable behavior, or otherwise "enabling" patients. It is about being kind and caring when you enforce treatment expectations and boundaries.

5. *Recognize differences among PTSD/SUD patients.* They vary in many ways, including the presence or absence of co-occurring personality disorders, physical health problems, financial concerns, and legal issues. They also differ in strengths, such as ability to get along with others and level of intelligence. Each patient's kaleidoscope of features will impact treatment. PTSD/SUD patients are not a homogeneous population.

6. *Severity of PTSD and SUD is key, not order of onset.* Some clinicians erroneously believe that if the PTSD occurred first (which it does in most cases), then addressing PTSD is primary. Yet rather than order of onset of PTSD and SUD, it is the *severity* of each that most determines the treatment plan. By the time the patient is sitting in front of you with both disorders, which came first is much less important than what happens next. Both disorders will need attention. And severe disorders will need the most immediate and strong help. Severity refers to both level of symptoms and also negative consequences, such as which disorder gets them in the most trouble, causes the most harm, etc. Some patients are equally severe on both disorders; others are more severe on one or the other. Use validated instruments to assess the severity of each to help determine the plan.

7. *Directly monitor substance use.* Good SUD care requires the clinician to actively inquire about substance use at every visit. Ideally, this will be verified by urinalysis, breathalyzer, or other biological methods. Even if those are not possible, which may be the case in private practice settings, it is crucial to use a valid self-report instrument and to have a clear written contract on substance use. The contract targets the goal per substance, such as "No more than 1 drink a day, measured with a shot glass," "No substance use at all," or whatever other goal is established. Inquire about substance use at each session, including

amount and frequency; patients will often not bring it up directly. PTSD symptoms should also be assessed ongoing.

8. *Do not push past-focused treatments.* Patients are sometimes overly strongly pushed into past-focused models with statements such as "You're avoiding if you don't do it," "This is the only way to really recover," and "If you do this work, it will get to the root of your problems and you won't need substances anymore." Even if well intentioned, these are not accurate for most PTSD/SUD patients, especially those with severe SUD. As reviewed earlier, scientific evidence at this point indicates that past- and present-focused approaches work equally well for PTSD/SUD patients. Be direct with patients about the evidence base and let them choose what is right for them without pressure. Some are ready for past-focused work, want to do it, and can benefit. Others do not.

9. *Attend to behavioral addictions as well as SUD.* There is increasing focus on behavioral addictions such as excessive gambling, work, exercise, internet, pornography, sex, etc. (Najavits et al. 2014; Freimuth 2005). Most are not in DSM-5 yet still warrant attention. Ask patients explicitly about these and offer options for help as needed.

10. *Choose PTSD/SUD models based on realistic factors.* Both the clinician and patient need models that fit for them. Factors such as preference for individual versus group work, past treatment experiences, appeal of various treatments, insurance coverage, and other factors will play a role.

11. *Provide up-to-date information.* Strive to stay current. Even if well intentioned, inaccurate messages can do more harm than good. See the beginning of this chapter for examples of such messages. Read updated books on PTSD/SUD. Reading on PTSD alone or SUD alone can be helpful but are not sufficient for the combination of PTSD/SUD combination. Get a broad understanding and seek training as needed.

16.4 Future Developments

Overall, as this review shows, various models have emerged to address the widespread suffering endured by PTSD/SUD patients. Such models have evidenced positive impact and can bring innovation and inspiration to clinical work. In the decades ahead, empirical efforts will, it is hoped, continue to expand understanding of how to best help these patients.

From a broader lens, it is also worth recognizing that no therapy model in and of itself is ever likely to quickly resolve what for many of these patients have been decades of abuse, neglect, violence, substance use, and associated problems, such as homelessness, criminal justice involvement, job problems, poverty, discrimination, and physical health problems. Many are multiply burdened (Brown et al. 1995), chronic in their PTSD and SUD, and come from generations of family who have also struggled with these issues. They often have few resources for care and receive treatment from some of the least trained clinical staff. They often end up in public health systems of care.

Thus it is worth considering options beyond therapy models per se and which may potentially boost the impact of models.

PTSD/SUD patients may need ongoing support rather than time-limited help. Some less severe patients may do well with a round of short-term treatment. But the clinical reality is that many cycle repeatedly through the revolving door of treatment. SUD in particular has been conceptualized as a disorder comparable to diabetes in needing long-term management rather than short-term models (Arria and McLellan 2012). This is reflected in the wisdom of 12-step approaches that provide free ongoing support to sustain abstinence from substances and which grew up as a grass-roots model by addicts themselves. For PTSD, there is as yet no widespread supportive resource of this type. Becoming creative about developing resources for chronic patients, beyond 12-step groups, may be an important public health goal. Some of the models identified in this article can perhaps be used in such ways.

The workforce treating these patients also needs support. Many clinicians have their own histories of trauma and addiction. They often handle large caseloads of complex patients without sufficient support or training. There is little research on how best to select and retain them and how to best support their work. Treatment models for PTSD/SUD are an important resource, but their professional needs go beyond models. Clinicians treating PTSD/SUD report notable gratification in the work but also significant stressors (Najavits et al. 2010).

Beyond the "horse race" of models, focus on cost, appeal, ease of implementation, and sustainability. Several decades of research indicate that well-constructed therapy models relevant to PTSD and SUD have positive impact but do not differ notably in their outcomes (Imel et al. 2008; Benish et al. 2007; Powers et al. 2010). However, they may differ in other important ways such as how much they cost, how easy they are to implement, and how sustainable they are. A model with slightly lower outcomes but greater strength in these factors may be an excellent choice. In the PTSD/SUD field, such factors have largely not yet been researched in relation to treatment models.

Case Example

To help highlight some of the themes in this chapter, the following case example is offered, using Seeking Safety as the treatment.

Implementation of Seeking Safety (SS). SS arose out of the need for a trauma intervention that could be used safely and effectively with substance abuse clients, most of whom have major trauma histories yet may not be able to tolerate emotionally intense past-focused PTSD therapies. SS is consistent with the stage-based approach to trauma recovery (Herman 1992), which is supported by PTSD experts (Cloitre et al. 2011). The first stage of work, *safety,* is present-focused, emphasizing stabilization and coping. SS focuses solely on this phase. Later work may include past-focused processing of trauma memories if needed.

SS provides education and coping skills for trauma survivors. It is optimistic, building hope through emphasis on ideals, humanistic language, inspiring quotations, and concrete strategies. Originally designed for co-occurring trauma and substance abuse, it is now used for either or both. SS is highly flexible: for males, females, all trauma types, adults, adolescents, groups, individuals, and any counselor, setting, and duration. It has been implemented successfully with numerous vulnerable populations including people who are homeless, living with HIV, incarcerated, suicidal, and cognitively impaired. Each SS topic offers a coping skill to build resilience, such as *Asking for Help, Honesty, Coping with Triggers, Self-Nurturing,* and *Healing from Anger.*

The case. Jolene is a 45-year-old African-American female veteran who served in the army 20 years ago. She survived a brutal sexual assault by a military commander, resulting in mild traumatic brain injury (mTBI) and severe PTSD. The mTBI resolved eventually, but the PTSD was so severe that she was virtually housebound for 20 years, living off of her benefits, unable to work, and in contact only with her siblings (her parents having died some years ago). She developed severe alcohol use disorder and came in for therapy on the advice of her primary care physician, who identified liver problems from the alcohol. She had never told anyone about the sexual assault until the SS therapy. In SS, patients can share the nature of their traumas, but we do not go into a detailed narrative of it. "Headlines, not details" is the guiding principle. Jolene expressed relief that she could work on her PTSD in SS without having to revisit the painful trauma narrative. She continually blamed herself for the trauma, saying "If I had been a better soldier, I would have been able to defend myself." She had had outstanding success in her military career until the assault but after it was unable to function and was discharged. "It's as if I was two different people: the person before and the person after."

The treatment. Jolene was hesitant to come to therapy and canceled the first several appointments. I encouraged her to try just one session. I let her know that it would be up to her whether or not she wanted to continue—thus striving from this first phone contact to empower her to choose what was best for her. Empowerment is a core aspect of SS. The model conveys that there are many ways to cope safely, and patients can choose what works for them, even if it is different than what others choose. "Safety" is a rich concept in SS, referring to safety in relationships, thinking, and behavior, with no harm to self or others.

Jolene ultimately attended a full course of SS with weekly sessions over 6 months. She was highly intelligent and conscientious, with military-style, responsible behavior—showing up on time, reading the handouts ahead of time, and following through on most of her therapy commitments (the latter is the SS term for homework). But emotionally she was all over the place—tearful, lacking focus, obsessing about small details, not taking care of her health (poor diet, no exercise), and drinking every day unable to stop.

Our primary focus in the work was threefold. First, we focused on coping—what she could do each week to move forward in her life, in any way possible. For example, the week that we covered the topic *Taking Good Care of Yourself,* she could see that her isolation was not healthy. That week she thus chose to attend an online AA meeting (an in-person meeting was not something she was willing to try). Another week we focused on *Setting Boundaries in Relationships*, and she was able to say no to her sister's request for money rather than giving into it as she had done too often in the past. Each session, we worked to relate the SS coping skills in meaningful yet also practical ways to her current struggles. Even small successes meant a lot to her—showing her that she was no longer stuck in the same old patterns but able to make new choices and to keep learning from them. SS, at its core, is all about learning—trying new strategies and adapting, refining, and changing them as needed to keep progressing. Such learning is both unique to each person yet also universal.

Our second major focus was reducing the alcohol use. Given the many years of daily drinking, her physician worked with her on the physiological aspects to prevent seizures that can occur with abrupt reduction of alcohol. In SS, I would gently bring up the alcohol either during the session, as part of our SS topic, weaving it in here and there to question, nudge, and guide her to see more clearly in its impact on her life and to explore alternative actions she could do when she had a craving to drink. I would ask questions such as, "Would you be willing to try drinking only every other day?" and we would explore that, always coming back to how the SS coping skills might help her to achieve that goal. Helping her see the linkages between her trauma and alcohol use was also a repeated theme. She said, "I can see it now much more clearly. I just wish I could have seen it 20 years ago." There was deep sadness with such statements, and her course of alcohol use had some ups and downs, but by the last third of the therapy, she had reduced her drinking by half and was moving toward abstinence.

Finally, our third major focus was bringing a compassionate approach to her self-hatred about her trauma. She had spent decades blaming and judging herself for not fighting off the attacker. We worked on SS topics such as *Compassion, Creating Meaning,* and *Integrating the Split Self* to help her respond to herself in kind ways when her inner critical voices arose. She was better able to get through her day with increased functionality as she learned to coach herself through her daily struggles rather than giving up. She was able to recognize too that there really had been no way for her to prevent the trauma—no matter how fine and strong a soldier she had been—and that her task now was to create a better future for herself rather than staying stuck in "beating herself up" about the past.

The case management component of SS also came into play, identifying referrals for any treatments that she would be willing to attend. She had limited social contact, often none in any given week, but was able to join a women-only therapy group and the online AA meetings. We also worked on referral to a nutrition consult to help with her poor diet.

She ended the SS therapy with greater hopefulness, even though there was still recovery work to do. "It has felt so healing to be able to start living more—to expand my world, to move forward."

16.5 Closing

The first generation of research on PTSD/SUD is impressive in attending to patients who were consistently excluded from most prior outcome research on PTSD. The development of new models tailored to this population has advanced the field, and at least one model thus far is established as evidence based (SS). However, there remains much to be done. There is a need for additional research to overcome methodology limitations of prior trials. Continued refinement of models is also needed. It is hoped that just as patients have often shown remarkable resilience, so too can this area of work continue to grow and expand.

References

Arria, A. M., & McLellan, A. T. (2012). Evolution of concept, but not action, in addiction treatment. *Substance Use and Misuse, 47*(8–9), 1041–1048.

Back, S. E., Waldrop, A. E., & Brady, K. T. (2009). Treatment challenges associated with comorbid substance use and posttraumatic stress disorder: Clinicians' perspectives. *The American Journal on Addictions, 18*(1), 15–20.

Baker, A., Kay-Lambkin, F., Lee, N. K., Claire, M., & Jenner, L. (2003). *A brief cognitive behavioural intervention for regular amphetamine users.* Canberra: Australian Government Department of Health and Ageing.

Benish, S., Imel, Z., & Wampold, B. (2007). The relative efficacy of bona fide psychotherapies for treating post-traumatic stress disorder: A meta-analysis of direct comparisons. *Clinical Psychology Review, 28,* 746–758.

Brady, K. T., Dansky, B. S., Back, S. E., Foa, E. B., & Caroll, K. M. (2001). Exposure therapy in the treatment of PTSD among cocaine-dependent individuals: Preliminary findings. *Journal of Substance Abuse Treatment, 21,* 47–54.

Brown, V. B., Huba, G., & Melchior, L. (1995). Level of burden: Women with more than one co-occurring disorder. *Journal of Psychoactive Drugs, 27,* 339–346.

Carroll, K. (1998). *A cognitive-behavioral approach: Treating cocaine addiction. NIH publication 98-4308.* Rockville: National Institute on Drug Abuse.

Chambless, D., & Hollon, S. (1998). Defining empirically supported therapies. *Journal of Consulting and Clinical Psychology, 66,* 7–18.

Cloitre, M., Courtois, C. A., Charuvastra, A., Carapezza, R., Stolbach, B. C., & Green, B. L. (2011). Treatment of complex PTSD: Results of the ISTSS expert clinician survey on best practices. *Journal of Traumatic Stress, 24*(6), 615–627.

Covington, S. S., Burke, C., Keaton, S., & Norcott, C. (2008). Evaluation of a trauma-informed and gender-responsive intervention for women in drug treatment. *Journal of Psychoactive Drugs, 40*(sup5), 387–398.

Emmelkamp, P. M. G., & Vedel, E. (2006). *Evidence-based treatments for alcohol and drug abuse: A practitioner's guide to theory, methods, and practice.* New York: Routledge.

Fallot, R. D., McHugo, G. J., Harris, M., & Xie, H. (2011). The trauma recovery and empowerment model: A quasi-experimental effectiveness study. *Journal of Dual Diagnosis, 7,* 74–89.

Foa, E. B., & Rothbaum, B. O. (1998). *Treating the trauma of rape: Cognitive-behavioral therapy for PTSD.* New York: Guilford.

Foa, E. B., Hembree, E. A., & Rothbaum, B. O. (2007). *Prolonged exposure therapy for PTSD: Emotional processing of traumatic experiences.* New York: Oxford University Press.

Foa, E. B., Yusko, D. A., McLean, C. P., Suvak, M. K., Bux, D. A., Jr., Oslin, D., O'Brien, C. P., Imms, P., Riggs, D. S., & Volpicelli, J. (2013). Concurrent naltrexone and prolonged exposure therapy for patients with comorbid alcohol dependence and PTSD: A randomized clinical trial. *JAMA, the Journal of the American Medical Association, 310*(5), 488–495.

Freimuth, M. (2005). *Hidden addictions: Assessment practices for psychotherapists, counselors, and health care providers.* Northvale: Jason Aronson.

Frisman, L., Ford, J., Hsui-Ju, L., Mallon, S., & Chang, R. (2008). Outcomes of trauma treatment using the TARGET model. *Journal of Groups in Addiction & Recovery, 3,* 285–303.

Garfield, S., & Bergin, A. (1994). *Handbook of psychotherapy and behavior change.* New York: John Wiley & Sons, Inc.

Gerger, H., Munder, T., & Barth, J. (2013). Specific and nonspecific psychological interventions for PTSD symptoms: A meta-analysis with problem complexity as a moderator. *Journal of Clinical Psychology, 70,* 601–615.

Herman, J. L. (1992). *Trauma and recovery.* New York: Basic Books.

Hoge CW, Grossman SH, Auchterlonie JL, Riviere LA, Milliken CS, Wilk JE. PTSD Treatment for Soldiers After Combat Deployment: Low Utilization of Mental Health Care and Reasons for Dropout. *Psychiatric Services,* 2014.

Imel, Z., Wampold, B., Miller, S., & Fleming, R. (2008). Distinctions without a difference: Direct comparisons of psychotherapies for alcohol use disorders. *Psychology of Addictive Behaviors, 22,* 533–543.

Imhof, J. (1991). Countertransference issues in alcoholism and drug addiction. *Psychiatric Annals, 21,* 292–306.

Kadden, R., Carroll, K., Donovan, D., Cooney, N., Monti, P., Abrams, D., Litt, M., & Hester, R. (1995). *Cognitive-behavioral coping skills therapy manual: A clinical research guide for therapists treating individuals with alcohol abuse and dependence* (Vol. 3). Rockville: U. S. Department of Health and Human Services.

McGovern, M. P., Lambert-Harris, C., Acquilano, S., Xie, H., Alterman, A. I., & Weiss, R. D. (2009). A cognitive behavioral therapy for co-occurring substance use and posttraumatic stress disorders. *Addictive Behaviors, 34*(10), 892–897.

Miller, W. R. (Ed.). (2004). *Combined behavioral intervention manual: A clinical research guide for therapists treating people with alcohol abuse and dependence (vol. 1, COMBINE monograph series): DHHS Publication No. (NIH) 04–5288.* Bethesda: NIAAA.

Miller, W. R., & Rollnick, S. (1991). *Motivational interviewing: Preparing people to change addictive behavior.* New York: Guilford.

Miller, W. R., Benefield, R. G., & Tonigan, J. S. (1993). Enhancing motivation for change in problem drinking: A controlled comparison of two therapist styles. *Journal of Consulting and Clinical Psychology, 61,* 455–461.

Mills, K. L., Teesson, M., Back, S. E., Brady, K. T., Baker, A. L., Hopwood, S., Sannibale, C., Barrett, E. L., Merz, S., Rosenfeld, J., & Ewer, P. L. (2012). Integrated exposure-based therapy for co-occurring posttraumatic stress disorder and substance dependence: A randomized controlled trial. *JAMA, the Journal of the American Medical Association, 308*(7), 690–699.

Najavits, L. M. (2004). Assessment of trauma, PTSD, and substance use disorder: A practical guide. In J. P. Wilson & T. M. Keane (Eds.), *Assessment of psychological trauma and PTSD* (pp. 466–491). New York: Guilford.

Najavits, L. (2013a). Creating change: A new past-focused model for PTSD and substance abuse. In P. Ouimette & J. P. Read (Eds.), *Handbook of trauma, PTSD and substance use disorder comorbidity.* Washington, DC: American Psychological Association Press.

Najavits, L. M. (2013b). Therapy for posttraumatic stress and alcohol dependence. *JAMA, the Journal of the American Medical Association, 310*(22), 2457–2458.

Najavits, L. M., & Hien, D. A. (2013). Helping vulnerable populations: A comprehensive review of the treatment outcome literature on substance use disorder and PTSD. *Journal of Clinical Psychology, 69,* 433–480.

Najavits, L. M., & Johnson, K. M. (2014a). Pilot study of creating change, a new past-focused model for PTSD and substance abuse. *The American Journal on Addictions.* doi:10.1111/j.1521-0391.2014.12127.x.

Najavits, L. M., Schmitz, M., Gotthardt, S., & Weiss, R. D. (2005). Seeking safety plus exposure therapy: An outcome study on dual diagnosis men. *Journal of Psychoactive Drugs, 37*, 425–435.

Najavits, L. M., Norman, S. B., Kivlahan, D., & Kosten, T. R. (2010). Improving PTSD/substance abuse treatment in the VA: A survey of providers. *The American Journal on Addictions, 19*(3), 257–263.

Najavits, L. M., Lung, J., Froias, A., Bailey, G. L., & Paull, N. (2014). A study of multiple behavioral addictions in a substance abuse sample. *Substance Use and Misuse, 49*, 479–484.

Ouimette, P., & Read, J. P. (Eds.). (2013). *Handbook of trauma, PTSD and substance use disorder comorbidity*. Washington, DC: American Psychological Association Press.

Pearlman, L. A., & Saakvitne, K. W. (1995). *Trauma and the therapist: Countertransference and vicarious traumatization in psychotherapy with incest survivors*. New York: WW Norton.

Powers, M. B., Halpern, J. M., Ferenschak, M. P., Gillihan, S. J., & Foa, E. B. (2010). A meta-analytic review of prolonged exposure for posttraumatic stress disorder. *Clinical Psychology Review, 30*(6), 635–641.

Read, J. P., Bollinger, A. R., & Sharansky, E. (2002). Assessment of comorbid substance use disorder and posttraumatic stress disorder. In P. Ouimette & P. J. Brown (Eds.), *Trauma and substance abuse: Causes, consequences, and treatment of comorbid disorders* (pp. 111–125). Washington, DC: American Psychological Association Press.

Sannibale, C. (2013). Randomized controlled trial of cognitive behaviour therapy for comorbid post-traumatic stress disorder and alcohol use disorders. *Addiction, 108*, 1397–1410.

Torchalla, I., Nosen, L., Rostam, H., & Allen, P. (2012). Integrated treatment programs for individuals with concurrent substance use disorders and trauma experiences: A systematic review and meta-analysis. *Journal of Substance Abuse Treatment, 42*(1), 65–77.

Triffleman, E. (2000). Gender differences in a controlled pilot study of psychosocial treatments in substance dependent patients with post-traumatic stress disorder: Design considerations and outcomes. *Alcoholism Treatment Quarterly, 18*(3), 113–126.

van Dam, D., Ehring, T., Vedel, E., & Emmelkamp, P. M. (2013). Trauma-focused treatment for posttraumatic stress disorder combined with CBT for severe substance use disorder: A randomized controlled trial. *BMC Psychiatry, 13*(1), 172.

van Emmerik, A. A. P., Kamphuis, J. H., & Emmelkamp, P. M. G. (2008). Treating acute stress disorder and posttraumatic stress disorder with cognitive behavioral therapy or structured writing therapy: A randomized controlled trial. *Psychotherapy and Psychosomatics, 77*(2), 93–100.

Volpicelli, J., Pettinati, H., McLellan, A., & O'Brien, C. (2001). *Combining medication and psychosocial treatments for addictions: The BRENDA approach*. New York: Guilford.

Treating PTSD and Borderline Personality Disorder

17

Melanie S. Harned and Kathryn E. Korslund

Borderline personality disorder (BPD) is a severe and complex psychological disorder characterized by pervasive emotion dysregulation, unstable relationships, impulsive behavior, and recurrent suicidal and non-suicidal self-injury (NSSI). PTSD is one of the most common co-occurring disorders among individuals with BPD, with comorbidity rates ranging from approximately 30 % in community samples (Grant et al. 2008; Pagura et al. 2010) to 50 % in clinical samples (Harned et al. 2010; Zanarini et al. 1998). There are several theoretical models to explain the high comorbidity between BPD and PTSD. Some models focus on the common etiological factors between the two disorders. For example, childhood abuse has been implicated in the development of both BPD and PTSD (Widom 1999; Widom et al. 2009). Other models propose that PTSD mediates the relationship between trauma exposure and BPD criterion behaviors. For example, PTSD symptoms of reexperiencing and avoidance/numbing have been found to mediate the relationship between childhood sexual abuse and NSSI (Weierich and Nock 2008). Finally, some models suggest a reciprocal relationship such that each disorder functions to maintain the other. For example, PTSD has been shown to exacerbate BPD criterion behaviors, such as emotion dysregulation, suicide attempts, and NSSI (Pagura et al. 2010; Harned et al. 2010; Marshall-Berenz et al. 2011) and to decrease the likelihood of achieving diagnostic remission from BPD over 6 and 10 years of naturalistic

M.S. Harned, PhD (✉) • K.E. Korslund, PhD
Department of Psychology, University of Washington, 355915,
Seattle, WA 98195, USA
e-mail: mharned@u.washington.edu

© Springer International Publishing Switzerland 2015
U. Schnyder, M. Cloitre (eds.), *Evidence Based Treatments for Trauma-Related Psychological Disorders: A Practical Guide for Clinicians*,
DOI 10.1007/978-3-319-07109-1_17

follow-up (Zanarini et al. 2004, 2006). Conversely, BPD is associated with high experiential avoidance (Iverson et al. 2012), which is likely to maintain PTSD (Shenk et al. 2014). Given the multiple and complex relationships between PTSD and BPD suggested by these models, successful treatment of both disorders is likely necessary to achieve optimal outcomes for individuals with this comorbidity. In this chapter, we will review research on treatment approaches for individuals with PTSD and BPD, discuss common challenges that arise during trauma-focused treatment with this population, and present a case example.

17.1 Treatment Approaches for Co-occurring PTSD and Borderline Personality Disorder

Three general approaches have been evaluated as treatments for PTSD among individuals with BPD, including (1) single-diagnosis treatments, (2) phase-based treatments, and (3) integrated treatments. Single-diagnosis treatments focus solely on treating PTSD, and any improvements in comorbid problems occur as a secondary result of targeting PTSD. Phase-based treatments include an initial treatment phase targeting comorbid problems followed by a second phase of trauma-focused treatment. Some phase-based treatments also include a third phase in which psychosocial functioning is typically addressed. Finally, integrated treatments are designed to provide comprehensive, idiographic treatment for individuals with PTSD and BPD by targeting the full range of problems with which clients may present, including but not limited to both of these disorders and the factors explaining the relationships between them. The present review will focus on treatments from each of these general approaches that have been evaluated in terms of their specific effectiveness for individuals with PTSD and BPD. While several other treatments for PTSD have included individuals with BPD (e.g., Cloitre et al. 2010; Mueser et al. 2008; Sachsse et al. 2006), they will not be reviewed here as they have not reported outcomes specific to this subgroup.

17.1.1 Single-Diagnosis Treatments

17.1.1.1 Cognitive Processing Therapy (CPT) (Chap. 10)

CPT is a brief, outpatient treatment for PTSD that is typically delivered in 12 weekly or biweekly individual sessions (Resick and Schnicke 1993). The treatment includes cognitive therapy to identify and challenge trauma-related beliefs and exposure in the form of writing and reading about the traumatic event. To date, one study has evaluated the effect of borderline personality characteristics (BPC) on outcomes in a randomized controlled trial (RCT) comparing CPT to prolonged exposure (PE) (Clarke et al. 2008). Participants included 131 female sexual assault survivors with PTSD, of whom 39 (25.2 %) were above the cutoff for a clinical level of BPC according to self-report. Women with serious suicidal intent, recent suicidal or self-injurious behavior, ongoing abuse, or current substance dependence, bipolar or psychotic disorders were excluded. Results indicated that BPC scores were unrelated to treatment dropout, and there was no evidence that BPC was related to worse outcomes in the rate of change in PTSD and other trauma-related symptoms (e.g., dissociation, depression, sexual concerns). The interaction between type of treatment (CPT or PE) and BPC score was not significant for any outcome, indicating that both treatments were comparably effective for individuals with BPC.

17.1.1.2 Prolonged Exposure (PE) (Chap. 8)

PE is a brief, outpatient treatment for PTSD that is typically delivered in 10–15 weekly or biweekly individual sessions (Foa et al. 2007). The primary PE treatment components include imaginal exposure to the trauma memory and in vivo exposure to feared but non-dangerous situations. In addition to the study of PE and CPT reviewed above (Clarke et al. 2008), a second study examined the impact of full or partial BPD on treatment outcome in an RCT comparing PE, stress inoculation training (SIT), and a combined PE/SIT treatment (Feeny et al. 2002). Treatment was delivered in 9 biweekly individual sessions. Participants were female assault survivors with a primary diagnosis of PTSD who were not acutely suicidal, had no recent history of suicidal or self-injurious behavior, were not currently involved in an abusive relationship, and did not meet criteria for substance dependence, bipolar, or psychotic disorders. Analyses were conducted using the treatment completer sample ($n=58$), of whom 9 (15.5 %) met full or partial criteria for BPD. Given the small number of participants with BPD, analyses were not conducted separately by treatment type. When the three treatments were combined, BPD was not significantly related to outcome. However, women with full or partial BPD were significantly less likely than those without BPD to achieve good end-state functioning (11 % vs. 51 %), which was defined as being below clinical cutoffs for PTSD, depression, and anxiety.

17.1.1.3 Narrative Exposure Therapy (NET) (Chap. 12)

NET is a short-term treatment for PTSD that is designed for survivors of multiple and complex traumas such as victims of organized violence and conflict (Schauer et al. 2011). NET is typically delivered in 5–10 weekly or biweekly individual sessions. The primary component of NET is the creation of a written, cohesive narrative that integrates traumatic events into the individual's larger life story. An open trial feasibility study evaluated NET among ten women with PTSD and co-occurring BPD (Pabst et al. 2012). Women actively engaging in NSSI were included, but those with acute suicidality, a recent suicide attempt, and other severe comorbidities (e.g., drug abuse, psychosis) were excluded. Treatment occurred primarily in inpatient settings, although three women were treated solely on an outpatient basis. The average duration of treatment was 14 sessions. From pretreatment to 6 months after therapy, there were large and significant improvements in PTSD, depression, and dissociation, but not BPD symptoms.

17.1.2 Phase-Based Treatments

17.1.2.1 Dialectical Behavior Therapy for PTSD (DBT-PTSD)

Bohus and colleagues (Bohus et al. 2013; Steil et al. 2011) have developed an adaptation of dialectical behavior therapy (DBT) for PTSD related to childhood sexual abuse. DBT-PTSD is delivered as a 12-week residential treatment that includes three treatment phases: (1) Weeks 1–4: psychoeducation; identification of typical cognitive, emotional, and behavioral strategies to escape emotions; and teaching of DBT skills to control these behaviors. (2) Weeks 5–10: trauma-focused cognitive and exposure-based interventions. (3) Weeks 11–12: radical acceptance of trauma-related facts and addressing psychosocial functioning. Clients receive biweekly individual sessions (23 sessions total) and several group interventions, including group skills training (11 sessions total), group focused on self-esteem (8 sessions total), and group mindfulness practice (3 sessions total). In addition, clients attend three nonspecific groups each week (e.g., music and art therapy). An RCT has evaluated the efficacy of DBT-PTSD for women with and without BPD in comparison to a treatment as usual-waitlist control (TAU-WL) (Bohus et al. 2013). Participants were 74 women with childhood sexual abuse-related PTSD, including 33 (44.6 %) who met criteria for BPD. Women actively engaging in NSSI were included, and those with a life-threatening behavior in the prior 4 months, current substance dependence, a lifetime diagnosis of schizophrenia, or a body mass index less than 16.5 were excluded. DBT-PTSD was superior to TAU-WL in improving PTSD, depression, and global functioning, but not global symptom severity, dissociation, or BPD symptoms. These results were comparable for the subgroup of women with BPD in each condition, and BPD severity was generally unrelated to treatment outcome. Among women with BPD who received DBT-PTSD, the rate of remission of PTSD was 41.2 %. There was no evidence of worsening of PTSD, NSSI, or suicidality in DBT-PTSD.

17.1.3 Integrated Treatments

17.1.3.1 Dialectical Behavior Therapy (DBT)

DBT is a comprehensive, principle-driven treatment for individuals with BPD that is rooted in behavior therapy and incorporates dialectical philosophy and elements of western contemplative and eastern Zen practices (Linehan 1993a, b). Standard DBT is typically provided as a 1-year outpatient treatment and includes 4 weekly treatment modes: individual therapy, group skills training, therapist consultation team, and telephone consultation (as needed). As an integrated treatment, DBT is designed to simultaneously treat multiple problems according to a hierarchy of treatment targets, including (1) life-threatening behaviors, (2) therapy-interfering behaviors, and (3) behaviors that interfere with quality of life. Within this target hierarchy, PTSD is considered a quality of life problem that is targeted once life-threatening and therapy-interfering behaviors are sufficiently controlled. Although the DBT manual recommends the use of exposure to treat PTSD, it does not include a protocol specifying exactly when or how to do so. Without a specific protocol for treating PTSD, 33–35 % of recently and recurrently suicidal and self-injuring women with BPD achieve remission from PTSD during 1 year of DBT and up to 1 year of follow-up (Harned et al. 2008, 2014). In addition, PTSD predicts less improvement in NSSI and suicidality during DBT (Barnicot and Priebe 2013; Harned et al. 2010).

17.1.3.2 DBT with the DBT Prolonged Exposure Protocol (DBT + DBT PE)

The DBT PE protocol was developed to improve the effects of standard DBT on PTSD, particularly for suicidal and self-injuring individuals with BPD (Harned 2013). The DBT PE protocol is based on PE, and the primary treatment components include imaginal and in vivo exposure. DBT strategies are incorporated into PE (e.g., to target problems that may occur during or as a result of trauma-focused treatment), and structured procedures are included to address complexities common in this client population (e.g., multiple, often fragmented trauma memories, intense shame, traumatic events that do not meet the standard definitions of trauma such as rejection, invalidation, and betrayal). The combined DBT and DBT PE protocol treatment lasts 1 year and begins with standard DBT focused on stabilizing life-threatening behaviors and other higher-priority targets. The DBT PE protocol is integrated into individual DBT therapy sessions if/when clients meet specified readiness criteria (e.g., not at imminent risk of suicide, no suicide attempts or NSSI for at least 2 months, no serious therapy-interfering behaviors, able and willing to experience intense emotions without escaping). Following completion of the DBT PE protocol, the rest of the treatment year uses standard DBT to address the client's remaining treatment goals, which often include improving psychosocial functioning.

To date, DBT + DBT PE has been evaluated in an open trial ($n = 13$) (Harned et al. 2012) and an RCT ($n = 26$) that compared DBT with and without the DBT PE protocol (Harned et al. 2014). Both studies included women with BPD, PTSD, and recent (past 2–3 months) suicidal behavior or NSSI and excluded those with bipolar or psychotic disorders. Across both studies, the DBT PE protocol was feasible to implement for 80–100 % of treatment completers who started the protocol after an average of 20 weeks of DBT; of these, 73 % completed the full protocol in an average of 13 sessions. DBT + DBT PE was highly acceptable to clients and therapists in terms of treatment expectancies and satisfaction, and a majority of clients (73.8 %) reported a preference for DBT + DBT PE compared to either DBT or PE alone (Harned et al. 2013). Across both studies, DBT + DBT PE clients in the intent-to-treat samples showed large and significant improvements in PTSD severity as well as high rates of reliable improvement (70.0–83.3 %) and remission of PTSD (58.3–60.0 %). In the RCT, clients who completed the DBT PE protocol were two times more likely than those who completed DBT to achieve remission from PTSD (80 % vs. 40 %) while simultaneously being 2.4 times less likely to attempt suicide (17 % vs. 40 %) and 1.5 times less likely to self-injure (67 % vs. 100 %). In both studies, clients in DBT + DBT PE also showed large pre-post improvements in dissociation, depression, anxiety, guilt, shame, and social and global functioning, and, in the RCT, these improvements were larger in DBT + DBT PE than in DBT. In the RCT, 80 % of DBT + DBT PE completers versus 0 % of DBT completers both reliably improved and reached a normative level of functioning in terms of global symptom severity at posttreatment.

17.1.4 Summary

In sum, five treatments for PTSD have been shown to be effective in reducing PTSD and associated problems for individuals with comorbid BPD. These treatments vary not only in their general approach (single diagnosis, phase based, and integrated) but also in the types of trauma-focused interventions used (exposure, cognitive therapy, narration), types of trauma they were designed to treat (adult assaults, childhood sexual abuse, and multiple traumas), length (ranging from 9 to 52 sessions), and treatment setting (inpatient, residential, and outpatient). Of particular note, although each of these treatments has been evaluated among clients with BPD/BPC, most have excluded individuals with problems common in severe BPD, such as acute suicidality (Clarke et al. 2008; Feeny et al. 2002; Pabst et al. 2012), recent life-threatening behavior (Bohus et al. 2013), recent suicidal behavior (Clarke et al. 2008; Feeny et al. 2002; Pabst et al. 2012), recent NSSI (Clarke et al. 2008; Feeny et al. 2002), ongoing abuse (Clarke et al. 2008; Feeny et al. 2002), and/or substance dependence (Clarke et al. 2008; Feeny et al. 2002; Pabst et al. 2012; Bohus et al. 2013). Thus, their generalizability to BPD clients with these co-occurring problems is unknown. To date, only one treatment has been developed specifically for individuals with co-occurring BPD and PTSD that has included clients with each of these severe co-occurring problems (Harned et al. 2012, 2014). However, research on treatments for co-occurring BPD and PTSD is generally limited, and additional research is needed to replicate and extend these findings in larger and more representative samples of clients with this challenging comorbidity.

17.2   Special Challenges

Treatment of clients with both PTSD and BPD is often complicated by a variety of factors. Although the issues described below are likely to interfere with effective treatment of any kind, these factors are highlighted as posing particular challenges to clinicians engaging in trauma-focused treatment.

17.2.1 Suicide and Self-Injury

Suicidal behavior and NSSI are often considered a "hallmark" feature of BPD, with 60–70 % reporting a history of multiple suicide attempts and NSSI episodes (Zanarini et al. 2008) and 8–10 % dying by suicide (Pompili et al. 2005). Among individuals with BPD, these behaviors are often precipitated by PTSD symptoms (Harned et al. 2010) and most often function to provide relief from unpleasant emotions (Brown et al. 2002). As trauma-focused treatments often elicit intense emotions and can cause initial increases in PTSD symptoms before improvement is seen (Nishith et al. 2002), it is understandable that clinicians and BPD patients may both be wary of the potential for a recurrence of these behaviors during PTSD treatment. Moreover, it is possible that fears of intense emotion may prevent therapists and clients alike from fully allowing trauma-related emotions to be experienced, thus potentially decreasing the effectiveness of treatment. Additionally, if suicidal and self-injurious behaviors function as an escape from trauma-related emotions, then the opportunity to learn that these painful emotions can be tolerated without escaping will likely be missed. To address these factors, all of the treatments reviewed above require clients to be abstinent from serious suicidal behavior for a period of 2–4 months before beginning trauma-focused treatment, and most also require abstinence from NSSI. In addition, several treatments include an initial stabilizing phase to help suicidal and self-injuring clients learn the skills necessary to control these behaviors prior to initiating trauma-focused interventions.

17.2.2 Emotion Dysregulation

The regulation of emotion is a complex process involving multiple components of the emotional system (e.g., cognitive interpretation, physiological sensation, behavioral expression). Dysregulation can occur at any point in the system. The biosocial theory of BPD proposed in DBT is that it is the transaction between an emotionally vulnerable biology and an invalidating environment (which may include childhood abuse and trauma) that leads to the pervasive disruption of the emotion regulation system that is central to BPD (Linehan 1993a). According to the theory, emotional vulnerability is defined as having a lowered threshold for emotionally salient cues, increased emotional reactivity, and a slow return to emotional baseline. The emotion dysregulation exhibited by BPD individuals is further intensified by the presence of PTSD (Harned et al. 2010; Marshall-Berenz et al. 2011) and can complicate PTSD treatment in several ways. Dysregulated emotions can lead to over-engagement during trauma-focused treatment, although more often the dysregulated emotional system yields emotional withdrawal and suppression of emotional experience. Either extreme deviates from optimal emotional engagement and is likely to interfere with treatment response. Emotion dysregulation of BPD patients is extensive and typically extends across the entire emotional spectrum. As such, intense non-fear emotions such as sadness, anger, and shame may equally interfere with treatment effectiveness. To address this, several treatments reviewed above teach clients behavioral skills (e.g., emotion regulation, distress tolerance) prior to beginning trauma-focused treatment and coach clients to use these skills as needed to increase or decrease emotional intensity during trauma-focused interventions.

17.2.3 Dissociation

Many clients with PTSD and BPD also experience dysregulation across cognitive processes. Dissociation can be thought of as a specific reaction to intense emotions or trauma-relevant cues that functions to reduce distress by disrupting attention and information processing. Like many maladaptive behaviors, the dissociative response is often outside the awareness of the client or occurs without intention. Dissociation can pose a significant challenge to successful implementation of trauma-focused treatment as it interferes with establishing optimal emotional engagement and reduces the opportunity for new learning. Given that more than two-thirds of BPD clients report moderate to high levels of dissociation (Zanarini et al. 2000), this is not a minor problem facing clinicians. Dissociation during trauma-focused treatment is typically addressed by coaching clients to use skills that increase awareness of the present moment (e.g., mindfulness, distraction with intense physical sensations).

Case Example

To provide an illustration of treatment for co-occurring PTSD and BPD, as well as strategies for addressing common challenges, we will present a case example of a client who received DBT + DBT PE.

Identifying Information and Relevant History

"Amanda" was a 19-year-old single, Caucasian woman who had recently moved to the area to live with her mother's extended family. She grew up in a small town in another part of the country with her mother, stepfather, and younger siblings. She described her mother as emotionally volatile and often depressed and her stepfather as strict and critical. From the ages of 8–12, Amanda was sexually molested by her grandfather, who convinced her the abuse was a "game" and made her feel special and loved for playing the game with him. The abuse stopped abruptly when Amanda was 12 years old after which she developed symptoms of dysthymic disorder, including persistent sadness, poor self-esteem, and low energy. At age 14, she began engaging in NSSI by cutting her arms and legs with a razor, a behavior that recurred every few months throughout high school. Despite these childhood adversities, Amanda was a good student, had several close friends, and was active in extracurricular activities.

After graduating from high school, Amanda attended a nearby college and lived on campus. Near the end of her first semester, she experienced a number of interpersonal stressors beginning with her boyfriend of 2 years breaking up with her unexpectedly. She became depressed, began cutting several times per week, and was eventually psychiatrically hospitalized due to suicidal ideation. After discharge, she returned to her family and began outpatient therapy. During this time, she disclosed her sexual abuse to her mother and stepfather for the first time. Her mother responded supportively but was intensely distressed, whereas her stepfather reacted by telling her never to speak of it again. Amanda also disclosed her abuse to her pastor and his wife. Soon, news of her allegations began to spread throughout the small community. Because her grandfather was prominent in the town, others disbelieved her, and she was shunned and criticized. Several months later Amanda moved across the country to escape the situation.

At intake, Amanda had been in the area for 6 months and was attending community college. She had no social supports beyond the relatives with whom she was living, was cutting herself weekly, had frequent suicidal ideation, and was binge eating several times per month. She met criteria for BPD, PTSD, major depressive disorder, dysthymic disorder, and generalized anxiety disorder and was subthreshold for binge eating disorder.

Treatment Process

DBT

The beginning sessions of DBT addressed pretreatment tasks, including identifying Amanda's treatment goals, orienting her to treatment, and obtaining and strengthening commitments to stay alive and stop self-injuring. Amanda's primary treatment goals were to stop self-injuring, increase her ability to experience and express emotions, and build more friendships. Amanda reported that her past sexual abuse had always "bothered" her, but did not identify it as a treatment goal, largely because she was not familiar with PTSD and did not know that it was treatable. In the second DBT session, her therapist oriented her to the PTSD diagnosis as well as the basic rationale and procedures of the DBT PE protocol. Amanda was ambivalent about treating her PTSD, saying that it sounded "scary" and her sexual abuse was "too embarrassing to talk about." Thus, she and her therapist agreed to wait and reassess her interest in treating PTSD as treatment progressed.

The first phase of treatment (weeks 4–12) focused primarily on helping Amanda gain control over NSSI. Diary cards were used to help Amanda track suicidal and non-suicidal urges and actions, the intensity of various emotions, and her use of DBT skills. In individual therapy, behavioral chain analyses of specific incidents of increased urges to self-injure were conducted, and solutions were generated. These solutions drew on the DBT skills Amanda was learning in her weekly skills group, and between-session phone calls were used to provide in vivo coaching on applying the solutions. In these initial weeks, a consistent pattern emerged in which urges to self-injure and commit suicide were reliably preceded by sadness. Amanda's initial response was to invalidate her emotion, believing that it was irrational, excessive, and/or a sign of incompetence. Thinking about self-injury and suicide functioned to distract her from the emotion and provide temporary relief. Thus, the key interventions were teaching Amanda skills to experience and tolerate emotion, while also increasing her ability to validate herself. With these interventions, Amanda succeeded in not self-injuring despite having frequent high urges to do so.

As treatment progressed, it became increasingly apparent that Amanda's sexual abuse as well as the rejection she had experienced after disclosing it was the cause of much of her emotional misery. As a result, Amanda's therapist began to actively work to increase her motivation for PTSD treatment. Her therapist highlighted the ways in which PTSD and trauma-related problems interfered in her life and linked her goals to the need to treat her PTSD. Although still quite ambivalent, Amanda agreed to consider PTSD treatment due to her strong connection to her therapist and her belief that it would ultimately help her, even if the process would be painful. After 12 weeks of DBT, when Amanda had been abstinent from self-injury for 13 weeks and was increasingly able to use skills to experience emotions without avoiding, she and her therapist agreed she was ready to start the DBT PE protocol. She completed the PTSD Checklist (PCL) (Weathers et al. 1993) at this session and scored a 62 (out of 85). Given Amanda's lengthy commute to the clinic, it was decided that the treatment would be implemented in one 2-h individual session per week (90 min of DBT PE and 30 min of DBT) in addition to her ongoing weekly skills group and between-session phone coaching.

The DBT PE Protocol

During Session 1, the therapist reviewed the treatment rationale and conducted a structured trauma interview to identify and prioritize Amanda's three most distressing memories. Amanda experienced high shame while thinking about her traumatic experiences, but managed to briefly describe each of the three memories. She elected to start treatment with her most distressing memory, which was the last time that her grandfather had sexually abused her. DBT commitment strategies were used to obtain and strengthen commitments to refrain from suicide and self-injury and to actively engage in the PTSD treatment. Finally, a postexposure skills plan was developed that consisted of DBT skills that she could use after exposure tasks as needed. Throughout this session, Amanda reported a number of concerns about beginning PTSD treatment (e.g., that she would not be able to tolerate it), which her therapist responded to with validation and encouragement.

At the beginning of Session 2, review of Amanda's DBT diary card indicated several days of higher suicide and self-injury urges, which she attributed to increased distress due to anticipation of beginning imaginal exposure the next week. Her PCL score had also increased to a 73. She remained firmly committed to not engaging in suicide and self-injury and was confident that she had the skills to do so. As such, her therapist proceeded with the planned DBT PE protocol tasks. These included psychoeducation about common reactions to trauma followed by a detailed rationale for in vivo exposure and the construction of an in vivo exposure hierarchy. Amanda had some difficulty identifying in vivo exposure tasks, as she did not report much behavioral avoidance. The resulting hierarchy primarily included tasks related to exposure to men, particularly men who reminded her of her grandfather, and activities that elicited unjustified shame (e.g., sharing personal information with friends). She was assigned her first in vivo exposure homework to sit one row removed from men on the bus two times and to sit next to men in three of her classes. Her therapist also asked her to make a specific plan for what she would do immediately following the first imaginal exposure session the next week.

At Session 3, Amanda reported that she had almost canceled the session due to a high desire to avoid the imaginal exposure. Her DBT diary card indicated that she had continued to have higher suicide and self-injury urges on several days. Her therapist responded by validating her distress, reinforcing her for coming, and expressing confidence in her ability to complete the exposure. After reviewing her in vivo homework, her therapist provided a detailed rationale for imaginal exposure and oriented her to the specific procedures. During this discussion, Amanda reported several common concerns, including fears that her therapist would think her abuse was "not a big deal" and that her memory was insufficiently detailed. Although she was reluctant to start, Amanda ultimately did very well in completing the imaginal exposure and repeated the trauma narrative multiple times. Immediately before and after the exposure, Amanda completed ratings of the probability and cost estimates of feared outcomes (0–100), urges (to commit suicide, self-injure, quit therapy, and use substances: 0–5), Subjective Units of Distress (SUDs: 0–100), and seven primary emotions (sadness, fear, guilt, shame, anger, disgust, and joy: 0–100). Although her SUDs began and ended at a 90, she reported a large decrease in fear (100 to 50). Her high SUDs were accounted for by sadness, guilt, shame, and disgust, all of which she rated as 100 at the end of the imaginal exposure. She also reported maximum urges to self-injure and quit therapy at the end of the exposure, as well as a moderate urge to commit suicide. Processing focused on her self-blame, particularly her beliefs that she should have disclosed the abuse at the time it was happening and known that it was "wrong." Homework included daily listening to the imaginal exposure recording and continued practice of the two in vivo exposure tasks from the prior week. At the end of the session, she and her therapist briefly reviewed her skills plan and confirmed her commitment to not self-injure. They also planned a check-in phone call for later that evening.

Sessions 4 and 5 involved continued imaginal exposure and processing of the full trauma memory. In Session 4, her SUDs remained elevated (90), largely due to new details she had remembered and added into the narrative. She also continued to report high urges to self-injure and quit therapy during the exposure, but no longer reported any suicide urges. Her fear was greatly reduced (10), but her sadness, guilt, shame, and disgust all remained at 100 after the exposure. Processing focused on her belief that she should have reacted differently at the time of the event and guilt about the impact of her disclosure on her mother. At the beginning of Session 5, review of Amanda's homework showed that she had not yet experienced any habituation (in terms of SUDs) to the imaginal exposure. Given this, her therapist briefly assessed if she was engaging in any avoidance, and Amanda acknowledged that she had been skipping one detail that she found particularly shameful. In addition, she said that she had been thinking about self-injury during the imaginal exposure as a way to make it less distressing. Her therapist encouraged her to add in the final detail and to stop distracting herself. Amanda agreed and completed the imaginal exposure without avoidance which facilitated habituation (post-SUDs =60). In addition, her guilt was significantly lower (60), which she attributed to no longer completely blaming herself for the abuse, and she reported no urges to commit suicide or self-injure. However, her shame, disgust, and sadness remained at 100. Processing continued to focus on the self-blame that was fueling her remaining guilt.

In Session 6, the focus switched to imaginal exposure and processing of a hotspot within the larger trauma memory. At the end of the exposure, Amanda reported moderate SUDs (60) and no fear, guilt, or urges to commit suicide or self-injure. Processing focused on her high shame, which was related to her belief that her experiences with her grandfather had made her dirty and unlovable. In this session, her therapist also discovered that Amanda had been avoiding contact with people and taking showers after completing her imaginal exposure homework. Her therapist coached her to use the DBT skill of opposite action for disgust and shame after listening to her exposure recording, which included interacting with her family members and not showering. Two days after this session, Amanda found out that her younger brother had made a potentially lethal suicide attempt. Given this, the DBT PE protocol was temporarily postponed to allow time to address and process this significant event via standard DBT.

After a 2-week break, and when Amanda's brother was medically stable, the DBT PE protocol was resumed. Sessions 7 and 8 focused on imaginal exposure and processing of the hotspot while practicing opposite action for shame (e.g., making eye contact with her therapist, sitting up straight, speaking confidently). In addition, she completed in vivo exposure homework that specifically targeted unjustified shame, including sharing aspects of her abuse history with supportive friends. These interventions resulted in reduced shame (30), continued reduction of overall distress (SUDs =40–50), and notable improvements on the PCL (score =53). In Session 7, processing focused primarily on her high self-directed disgust (60), including a discussion of whether it was justified or unjustified, and how it was impacting her ability to pursue romantic relationships. Her in vivo exposure homework focused on situations that would provide her with corrective feedback about whether she was "disgusting," including tasks such as interacting with male peers and flirting with men she found attractive. In Session 8, only the justified emotions of sadness and anger remained elevated (both were 100). Processing focused on both emotions, particularly anger toward her grandfather, and included discussion of DBT skills for reducing the intensity of unwanted anger. As Amanda had planned a trip to her hometown for the next week to visit her family, she and her therapist took advantage of the opportunity to plan a number of in vivo exposure tasks to locations in which she had experienced the abuse.

At Session 9, Amanda reported greatly reduced distress about the trauma memory. In this session she completed imaginal exposure to the full memory, during which her SUDs peaked at a 10. Amanda and her therapist then discussed if there were any other memories that continued to cause her distress. Amanda reported that she still experienced distress about a memory in which she had initiated sexual contact with her grandfather outside the context of their typical "game." In Session 10, Amanda completed imaginal exposure to this second memory. She reported peak SUDs of 80 that decreased to 60. Processing focused on shame and disgust caused by her belief that she had "sexually pleasured" her grandfather. At Session 11, the second memory was again targeted via imaginal exposure, and Amanda reported a large reduction in SUDs (post-SUDs =30) as well as the unjustified emotions of fear, shame, guilt, and disgust (all <30). At Session 12, Amanda reported that her SUDs had been very low (<30) during all of her imaginal exposure homework practice, and it was agreed that no further exposure to her childhood sexual abuse was needed. Instead, she decided to target a third event, which was the memory of her boyfriend breaking up with her. This exposure elicited only a peak SUDs of 10, and in Session 13 Amanda and her therapist agreed that no further PTSD treatment was needed, as she no longer reported significant distress about any past traumatic event, and her score on the PCL had decreased to 30. This final session focused on review of her progress and relapse prevention, including completing structured worksheets on how to continue practicing exposure, adopt an exposure lifestyle, plan for high-risk situations, and manage potential future relapses.

DBT After the DBT PE Protocol

The remainder of the treatment year (months 8–12) consisted of standard DBT focused on Amanda's remaining treatment goals, including building her network of friends, pursuing a romantic relationship, increasing self-validation, and practicing her assertiveness skills. In the 10th month of treatment, Amanda engaged in the only episode of non-suicidal cutting that occurred during treatment. She experienced the cutting as so non-reinforcing that it had the effect of cementing her commitment to never engage in the behavior again. By the end of treatment, she remained in remission from PTSD and major depression, had been accepted into a 4-year college, had developed a strong network of friends, and reported that she felt confident in her ability to skillfully manage life stressors.

17.3   Future Directions

Over the past decade, there have been several promising new developments in evidence-based treatment for individuals with co-occurring PTSD and BPD. Despite common clinical lore suggesting that trauma-focused treatment is contraindicated for individuals with BPD, it is now clear that PTSD can be safely and effectively treated in this complex client population. As research in this area progresses, an important issue to address will be to determine which treatments are most appropriate and effective for BPD individuals with various levels of disorder. Based on the existing research, it may be the case that brief (9–12-session) single-diagnosis treatments focused solely on PTSD may be appropriate for clients with a primary diagnosis of PTSD and a mild level of BPD-related disorder (e.g., without suicidal and self-injurious behavior or other severe comorbidities) (Clarke et al. 2008; Feeny et al. 2002; Pabst et al. 2012). BPD clients with a moderate level of disorder (e.g., NSSI without acute suicidality, one or more significant comorbidities) may benefit from longer (12–16-week) and/or more intensive (e.g., residential) phase-based treatments that implement strategies from BPD treatments (e.g., skills training) prior to targeting PTSD (Bohus et al. 2013). Finally, longer-term treatment (e.g., 1 year) that provides integrated treatment for BPD, PTSD, and other co-occurring problems may be necessary for BPD clients with a severe level of disorder (e.g., recent serious suicidal and/or self-injurious behaviors, multiple severe comorbidities) (Harned et al. 2012, 2014). In addition, more research is needed to develop empirically derived criteria for determining readiness to engage in trauma-focused treatment for BPD individuals. For example, it is not yet clear whether PTSD can be safely and effectively treated among BPD clients who are actively engaging in NSSI, particularly in outpatient settings. Finally, although it is now clear that effective treatments for co-occurring PTSD and BPD exist, few therapists are trained to provide them. Moreover, no research has examined effective methods of training therapists to provide these treatments for individuals with BPD, nor has it evaluated the effectiveness of these treatments when delivered by community clinicians to BPD clients in routine practice settings. Thus, there is a clear need for implementation and effectiveness research to determine how to make these treatments more widely available to the clients who need them.

References

Barnicot, K., & Priebe, S. (2013). Post-traumatic stress disorder and the outcome of dialectical behaviour therapy for borderline personality disorder. *Personality and Mental Health, 7*(3), 181–190.

Bohus, M., Dyer, A. S., Priebe, K., Kruger, A., Kleindienst, N., Schmahl, C., et al. (2013). Dialectical behaviour therapy for post-traumatic stress disorder after childhood sexual abuse in patients with and without borderline personality disorder: A randomised controlled trial. *Psychotherapy and Psychosomatics, 82*(4), 221–233.

Brown, M., Comtois, K. A., & Linehan, M. M. (2002). Reasons for suicide attempts and nonsuicidal self-injury in women with borderline personality disorder. *Journal of Abnormal Psychology, 111*(1), 198–202.

Clarke, S. B., Rizvi, S., & Resick, P. A. (2008). Borderline personality characteristics and treatment outcome in cognitive-behavioral treatments for PTSD in female rape victims. *Behavior Therapy, 39,* 72–78.

Cloitre, M., Stovall-McClough, K. C., Nooner, K., Zorbas, P., Cherry, S., Jackson, C. L., et al. (2010). Treatment for PTSD related to childhood abuse: A randomized controlled trial. *The American Journal of Psychiatry, 167*(8), 915–924.

Feeny, N. C., Zoellner, L. A., & Foa, E. B. (2002). Treatment outcome for chronic PTSD among female assault victims with borderline personality characteristics: A preliminary examination. *Journal of Personality Disorders, 16*(1), 30–40.

Foa, E., Hembree, E., & Rothbaum, B. (2007). *Prolonged exposure therapy for PTSD: Emotional processing of traumatic experiences.* New York: Oxford University Press.

Grant, B. F., Chou, S. P., Goldstein, R. B., Huang, B., Stinson, F. S., Saha, T. D., et al. (2008). Prevalence, correlates, disability, and comorbidity of DSM-IV borderline personality disorder: Results from the Wave 2 National Epidemiologic Survey on Alcohol and Related Conditions. *The Journal of Clinical Psychiatry, 69*(4), 533–545.

Harned, M. S. (2013). Treatment of posttraumatic stress disorder with comorbid borderline personality disorder. In D. McKay & E. Storch (Eds.), *Handbook of treating variants and complications in anxiety disorders.* New York: Springer Press.

Harned, M. S., Chapman, A. L., Dexter-Mazza, E. T., Murray, A., Comtois, K. A., & Linehan, M. M. (2008). Treating co-occurring Axis I disorders in recurrently suicidal women with borderline personality disorder: A 2-year randomized trial of dialectical behavior therapy versus community treatment by experts. *Journal of Consulting and Clinical Psychology, 76*(6), 1068–1075.

Harned, M. S., Rizvi, S. L., & Linehan, M. M. (2010a). The impact of co-occurring posttraumatic stress disorder on suicidal women with borderline personality disorder. *The American Journal of Psychiatry, 167*(10), 1210–1217.

Harned, M. S., Jackson, S. C., Comtois, K. A., & Linehan, M. M. (2010b). Dialectical behavior therapy as a precursor to PTSD treatment for suicidal and/or self-injuring women with borderline personality disorder. *Journal of Traumatic Stress, 23*(4), 421–429.

Harned, M. S., Korslund, K. E., Foa, E. B., & Linehan, M. M. (2012). Treating PTSD in suicidal and self-injuring women with borderline personality disorder: Development and preliminary evaluation of a Dialectical Behavior Therapy Prolonged Exposure Protocol. *Behaviour Research and Therapy, 50*(6), 381–386.

Harned, M. S., Tkachuck, M. A., & Youngberg, K. A. (2013). Treatment preference among suicidal and self-injuring women with borderline personality disorder and PTSD. *Journal of Clinical Psychology, 69*(7), 749–761.

Harned, M. S., Korslund, K. E., & Linehan, M. M. (2014). A pilot randomized controlled trial of Dialectical Behavior Therapy with and without the Dialectical Behavior Therapy Prolonged Exposure protocol for suicidal and self-injuring women with borderline personality disorder and PTSD. *Behaviour Research and Therapy, 55,* 7–17.

Iverson, K. M., Follette, V. M., Pistorello, J., & Fruzzetti, A. E. (2012). An investigation of experiential avoidance, emotion dysregulation, and distress tolerance in young adult outpatients with borderline personality disorder symptoms. *Personality Disorders: Theory, Research and Treatment, 3,* 415–422.

Linehan, M. M. (1993a). *Cognitive-behavioral treatment of borderline personality disorder.* New York: Guilford Press.

Linehan, M. M. (1993b). *Skills training manual for treating borderline personality disorder.* New York: Guilford Press.

Marshall-Berenz, E. C., Morrison, J. A., Schumacher, J. A., & Coffey, S. F. (2011). Affect intensity and lability: The role of posttraumatic stress disorder symptoms in borderline personality disorder. *Depression and Anxiety, 28*(5), 393–399.

Mueser, K. T., Rosenberg, S. D., Xie, H., Jankowski, M. K., Bolton, E. E., Lu, W., et al. (2008). A randomized controlled trial of cognitive-behavioral treatment for posttraumatic stress disorder in severe mental illness. *Journal of Consulting and Clinical Psychology, 76*(2), 259–271.

Nishith, P., Resick, P. A., & Griffin, M. G. (2002). Pattern of change in prolonged exposure and cognitive processing therapy for female rape victims with posttraumatic stress disorder. *Journal of Consulting and Clinical Psychology, 70*, 880–886.

Pabst, A., Schauer, M., Bernhardt, K., Ruf, M., Goder, R., Rosentraeger, R., et al. (2012). Treatment of patients with borderline personality disorder and comorbid posttraumatic stress disorder using narrative exposure therapy: A feasibility study. *Psychotherapy and Psychosomatics, 81*(1), 61–63.

Pagura, J., Stein, M. B., Bolton, J. M., Cox, B. J., Grant, B., & Sareen, J. (2010). Comorbidity of borderline personality disorder and posttraumatic stress disorder in the U.S. population. *Journal of Psychiatric Research, 44*(16), 1190–1198.

Pompili, M., Girardi, P., Ruberto, A., & Tatarelli, R. (2005). Suicide in borderline personality disorder: A meta-analysis. *Nordic Journal of Psychiatry, 59*(5), 319–324.

Resick, P. A., & Schnicke, M. K. (1993). *Cognitive processing therapy for rape victims: A treatment manual.* Newbury Park: Sage.

Sachsse, U., Vogel, C., & Leichsenring, F. (2006). Results of psychodynamically oriented trauma-focused inpatient treatment for women with complex posttraumatic stress disorder (PTSD) and borderline personality disorder (BPD). *Bulletin of the Menninger Clinic, 70*(2), 125–144.

Schauer, M., Neuner, F., & Elbert, T. (2011). *Narrative exposure therapy: A short-term intervention for traumatic stress disorders* (2nd ed.). Cambridge, MA: Hogrefe Publishing.

Shenk, C. E., Putnam, F. W., Rausch, J. R., Peugh, J. L., & Noll, J. G. (2014). A longitudinal study of several potential mediators of the relationship between child maltreatment and posttraumatic stress disorder symptoms. *Development and Psychopathology, 26*, 81–91.

Steil, R., Dyer, A., Priebe, K., Kleindienst, N., & Bohus, M. (2011). Dialectical behavior therapy for posttraumatic stress disorder related to childhood sexual abuse: A pilot study of an intensive residential treatment program. *Journal of Traumatic Stress, 24*(1), 102–106.

Weathers, F. W., Litz, B. T., Herman, D. S., Huska, J. A., & Keane, T. M. (1993). *The PTSD checklist: Reliability, validity, and diagnostic utility.* Paper presented at the annual meeting of the Association for the Advancement of Behavior Therapy, Washington, DC.

Weierich, M. R., & Nock, M. K. (2008). Posttraumatic stress symptoms mediate the relations between childhood sexual abuse and nonsuicidal self-injury. *Journal of Consulting and Clinical Psychology, 76*, 39–44.

Widom, C. S. (1999). Posttraumatic stress disorder in abused and neglected children grown up. *The American Journal of Psychiatry, 156*, 1223–1229.

Widom, C. S., Czaja, S. J., & Paris, J. (2009). A prospective investigation of borderline personality disorder in abused and neglected children followed up into adulthood. *Journal of Personality Disorders, 23*, 433–446.

Zanarini, M. C., Frankenburg, F. R., Dubo, E. D., Sickel, A. E., Trikha, A., Levin, A., et al. (1998). Axis I comorbidity of borderline personality disorder. *The American Journal of Psychiatry, 155*(12), 1733–1739.

Zanarini, M. C., Ruser, T., Frankenburg, F. R., & Hennen, J. (2000). The dissociative experiences of borderline patients. *Comprehensive Psychiatry, 41*, 223–227.

Zanarini, M. C., Frankenburg, F. R., Hennen, J., Reich, D. B., & Silk, K. R. (2004). Axis I comorbidity in patients with borderline personality disorder: 6-year follow-up and prediction of time to remission. *The American Journal of Psychiatry, 161*(11), 2108–2114.

Zanarini, M. C., Frankenburg, F. R., Hennen, J., Reich, D. B., & Silk, K. R. (2006). Prediction of the 10-year course of borderline personality disorder. *The American Journal of Psychiatry, 163*(5), 827–832.

Zanarini, M. C., Frankenburg, F. R., Reich, D. B., Fitzmaurice, G., Weinberg, I., & Gunderson, J. G. (2008). The 10-year course of physically self-destructive acts reported by borderline patients and axis II comparison subjects. *Acta Psychiatrica Scandinavica, 117*(3), 177–184.

The Complexity of Chronic Pain in Traumatized People: Diagnostic and Therapeutic Challenges

18

Naser Morina and Niklaus Egloff

18.1 Chronic Pain

Posttraumatic stress is more than having intrusions, avoidance and numbing, negative alterations in cognitions and mood, and hyperarousal symptoms. Another consequence of severe traumatic events is physical symptoms. Physical complaints, in particular, pain, have been found to be among the most frequently reported symptoms in individuals with PTSD (McFarlane et al. 1994). Pain symptoms are particularly often seen in the veteran population (Otis et al. 2003; Shipherd et al. 2007), and they have been found to be the most common complaint among torture victims (Olsen et al. 2006). Pain symptoms seem to play an important role in the aftermath of a traumatic event as pain has been identified as a predictor for development of posttraumatic stress symptoms (Norman et al. 2008).

Pain is a multidimensional, complex, and subjective perceptual experience. It often results from injuries related to events, such as occupational injuries, motor vehicle accidents, military combat/war situations, and torture. According to the International Association for the Study of Pain, pain is defined as an unpleasant sensory and emotional experience associated with actual or potential tissue damage or described in terms of such damage (Merskey and Bogduk 1994). It is known that after a traumatic event involving physical injury, pain may be a direct consequence of the injury but may become chronic over time via several steps and pathways, with

N. Morina (✉)
Department of Psychiatry and Psychotherapy,
University Hospital Zurich,
Zurich, Switzerland
e-mail: naser.morina@usz.ch

N. Egloff
Division of Psychosomatic Medicine,
Bern University Hospital,
Bern, Switzerland

© Springer International Publishing Switzerland 2015
U. Schnyder, M. Cloitre (eds.), *Evidence Based Treatments for Trauma-Related Psychological Disorders: A Practical Guide for Clinicians*,
DOI 10.1007/978-3-319-07109-1_18

psychological factors increasingly playing a role in pain maintenance (Casey et al. 2008). Chronic pain is described as pain with a duration of 3–6 months or more, persisting after the injury has resolved. Chronic pain is often associated with functional and psychosocial problems, which can negatively impact on patients' lives. Chronic persisting pain is frequently associated with functional disturbance, emotional distress, reduced quality of life, and a high utilization of medical services. It also results in absenteeism and reduced work performance and is a frequent subject of litigation and high-cost insurance claims.

Millions of people all over the world experience chronic pain. In a large general population over 17 countries around the world, prevalence rates of chronic pain between 10 and 42 % were found (Demyttenaere et al. 2007). Around one in three US Americans suffer from some kind of persistent pain in their lifetimes and many of them are seriously disabled from their chronic pain symptoms. Data from the 2010 National Health Interview Survey indicate that during a 3-month period approximately 19 % of adults in the United States report chronic pain (Schiller et al. 2012). Consequently, clinically significant chronic pain is an increasingly costly and debilitating medical condition in industrialized countries with costs over billions annually (Dersh et al. 2002).

18.2 Relationship of Chronic Pain and PTSD

Clinically significant pain symptoms are highly prevalent in PTSD patients. For example, Mayou and Bryant (2001) found that 36 % of seriously injured and 20 % of less seriously injured motor vehicle accident survivors suffered from persistent pain one year after their accident. The prevalence of pain has been estimated to range from 45 to 87 % in patients referred for the treatment of PTSD (Asmundson et al. 2002; Otis et al. 2003). Conversely, the prevalence of PTSD has been estimated to be between 20 and 34 % in patients referred for the treatment of chronic pain (Otis et al. 2003). The high occurrence of PTSD and chronic pain as comorbid conditions is not surprising and is related to a range of traumatic events including natural disasters, military combat situations, torture, and rape.

Though chronic pain and PTSD are conditions that may co-occur, their association to one another is not always evident and is often overlooked. People suffering from chronic pain often have symptoms very similar to PTSD symptoms. For example, they frequently experience anxiety and depression symptoms. Further, they are often grumpy, disinterested and withdrawn, and angry or unhappy and suffer from nightmares and sleeplessness. In light of the strong relationship between chronic pain and PTSD, they have been described as "mutually maintaining" disorders. Several theoretical models have been proposed, including shared vulnerability (Asmundson et al. 2002), where individual factors predispose certain subjects to develop both chronic pain and PTSD when exposed to certain life events. Another theoretical model is the mutual maintenance model (Sharp and Harvey 2001) in which components of PTSD maintain and exacerbate symptoms of pain and vice versa. Because PTSD symptoms can heighten arousal, which leads to increased muscle tension and muscular pain, this can subsequently function as reminders of traumatic experiences. These reminders can in turn elicit further PTSD re-experiencing reactions (Carty et al. 2011). Some authors assume a common neuro-physiological basis of the phenomena of persistence of pain, persistence of stress, and persistence of anxiety by imprinting and hypersensitivity (Egloff et al. 2013). In the imprinting model, a potentially traumatic event is capable of fixating emotional as well as somatosensory or nociceptive experiences. Imprinting is an extremely long-lasting and robust form of preserving experiences. Threat-induced hypersensitivity describes the hyperexcitability with regard to internal or external signals, such as stress, anxiety, and pain. Imprinting and hypersensitivity are well-proven and protective mechanisms in numerous everyday situations of minor threats. The symptoms and sufferings of patients with PTSD are based on the same mechanisms connected with major threat. In this as in other models, the relationship between the development of persistent pain conditions and posttraumatic stress in the aftermath of a traumatic event is still poorly understood. However, understanding the mechanisms which link these two conditions requires, at minimum, a systematic investigation and understanding of temporal relationships among different elements, such as the injury, psychological distress, pain, PTSD, etc.

18.3 Neurobiology of Chronic Pain in Traumatized People

Beyond the phenomenological relationships described above, neurobiological mechanisms play a major role in the development and maintenance of chronic pain. In the following, we distinguish between the neurobiological mechanisms of *sensitization*, *imprinting*, *pain enhancement by the anxiety system*, and *pain-numbing* mechanisms.

18.3.1 Neuronal Pain Sensitization Mechanisms

Pain disorders in traumatized persons often have in common that they are not or not sufficiently explained by structural somatic injury. This fact could mislead an observer to rush to the conclusion that the pain reported by a patient is of "virtual" origin. In order to be able to understand this type of pain disorder, one must differentiate between the somatic injury that triggers pain and the neuroperceptive process of perceiving pain. If traumatization occurs, both of these are generally affected. Many traumatized people suffer from a local physical trauma as well as from a massive disturbance of the structures processing pain stimuli. Generally, every persistent or severe local physical injury can cause a neurofunctional enhancement of the pain-transmitting structures (McLean et al. 2005; Sandkuhler 1996). The mechanism of chronification by an enhancement of synaptic pain transmission at the spinal level of the central nerve system is in general referred to as "central sensitization." Secondly, it has to be stressed that certain local injuries themselves can directly provoke persistent neurogenic pain. A typical example of neurogenic pain is burning sensations of the soles after flogging torture, named falanga (see Case Report) (Prip and Persson 2008). Thirdly, animal experiments have shown that repeated high stress itself can lead to peripheral enhancement of pain stimuli: under the influence of the stress hormones (cortisol and epinephrine), the intracellular signal pathway in the nociceptive nerve fibers (nociceptors) is altered and leads to enhancement and prolongation of pain signals (Khasar et al. 2009).

Apart from the peripheral and spinal sensitization, increased pain sensitivity can also be of central, i.e., cerebral, origin. The continued and intense experience of stress leads to an increase in pain sensitivity on the level of the brain via multiple neurofunctional mechanisms (Egle et al. 2002; Felitti et al. 1998; Khasar et al. 2009; Kivimaki et al. 2004; McBeth et al. 2001). The resulting sensitization is a form of implicit learning that was demonstrated in individual nerve cells as well as entire organisms (Imbierowicz and Egle 2003; Kandel 2006). Sensitization brings about an increased reaction to painful stimuli (hyperalgesia) and an increased reaction even towards neutral stimuli (e.g., allodynia) (Holzl et al. 2005; Yunus 2008). At the neurotransmitter level, traumatization is associated with massive glutamate release induced by the amygdala (Nair and Singh Ajit 2008). Glutamate is a classical neuronal stimulus enhancer that generally plays a role in the sensitization and long-term potentiation (chronification) of synaptic signals (Blair et al. 2001).

18.3.2 Imprinting as a Factor of Pain Chronification

Imprinting is an extremely lasting form of preserving experiences in the memory networks. As early as in the late 1980s, it was assumed that excessive neuroendocrine stress responses may lead to an over consolidated memory of trauma (Pitman 1989). Furthermore, imprinting is the basis for subsequent mnestic reactivations. Pain experiences in traumatized individuals are typically reactivated by stimuli associatively linked to the traumatic experience. The associative chains involved work both ways: trauma associations can evoke pain experiences and pain experiences can evoke trauma associations (Whalley et al. 2007).

In clinical terms, we distinguish two types of memory-associated pain: firstly, "pain intrusions," i.e., transient somatosensory flashbacks with the pain quality of the initial traumatic event (Salomons et al. 2004), and, secondly, "chronic memory pain" which is characterized by its persistent nature. Often there is a direct anatomical relationship to the initial pain-evoking event (Williams et al. 2010). For both types of pain, it seems that the central nervous system has irreversibly frozen the sensations of the primary pain impression by mechanisms of hypermnesia.

18.3.3 Synergisms Between Pain System and the Anxiety System

Anxiety is one of the most decisive factors in relation to the risk of traumatization. Pain and anxiety are closely related physiologically. Whereas anxiety is a psychophysiological alarm function that signals a situational threat to integrity, pain is a psychophysiological alarm function that signals a physical threat to integrity. Even in animal experiments, it has been shown that with respect to neuroperception, an additive effect takes place if both alarm systems are activated (Colloca and Benedetti 2007; Williams et al. 2010). Neugebauer et al. (2004) imply a relationship with some direct modulation by the laterocapsular division of the central nucleus of the amygdala, assuming this to be of major importance in traumatogenic pain genesis.

18.3.4 Pain-Numbing Mechanisms

Besides the aforementioned pain-intensifying mechanisms related to trauma, there are also several mechanisms of endogenous-reactive pain-numbing mechanisms in situations of serious threat: trauma-associated situations exceeding the maximal subjective tolerance give rise to dissociative processes. The latter can be followed by clouding of consciousness, e.g., through the effect of endorphins (self-narcotization), or by emotional and physical numbness (auto-anesthesia) (Pitman et al. 1990). These neurofunctional losses reflect an attempt to turn a desperate situation that is intolerable into one that is "survivable."

Furthermore, chronic pain in traumatized persons is often associated with cutaneous numbness. Normally the areas with reduced sensitivity to touch and temperature do not correspond with the anatomical distribution of peripheral nerves. These nondermatomal somatosensory deficits are of central origin (Egloff et al. 2009; Mailis-Gagnon and Nicholson 2011). Possibly, investigations showing reduced pain sensitivity in posttraumatic stress disorder are explained by such pain-numbing mechanisms (Moeller-Bertram et al. 2012). It is important to note that trauma-induced hyperalgesia and pain-numbing mechanisms do not exclude each other since intense pain is typically a prerequisite for the triggering of dissociative pain-numbing processes. Typically, chronic pain and reduced superficial sensitivity appear concomitantly (Mailis-Gagnon and Nicholson 2011). This "paradoxical" situation is observed in the clinician's workaday life, i.e., patients complain about increased pain although the limbs in question show a reduced superficial sensitivity to touch and temperature (Egloff et al. 2009; Mailis-Gagnon and Nicholson 2011).

18.4 Diagnosis and Differential Diagnosis

As described, clinically significant chronic pain is a complex phenomenon with substantial biological, psychological, and social interactions which must be given attention diagnostically. However, chronic pain can be a critically challenging aspect for both assessment and treatment of PTSD. Psychological assessments of patients with PTSD do not typically focus on clinically significant pain symptoms. Usually patients consult one health-care provider with their posttraumatic stress symptoms and another specialist for support with their pain symptoms. Clinicians treating patients with PTSD should consider including pain assessment into their standard clinical routine to facilitate case conceptualization for the patients with chronic pain. Hence, a successful treatment of the pain syndromes in traumatized patients requires a careful history taking and a detailed physical assessment including neurological, orthopedic, and psychiatric aspects of pain (Rasmussen et al. 2006).

The clinical differential diagnosis of pain in traumatized people should include the following possibilities of pain origin:

(a) Acute nociceptive pain (pain in relation with a concrete physical lesion, e.g., an injury in a car accident)
(b) Persistent chronic nociceptive pain (long-lasting pain resulting from an initial or persistent physical lesion, often leading to secondary pain enhancement effects, depression, and insufficient pharmacological treatment effects)
(c) Neuropathic pain (structural lesion of nerves, e.g., neuropathic pain following torture)
(d) Complex regional pain syndromes type I or type II (reactive persistent local pain syndrome with additive neuroinflammatory and neurovascular symptoms, including peripheral and central pain mechanisms)
(e) Stress-associated myofascial pain syndromes (chronic muscular pain syndrome, e.g., in the context of stress-induced tension headache)
(f) Pain symptoms resulting from enhanced pain sensitivity (e.g., generalized hyperalgesia in fibromyalgia-like disorders)
(g) Chronic memory pain (long-lasting local pain syndromes at the anatomical location of earlier physical traumatization, without any explanation of persistent local injuries)
(h) Pain flashbacks (e.g., transient memory-based somatosensory pain experience triggered by associations)
(i) Drug-associated pain syndromes (e.g., analgesic-induced headache or opioid-induced hyperalgesia)
(j) Combinations of (a)–(i)

In addition to a detailed physical assessment, it is critical that the examination includes a detailed history taking concerning psychological and social aspects. A pain assessment should also focus on the following key elements (Asmundson et al. 2011): (a) pain severity and stability, (b) pain location, (c) pain-related attitudes, (d) pain-related beliefs, (e) pain-specific emotional distress, (f) pain-related coping styles, and (g) pain-related functional capacity. To facilitate the examination of clinically significant pain characteristics, screening open-ended questions can be asked, e.g.: "Where do you feel pain?" "On a scale from '0=not at all' to '10=worst pain imaginable,' how bad is your pain right now?" "Is your pain present all the time?" "What makes your pain symptoms worse?" "What makes the pain better?" "What daily/work activities does your pain interfere with?" These key questions can be followed by self-report instruments to assess the pain symptoms.

Having said that, not all health-care providers are aware of and trained in the assessment of people suffering from posttraumatic stress symptoms when assessing patients presenting with clinically significant pain symptoms. The presence of an undiagnosed PTSD can lead to complications, more pain, and insufficient treatment. The reverse is true as well: psychologists treating traumatized patients should bear in mind the broad spectrum of different pain origins.

18.5 Treatment for Comorbid PTSD and Chronic Pain

Dealing with chronic pain is a challenging struggle that requires a life management approach focused on caring for physiology and psychology. This can be even more difficult when the source of pain encompasses (psychological) trauma. Given the high occurrence of chronic pain and PTSD among traumatized persons and the negative impact this relationship can have on quality of life, it is important that treatments address these conditions in an effective manner. Patients with comorbid pain and PTSD experience more intense pain, more emotional distress, higher levels of life interference, and greater disability than pain patients without PTSD or PTSD patients without pain symptoms. There are good evidence-based treatments for each of the two conditions (Foa et al. 1999; Hoffman et al. 2007).

As described in this book, cognitive behavioral therapy is the most effective treatment for PTSD. As is true for every PTSD treatment approach, psychoeducation should be an integral part of the treatment PTSD and chronic pain. During the treatment, the patient and the therapist collaborate to develop an individual model of the patient's current complaints and possible ways to recovery. Many of the cognitive behavioral therapy tools can also be used for the adaptive chronic pain management. These tools, for example, can be used not only to specifically address how fears and avoidance of the trauma may lead to maintain the symptoms and decrease the ability to function but also to discuss how pain may be a trigger of reminders of the trauma and increase the arousal, anxiety, and avoidance. By gradually increasing coping and management skills and thereby the activity level, the patients may also be able to decrease their focus on pain and engage more in life again. One very important issue in dealing with chronic pain and PTSD patients is to be aware of feelings of being out of control and helpless. It is very important for health-care providers to understand that patients try to regain a sense of control over their lives.

Another evidence-based therapeutic approach for lessening pain-related distress is a biofeedback-oriented intervention. Biofeedback is a treatment method by which patients learn how to change psychophysiological parameters to improve their health by using signals from their own bodies. There is evidence demonstrating effects of biofeedback on posttraumatic stress symptoms (Tatrow et al. 2003). However, biofeedback should only be used as an additional treatment tool in conjunction with a state-of-the-art intervention for PTSD and chronic pain.

In the scientific literature, pain specialists are increasingly recognizing the need for a multimodal approach to pain management and some pilot studies have already demonstrated this. For example, Otis and colleagues (2009) have presented an integrated treatment for traumatized people with chronic pain and posttraumatic stress disorder (Table 18.1).

Table 18.1 Overview of treatment approaches for PTSD and chronic pain

Level of intervention	Potential key issues and intervention methods
Level 1: peripheral nociception	In many trauma-associated pain disorders, an additional somatic nociceptive partial problem exists (e.g., painful muscular tension). The therapeutic goal is to limit the action of this peripheral-nociceptive input through interventions such as muscle-relaxing biofeedback, local heat, heating pads, warming ointment, and warm baths
	Sometimes conventional analgesics are employed. Since supportive long-term therapies are often of concern, its usage is restricted due to concern for side effects of drugs, such as nonsteroidal anti-inflammatory drugs (NSAIDs) and opiates. Each analgesic prescription must be critically checked regarding its effectiveness and side effects
	On the behavioral level, an important component concerns dosaging of the individual's physical capacity, e.g., taking regular breaks, physiotherapeutic posture training, and activating movement therapy
Level 2: autonomic imbalance	Stress promotes the development of pain-processing disorders; stress acutely amplifies pain. Reciprocally, pain generates vegetative and emotional stress
	Interventions include the correction of sympathovagal imbalance by strengthening the parasympathetic nervous system through practice and regular exercise of a relaxation method (progressive muscle relaxation according to Jacobson, yoga, meditation, autogenic training, biofeedback)
	Analysis of the individual biographical stress profile along with the creation of individual orientated stress relief measures
	Sleep hygiene measures
Level 3: perceptual processing of pain	Use of central pain-modulating drugs, such as serotonin reuptake inhibitors or tricyclic antidepressants
	Body awareness therapy: defocusing on pain training instead of pain scanning, enjoyment and pleasure training, mindfulness exercises, autosuggestion
	Distraction strategies: music, media, occupational therapy, excursions, contacts, meaningful everyday tasks
	Planning of an individualized home program
Level 4: emotional pain amplification	Anxiety management and disorder-specific cognitive behavioral therapy, antidepressant medication
	Conflict resolution therapy to relieve biographic and daily stressors. Important is a distinction between pain-causing distress and pain-maintaining emotional stressors
	Awareness regarding the handling of emotions and emotional self-efficacy training
	Participation in pleasurable group therapy dealing with drama, music, humor
	Personal diary, rituals
Level 5: mental pain amplification	Restructuring of dysfunctional cognitions ("I have an unknown cause of pain," "I'm going crazy," "I will end up in a wheelchair," "I must not move," "Illness is punishment," etc.)
	Pain group therapy; goal: learn one's own self-competence and self-efficacy; from "pain victim" to "pain manager"
	Restructuring of dysfunctional behavior (e.g., excessive activity due to self-esteem deficit, fear-avoidance behavior)
	Involvement in pain information training (=patient education) through presentations, leaflets, movies

(continued)

Table 18.1 (continued)

Level of intervention	Potential key issues and intervention methods
Level 6: social consequences	Chronic pain and trauma always have an effect on partnership, family, and friends: involvement and information of the partner and possibly the children. Seek relief solutions that are viable for everyone. Note if the disease has taken on a relationship regulatory influence
	Problems with health/social insurances: in many cases patients with pain disorders make frustrating experiences with insurances. Involve professional consultants
	Generally: social impacts can become an independent disease-maintaining stressor. Integrating these secondary social effects of the disease is an important part of the multimodal pain therapy

Pain disorders in traumatized people are usually multi-causal. Consequently, the therapeutic measures are applied on various levels. One speaks of an individualized multimodal therapy

Case Report

A 54-year-old woman presented chronic pain disorder at our tertiary pain clinic. The patient suffered from whole body pain, especially in the area of the back and the thighs. Her constant pain was increased by stress and anxiety as well as by physical activities, such as standing for some time, walking, or lying down. Additionally, the patient complained about numbness on the right side of the body as well as burning sensations in the area of the foot soles. The pain was associated with disturbed sleep onset and sustained insomnia accompanied by nightmares and fear of the "dark and bad thoughts." She was easily startled and felt immediately "paralyzed" if she heard certain noises.

A detailed psychosocial exploration revealed the following history: the patient, a professor of history, had been a human rights activist in her native country in the Middle East. Due to her political activities, she was persecuted by the police and jailed. There were several methods used to wear the patient down and to torture confessions from her. The patient saw the origin of the back pain as well the pain in the area of the thighs in her forced fixation in a tire during several days (Fig. 18.1).

Diagnostically speaking, the patient fulfilled all the criteria for a posttraumatic stress disorder. The clinical examination showed visible results of the physical torture in the form of 18 stab wound scars in the area of the sacral lumbar spine. The neurological examination additionally revealed a superficial hyperesthesia of the right side of the body. Such nondermatomal somatosensory deficits (NDSDs), typically with hemibody distribution, are known in individuals with high levels of adverse life events in combination with somatic pain events (Egloff et al. 2012). The burning foot sole pain was a result of the lashing (falanga). This form of torture typically leaves a burning and neuropathic-like pain which often increases during the winter months (Prip and Persson 2008). X-rays and MRI of the back and pelvis did not reveal any structural explanations for the pain (e.g., fractures, discopathies). Although there were hardly any visible marks and scars left, the physically abused parts of the body were irreversibly imprinted in her pain perception system (Fig. 18.1).

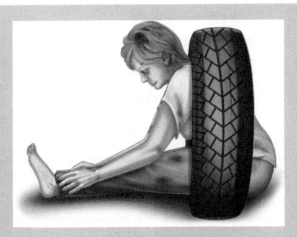

Fig. 18.1 Torture of a 54-year-old woman who was politically persecuted. The drawing is based on explanation and a draft by the patient

The patient went through several treatment phases. From the very beginning, it was important for her that the therapist was familiar with trauma-induced bodily pain as well as the psychological sequelae of the traumatization. The pain interview and the examinations were performed very carefully with respectful attention to any signals of stress or dissociation. The formulation of the questions allowed the patient to reveal what and as much as she wanted of her traumatic past. Nevertheless, a coherent story began to develop after a short time.

At the beginning of the treatment, the therapist explained that it is typical that many forms of pain cannot be made visible by MRI or X-rays, noting that, in any case, X-rays never reveal the pain but only marks of physical injuries. The fact that the MRI and X-ray imaging in her case showed no persistent structural lesions was a relief for the patient. The patient's observation that her type of body pain was of the type that increased in stress situations allowed a change in her pain model: her body developed an "alarm mechanism" with hypersensitivity to any form of threat and stress, including pain. Additionally, these memories were experienced and expressed in her body (hypermnesia). The traumatized organism cannot forget the sufferings. These typical aspects of trauma-associated pain were explained and illustrated to the patient with the help of easily understandable educational pictures (www. hklearning.net/CLIP/Trauma.pdf). These didactic metaphors supported her development of a pain model with which she could identify. She realized that hyperalgesia as well as hypermnesia had developed as essential mechanisms of "protection" for her body.

After having explained the pain sufficiently for the patient, she was also ready for psychotherapeutic sessions focusing on the strengthening of her resources, the treatment of her trauma, as well as the reduction of stress.

Her resources luckily included a very strong and intact sense of self-respect that proved to be important and meaningful in her recovery. Her belief in human rights and her ability to express her personal feelings and thoughts facilitated the psychotherapeutic process. Reinforcement of her sense of self-respect as well as her growing understanding of psychophysical nature of her symptoms played an important stabilizing role in her treatment as well as in her personal development and the management of her everyday life. With the help of an additional behavioral therapy, focused mainly on reducing flash-back-inducing triggers, the patient succeeded in gaining also more and more control over the other trauma-associated stress symptoms and she overcame the existing "fear-avoidance behavior" step by step. Additionally, treatment for her bodily pain symptoms included a carefully tailored daily (home) program of physical reconditioning and music-supported exercise therapy. With the exception of intermittent use of medication, paracetamol, this patient did not need any long-lasting medical therapy anymore.

18.6   Conclusion

As stated above, there is considerable clinical and empirical evidence regarding the comorbidity of chronic pain and trauma-related disorders. Patients with PTSD have higher rates of numerous clinically significant chronic pain conditions. Likewise, patients with chronic pain are often diagnosed with posttraumatic-related stress disorders. Accordingly, patients with comorbid chronic pain and PTSD are more distressed and impaired than those with only one or the other type of disorder. Due to the interaction of these conditions, patients can also be more complex and challenging to treat, especially if there is the need to convey to them that it is likely that they will need to "live with the pain" and "manage it" for the rest of their lives. The assessment of chronic pain in traumatized patients requires consideration of broad etiological factors. It is important to work out with the patient a "model of the pain," which allows a proper understanding and action perspective.

Interdisciplinary diagnostics and therapy seem to be crucial for therapists and physicians, including psychological therapists and physicians experienced in pain diagnostic and therapy and therefore favor a tailored individualized multimodal and integrative intervention addressing clinically significant pain and posttraumatic stress symptoms. The best way to do so would be to work in interdisciplinary teams in either inpatient, outpatient, or day hospital settings.

References

Asmundson, G. J. G., Coons, M. J., Taylor, S., & Katz, J. (2002). PTSD and the experience of pain: Research and clinical implications of shared vulnerability and mutual maintenance models. *Canadian Journal of Psychiatry, 47*(10), 930–937.

Asmundson, G. J. G., McMillan, K. A., & Carleton, K. A. (2011). Understanding and managing clinically significant pain in patients with an anxiety disorder. *FOCUS, 9*, 264–272.

Blair, H. T., Schafe, G. E., Bauer, E. P., Rodrigues, S. M., & LeDoux, J. E. (2001). Synaptic plasticity in the lateral amygdala: A cellular hypothesis of fear conditioning. *Learning and Memory, 8*(5), 229–242. doi:10.1101/lm.30901.

Carty, J., O'Donnell, M., Evans, L., Kazantzis, N., & Creamer, M. (2011). Predicting posttraumatic stress disorder symptoms and pain intensity following severe injury: The role of catastrophizing. *European Journal of Psychotraumatology, 2.* doi: 10.3402/ejpt.v2i0.5652.

Young Casey, C., Greenberg, M. A., Nicassio, P. M., Harpin, R. E., & Hubbard, D. (2008). Transition from acute to chronic pain and disability: A model including cognitive, affective, and trauma factors. *Pain, 134*(1), 69–79.

Colloca, L., & Benedetti, F. (2007). Nocebo hyperalgesia: How anxiety is turned into pain. *Current Opinion in Anaesthesiology, 20*(5), 435–439. doi:10.1097/ACO.0b013e3282b972fb.

Demyttenaere, K., Bruffaerts, R., Lee, S., Posada-Villa, J., Kovess, V., Angermeyer, M. C., Levinson, D., de Girolamo, G., Nakane, H., Mneimneh, Z., Lara, C., de Graaf, R., Scott, K. M., Gureje, O., Stein, D. J., Haro, J. M., Bromet, E. J., Kessler, R. C., Alonso, J., & Von Korff, M. (2007). Mental disorders among persons with chronic back or neck pain: Results from the world mental health surveys. *Pain, 129*(3), 332–342.

Dersh, J., Polatin, P. B., & Gatchel, R. J. (2002). Chronic pain and psychopathology: Research findings and theoretical considerations. *Psychosomatic Medicine, 64*(5), 773–786. doi:10.1097/01.psy.0000024232.11538.54.

Egle, U. T., Hardt, J., Nickel, R., Kappis, B., & Hoffmann, S. O. (2002). Long-term effects of adverse childhood experiences – Actual evidence and needs for research1/2. *Zeitschrift für Psychosomatische Medizin und Psychotherapie, 48*(4), 411–434.

Egloff, N., Hirschi, A., & von Kanel, R. (2013). Traumatization and chronic pain: A further model of interaction. *Journal of Pain Research, 6*, 765–770. doi:10.2147/JPR.S52264.

Egloff, N., Maecker, F., Stauber, S., Sabbioni, M. E., Tunklova, L., & von Kanel, R. (2012). Nondermatomal somatosensory deficits in chronic pain patients: Are they really hysterical? *Pain, 153*(9), 1847–1851. doi:10.1016/j.pain.2012.05.006.

Egloff, N., Sabbioni, M. E., Salathe, C., Wiest, R., & Juengling, F. D. (2009). Nondermatomal somatosensory deficits in patients with chronic pain disorder: Clinical findings and hypometabolic pattern in FDG-PET. *Pain, 145*(1–2), 252–258. doi:10.1016/j.pain.2009.04.016.

Felitti, V. J., Anda, R. F., Nordenberg, D., Williamson, D. F., Spitz, A. M., Edwards, V., Koss, M. P., & Marks, J. S. (1998). Relationship of childhood abuse and household dysfunction to many of the leading causes of death in adults. The Adverse Childhood Experiences (ACE) Study. *American Journal of Preventive Medicine, 14*(4), 245–258.

Foa, E. B., Davidson, J. R. T., Frances, A., Culpepper, L., Ross, R., & Ross, D. (1999). The expert consensus guideline series: Treatment of posttraumatic stress disorder. *Journal of Clinical Psychiatry, 60*(Suppl 16), 4–76.

Hoffman, B. M., Papas, R. K., Chatkoff, D. K., & Kerns, R. D. (2007). Meta-analysis of psychological interventions for chronic low back pain. *Health Psychology, 26*(1), 1–9. doi:10.1037/0278-6133.26.1.1.

Holzl, R., Kleinbohl, D., & Huse, E. (2005). Implicit operant learning of pain sensitization. *Pain, 115*(1–2), 12–20. doi:10.1016/j.pain.2005.01.026.

Imbierowicz, K., & Egle, U. T. (2003). Childhood adversities in patients with fibromyalgia and somatoform pain disorder. *European Journal of Pain, 7*(2), 113–119. doi:10.1016/s1090-3801(02)00072-1.

Kandel, E. R. (2006). *In search of memory: The emergence of a new science of mind.* New York: Norton & Co.

Khasar, S. G., Dina, O. A., Green, P. G., & Levine, J. D. (2009). Sound stress-induced long-term enhancement of mechanical hyperalgesia in rats is maintained by sympathoadrenal catecholamines. *The Journal of Pain, 10*(10), 1073–1077. doi:10.1016/j.jpain.2009.04.005.

Kivimaki, M., Leino-Arjas, P., Virtanen, M., Elovainio, M., Keltikangas-Jarvinen, L., Puttonen, S., Vartia, M., Brunner, E., & Vahtera, J. (2004). Work stress and incidence of newly diagnosed fibromyalgia: Prospective cohort study. *Journal of Psychosomatic Research, 57*(5), 417–422. doi:10.1016/j.jpsychores.2003.10.013.

Mailis-Gagnon, A., & Nicholson, K. (2011). On the nature of nondermatomal somatosensory deficits. *The Clinical Journal of Pain, 27*(1), 76–84. doi:10.1097/AJP.0b013e3181e8d9cc.

Mayou, R., & Bryant, B. (2001). Outcome in consecutive emergency department attenders following a road traffic accident. *The British Journal of Psychiatry, 179*(6), 528–534. doi:10.1192/bjp.179.6.528.

McBeth, J., Morris, S., Benjamin, S., Silman, A. J., & Macfarlane, G. J. (2001). Associations between adverse events in childhood and chronic widespread pain in adulthood: Are they explained by differential recall? *The Journal of Rheumatology, 28*(10), 2305–2309.

McFarlane, A. C., Atchison, M., Rafalowicz, E., & Papay, P. (1994). Physical symptoms in posttraumatic stress disorder. *Journal of Psychosomatic Research, 38*(7), 715–726.

McLean, S. A., Clauw, D. J., Abelson, J. L., & Liberzon, I. (2005). The development of persistent pain and psychological morbidity after motor vehicle collision: Integrating the potential role of stress response systems into a biopsychosocial model. *Psychosomatic Medicine, 67*(5), 783–790. doi:10.1097/01.psy.0000181276.49204.bb.

Merskey, H., & Bogduk, N. (Eds.). (1994). *Classification of chronic pain. IASP task force on taxonomy* (2nd ed.). Seattle: IASP Press.

Moeller-Bertram, T., Keltner, J., & Strigo, I. A. (2012). Pain and post traumatic stress disorder – Review of clinical and experimental evidence. *Neuropharmacology, 62*(2), 586–597. doi:10.1016/j.neuropharm.2011.04.028.

Nair, J., & Singh Ajit, S. (2008). The role of the glutamatergic system in posttraumatic stress disorder. *CNS Spectrums, 13*(7), 585–591.

Neugebauer, V., Li, W., Bird, G. C., & Han, J. S. (2004). The amygdala and persistent pain. *The Neuroscientist, 10*(3), 221–234. doi:10.1177/1073858403261077.

Norman, S. B., Stein, M. B., Dimsdale, J. E., & Hoyt, D. B. (2008). Pain in the aftermath of trauma is a risk factor for post-traumatic stress disorder. *Psychological Medicine, 38*(04), 533–542. doi:10.1017/S0033291707001389.

Olsen, D. R., Montgomery, E., Bøjholm, S., & Foldspang, A. (2006). Prevalent musculoskeletal pain as a correlate of previous exposure to torture. *Scandinavian Journal of Public Health, 34*(5), 496–503. doi:10.1080/14034940600554677.

Otis, J. D., Keane, T. M., & Kerns, R. D. (2003). An examination of the relationship between chronic pain and post-traumatic stress disorder. *Journal of Rehabilitation Research and Development, 40*(5), 397–405.

Otis, J. D., Keane, T. M., Kerns, R. D., Monson, C., & Scioli, E. (2009). The development of an integrated treatment for veterans with comorbid chronic pain and posttraumatic stress disorder. *Pain Medicine, 10*(7), 1300–1311. doi:10.1111/j.1526-4637.2009.00715.x.

Pitman, R. K. (1989). Post-traumatic stress disorder, hormones, and memory. *Biological Psychiatry, 26*(3), 221–223.

Pitman, R. K., van der Kolk, B. A., Orr, S. P., & Greenberg, M. S. (1990). Naloxone-reversible analgesic response to combat-related stimuli in posttraumatic stress disorder. A pilot study. *Archives of General Psychiatry, 47*(6), 541–544.

Prip, K., & Persson, A. L. (2008). Clinical findings in men with chronic pain after falanga torture. *The Clinical Journal of Pain, 24*(2), 135–141. doi:10.1097/AJP.0b013e31815aac36.

Rasmussen, O. V., Amris, S., Blaauw, M., & Danielsen, L. (2006). Medical physical examination in connection with torture. *Torture, 16*(1), 48–55.

Salomons, T. V., Osterman, J. E., Gagliese, L., & Katz, J. (2004). Pain flashbacks in posttraumatic stress disorder. *The Clinical Journal of Pain, 20*(2), 83–87.

Sandkuhler, J. (1996). Neurobiology of spinal nociception: New concepts. *Progress in Brain Research, 110*, 207–224.

Schiller, J. S., Lucas, J. W., Ward, B. W., & Peregoy, J. A. (2012). Summary health statistics for U.S. adults: National Health Interview Survey, 2010. *Vital and Health Statistics, 10*(252), 1–207.

Sharp, T. J., & Harvey, A. G. (2001). Chronic pain and posttraumatic stress disorder: Mutual maintenance? *Clinical Psychology Review, 21*(6), 857–877.

Shipherd, J. C., Keyes, M., Jovanovic, T., Ready, D. J., Baltzell, D., Worley, V., Gordon-Brown, V., Hayslett, C., & Duncan, E. (2007). Veterans seeking treatment for posttraumatic stress disorder: What about comorbid chronic pain? *Journal of Rehabilitation Research and Development, 44*(2), 153–166.

Tatrow, K., Blanchard, E. B., & Silverman, D. J. (2003). Posttraumatic headache: An exploratory treatment study. *Applied Psychophysiolgy and Biofeedback, 28*(4), 267–278.

Whalley, M. G., Farmer, E., & Brewin, C. R. (2007). Pain flashbacks following the July 7th 2005 London bombings. *Pain, 132*(3), 332–336. doi:10.1016/j.pain.2007.08.011.

Williams, A. C., Pena, C. R., & Rice, A. S. (2010). Persistent pain in survivors of torture: A cohort study. *Journal of Pain and Symptom Management, 40*(5), 715–722. doi:10.1016/j.jpainsymman.2010.02.018.

Yunus, M. B. (2008). Central sensitivity syndromes: A new paradigm and group nosology for fibromyalgia and overlapping conditions, and the related issue of disease versus illness. *Seminars in Arthritis and Rheumatism, 37*(6), 339–352. doi:10.1016/j.semarthrit.2007.09.003.

Part V

Treating Special Populations

Evidence-Based Treatments for Children and Adolescents

19

Markus A. Landolt and Justin A. Kenardy

19.1 Introduction/Background

19.1.1 Epidemiology of Trauma and Trauma-Related Disorders in Children and Adolescents

Trauma can affect all ages: similar to adults, children and adolescents may experience a wide range of potentially traumatic events and develop trauma-related psychological disorders. Indeed, exposure to trauma seems to be a rather common phenomenon in childhood. Epidemiological studies confirmed that the number of children and adolescents experiencing potentially traumatic events is astonishingly high with lifetime prevalence rates between 50 and 90 % (Copeland et al. 2007; Elklit 2002; Kilpatrick et al. 2003; Landolt et al. 2013). For example, a recent population-based study in almost 7,000 Swiss adolescents found that 56.6 % of the girls and 55.7 % of the boys reported that they had experienced at least one traumatic event in their life (Landolt et al. 2013). Experiences of physical and sexual

M.A. Landolt, PhD (✉)
Department of Psychosomatics and Psychiatry,
University Children's Hospital, University of Zurich,
Zurich, Switzerland
e-mail: markus.landolt@kispi.uzh.ch

Department of Child and Adolescent Health Psychology,
Institute of Psychology, University of Zurich,
Zurich, Switzerland

J.A. Kenardy, PhD
School of Psychology,
University of Queensland,
St Lucia, QLD, Australia

Centre of National Research on Disability and Rehabilitation Medicine,
University of Queensland,
St Lucia, QLD, Australia

© Springer International Publishing Switzerland 2015
U. Schnyder, M. Cloitre (eds.), *Evidence Based Treatments for Trauma-Related Psychological Disorders: A Practical Guide for Clinicians*,
DOI 10.1007/978-3-319-07109-1_19

abuse and other types of violence, war, natural disasters, severe illness, accidents and emotional and physical neglect are among the most frequent events that traumatise youth. While many epidemiological studies confirmed that the experience of potentially traumatic events is quite common in childhood and adolescence, the lifetime prevalence rates of PTSD itself varied between 0.5 and 9 %. PTSD, however, is not the only psychological disorder that can develop after experiencing a traumatic event. Frequent comorbid disorders include anxiety and depression (Copeland et al. 2007). In preschool children, oppositional defiant disorder and separation anxiety disorder are the most common comorbid disorders (Scheeringa and Zeanah 2008). Moreover, traumatised children and adolescents report a considerably impaired health-related quality of life, thus showing that trauma negatively impacts general functioning and well-being of children and adolescents (Alisic et al. 2008; Landolt et al. 2009).

19.1.2 Assessment of Child Trauma and Validity of Diagnostic Criteria for Children

Case Example

Seven-year-old Peter, his 2-year-old sister Mary and his parents were eating lunch at home on a Sunday when a truck loaded with barrels of gasoline crashed just in front of the house. After initial impact, some of the barrels exploded, setting the family's house on fire within seconds. The parents immediately took their children out of the house through the back door. Fortunately, no one was hurt. The house, however, burnt down and was completely destroyed.

All family members developed acute stress symptoms in the immediate aftermath of the event. Peter had difficulties sleeping because of recurring nightmares and displayed many symptoms of hyperarousal. Mary became very reluctant to leave her mother, cried a lot, became very distressed when her mother took her to day care and insisted sleeping in the parents' bed. Peter's mother and father both had sleeping problems and intrusive thoughts and were hyperalert.

Around 4 months later, Peter's father's symptoms had resolved; he was back at work and showed no functional impairment. The two children, however, still had many symptoms. Peter met full DSM-5 criteria for PTSD. He had nightmares and flashbacks which were triggered by trauma-related cues (criterion B); he did not want to talk about the accident, persistently avoided going near the burned house, would not go into any room with a burning fireplace and became very distressed if he saw a fire on television (criterion C); he showed changes in his thoughts and mood since the fire, in that he became more negative and pessimistic, and less interested in playing with his friends (criterion D); he was hypervigilant, had concentration problems in school and showed an exaggerated startle response (criterion E).

Two-year-old Mary was also symptomatic and considerably impaired in her daily functioning. She had developed a strong separation anxiety and refused to attend day care. She was often very irritable and showed aggressive behaviour towards both parents. Mary also continued to not sleep alone, she withdrew from other children and relatives and she showed regressive behaviour (thumb sucking). There were no explicit indications that she experienced intrusions. In contrast to her school-age brother, young Mary did not meet criteria for any of the common trauma-related diagnoses, her symptoms being less specific. Still, she was clearly symptomatic and impaired in her function.

Peter's mother also developed PTSD which required treatment. If a person with PTSD has children, it is very common that parenting capacities are negatively affected, and this in turn may have a detrimental effect on the child. While Peter's father attempted to maintain the pre-trauma parenting style, these attempts were often undermined by the mother who had become very overprotective and more lenient and inconsistent with behaviour management. This contributed to the development of problematic behaviours including avoidance, aggression and distress in the children. Furthermore, if one parent is symptomatic and the other is not, there is often conflict about different parenting strategies.

This example highlights the differential impact of a traumatic event on children in different ages and shows the importance of the family system in understanding the child's symptomatology.

19.1.2.1 Diagnostic Issues

Research has confirmed that children's reactions to traumatic events differ to some extent from those of adolescents and adults, as shown in the previous case example. Particularly, preschool-age children's posttraumatic stress symptoms are very often less specific than those of older children and adolescents, making the diagnostic criteria less valid for this age group (Scheeringa 2011). Since the DSM-III-R has been published, diagnostic criteria for PTSD have therefore included developmental considerations for children and adolescents such as repetitive play. However, it was only recently with the publication of the DSM-5 (American Psychiatric Association 2013) that a separate PTSD subtype for preschool-age children (<6 years) has been defined. Still, however, conceptualisation of trauma-related disorders in the youngest children (<2 years) remains unclear.

When conducting diagnostic assessments with children, developmentally sensitive measures must be used. Assessment needs to involve a comprehensive diagnostic interview with the caregiver and, if the child is older than 7 years, the child itself. Fortunately, several well-validated standardised measures are available (see Table 19.1). However, many of them have not yet been revised according to the new DSM-5 criteria.

Table 19.1 Standardised measures of PTSD for children and adolescents

Measure	Authors	Specifics
Clinician-Administered PTSD Scale for Children and Adolescents (CAPS-CA)	Nader et al. (2002)	Structured clinical interview for ages 8–18 years; assessment of PTSD according to DSM-IV
UCLA PTSD Reaction Index for DSM-5	Pynoos and Steinberg (2013)	Self-report measure; version for preschool-age and school-age children and parents (proxy rating). Assessment of PTSD symptoms according to DSM-5
Child PTSD Symptom Scale (CPSS)	Foa et al. (2001)	Self-report measure for ages 8–16 years; assessment of PTSD according to DSM-IV
Trauma Symptom Checklist for Children (TSCC)	Briere (1996)	Self-report measure for ages 8–16 years; broadband measure of posttraumatic symptoms (anxiety, depression, PTSS, dissociation, etc.); norms available
Trauma Symptom Checklist for Young Children (TSCYC)	Briere (2005)	Caregiver report; broadband measure of posttraumatic symptoms; norms available
PTSD module of the Diagnostic Infant and Preschool Assessment (DIPA)	Scheeringa (2004), Scheeringa and Haslett (2010)	Structured interview with the caregiver; for children ages 1–6 years; assessment of preschool type PTSD according to DSM-5

19.2 Early Intervention: Treatment of Acute Stress and Prevention of PTSD

19.2.1 Rationale

Although the majority of children exposed to trauma will recover from initial stress symptoms, a significant proportion will not and will experience clinically significant ongoing difficulties. If left untreated, symptoms can follow a chronic and unremitting course. The impact of having untreated PTSD starting in childhood is likely to be life changing and lifelong for an individual. Longer-term effects include social and emotional development problems, academic problems, psychiatric disorders, alcohol abuse and drug-related problems, risk-taking behaviours, problems with the law and impaired physical health (Mersky et al. 2013). Whenever the trauma occurs on the development trajectory of the child, it is likely to negatively affect the trajectory so that development is either delayed or regression in the developmental stage occurs. However it must be noted that the impact of such a delay can be ongoing if remission does not occur, either naturally or through intervention.

The impact and cost of PTSD in childhood to the community is likely to be much greater than for adult PTSD since the effects are potentially lifelong. For this reason, early intervention should be prioritised especially where children who are at higher risk can be identified and targeted for intervention. In this way, the cost effectiveness of such early intervention is optimised.

19.2.2 Intervention Programmes and Components

There are a number of different protocols and manuals for early interventions in acutely traumatised children. A programme for use in the immediate aftermath after trauma is *Psychological First Aid* (PFA), which has been developed in the United States (Ruzek et al. 2007). It consists of specific components adapted for use with children and can be employed as an immediate care model following exposure to all types of traumatic events. However, it is crucial that it is delivered within a framework that includes access to specialised care.

Many early intervention protocols and manuals include components based on cognitive-behavioural therapy (e.g. trauma narrative, some kind of exposure, training of coping skills), and most of them include the child's caregivers in the intervention. An almost universally used component of early interventions in children is information provision (psychoeducation). Hereby, the content should be oriented to the events and the age group. Information given following trauma should include:

- Likely outcomes, especially emphasising positive outcomes
- Use of effective coping strategies
- Further avenues of care if required
- How to decide if further care may be required

Information can also include information for and about caregivers, siblings and teachers who may also be affected by the trauma or the child's symptoms. Ideally information provision should be part of an overall stepped care approach that includes screening and ongoing assessment together with appropriate levels of intervention, specifically to those children who based on the screening are at risk for PTSD.

There are several validated screening tools available for children following trauma. These include the *Screening Tool for Early Predictors of PTSD* (STEPP) (Winston et al. 2003) and an Australian adaptation called the STEPP-AUS (Nixon et al. 2010), the CTSQ (Kenardy et al. 2006) for school-aged children and the *Pediatric Emotional Distress Scale – Early Screener* (PEDS-ES) (Kramer et al. 2013) for preschool children.

19.2.3 State of Evidence

There is not a strong evidence base available on very early interventions in children (Kramer and Landolt 2011). Only a handful of studies exist. Overall, these studies indicate some benefit of early intervention although there is an urgent need for more work using larger samples and more robust designs. A promising study by Berkowitz et al. (2011) that examined the effects of the *Child and Family Traumatic Stress Intervention* which targets child–caregiver relationship found some good benefits. Notably, studies with preschool-age children are completely missing to date.

19.2.4 Current Recommendations

Children of all ages, from infants and preschoolers to older children and adolescents, are commonly affected by exposure to traumatic events. In the case of sexual abuse and accidental injury, these rates of exposure can be higher than for adults. Clinicians and healthcare providers should therefore assess psychological impact routinely, will need to be able to provide the care required and if unavailable seek referral to specialist services. Use of screening and a stepped care approach in combination with an appropriate intervention and referral as needed is recommended. There is some evidence emerging about possible early intervention following trauma, although the currently available evidence is insufficient to make a firm recommendation.

19.3 Treatment of PTSD and Other Trauma-Related Disorders

19.3.1 Fundamentals of Therapy

Many different treatment approaches and techniques are used with traumatised children and adolescents. To meet the specific needs of the individual child and to consider the severity and the degree of impairment of the child's PTSD symptoms, these approaches and techniques are very often combined by practitioners (multimodal treatment approach). Yet, although there are considerable differences between approaches, the following fundamental aspects are considered to be important, independent of the specific approach (e.g. American Academy of Child and Adolescent Psychiatry 2010):

- There is nowadays very convincing evidence for children across all ages that trauma-specific treatment approaches that directly address the traumatic experience are superior to nonspecific therapies in reducing PTSD symptoms.
- Involvement of caregivers: Since a child, especially a younger child, is highly dependent on caregivers, treatment approaches have to include the child's caregivers, if available. Studies have shown that the inclusion of parents in treatment is associated with a greater reduction of symptoms.
- Since children with PTSD often have comorbid disorders such as depression, ADHD or anxiety disorders, treatment of such conditions should be integrated.
- Treatment approaches should not only focus on symptoms but also on enhancing daily functioning, development and resiliency.
- Age specificity of the treatment: Trauma therapies need to consider developmental issues.
- Consideration of the child's and family's cultural and social background.
- Trauma therapy is usually based on a phase model. Most treatment approaches are implicitly or explicitly based on a phase model of trauma therapy which includes three different stages: (1) safety and stabilisation (physical, psychologi-

cal, social), (2) processing of traumatic memories (exposure, trauma narrative) and (3) a phase of reintegration and reconnection (transition from being a victim to being a survivor).

19.3.2 Cognitive-Behavioural Therapy

19.3.2.1 Background

Cognitive-behavioural therapy (CBT) combines two well-established types of psychotherapy which have been shown to be very effective in treating anxiety and stress-related disorders: behaviour therapy and cognitive therapy. The CBT model explains the development of trauma symptoms based on principles of learning theories (e.g. classical and instrumental learning) and cognitive theories (e.g. dysfunctional thoughts, beliefs and assumptions about the traumatic event and oneself). CBT then aims at changing behaviours, thoughts and emotions of traumatised children and adolescents through specific treatment components.

19.3.2.2 Procedure/Components

Many variations of trauma-specific CBT exist; most of them, however, share the following components and combine both individual sessions with the child and the parent and conjoint parent–child sessions:

- Psychoeducation about trauma-related symptoms and the CBT approach
- Affective modulation skills for managing physiological and emotional distress (used in preparation for the exposure-based part of the therapy)
- Training of coping skills
- Cognitive processing and restructuring of dysfunctional cognitions
- Creation of a trauma narrative
- In vivo exposure to traumatic reminders (graduated exposure to trauma-related stimuli)

Not all CBT models for traumatised children include all of these components (e.g. trauma narrative or cognitive restructuring missing). Others, however, add additional components such as training of parental skills or standardised inclusion of important systems such as the school. As Dorsey et al. (2011) highlight, CBT treatment approaches also include common structural components, including modelling, coached practice of new skills during and in between sessions.

The most widely used and best researched CBT approach to treat PTSD in children and adolescents is the trauma-focused CBT (TF-CBT) protocol (Cohen et al. 2006) which has initially been developed for treating sexually abused school-age children and their nonperpetrating parents. In the last decade, the method has now successfully been applied to a wide variety of children with different traumatic experiences. Moreover, Scheeringa et al. have shown that TF-CBT with some minor adaptations is also effective in preschoolers (Scheeringa et al. 2011). TF-CBT has also been adapted for different cultural backgrounds and for childhood traumatic grief. Besides the TF-CBT, there are currently several other manualised CBT protocols for child PTSD being used and studied, among them, for example, Narrative Exposure Therapy for Kids (KIDNET) (Ruf et al. 2010), a childhood version of Prolonged Exposure Therapy (Aderka et al. 2011), Skills Training in Affect and Interpersonal Regulation for Adolescents STAIR-A (Gudiño et al. 2014) or the Seeking Safety Therapy (Najavits 2002). The website of the Child Traumatic Stress Network lists many of these protocols (www.nctsnet.org).

19.3.2.3 Evidence

There are many randomised controlled trials showing that CBT, in particular TF-CBT, is highly effective in reducing symptoms of PTSD, depression and behaviour problems in children and adolescents after different types of single or multiple (complex) trauma in an individual or group setting (for an overview see Dorsey et al. 2011). TF-CBT has both proven to be superior to a child-centred, supportive treatment and to a waiting list control group. The current Cochrane Review (Gillies et al. 2012) and the current treatment guidelines for the treatment of child PTSD from the International Society of Traumatic Stress Studies (Foa 2009) and from the American Academy of Child and Adolescent Psychiatry (2010) all conclude that CBT has the highest level of evidence for the treatment of child PTSD. Therefore, the use of CBT to treat child and adolescent PTSD is highly recommended. However, evidence for preschool-age children, for specific ethnic minorities and for certain types of trauma (e.g. medical trauma) is still limited, and more research is needed.

19.3.3 Eye Movement Desensitisation and Reprocessing (EMDR)

19.3.3.1 Background

Developed by Francine Shapiro in the 1980s, Eye Movement Desensitisation and Reprocessing (EMDR) is based on the premise that adaptive information processing following a traumatic event is adversely affected by emotions and dissociation, leading to incomplete processing of experience in memory. Through the use of a dual-attention task, recall of thoughts, images and sensation at the same time as attending to the visual stimulus of a moving finger or equivalent is the core technique in EMDR. The proposed mechanism of change is that the dual attention facilitates more complete information processing of the traumatic memory.

19.3.3.2 Procedure/Components

EMDR is usually delivered in the following eight phases: history taking and treatment planning, preparation, assessment, desensitisation, installation, body scan, closure and re-evaluation. The main part of the intervention involves moving through the assessment to the body scan phases repeatedly until the traumatic experience is processed.

EMDR has been applied with traumatised school-aged children. There are age-appropriate modifications to the method (Tinker and Wilson 1999), and the intervention is directed at the child without formal involvement of parents, although parents are provided with support and psychoeducation.

19.3.3.3 Evidence

There is sufficient evidence to support EMDR as an evidence-based intervention for adults (Bisson et al. 2007, Chap. 11). This evidence comes from multiple randomised controlled trials and meta-analyses. However there is much less evidence supporting the application of EMDR with children. A recent meta-analysis (Rodenburg et al. 2009) identified studies that compared EMDR to a waiting list control, to treatment as usual and to CBT. Since then, there have been several other trials (e.g. Farkas et al. 2010; Kemp et al. 2010); however, the picture is still unclear. Overall, the evidence indicates that there is little or no support for the effectiveness of EMDR in reducing PTSD in those studies that compare it to waiting list or usual care controls. However, this may be due to the quality of the methodology of these studies. There is some support for EMDR, in that the two studies that compared EMDR and CBT directly (de Roos et al. 2011; Jaberghaderi et al. 2004) demonstrated equivalence between the two and, in the case of De Roos et al. (2011), with fewer sessions of treatment. However, neither study was of high quality nor provided support for clinically significant change as a result of EMDR, and this is a need in future research. There is also no available evidence on EMDR with preschool children.

19.3.4 Psychodynamic Therapy

19.3.4.1 Background

The focus of psychodynamic treatment models are the emotional conflicts which are caused by the traumatic experience, particularly as they relate to the individual's early life experiences. Psychodynamic therapies do not focus on the symptoms alone but on the meaning and the effects of the traumatic events for the individual child and his development. Importantly, trauma and its effects are considered as different across individuals and one has to understand the individual child to provide appropriate treatment. Therefore, modern psychodynamic therapies may include different modalities, such as talk therapy, trauma-focused play therapy, parental counselling and interventions in schools. In younger children, based on theories of attachment, the focus of intervention is the mother (parent)–child relationship. Psychodynamic therapists also conceptualise issues of transference and counter-transference and consider them in the planning of their therapies (Terr 2013).

19.3.4.2 Procedure/Components

Procedures and components of psychodynamic treatment of traumatised youth differ enormously dependent on the specific protocol or manual used, making it impossible to describe a typical procedure. Usually, however, psychodynamic therapy has a longer duration compared to other methods and does not solely focus on the child's symptoms.

The Child–Parent Psychotherapy (CPP; (Lieberman and Van Horn 2005), for example, is conducted over 50 weekly sessions in a dyadic setting with the parent and the child (>7 years). Based on the observation and modification of the child-parent interaction during the therapy sessions, CPP aims at strengthening the child–parent relationship in order to allow the child a healthy development. Parents are provided with assistance to better interpret their child's behaviours and feelings and to provide age-appropriate emotional support. Because CPP is usually provided in the context of domestic violence, a joint child-parent trauma narrative is developed.

A quite different treatment protocol was described by Trowell et al. (2002) with sexually abused school-aged girls. These authors' psychodynamic therapy involved 30 sessions consisting of three different phases: engagement, focus on issues relevant to the traumatised child and ending.

Lenore Terr, one of the pioneers of child psychotraumatology, who works with a strong psychodynamic background, describes three principles of healing in working with traumatised children (Terr 2013): abreaction (emotional expression), context (cognitive understanding) and correction (behavioural or fantasised change). Above all, attachment is seen as a crucial issue in traumatised children.

19.3.4.3 Evidence

Efficacy of psychodynamic methods is supported by several randomised controlled trials as well as a high number of clinical case studies (American Academy of Child and Adolescent Psychiatry 2010; Foa 2009). Most of the controlled studies have examined the effects of long-term relationship-based interventions for traumatised young children and their caregivers affected by domestic violence. Currently, Child–Parent Psychotherapy (CPP) is the best studied method (Lieberman and Van Horn 2005). In sum, available studies show that CPP effectively reduces child and parent symptomatology and enhances the quality of attachment between child and parents.

19.3.5 School-Based Interventions

19.3.5.1 Background

Schools can serve a key role in assisting children during a traumatic stress. Schools are often the haven of consistency and safety in the lives of children who have been exposed to traumatic stress to the community such as disasters or interpersonal trauma such as abuse or violence. The routine and predictability of schools combined with the longer-term oversight and care of students by teachers provides an excellent opportunity to bolster and support existing coping and resilience but also to identify students in need of further care that may not be within the school's capacity or capability. Schools provide a natural opportunity to engage, inform and resource children and their families in the face of community trauma. They also can act as the conduit to appropriate levels of care for children. However, in order for this process to be effective, there must be a close liaison between the school and specialist healthcare providers.

Schools have also been employed as the setting for intervention directly with children exposed to traumatic events with the goal of reducing the traumatic stress. This involves the direct delivery of psychological care within the school to students by therapists. Why should delivery within schools as opposed to other more usual settings be important? Jaycox et al. (2010) have demonstrated that following a community trauma an intervention delivered within a school is not only as effective as one delivered in a standard clinical setting, but more crucially the uptake rate of the school-based intervention was significantly greater than in the clinical setting.

19.3.5.2 Procedure and Components

Of interventions that have been delivered within schools for posttraumatic stress, those that have the most evidence are the ones based on trauma-focused CBT; however, a number of other interventions have been successfully applied employing CBT and other components. Typically the interventions are aimed primarily at students but can incorporate teachers, where the focus is on classroom management and support of students with posttraumatic stress. Jaycox et al. (2009) did demonstrate that teachers can be effective in helping to deliver the intervention in schools; however, the size of the effect of the intervention was considerably lower than those where a therapist was the primary treatment provider (Rolfnes and Idsoe 2011). Cognitive-Behavioural Intervention for Trauma in Schools (C-BITS) (Jaycox et al. 2009) is distinct from standard trauma-focused CBT in that it is largely offered in group format, does not include parents and can be slightly shorter in duration (10 sessions plus 1–3 individual sessions). As with trauma-focused CBT, C-BITS includes psychoeducation, relaxation, development of a trauma narrative and exposure to trauma reminders, anxiety and distress management skills.

19.3.5.3 Evidence

School-delivered interventions have been evaluated by a number of good-quality randomised controlled trials and several uncontrolled trials (Rolfnes and Idsoe 2011). The strongest evidence comes from the work of Jaycox and colleagues (2009) with C-BITS and variants, which demonstrate medium to large effect size for posttraumatic stress symptoms. One study of note was a large randomised controlled trial by Jordans et al. (2010). Here a CBT-based intervention was delivered in schools to children in Nepal exposed to armed conflict. This study found medium-size effects on PTSD symptoms.

19.3.6 Pharmacological Treatment

19.3.6.1 Background

PTSD and other trauma-related disorders have been shown to be associated with a variety of neurobiological alterations, such as dysregulations of catecholamine secretion and the hypothalamic–pituitary–adrenal axis. Moreover, structural and functional changes of the central nervous system (e.g. prefrontal cortex, amygdala, hippocampus, corpus callosum) have been found in traumatised individuals.

While such research in children is still in its infancy, it is widely accepted that such alterations are also present in children and may have a very deleterious effect on their development. Pharmacological treatment aims at influencing some of these physiological dysregulations by trying to decrease adrenergic responsiveness and dopaminergic activity and to increase availability of serotonin (Stamatokos and Campo 2010). Targeted symptoms mainly include hyperarousal, irritability, severe sleep problems, nightmares and concentration problems. Also, in children with comorbid disorders that are known to be responsive to pharmacological treatment, the use of medication can be considered. The goal of medication in traumatised children is to treat specific symptoms that interfere with normal development and to help the child tolerate a psychological treatment.

Although there is very limited evidence for the effectiveness of pharmacological treatment in children and adolescents with PTSD and although no medication is currently approved by the Food and Drug Administration (FDA) for treatment of childhood PTSD, medication is widely used to treat PTSD symptoms in youth. The current treatment guidelines of the *International Society for Traumatic Stress Studies* (Foa 2009) recommend the use of medication for the treatment of child PTSD if comorbid psychiatric conditions are present that respond to pharmacological treatment (major depressive disorder, obsessive-compulsive disorder, ADHD, general anxiety disorder), if the intensity of the child's traumatic stress symptoms limits a child's ability to engage in psychotherapy and if there is no access to psychotherapy.

19.3.6.2 Procedure

If pharmacological treatment is considered, the first step is education of the child and his caregivers about the specific agent and potential short- and long-term adverse effects. The choice of medication depends on the individual symptoms and comorbid conditions. If informed consent is given and no significant comorbidity is present, selective serotonin reuptake inhibitors (SSRIs) which are approved for use in adult PTSD are a good first option because a variety of traumatic stress symptoms are associated with serotonergic dysregulation (American Academy of Child and Adolescent Psychiatry 2010). Some evidence from adults and from open clinical trials in children and adolescents with PTSD suggest that medications other than SSRIs may be helpful (α- and β-adrenergic blocking agents, tricyclic antidepressants, serotonin–norepinephrine reuptake inhibitors, opiates, atypical antipsychotic agents). Also, there are interesting pilot data on the use of pharmacological interventions in secondary prevention of child PTSD which suggest that specific pharmacological agents may help to prevent PTSD if applied early after a traumatic event (Maccani et al. 2012).

19.3.6.3 Evidence

Current systematic reviews of the effectiveness of psychopharmacological treatment of childhood PTSD can be found in Huemer et al. (2010), Strawn et al. (2010) and Stamatokos and Campo (2010). In sum, the authors conclude that current research data are very limited and do not support the use of any pharmacological agent as a first-line treatment for PTSD in children and adolescents. Therefore, available research does not support the use of medication alone for the treatment of childhood PTSD (American Academy of Child and Adolescent Psychiatry 2010).

19.3.7 Young Children

Young children under the age of 6 years do present with PTSD symptoms such as re-experiencing (e.g. through nightmares, posttraumatic play), avoidance of reminders of the event and physiological hyperarousal (e.g. irritability, sleep disturbance, exaggerated startle) (Scheeringa et al. 2003). However, DSM-IV PTSD criteria did not adequately describe the symptoms in infants and preschool children. Therefore, the prevalence of PTSD in young children has largely been underestimated to date (Scheeringa et al. 1995). This has led to the addition of a preschool subtype for PTSD in the DSM-5 (American Psychiatric Association 2013).

Prevalence of PTSD assessed using developmentally sensitive methods in young children exposed to physical or sexual abuse rates is between 26 and 60 % (De Young et al. 2011). De Young et al. (2012) have shown that young children also develop depression, separation anxiety disorder (SAD), oppositional defiant disorder (ODD) and specific phobias following traumatic events. These disorders are highly comorbid with PTSD and may become the focus of intervention, where the root cause for these disorders may in fact be posttraumatic stress.

Research into interventions for young children is not well developed. For example, there are currently no known published studies examining the effectiveness of preventive psychological interventions following trauma. There are, however, several randomised controlled trails that have focused intervention on young children with posttraumatic stress. All of these studies have either focused on or included children exposed to abuse. However two of these provided treatment only to young children exposed to abuse (Cohen and Mannarino 1996; Deblinger et al. 2001). The study by Cohen and Mannarino (1996) compared TF-CBT to a supportive therapy in 39 children aged 3–6, where they found that the TF-CBT was associated with reduction in internalising problems on the CBCL; however, they failed to measure PTSD. In contrast, Deblinger et al. (2001) found that, compared to a supportive therapy, TF-CBT did not produce a benefit in 44 children aged 2–8. Recently, Scheeringa et al. (2011) did find a specific benefit for a 12-session TF-CBT compared to a waiting list control in 64 children aged between 3 and 6 years.

Parents are key to intervening with young children. Many parents will be experiencing symptoms of stress following trauma in the child either because of shared direct exposure or secondary stress associated with circumstances of the trauma and the child's responses. Approximately 25 % of parents will experience clinical levels of distress after a young child's trauma (Landolt et al. 2012). Parental traumatic stress is a predictor for subsequent traumatic stress in the young child, indicative of a directional relationship (De Young et al. 2014). In cases of abuse or neglect, parents or close relatives may be directly involved as perpetrators or by being complicit in the abuse. In these cases, consideration of the role of parents in recovery is complex but essential.

Parenting and attachment are also likely to be crucial influences for the young child's adjustment following trauma. The parent–child relationship helps to assist the child regulate their distress and generally buffer the child from the impact of stressors (Lieberman 2004). Parents also provide the most important model for coping with stress and stressors. Where a parent is emotionally affected by the circumstances of the child's trauma, their lack of coping will be modelled to the child (Nugent et al. 2007). This suggests that intervention for parents' distress should precede or co-occur with any intervention for children (e.g. Cobham et al. 1998).

In a study that examined the effects of early intervention for parents of young children exposed to trauma, Melnyk et al. (2004) employed a coping-based support and psychoeducation for parents of children (2–7 years) who were admitted to a paediatric intensive care unit. They found that parents in the intervention group had significantly lower stress, depression and PTSD symptoms.

In the very young children, there have been some developments in attachment-focused intervention. While these have not targeted PTSD, they have addressed problematic attachment that is present in children exposed to abuse. The Circle of Security model (Hoffman et al. 2006) is one such model that does have some limited empirical support. Using a pre-post design, the model was shown to significantly change attachment styles in 65 preschool children. This 20-week intervention is costly but has the potential to inform trauma-focused treatments for this age group.

19.4 Summary and Conclusion

While the evidence with regard to trauma therapy in adults is quite good, this is still not the case in children due to the unsatisfactory quality of many treatment studies. Establishing such evidence requires standardised treatment protocols and randomised controlled trials.

Although various guidelines (e.g. NICE guidelines, AACAP practice parameters, ISTSS guidelines, etc.), reviews and meta-analyses (e.g. Gillies et al. 2012; Leenarts et al. 2013) on effectiveness of child trauma therapy are currently available, recommendations across these documents are quite inconsistent. This is largely due to different definitions of evidence levels and different inclusion and exclusion criteria for studies.

Nevertheless, the evidence clearly suggests that psychotherapy is considered the first choice of treatment. Medication may be used as a second line if psychotherapy is not available or if the child has a comorbid condition. One psychotherapeutic treatment that is recommended in all guidelines and that has been found to be effective in all meta-analyses is CBT, specifically trauma-focused CBT (TF-CBT), and to some extent Child–Parent Psychotherapy, a psychodynamic treatment approach for young children (Lieberman and Van Horn 2005). Current evidence is insufficient to determine the effectiveness of EMDR, play therapy, family therapy and pharmacological therapy in children and adolescents.

Notably, all current treatments that proved to be effective employ methods such as behavioural and emotional regulation, cognitive processing and coping strategies, and they all directly address the traumatic experience (mostly through exposure and creation of a narrative) and include caregivers. Currently, there is no evidence to conclude that children and adolescents with particular types of trauma are more or less likely to respond to psychological therapies than others (Gillies et al. 2012). However, evidence regarding specific treatments of children with complex trauma is still lacking. Future studies are needed to clarify how these children can be effectively treated. Also we need more studies on preschool-age children, specifically below the age of 4 years. Finally, as highlighted by Carrion and Kletter (2012), future treatment protocols should better integrate current findings on neurobiological mechanisms in trauma with psychotherapy. This may especially be promising with regard to early interventions after trauma.

References

Aderka, I. M., Appelbaum-Namdar, E., Shafran, N., & Gilboa-Schechtman, E. (2011). Sudden gains in prolonged exposure for children and adolescents with posttraumatic stress disorder. *Journal of Consulting and Clinical Psychology, 79*, 441–446.

Alisic, E., van der Schoot, T. A., van Ginkel, J. R., & Kleber, R. J. (2008). Looking beyond posttraumatic stress disorder in children: Posttraumatic stress reactions, posttraumatic growth, and quality of life in a general population sample. *Journal of Clinical Psychiatry, 69*, 1455–1461.

American Academy of Child and Adolescent Psychiatry. (2010). Practice parameter for the assessment and treatment of children and adolescents with posttraumatic stress disorder. *Journal of the American Academy of Child and Adolescent Psychiatry, 49*, 414–430.

American Psychiatric Association. (2013). *Diagnostic and statistical manual of mental disorders* (5th ed.). Arlington: American Psychiatric Association.

Berkowitz, S., Smith Stover, C., & Marans, S. R. (2011). The Child and Family Traumatic Stress Intervention: Secondary prevention for youth at risk of developing PTSD. *Journal of Child Psychology and Psychiatry, 52*, 676–685.

Bisson, J. I., Ehlers, A., Matthews, R., Pilling, S., Richards, D., & Turner, S. (2007). Psychological treatments for chronic post-traumatic stress disorder. Systematic review and meta-analysis. *The British Journal of Psychiatry: the Journal of Mental Science, 190*, 97–104.

Briere, J. (1996). *Trauma symptom checklist for children (TSCC), professional manual.* Odessa: Psychological Assessment Resources.

Briere, J. (2005). *Trauma symptom checklist for young children (TSCYC): Professional manual.* Lutz: Psychological Assessment Resources Inc.

Carrion, V. G., & Kletter, H. (2012). Posttraumatic stress disorder: Shifting toward a developmental framework. [Review]. *Child and Adolescent Psychiatric Clinics of North America, 21*, 573–591.

Cobham, V. E., Dadds, M. R., & Spence, S. H. (1998). The role of parental anxiety in the treatment of childhood anxiety. *Journal of Consulting and Clinical Psychology, 66*, 893–905.

Cohen, J. A., & Mannarino, A. P. (1996). A treatment outcome study for sexually abused preschool children: Initial findings. *Journal of the American Academy of Child and Adolescent Psychiatry, 35*, 42–50.

Cohen, J. A., Mannarino, A. P., & Deblinger, E. (2006). *Treating trauma and traumatic grief in children and adolescents.* New York: Guilford Press.

Copeland, W. E., Keller, G., Angold, A., & Costello, E. J. (2007). Traumatic events and posttraumatic stress in childhood. *Archives of General Psychiatry, 64*, 577–584.

de Roos, C., Greenwald, R., den Hollander-Gijsman, M., Noorthoorn, E., von Buuren, S., & de Jong, A. (2011). A randomised comparison of cognitive behavioural therapy (CBT) and eye movement desensitisation and reprocessing (EMDR) in disaster- exposed children. *European Journal of Psychotraumatology, 2*, 5881. doi: 10.3402/ejpt.v2i0.5881.

De Young, A. C., Kenardy, J. A., & Cobham, V. E. (2011). Trauma in early childhood: A neglected population. *Clinical Child and Family Psychology Review, 14,* 231–250.

De Young, A. C., Kenardy, J. A., Cobham, V. E., & Kimble, R. (2012). Prevalence, comorbidity and course of trauma reactions in young burn injured children. *Journal of Child Psychology and Psychiatry, 53,* 56–63.

De Young, A. C., Hendrikz, J., Kenardy, J. A., Cobham, V. E., & Kimble, R. M. (2014). Prospective evaluation of parent distress following paediatric burns and identification of risk factors for young child and parent PTSD. *Journal of Child and Adolescent Psychopharmacology, 24,* 9–17.

Deblinger, E., Stauffer, L. B., & Steer, R. A. (2001). Comparative efficacies of supportive and cognitive behavioral group therapies for young children who have been sexually abused and their nonoffending mothers. *Child Maltreatment, 6,* 332–343.

Dorsey, S., Briggs, E. C., & Woods, B. A. (2011). Cognitive-behavioral treatment for posttraumatic stress disorder in children and adolescents. *Child and Adolescent Psychiatric Clinics of North America, 20,* 255–269.

Elklit, A. (2002). Victimization and PTSD in a Danish national youth probability sample. *Journal of the American Academy of Child and Adolescent Psychiatry, 41,* 174–181.

Farkas, L., Cyr, M., Lebeau, T. M., & Lemay, J. (2010). Effectiveness of MASTR/EMDR therapy for traumatized adolescents. *Journal of Child and Adolescent Trauma, 3,* 125–142.

Foa, E. B. (Ed.). (2009). *Effective treatments for PTSD.* New York: Guilford Press.

Foa, E. B., Johnson, K. M., Feeny, N. C., & Treadwell, K. R. H. (2001). The Child PTSD Symptom Scale: A preliminary examination of its psychometric properties. *Journal of Clinical Child Psychology, 30,* 376–384.

Gillies, D., Taylor, F., Gray, C., O'Brien, L., & D'Abrew, N. (2012). Psychological therapies for the treatment of post-traumatic stress disorder in children and adolescents (review). *Cochrane Database Syst Rev,* (12):CD006726.

Gudiño, O. G., Weiss, R. J., Havens, J. F., Biggs, E. A., Diamond, U. N., Marr, M., Jackson, C., & Cloitre, M. (2014). Group trauma-informed treatment for adolescent psychiatric inpatients: A preliminary uncontrolled trial. *Journal of Traumatic Stress, 27,* 1–5.

Hoffman, K. T., Marvin, R. S., Cooper, G., & Powell, B. (2006). Changing toddlers' and preschoolers' attachment classifications: The circle of security intervention. *Journal of Consulting and Clinical Psychology, 74,* 1017–1026.

Huemer, J., Erhart, F., & Steiner, H. (2010). Posttraumatic stress disorder in children and adolescents: A review of psychopharmacological treatment. *Child Psychiatry and Human Development, 41,* 624–640.

Jaberghaderi, N., Greenwald, R., Rubin, A., Zand, S. O., & Dolatabadi, S. (2004). A comparison of CBT and EMDR for sexually-abused Iranian girls. *Clinical Psychology and Psychotherapy, 11,* 358–368.

Jaycox, L. H., Langley, A., Stein, B., Wong, M., Sharma, P., Scott, M., & Schonlau, M. (2009). Support for students exposed to trauma: A pilot study. *School Mental Health, 1,* 49–60.

Jaycox, L. H., Cohen, J. A., Mannarino, A. P., Walker, D. W., Langley, A. K., Gegenheimer, K. L., Scott, M., & Schonlau, M. (2010). Children's mental health care following Hurricane Katrina: A field trial of trauma-focused psychotherapies. *Journal of Traumatic Stress, 23,* 223–231.

Jordans, M. J. D., Komproe, I. H., Tol, W. A., Kohrt, B. A., Luitel, N. P., Macy, R. D., & de Jong, J. T. V. M. (2010). Evaluation of a classroom-based psychosocial intervention in conflict-affected Nepal: A cluster randomized controlled trial. *Journal of Child Psychology and Psychiatry, 51,* 818–826.

Kemp, M., Drummond, P., & McDermott, B. (2010). A wait-list controlled pilot study of eye movement desensitization and reprocessing (EMDR) for children with post-traumatic stress disorder (PTSD) symptoms from motor vehicle accidents. *Clinical Child Psychology and Psychiatry, 15,* 5–25.

Kenardy, J. A., Spence, S. H., & Macleod, A. C. (2006). Screening for posttraumatic stress disorder in children after accidental injury. *Pediatrics, 118,* 1002–1009.

Kilpatrick, D. G., Rugierro, K. J., Acierno, R., Saunders, B. E., Resnick, H. S., & Best, C. L. (2003). Violence and risk of PTSD, major depression, substance abuse/dependence, and comorbidity: Results from the National Survey of Adolescents. *Journal of Consulting and Clinical Psychology, 71*, 692–700.

Kramer, D. N., & Landolt, M. A. (2011). Characteristics and efficacy of early psychological interventions in children and adolescents after single trauma: A meta-analysis. *European Journal of Psychotraumatology, 2*, 1–24.

Kramer, D. N., Hertli, M. B., & Landolt, M. A. (2013). Evaluation of an early risk screener for PTSD in preschool children after accidental injury. *Pediatrics, 132*(4), e945–e951.

Landolt, M. A., Buehlmann, C., Maag, T., & Schiestl, C. (2009). Quality of life is impaired in pediatric burn survivors with posttraumatic stress disorder. *Journal of Pediatric Psychology, 34*, 14–21.

Landolt, M. A., Ystrom, E., Sennhauser, F. H., Gnehm, H. E., & Vollrath, M. E. (2012). The mutual prospective influence of child and parental posttraumatic stress symptoms in pediatric patients. *Journal of Child Psychology and Psychiatry, 53*, 767–774.

Landolt, M. A., Schnyder, U., Maier, T., Schoenbucher, V., & Mohler-Kuo, M. (2013). Trauma exposure and posttraumatic stress disorder in adolescents: A national survey in Switzerland. *Journal of Traumatic Stress, 26*, 209–216.

Leenarts, L. E., Diehle, J., Doreleijers, T. A., Jansma, E. P., & Lindauer, R. J. (2013). Evidence-based treatments for children with trauma-related psychopathology as a result of childhood maltreatment: A systematic review. *European Child & Adolescent Psychiatry, 22*, 269–283.

Lieberman, A. F. (2004). Traumatic stress and quality of attachment: Reality and internalization in disorders of infant mental health. *Infant Mental Health Journal, 25*, 336–351.

Lieberman, A. F., & Van Horn, P. (2005). *Don't hit mummy! A manual for child – parent psychotherapy for young witnesses of family violence*. Washington, DC: Zero to Three Press.

Maccani, M. A., Delahanty, D. L., Nugent, N. R., & Berkowitz, S. J. (2012). Pharmacological secondary prevention of PTSD in youth: Challenges and opportunities for advancement. *Journal of Traumatic Stress, 25*, 543–550.

Melnyk, B. M., Corbo-Richert, B., Alpert-Gillis, L., Feinstein, N. F., Crean, H. F., Johnson, J., Fairbanks, E., Small, L., Rubenstein, J., & Slota, M. (2004). Creating opportunities for parent empowerment: Program effects on the mental health/coping outcomes of critically ill young children and their mothers. *Pediatrics, 113*, e597–e607.

Mersky, J. P., Topitzes, J., & Reynolds, A. J. (2013). Impacts of adverse childhood experiences on health, mental health, and substance use in early adulthood: A cohort study of an urban, minority sample in the U.S. *Child Abuse and Neglect, 37*, 917–925.

Nader, K. O., Kriegler, J. A., Blake, D. D., Pynoos, R. S., Newman, E., & Weather, F. W. (2002). *The clinician-administered PTSD scale, child and adolescent version (CAPS-CA)*. White River Junction: National Center for PTSD.

Najavits, L. M. (2002). *Seeking safety: A treatment manual for PTSD and substance abuse*. New York: Guilford Press.

Nixon, R., Ellis, A. A., Nehmy, T. J., & Ball, S. A. (2010). Screening and predicting posttraumatic stress and depression in children following single-incident trauma. *Journal of Clinical Child and Adolescent Psychology, 39*, 588–596.

Nugent, N. R., Ostrowski, S., Christopher, N. C., & Delahanty, D. L. (2007). Parental posttraumatic stress symptoms as a moderator of child's acute biological response and subsequent posttraumatic stress symptoms in pediatric injury patients. *Journal of Pediatric Psychology, 32*, 309–318.

Pynoos, R. S., & Steinberg, A. M. (2013). *UCLA PTSD reaction index for children/adolescents – DSM-5*. Los Angeles: National Center for Child Traumatic Stress.

Rodenburg, R., Benjamin, A., de Roos, C., Meijer, A. M., & Stams, G. J. (2009). Efficacy of EMDR in children: A meta-analysis. *Clinical Psychology Review, 29*, 599–606.

Rolfnes, E. S., & Idsoe, T. (2011). School-based intervention programs for PTSD symptoms: A review and meta-analysis. *Journal of Traumatic Stress, 24*, 155–165.

Ruf, M., Schauer, M., Neuner, F., Catani, C., Schauer, E., & Elbert, T. (2010). Narrative exposure therapy for 7- to 16-year-olds: A randomized controlled trial with traumatized refugee children. *Journal of Traumatic Stress, 23*, 437–445.

Ruzek, J. I., Brymer, M. J., Jacobs, A. K., Layne, C. M., Vernberg, E. M., & Watson, P. J. (2007). Psychological first aid. *Journal of Mental Health Counseling, 29*(1), 17–49.

Scheeringa, M. S. (2004). *Diagnostic infant and preschool assessment (DIPA) (version 7/27/13)*. *Unpublished instrument.* Retrieved from: http://www.infantinstitute.com/. 3 Dec 2013.

Scheeringa, M. S. (2011). PTSD in children younger than the age of 13: Toward developmentally sensitive assessment and management. *Journal of Child and Adolescent Trauma, 4*, 181–197.

Scheeringa, M. S., & Haslett, N. (2010). The reliability and criterion validity of the diagnostic Infant and Preschool Assessment: A new diagnostic instrument for young children. *Child Psychiatry and Human Development, 41*(3), 299–312.

Scheeringa, M. S., & Zeanah, C. (2008). Reconsideration of harm's way: Onsets and comorbidity patterns of disorders in preschool children and their caregivers following Hurricane Katrina. *Journal of Clinical Child & Adolescent Psychology, 37*, 508–518.

Scheeringa, M. S., Zeanah, C. H., Drell, M. J., & Larrieu, J. A. (1995). Two approaches to the diagnosis of posttraumatic stress disorder in infancy and early childhood. *Journal of the American Academy of Child and Adolescent Psychiatry, 34*, 191–200.

Scheeringa, M. S., Zeanah, C. H., Myers, L., & Putnam, F. W. (2003). New findings on alternative criteria for PTSD in preschool children. *Journal of the American Academy of Child and Adolescent Psychiatry, 42*, 561–570.

Scheeringa, M. S., Weems, C. F., Cohen, J. A., Amaya-Jackson, L., & Guthrie, D. (2011). Trauma-focused cognitive-behavioral therapy for posttraumatic stress disorder in three through six year-old children: A randomized clinical trial. *Journal of Child Psychology and Psychiatry, 52*, 853–860.

Stamatokos, M., & Campo, J. V. (2010). Psychopharmacologic treatment of traumatized youth. *Current Opinion in Pediatrics, 22*, 599–604.

Strawn, J. R., Keeshin, B. R., DelBello, M. P., Geracioti, T. D., & Putnam, F. W. (2010). Psychopharmacologic treatment of posttraumatic stress disorder in children and adolescents: A review. *Journal of Clinical Psychiatry, 71*, 932–941.

Terr, L. C. (2013). Treating childhood trauma. *Child and Adolescent Psychiatric Clinics of North America, 22*, 51–66.

Tinker, R. H., & Wilson, S. A. (1999). *Through the eyes of a child: EMDR with children.* New York: Norton & Co.

Trowell, J., Kolvin, I., Weeramanthri, T., Sadowski, H., Berelowitz, M., Glasser, D., & Leitch, I. (2002). Psychotherapy for sexually abused girls: Psychopathological outcome findings and patterns of change. *British Journal of Psychiatry, 180*, 234–247.

Winston, F. K., Kassam-Adams, N., Garcia-Espana, F., Ittenbach, R., & Cnaan, A. (2003). Screening for risk of persistent posttraumatic stress in injured children and their parents. *Journal of the American Medical Association, 290*, 643–649.

Treating PTSD Symptoms in Older Adults

20

Maja O'Connor and Ask Elklit

We live in a society that idealizes youth. Every day we are exposed to advertisements, social media, and TV programs casting the young and beautiful. In our careers, social arenas, and health systems, we are encouraged to be fit, healthy, strong, slim, beautiful, efficient, exciting, quick, etc. These are all qualities that are more pronounced in youth and decrease in old age. At the same time, fewer children are being born in the Western world, and people live longer. This leads to a growing proportion of older people in society, who lived long lives and who are likely to have experienced many losses or even traumas. Older people are not as fast, efficient, or healthy as the young ideal, and they are often seen as rigid and predictable: "When you know one old person, you know them all." Following this line of thought, it is often presumed that older people are neither willing nor able to change their ways. But is that really so? This chapter investigates trauma reactions in older people, the efficacy of psychotherapy with older people in general, and the treatment of posttraumatic stress reactions in older people in particular.

M. O'Connor (✉)
Unit for psychooncology and health psychology (EPoS), Department of Psychology,
School of Business and Social Sciences, Aarhus University,
Aarhus, Denmark
e-mail: maja@psy.au.dk

A. Elklit
Department of Psychology,
National Center for Psychotraumatology, University of Southern Denmark,
Odense, Denmark

© Springer International Publishing Switzerland 2015
U. Schnyder, M. Cloitre (eds.), *Evidence Based Treatments for Trauma-Related Psychological Disorders: A Practical Guide for Clinicians*,
DOI 10.1007/978-3-319-07109-1_20

20.1 PTSD in Older Populations

The prevalence of PTSD in Western adult populations is relatively well established. In such adult populations, we see PTSD prevalence identified by clinical interview ranging from approximately 7–8 % for lifetime PTSD (Breslau et al. 1991; Kessler and Wang 2008) and ranging from 3 to 4 % for the past 12 months (Gadermann et al. 2012; Kessler et al. 2012). The prevalence of PTSD, similar to anxiety, mood, and substance disorders, is highest in middle adulthood (8–9 %), somewhat lower in young adults (6 %), and approximately half as frequent in older adults (3 %) compared to 7 % in the total population (Ditlevsen and Elklit 2010; Kessler and Wang 2008). Two European studies investigated posttraumatic stress reactions in general older populations mainly by self-report questionnaires with high correspondence with the DSM-IV diagnostic classification of PTSD (Glaesmer et al. 2012; Maercker et al. 2008). In the above studies, self-reported posttraumatic stress, or what we will call posttraumatic stress disorder (PTSD) symptoms, was identified in 4–5 % of the older participants (Glaesmer et al. 2012; Maercker et al. 2008). Other studies with similar research methods found equal levels of PTSD symptoms in younger and older populations (Spitzer et al. 2008). Although possibly not as common as in younger adult populations (Creamer and Parslow 2008), we can conclude that PTSD symptoms are present in a significant minority of general older populations.

Studies on PTSD symptoms in older samples generally fall within two main groups: those that focus on acute reactions to recent traumatic experiences and those that describe chronic PTSD symptoms from past and often sustained traumatic experiences. Recent traumatic reactions have mainly been studied in older populations who experienced natural disasters such as floods and earthquakes, accidents, or physical injuries (Averill and Beck 2000; Chung et al. 2006; Elklit and O'Connor 2005; O'Connor 2010b; Ruskin and Talbott 1996; Yang et al. 2003). Older people are in general less exposed to accidents, assaults, and combat than younger populations but are confronted with a wide variety of potentially traumatic age-related challenges such as loss of physical functioning, death of close relatives, siblings, and/or partners, or chronic and life-threatening illness (Carr 2004; O'Connor 2010b; Silverman et al. 2000). The above studies indicate that older people respond to acute trauma with similar magnitude and pattern of PTSD symptoms as younger adults, with a PTSD symptoms prevalence of 4–18 % in older populations (Carr 2004; O'Connor 2010a; Silverman et al. 2000). Both major and minor traumatic events can potentially lead to PTSD symptoms in older people (Lapp et al. 2011; Ruskin and Talbott 1996), and a mix of multiple long-term and recent losses are common in old people, as seen in the case of Alice in the textbox below.

Alice, 82 years old, is referred to mindfulness-based cognitive therapy for depression (MBCT). Three years earlier, her husband, Henry, passed away after a long battle with multiple sclerosis. Alice is grief-stricken and physically exhausted after Henry's death. But, after some months, she starts enjoying life again going to church, taking trips abroad with her youngest daughter Sue, and attending her yoga classes. Then she has a cerebral hemorrhage. She is in rehabilitation for 2 months, and when she finally comes home, she has a constant tremor in her right hand and has difficulties concentrating on anything for long. While she gradually regains most of her previous physical function, her mood deteriorates, and she finally contacts her doctor for help. After diagnosing a moderate depression, he refers her to us. When she arrives for the first class, her eyes are dim and she is very quiet. As the 8-week course progress, she, little by little, starts speaking up in class. The daily exercises remind her of her yoga training and are a great help to her when the negative thoughts take over, and she enjoys coming to class. She tells the group that she is starting to feel more patient and forgiving with herself and generally appears less depressed. Alice also talks about her worries for her daughter, Sue, who suffers greatly from unexplainable back pain. Around the 6th week of MBCT, Sue is diagnosed with an aggressive and terminal type of bone cancer. Sue has called Alice and told her the bad news over the phone. Alice is shocked by the news. Now, every time the phone rings, she feels caught in the chest and sick to her stomach and experiences a strong emotional reaction. Alice begins having intrusive memories about the call. She has trouble sleeping because she has recurrent nightmares about Sue calling with the bad news. Soon Alice starts feeling permanently uneasy and at guard, not really trusting that life will ever be okay again. She cancels her lifelong subscription to the cancer association because receiving their newsletter reminds her of Sue's illness and makes her feel bad, and she has difficulties falling asleep at night because she worries about what is going to happen. During the daytime, she finds it difficult to concentrate on her daily activities, but she still comes to class throughout the rest of the course.

In a short span of years, Alice experiences a number of potentially traumatic events. First, the death of her husband which Alice appears to react to with what can be characterized as a natural grieving process (Stroebe et al. 2013). Throughout the last couple of decades, substantial work has been done to develop a set of diagnostic criteria to identify prolonged grief reactions that are complicated enough to be considered pathological (Bryant 2014; Maercker et al. 2013; Shear et al. 2011). In DSM-5, a prolonged grief disorder named persistent complex bereavement disorder has been included as a condition for further study (American Psychiatric Association 2013, for further details see Chap. 6). This disorder has some symptoms in common with PTSD, but in prolonged grief intrusion is often related to many different aspects of the loss, including positive aspects of the lost relationship, while intrusion in PTSD is usually consistently negative and related to the traumatic event. Further, where PTSD is usually characterized by consistent avoidance of trauma-related stimuli, in prolonged grief avoidance symptoms are combined with symptoms of persistent yearning for the deceased and difficulties accepting the reality of the loss (American Psychiatric Association 2013).

After the loss of her husband, Alice has a cerebral hemorrhage that leads to a clinical depression, which apparently is successfully treated with MBCT. Finally, Alice's daughter receives a terminal diagnosis of an aggressive cancer. Alice now reacts with a number of PTSD symptoms as defined in the DSM-5 (American Psychiatric Association 2013). She has recurrent, involuntary thoughts and nightmares about the call from Sue (intrusion symptoms), and she reacts to this confrontation with the traumatic event with prolonged somatic and emotional distress. She cancels her cancer newsletter because receiving it makes her feel bad (avoidance symptoms), she feels that life will never be okay again (negative alterations in cognitions/dysphoria), and she has problems concentrating and falling asleep combined with a constant feeling of being at guard (arousal symptoms). The case of Alice illustrates how cumulative stressors are common in old age and how an older person can cope successfully with certain stressors.

On this basis, the PTSD symptoms in older people can be divided into two types:

1. Chronic PTSD symptoms

    PTSD symptoms often develop into a chronic condition with many individuals having a fluctuating course where intermittent exposure to new stressors leads to an exacerbation of symptoms. The posttraumatic symptoms have often been present in varying degree since the traumatic event, and due to the many years the individuals have lived with this condition, chronic PTSD symptoms will often have an impact on the personality, physical health, and quality of life.

2. Recent PTSD symptoms

    PTSD symptoms emerge in response to one or more traumatic experiences in the relatively recent past. This includes all events that fulfill the A1 criterion of PTSD (See Part II of this volume for further elaboration of the A1 and other PTSD criteria) such as the death of spouse, critical illness in self or close relative, exposure to natural or man-made disasters, interpersonal violence, etc.

Older people with PTSD symptoms often experience extensive impairments in their daily live functioning with serious physical and mental health problems and lower life satisfaction than older persons without such symptoms (Yaffe et al. 2010). In addition, PTSD symptoms in older people are associated with increased health service costs (Van Zelst et al. 2006). PTSD symptoms are related to increased risk of comorbid depression or anxiety (Spitzer et al. 2008), impairments in memory and attention function (Yaffe et al. 2010), and increased risk of coronary heart disease in older men (Kubzansky et al. 2007). Some argue that PTSD symptoms in older people may be related to accelerated age-related decline (Yaffe et al. 2010). For example, it has been identified that PTSD symptoms in older people are associated with a more significant reduction of memory and overall learning ability than what can be attributed to expected age-related changes (Lapp et al. 2011).

20.2 Physical, Mental, and Social Aspects of Aging: Describing the Target Group

In most Western countries, older persons are defined as 65 years or older. The aging population is growing rapidly worldwide, and over the next 40 years, we can expect a threefold increase, from 580 million people 65 and older in 2014 to more than two billion in 2045 (Laidlaw et al. 2003). Around the turn of the millennium, people aged 65 and over accounted for 13 % of the population; by 2030, it is estimated that it will include 20 % of the world population (Laidlaw et al. 2003). Consequently, we can expect to meet more old people in our daily lives and, thus, must be prepared to meet and effectively treat a greater number of older people in psychotherapy settings.

A number of age-related changes can be expected. Before the age of 70, observed age-related reductions in perceptual speed, vision, and hearing, reserve capacity, and quicker fatigue can be identified, but these changes are limited and can usually be compensated for by external aids such as spectacles, hearing aids, reducing background noise, and taking more time (Schaie 1994). From approximately the age of 70 going forward, the age-related changes will often be more extensive and eventually result in changes of a more qualitative nature that no longer can be fully compensated for by external aids. Perceptual and cognitive changes lead to reduction in ability to freely recall from long-term memory, and thus abstract problem solving becomes more difficult, while the ability for more concrete problem solving where free recall is not necessary remains at the same level into old age (Birren 1996). Decline in more complex mental functions such as working memory and executive functioning is therefore common with increasing age (James 2010).

Starting between the ages of 25 and 30, reductions in muscular strength, reaction time, and perceptual speed can be observed (Schaie 1994). By the age of 60, muscular strength is typically reduced by 20–40 % in both men and women (Spirduso and MacRae 1990). Age-related physiological decline can be observed from the age of 75 years with decrease in blood flow and lung and kidney function. The frequency of physical disorders such as cardiovascular diseases, cancer, respiratory illnesses, arthritis, and muscular diseases is several times higher than in younger populations (Morrison 2008). The ability to perform activities of daily living such as walking, cooking, climbing stairs, and personal hygiene is usually not significantly diminished until after the age of 85 years (Ruskin and Talbott 1996).

This may sound bleak, but although there is significant overall age-related decline on specific parameters, the majority of older people both manage their daily lives well and have high satisfaction with life (Mehlsen 2005). This may be because most of the challenges that people aged 70 plus need to handle are closely related to their daily lives and do not depend on quick reaction time and abstract problem-solving skills. Thus, as long as the challenges in old age do not significantly exceed the individual abilities, most old people appear able to successfully manage and enjoy their daily lives, in spite of reduced functional levels (Baltes and Baltes 1990).

With the exception of dementia (Oliver et al. 2008), most mental disorders are less prevalent in old than in younger age (Coleman and O'Hanlon 2008; Kessler and Wang 2008). This is in contrast with the common age-related trajectory for physical health problems where most people have at least one chronic medical condition by the age of 65 and experience an increasing number of chronic medical conditions with increasing age (Laidlaw et al. 2003). The majority of older people have one or more medical prescriptions, and more than 50 % of those 80 years and above have 6 prescriptions or more (Hajjar et al. 2007). Accordingly, assessments of older adults must include awareness and recognition of the potential negative effects of polypharmacy (the use of multiple medications by a patient) such as drug-drug interactions, increased side effects, decreased quality of life, decreased mobility, and decreased cognition (Hajjar et al. 2007). Older people generally consider long-standing illness as an expected part of life, and both satisfaction with own health and with life in general is usually high in this population (Laidlaw et al. 2003).

Although many age-related characteristics can be identified among older adults, there are substantial individual differences, and geriatric psychology emphasizes sensitivity to large inter- and intrapersonal variability on physical, cognitive, and personality-related characteristics in older people. Indeed individual differences are much more pronounced in older than in younger populations (Fromholt and Bruhn 1998; Johansson 2008). For example, some older people will have stable cognitive function throughout life until death, while others experience significant cognitive decline even in the early days of old age. Conversely, other older persons may have high physical functioning but low cognitive functioning (Lupien et al. 2005). In addition, individual differences among older adults become more pronounced with increasing age in regard to personality, coping, and psychopathology. This large individual variability has implications for mental health services. Clinicians providing services to the elderly, in contrast to younger individuals, will have relatively less ability to predict the specific needs of the individual client based on age alone. Older people simply are more diverse than younger people. Therefore, one must be especially careful not to make assumptions about age-related decline or physical illnesses across elderly persons or about typical patterns of decline across time for any specific individual.

20.3 Psychotherapy for the Aging Client

Different types of psychological intervention including cognitive-behavioral therapy (CBT), psychodynamic approaches, and systemic approaches have similar efficacy in older as in younger clients (Davenhill 2008; Laidlaw 2008; Roper-Hall 2008), but most efficacy studies of psychotherapy with older people evaluated CBT for depression and anxiety disorders, and thus CBT appears to be the best validated form of psychotherapy with older clients (Aspnes and Lynch 2007; James 2010; Laidlaw et al. 2003). This information, combined with the significantly increased risk of negative effects of polypharmacy in the aging client, suggests that evidence-based psychotherapeutic interventions should be preferred over psychotropic medications for the older person with mental health problems. Among people identified with psychiatric problems in primary care and motivated for psychotherapy, a relevant option is to provide psychotherapy combined with drug treatment.

In the light of the expected age-related changes in physical functioning and cognition, some of the identified advantages of CBT with older clients are the structured nature of CBT and its focus on specific skills to manage concrete, individual problems (Laidlaw 2008). Furthermore, CBT focuses on problems in the here-and-now, challenges automatic and stereotyped thinking, and contains individually adapted psychoeducation. These are all treatment strategies that are relevant to and effective in combination with natural age-related decline in cognition (Laidlaw 2008).

However, a recent study reported that only 10 % of older adults with mental problems requiring professional care seemed to receive the needed treatment (Aspnes and Lynch 2007). Negative attitudes and inaccurate beliefs among medical and mental health professionals and even by older people themselves may limit the use of CBT or other types of psychotherapy (Laidlaw et al. 2003). One potential inaccurate belief is that "depression in old age is a normal and expected reaction to the negative aspects of getting old." Indeed, we know that fewer older people have mental disorders relative to younger people and, moreover, that mental disorders such as mood and anxiety disorders in old age are reversible when treated adequately (Aspnes and Lynch 2007; Kessler and Wang 2008). Another assumption that contrasts with the above but is equally inaccurate is a belief that "old people with mental disorders are not able to benefit from and do not want psychotherapy" or that "you can't teach an old dog new tricks" (Laidlaw et al. 2003). The many efficacy studies of psychotherapy among older clients disconfirm this notion (e.g., Kessler and Wang 2008). Some studies even indicate that older people generally prefer psychotherapy to medical treatment (Aspnes and Lynch 2007).

Another type of negative belief that may have adverse effects on engaging mental health professionals in treating older people with mental health issues is that "it is terrible to get old" and that therefore therapy which focuses on increasing well-being and a positive outlook will do little good (Laidlaw et al. 2003). In reality, older people are generally happy with their lives and health, often more so than younger people (Laidlaw 2008). Finally, some clinicians, physicians, and older people may believe that there is "too little to gain at too high individual or socio-economic costs when investing in clients with such a short potential future life-span" (Laidlaw et al. 2003). This belief can be disconfirmed based on the fact that untreated depression, anxiety, or prolonged grief comes at great personal and socio-economic costs, while successful treatment reduces these costs (Laidlaw 2008).

Another complication is that older people have a tendency to present with psychosomatic complaints and symptoms rather than psychological symptoms in relation to mental disorders including PTSD (Kuwert et al. 2012; Nordhus 2008). Often, older people with mental problems bring up specific somatic symptoms such as aches, sleep disturbances, or weight loss rather than psychological symptoms such as depressed mood, anxiety, or suicidal ideation as the reason for paying the first visit to the local physician, who is often the first professional the older patients turn to (Nordhus 2008). Careful assessment via clinical interviews is necessary in order to identify that a mental rather than a somatic disorder may be the source of these symptoms (Laidlaw et al. 2003; Nordhus 2008).

The potential mix of somatic symptoms caused by mental problems and those caused by actual somatic disorders in older people sets high demands on the local physicians' ability to separate mental from somatic origins of the symptoms presented and to diagnose the fundamental disorder correctly. Because of these diagnostic challenges, the responsibility of getting the right type of help for the problem in question cannot rest on the physician alone. Older people themselves and their close relatives must keep in mind that mental health problems in older people such as depression have a tendency to be expressed via somatic symptoms including sleep disturbances, unexplainable aches and pains, or even constipation (Nordhus 2008). If the symptoms in question arise suddenly and without a clear somatic source and especially if the symptoms arise in the aftermath of spousal bereavement or other major, negative life events, there is reason to investigate potential psychological explanations for the symptoms in greater detail.

20.4 Guidelines for the Treatment of Older Adults

There are certain adaptations that can be considered when working clinically with older people. A basic consideration is designing and organizing the physical environment in the clinical setting for potential reductions in the client's sensory abilities such as hearing, vision, and physical perseverance and for reductions in cognitive abilities. Improved lighting and reduced background noise can help as can creating high contrast between foreground and background in pen-and-paper forms or computer-based assessments (Aspnes and Lynch 2007). Similarly, the structure, tasks, and process of treatment should take into account factors such as lower reserve capacity, mental perseverance, and abstract problem-solving ability as they are expressed in the specific client. This may be done by shortening sessions and home exercises due to quicker fatigue and limited cognitive reserve capacity in older clients and by including more breaks. Also, it may be beneficial to speak more slowly and clearly and, generally, be more patient than when working with younger clients.

The clinician can potentially enhance the effectiveness of psychotherapy by using less abstract problem solving in therapy (James 2010). Some studies indicate that older people may benefit more from psychotherapy with a focus on concrete problem solving than from supportive counseling (Alexopoulos et al. 2011). This finding underlines the benefits of choosing cue-based interventions relevant to the specific challenges or problems that currently exist in the older client's life and that are identified and defined by the client. For example, physical or verbal role play can incorporate meaningful concrete or sensory reminders from the client's own life such as photographs, physical objects, and diaries. A similar strategy can be applied with in vivo exposure where specific potential trauma-related cues are incorporated.

This strategy can help the older client to identify and retrieve the requested information/knowledge from memory (Alexopoulos et al. 2011) and can be compared to standard exposure in trauma treatment. Home-delivered therapy, in whole or part, is another way of creating access to a variety of cues for both client and clinician to lean on to enhance recall in the therapeutic process (Kiosses et al. 2011). This strategy is especially relevant in cases of significant cognitive decline such as the early stages of Alzheimer's disease or other types of dementia (Kiosses et al. 2011).

When working with older clients, the clinician must also generally expect to be somewhat more active and well structured than when working with younger clients. Older clients often improve more slowly in therapy than younger adult clients (Gallagher-Thompson and Thompson 1996). This latency may be reflected in the relatively long time it appears to take for symptoms of psychological distress following old age bereavement to decline naturally without intervention (O'Connor 2010a).

Although the known age-related changes may give an indication of the special considerations that often must be taken when working with older clients, the extensive individual variability in older people poses an extra challenge in adaptations of validated treatments to the individual older client. In addition, cohort differences – differences between age-groups due to the sociocultural characteristics of their generation – are in play when different generations meet. Cohort/generational effects may create a fundamental and unseen gap in cultural norms between client and clinician that will require identification by the clinician so that therapeutic strategies and interventions are sensitive to the patient's attitudes and values. Cohort differences are considerable and are even believed to be as large as age-related differences in intellectual domains (James 2010).

20.5 Treating PTSD Symptoms in Older People

The efficacy of CBT with older people is well established (James 2010; Laidlaw et al. 2003; Laidlaw 2008), and lessons learned from this work may be useful in relation to psychological interventions with older people more generally. One aspect of cognitive therapy when applied to older people is the necessity of obtaining a detailed background history and a thorough cognitive and symptom assessment during the first sessions of the treatment. Substantial time and attention may be required to complete this task because older people have had relatively long and often complex lives and thus have long and complex life stories that may be difficult for both the therapist and the client to track and use meaningfully in the treatment. Furthermore, older people tend to "drift" in their conversation in directions that might not be relevant enough to the target or problem formulation of the therapy. This conversational drift may be the result of a combination of reduced executive functioning and complex life story (Laidlaw et al. 2003). Keeping track of both the primary target of the therapy and relevant information from the life history poses a special challenge when working with older clients. In addition, older generations may try to please the clinician by going along with his/her suggestions as might be

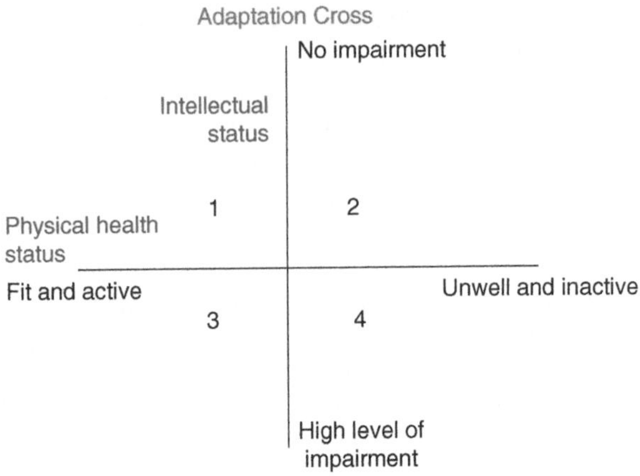

Fig. 20.1 Framework for clarifying patients' overall health status by James (2010)

Adaptation Cross

No impairment

Intellectual status

Physical health status

Fit and active | 1 | 2 | Unwell and inactive

                      3 | 4

High level of impairment

done in ordinary nontherapeutic conversation with consequence that the issues discussed are not the most relevant to the client.

James (2010) provides a framework to help clinicians identify useful age-related adaptations to treatment. The model organizes the client's overall health status along two dimensions, one with high versus low intellectual functioning and the other with high versus low physical health status (see Fig. 20.1).

For clients with high physical and high intellectual functioning (Fig. 20.1, quadrant 1), James suggests that any evidence-based intervention strategy that fits both client and clinician well generally can be applied successfully. For clients with high intellectual but low physical functioning (quadrant 2), the same applies but with a special obligation for the clinician to learn about the specific physical illness in question as this may affect which therapeutic strategies are the most relevant in the given situation. Information about these illnesses should be obtained from both the clients, their physicians, and from scientific sources, as needed. For clients with low intellectual but high physical functioning (quadrant 3), behavioral techniques combined with a cue-based approach are suggested. The same is recommended for clients with both low physical and low intellectual functioning (quadrant 4), but here home visits may be a helpful or even necessary next step (James 2010).

When planning and performing CBT with older people, James (2010) recommends spending the first few sessions thoroughly assessing and evaluating the clients' functional level with neuropsychological tests and life history information. This information, along with as much client involvement as possible, will contribute to the development of an engaging and effective treatment plan (James 2010). Client involvement and empowerment is especially important when working with older clients as this helps avoid falling into the trap of the client "drifting" into irrelevant subjects or staying on a topic to please the clinician (James 2010).

An interesting theory that may guide therapeutic work with older clients across mental disorders and therapeutic models is *the theory of selective optimization with compensation* (SOC) by Baltes and Baltes (1990). This framework aims to maintain a satisfying level of functioning in the areas most important to the individual when the limits of personal capacity are reached or exceeded. The SOC model guides older people with functional loss or other acquired disability to *select* the areas or functions that are most important to the individual because they relate to the individual identity, meaning-making, and experience of pleasure. Selection includes evaluation or reevaluation of personal goals both as a consequence to functional age-related loss and as a pro-action to deal with expected losses. *Optimization* is the effort to enhance the selected area and to compensate for unreachable wishes, on the intra-psychological level, for example, by reducing personal ambitions, and on the external level, for example, by simplifying the task as much as possible in a way that preserves the meaning of the selected area to the individual. *Compensation* involves the use of alternative means to reach the goal, for example, by taking counter steps to lessen or even prevent the potential loss (Baltes and Baltes 1990). One example of the SOC model applied can be seen with Alice, who was introduced at the beginning of this chapter.

Alice's daughter, Sue, dies about 2 months after the MBCT course ended. It is a hard blow for Alice, and although Sue rarely is out of her mind, Alice still keeps going and is able to find joy in life. Alice used to love traveling, usually with Sue, to Australia, the Caribbean, Greenland, and other exotic places. She sees herself as a bit of a "globe-trotter" and decides to keep traveling, but she chooses closer destinations that are easier to reach (an example of "selection"). Alice is aware that traveling alone is no longer an option for her, so she arranges to go with an old friend. They plan the trip carefully to reduce the risks of unexpected challenges as much as possible. Often the trips now go to places she can reach by bus, so the hassles and challenges of international airports are avoided (an example of "optimization"). Enjoying high-quality foreign food in well-regarded local restaurants used to be an essential part of these trips. However, finding good, local restaurants takes an effort, and independent traveling outside the arranged trips is becoming too stressful for Alice. Instead, she and her friend join the rest of the travelers for the arranged meals, and she decides to enjoy the company and getting to see a bit of the world, if not the food (an example of "compensation").

Using the SOC framework may be valuable in identifying goals for therapy for older clients and developing strategies for how to reach them.

20.5.1 Mindfulness-Based Cognitive Therapy

Mindfulness-based cognitive therapy (MBCT) and other systematic mindfulness training programs have been shown to reduce psychological distress such as depression and anxiety among both younger (Hofmann et al. 2010) and older adults (Smith et al. 2007; Splevins et al. 2009; Young and Baime 2010). MBCT is a group-based clinical intervention originally used for depressive relapse prevention that integrates elements of cognitive-behavioral therapy (Beck 1976) with systematic and extensive training in mindfulness meditations in class and as home exercises (Kabat-Zinn 2005). The aim of MBCT is to teach participants to become more aware of and relate differently to their thoughts, feelings, and bodily sensations (Segal et al. 2013). Through mindfulness exercises, the participants are taught to turn towards and accept intense emotional distress and bodily sensations in a nonjudgmental way. Specifically, the participants are taught to discover automatic reactions and thoughts as they arise, to detach their attention from the content of these reactions, and to regulate the attention back to experiences in the present moment, such as the breath or bodily sensations (Segal et al. 2013).

Our own clinical experience from MBCT-based group therapy with older people (mean age 77 years) with bereavement-related distress (O'Connor et al. 2014) is that adaptation of the physical setting of the therapy for the aging population can support the effectiveness of the intervention. For example, we provided the treatment at an optimal time (late enough for the participants to get there after breakfast, but not so late that the sessions would collide with afternoon napping), in a location with low background noise, a relatively small number of members (10–12 persons), and a short break during the session. The clinician spoke loudly and more slowly and provided clear information on the timeframe of the session and the homework. On the therapeutic level, we aimed to support intervention effectiveness by clear management of the psychological "classroom." For example, we actively created a culture where only one person spoke at a time, presented home exercises early in the session, and double-checked several times that everyone had understood the task. We also introduced more personally relevant cues than is traditionally the case in MBCT. For example, the therapist explored the experiences of a group member in greater detail than usual and explicitly related what was being said to similar events discussed in the participant's home exercise or to similar experiences presented by other group members. However, it is often a challenge to meet everyone's needs when instructing a group, as can be seen in the case in the textbox below.

> In the second session of this MBCT with women with chronic pain (mean age 58 years), the participants were presented with the cognitive ABC model of connections between triggers, thoughts, and feelings and subsequently worked with identifying triggers for both positive and negative emotional experiences and how mood may affect the experience of a situation (Segal et al. 2013). Karen aged 79 and Nora aged 75 really feel they learned something from these exercises and the class in general. Now, in week 6 of MBCT, the participants are asked to identify the first signs of relapse into depression or negative mood: the participants are asked to consider the types of events that may typically trigger negative moods for them, thoughts that run through their minds when there is a mood drop, and the emotions and bodily sensations that arise.

The participants are paired up to discuss these questions, and most of the younger participants start talking vigorously and writing on their worksheets. Karen and Nora just sit there looking at each other with their hands in their laps. The instructor comes over and asks if they have any questions. "We don't know what we are supposed to do" they say. The instructor explains: "Nora, remember last week when we had that meditation where we introduced a difficult experience and you told the class about that you noticed that sinking feeling in your stomach, and that you know that feeling very well from other bad times in your life?" "Yes" Nora says. "Well, today we are trying to identify and write down bodily sensations, feelings, and thoughts that we often have when we are feeling down, just like you often have a sinking feeling in your stomach at bad times. If we become good at noticing these signs of negative mood, it will make it easier for us to do something about it before the bad mood takes over in the future. This is what I would like you to do now." Nora nods, turns to Karen, and starts talking.

20.6   Advice to Clinicians Working with Older People with PTSD Symptoms

To date, no evidence-based protocol for treating PTSD symptoms in older people is available. However, the clinical literature indicates that minor adaptations of current protocols, mindful of the special needs of older adults, are likely to provide effective treatment. Clinicians must draw on their own clinical experience and evidence from treatment of PTSD symptoms in other adult populations. Part III of this volume outlines a number of evidence-based psychological treatments for trauma-related disorders that are likely to apply to older clients as well as they do for younger people. This gives room for the clinician to select a treatment method that fits with his or her experience and preferences and with the preferences and motivation of the client. Several observations and recommendations are provided below to guide the clinician in providing effective psychotherapy with older adults.

First, evidence-based psychotherapy protocols for depression in older people are available. Much can be gained from studying and incorporating knowledge from this work into the selected protocol or framework for treating adults for PTSD symptoms. Relevant suggestions on how to do this can be found in the work by James (2010) in advance of selecting the therapeutic strategies for the following course of treatment.

Second, a key aspect of therapy with older populations is empowerment of the client, an experience that is relevant and applicable across different evidence-based treatment protocols. The SOC model may support empowerment and help the clinician stay in tune with and focused on areas of functioning that are most important to the individual older client.

Third, supervision and training from clinicians with experience in working with older clients are strongly recommended for therapists who are not used to working with this population (James 2010). This may be particularly important in relation to handling the therapist's own impatience and irritation when working with older clients with especially pronounced tendency to progress and develop slowly in therapy.

Lastly, we will summarize strategies for responding to some of the special challenges of treating older clients, particularly individuals with PTSD symptoms. Certainly, there is an increasing frequency of intellectual disabilities beyond expected age-related changes resulting in dementia (Oliver et al. 2008), and many older people worry that the memory problems they are experiencing are signs of dementia. Since both expected age-related changes and PTSD symptoms often result in reduced memory function, this type of worry is based on actual experiences of memory problems, but may not be related to dementia. Intellectual functioning must be assessed before treatment begins, and if changes in cognitive functioning are detected during the course of treatment, assessment must be reapplied to identify their source. If there is a mild degree of dementia (e.g., Alzheimer's disease) present at the start of therapy, further cognitive decline can often be expected, and the treatment must be adapted accordingly during the course of treatment. New losses sometimes come thick and fast in old age, and it can be a challenge for the clinician and client to determine which issue is more important and should be dealt with first. Clinician and client will need to explicitly collaborate and agree on goals and process repeatedly throughout the course of treatment. The older client will present with somatic complaints, and it may be difficult to identify their source. Careful assessment of physical complaints, including review of health history and contact with health provider, is often necessary. This is particularly important because old people typically have several and constantly develop more somatic disorders that, if overlooked, can be detrimental for the client. Finally, the potential risk of cohort or generational effects between clients and clinicians should also be mentioned as a challenge. We have a tendency to be somewhat blind to our own cultural heritage, and it can be difficult to discover when cohort effects create a potentially destructive gap between client and clinician. Some of the assumptions clinicians make about aging may be cultural artifacts rather than true, age-related differences. Keeping a watch out for and an open mind to cohort effects is therefore important when doing psychotherapy with older people.

References

Alexopoulos, G. S., Raue, P. J., Kiosses, D. N., Mackin, R. S., Kanellopoulos, D., McCulloch, C., & Areán, P. A. (2011). Problem-solving therapy and supportive therapy in older adults with major depression and executive dysfunction. *Archives of General Psychiatry, 68*(1), 33–41.

American Psychiatric Association. (2013). *Diagnostic and statistical manual of mental disorders: DSM-5TM* (5th ed.). Arlington: American Psychiatric Publishing, Inc.

Aspnes, A. K., & Lynch, T. R. (2007). Individual and group psychotherapy. In *Essentials of geriatric psychiatry* (pp. 337–356). Arlington: American Psychiatric Publishing, Inc.

Averill, P. M., & Beck, J. G. (2000). Posttraumatic stress disorder in older adults: A conceptual review. *Journal of Anxiety Disorders, 14*, 133–156.

Baltes, P. B., & Baltes, M. M. (1990). Psychological perspectives on successful aging: The model of selective optimization with compensation. In *Successful aging: Perspectives from the behavioral sciences* (pp. 1–34). New York: Cambridge University Press.

Beck, A. T. (1976). *Cognitive therapy and the emotional disorders*. Oxford: International Universities Press.

Birren, J. E. (1996). *Encyclopedia of gerontology: Age, aging, and the aged* (Vol. 1 & 2). San Diego: Academic.

Breslau, N., Davis, E. C., Andreski, P. & Peterson, E. (1991). Traumatic events and posttraumatic stress disorder in an urban population of young adults *Archives of General Psychiatry, 48*(3), 216–222.

Bryant, R. A. (2014). Prolonged grief: Where to after diagnostic and statistical manual of mental disorders, 5th edition? *Current Opinion in Psychiatry, 27*(1), 21–26.

Carr, D. (2004). Gender, preloss marital dependence, and older adults' adjustment to widowhood. *Journal of Marriage and Family, 66*, 220–235.

Chung, M. C., Preveza, E., Papandreou, K., & Prevezas, N. (2006). Spinal cord injury, posttraumatic stress, and locus of control among the elderly: A comparison with young and middle-aged patients. *Psychiatry Interpersonal and Biological Processes, 69*(1), 69–80.

Coleman, P. G., & O'Hanlon, A. (2008). *Ageing and adaptation*. New York: Wiley.

Creamer, M., & Parslow, R. (2008). Trauma exposure and posttraumatic stress disorder in the elderly: A community prevalence study. *The American Journal of Geriatric Psychiatry, 16*(10), 853–856.

Davenhill, R. (2008). *Psychoanalysis and old age*. New York: Wiley.

Ditlevsen, D. N., & Elklit, A. (2010). The combined effect of gender and age on post traumatic stress disorder: Do men and women show differences in the lifespan distribution of the disorder? *Annals of General Psychiatry, 9*.

Elklit, A., & O'Connor, M. (2005). Post-traumatic stress disorder in a Danish population of elderly bereaved. *Scandinavian Journal of Psychology, 46*(5), 439–445.

Fromholt, P., Bruhn, P., & Bruhn, P. (1998). Cognitive dysfunction and dementia. In *Clinical geropsychology* (pp. 183–188). Washington: American Psychological Association.

Gadermann, A. M., Alonso, J., Vilagut, G., Zaslavsky, A. M., & Kessler, R. C. (2012). Comorbidity and disease burden in the national comorbidity survey replication (NCS-R). *Depression and Anxiety, 29*(9), 797–806.

Gallagher-Thompson, D., & Thompson, L. W. (1996). Applying cognitive-behavioral therapy to the psychological problems of later life. In *A guide to psychotherapy and aging: Effective clinical interventions in a life-stage context* (pp. 61–82). Washington: American Psychological Association.

Glaesmer, H., Kaiser, M., Bräehler, E., Freyberger, H., & Kuwert, P. (2012). Posttraumatic stress disorder and its comorbidity with depression and somatisation in the elderly—A German community-based study. *Aging & Mental Health, 16*(4), 403–412.

Hajjar, E. R., Cafiero, A. C., & Hanlon, J. T. (2007). Polypharmacy in elderly patients. *American Journal of Geriatric Pharmacotherapy, 5*(4), 345–351.

Hofmann, S. G., Sawyer, A. T., Witt, A. A., & Oh, D. (2010). The effect of mindfulness-based therapy on anxiety and depression: A meta-analytic review. *Journal of Consulting and Clinical Psychology, 78*(2), 169–183.

James, I. A. (2010a). *Cognitive behavioural therapy with older people. Interventions for those with and without dementia* (1st ed.). London: Jessica Kingsley Publishers.

Johansson, B. (2008). *Memory and cognition in ageing*. New York: Wiley.

Kabat-Zinn, J. (2005). *Full catastrophe living: Using the wisdom of your body and mind to face stress, pain, and illness* (15 anniversaryth ed.). New York: Delta Trade Paperback/Bantam Dell.

Kessler, R. C., & Wang, P. S. (2008). The descriptive epidemiology of commonly occurring mental disorders in the United States. *Annual Review of Public Health, 29*, 115–129.

Kessler, R. C., Petukhova, M., Sampson, N. A., Zaslavsky, A. M., & Wittchen, H. (2012). Twelve-month and lifetime prevalence and lifetime morbid risk of anxiety and mood disorders in the United States. *International Journal of Methods in Psychiatric Research, 21*(3), 169–184.

Kiosses, D. N., Teri, L., Velligan, D. I., & Alexopoulos, G. S. (2011). A home-delivered intervention for depressed, cognitively impaired, disabled elders. *International Journal of Geriatric Psychiatry, 26*(3), 256–262.

Kubzansky, L. D., Koenen, K. C., Spiro, A., III, Vokonas, P. S., & Sparrow, D. (2007). Perspective study of posttraumatic stress disorder symptoms and coronary heart disease in the normative aging study. *Archives of General Psychiatry, 64*(1), 109–116.

Kuwert, P., Braehler, E., Freyberger, H. J., & Glaesmer, H. (2012). More than 60 years later: The mediating role of trauma and posttraumatic stress disorder for the association of forced displacement in world war II with somatization in old age. *Journal of Nervous and Mental Disease, 200*(10), 911–914.

Laidlaw, K. (2008). *Cognitive behaviour therapy with older people*. New York: Wiley.

Laidlaw, K., Thompson, L. W., Dick-Siskin, L., & Gallagher-Thompson, D. (2003). *Cognitive behaviour therapy with older people*. New York: Wiley.

Lapp, L. K., Agbokou, C., & Ferreri, F. (2011). PTSD in the elderly: The interaction between trauma and aging. *International Psychogeriatrics, 23*(6), 858–868.

Lupien, S. J., Wan, N., Huppert, F. A., Baylis, N., & Keverne, B. (2005). Successful ageing: From cell to self. In *The science of well-being* (pp. 75–103). New York: Oxford University Press.

Maercker, A., Forstmeier, S., Enzler, A., Krüsi, G., Hörler, E., Maier, C., & Ehlert, U. (2008). Adjustment disorders, posttraumatic stress disorder, and depressive disorders in old age: Findings from a community survey. *Comprehensive Psychiatry, 49*(2), 113–120.

Maercker, A., Brewin, C. R., Bryant, R. A., Cloitre, M., Reed, G. M., van Ommeren, M., Humayun, A., Jones, L. M., Kagee, A., Llosa, A. E., Rousseau, C., Somasundaram, D. J., Souza, R., Suzuki, Y., Weissbecker, I., Wessely, S. C., First, M. B., & Saxena, S. (2013). Proposals for mental disorders specifically associated with stress in the international classification of diseases-11. *The Lancet, 381*(9878), 1683–1685.

Mehlsen, M. Y. (2005). Den paradoksale livstilfredshed i alderdommen. *Psyke and Logos, 26*(2), 609–628.

Morrison, V. (2008). *Ageing and physical health*. New York: Wiley.

Nordhus, I. H. (2008). *Manifestations of depression and anxiety in older adults*. New York: Wiley.

O'Connor, M. (2010a). "A longitudinal study of PTSD in the elderly bereaved: Prevalence and predictors": Erratum. *Aging & Mental Health, 14*(5), 3.

O'Connor, M. (2010b). PTSD in older bereaved people. *Aging & Mental Health, 14*(6), 670–678.

O'Connor, M., Piet, J., & Hougaard, E. (2014). The effects of mindfulness-based cognitive therapy on depressive symptoms in elderly bereaved people with loss-related distress: A controlled pilot study. *Mindfulness 5*, 400–409. http://dx.doi.org.ez.statsbiblioteket.dk:2048/10.1007/s12671-013-0194-x

Oliver, C., Adams, D., & Kalsy, S. (2008). *Ageing, dementia and people with intellectual disability*. New York: Wiley.

Roper-Hall, A. (2008). *Systemic interventions and older people*. New York: Wiley.

Ruskin, P. E., & Talbott, J. A. (1996). *Aging and posttraumatic stress disorder* (1st ed.). Washington: American Psychiatric Association.

Schaie, K. W. (1994). The course of adult intellectual development. *American Psychologist, 49*(4), 304–313.

Segal, Z. V., Williams, J. M. G., & Teasdale, J. D. (2013). *Mindfulness-based cognitive therapy for depression* (2nd ed.). New York: Guilford Press.

Shear, M. K., Simon, N., Wall, M., Zisook, S., Neimeyer, R., Duan, N., Reynolds, C., Lebowitz, B., Sung, S., Ghesquiere, A., Gorscak, B., Clayton, P., Ito, M., Nakajima, S., Konishi, T., Melhem, N., Meert, K., Schiff, M., O'Connor, M. F., First, M., Sareen, J., Bolton, J., Skritskaya, N., Mancini, A. D., & Keshaviah, A. (2011). Complicated grief and related bereavement issues for DSM-5. *Depression and Anxiety, 28*(2), 103–117.

Silverman, G. K., Jacobs, S. C., Kasl, S. V., Shear, M. K., Maciejewski, P. K., Noaghiul, F. S., & Prigerson, H. G. (2000). Quality of life impairments associated with diagnostic criteria for traumatic grief. *Psychological Medicine, 30*, 857–862.

Smith, A., Graham, L., & Senthinathan, S. (2007). Mindfulness-based cognitive therapy for recurring depression in older people: A qualitative study. *Aging & Mental Health, 11*(3), 346–357.

Spirduso, W. W., & MacRae, P. G. (1990). *Motor performance and aging.* San Diego: Academic Press.

Spitzer, C., Barnow, S., Völzke, H., John, U., Freyberger, H. J., & Grabe, H. J. (2008). Trauma and posttraumatic stress disorder in the elderly: Findings from a German community study. *Journal of Clinical Psychiatry, 69*(5), 693–700.

Splevins, K., Smith, A., & Simpson, J. (2009). Do improvements in emotional distress correlate with becoming more mindful? A study of older adults. *Aging & Mental Health, 13*(3), 328–335.

Stroebe, M., Schut, H., & van den Bout, J. (2013). *Complicated grief: Assessment of scientific knowledge and implications for research and practice* (pp. 295–311). New York: Routledge/ Taylor & Francis Group.

Van Zelst, W. H., De Beurs, E., Beekman, A. T. F., Van Dyck, R., & Deeg, D. D. H. (2006). Well-being, physical functioning, and use of health services in the elderly with PTSD and subthreshold PTSD. *International Journal of Geriatric Psychiatry, 21*(2), 180–188.

Yaffe, K., Vittinghoff, E., Lindquist, K., Barnes, D., Covinsky, K. E., Neylan, T., Kluse, M., & Marmar, C. (2010). Posttraumatic stress disorder and risk of dementia among US veterans. *Archives of General Psychiatry, 67*(6), 608–613.

Yang, Y. K., Yeh, T. L., Chen, C. C., Lee, C. K., Lee, I. H., Lee, L., & Jeffries, K. J. (2003). Psychiatric morbidity and posttraumatic symptoms among earthquake victims in primary care clinics. *General Hospital Psychiatry, 25*(4), 253–261.

Young, L. A., & Baime, M. J. (2010). Mindfulness-based stress reduction: Effect on emotional distress in older adults. *Complementary Health Practice Review, 15*(2), 59–64.

Selected References

Baltes, P. B., & Baltes, M. M. (1990). Psychological perspectives on successful aging: The model of selective optimization with compensation. In *Successful aging: Perspectives from the behavioral sciences.* New York: Cambridge University Press.

James, I. A. (2010). *Cognitive behavioural therapy with older people. Intervnentions for those with and without dementia* (1st ed.). London: Jessica Kingsley Publishers.

Woods, B., & Clare, L. (2008). *Psychological interventions with people with dementia.* New York: Wiley.

Treatment of Traumatized Refugees and Immigrants

21

Thomas Maier

21.1 Introduction

Since humankind's expulsion from paradise, murder, violence, and warfare have always been our haunting companions. The dark sides of our character seem to follow us across history and generate evil in different forms: rivalry, hatred, envy, rage, anger, and violence. Even the great humanistic projects of civilization such as religion, democracy, and universal human rights apparently cannot effectively and permanently repress these manifestations of our inner demons (Modvig and Jaranson 2004). When we look at certain regions of the world today, it even seems doubtful that humankind has made any progress at all since our earliest history. What has definitely changed, however, is the perception and acknowledgment of the damage that human aggression causes. Indeed, interpersonal violence, especially in its most cruel form of physical violence, has severe psychological consequences for the victims and detrimental effects at various levels: not only individuals but also the victim's social environment and the society as a whole are affected. Even for the perpetrators, committed violence is often eventually destructive. A study of the effects of human aggression, on the other hand, makes obvious the fact that most humans are equally capable of immense compassion and have the strong wish to repair and restore what evil destroys (Volkan 2004).

Migration – the intentional but often not voluntary dislocation of people from one place to another – is equally a constant in the history of humankind (Silove 2004). Since the earliest times, people have permanently moved and migrated in search of a better life. The motives for emigration are as diverse as people themselves; however, escape from poverty, starvation, war, and persecution have always

T. Maier
Psychiatric Services of St. Gallen North,
Zurcherstrasse 30, CH-9501 Wil St. Gallen, Switzerland
e-mail: thomas.maier@gd-kpdw.sg.ch

U. Schnyder, M. Cloitre (eds.), *Evidence Based Treatments for Trauma-Related Psychological Disorders: A Practical Guide for Clinicians*,
DOI 10.1007/978-3-319-07109-1_21

been important reasons for relinquishing a home and homeland. At this very moment, several million people are in flight, and many more millions already live in exile. The UN estimates that some 3 % of the world's population – i.e., more than 200 million people – are international migrants (United Nations 2011). Several more millions are so-called internally displaced persons, people who migrate within the borders of their home countries. Many of them are refugees in the truest sense of the word, but the term "refugee" as defined by the UN refugee convention of 1951 does not apply to people migrating within their home country. Some of those who emigrate find a new and fruitful home in their hosting country, but many are less lucky and live in despair and marginalization. Hundreds of thousands of poor and desperate exiles constantly try to find a way into the promised land, i.e., the wealthy countries of the northern hemisphere. As a consequence, these countries tighten their immigration legislation and try to discourage people from immigration. Only well-educated and healthy individuals are welcome while moneyless and stranded exiles are kept out of the boat.

Global economic disparities and human rights violations in the forms of extreme poverty, famine, displacement, persecution, unlawful confinement, torture, and war produce an immense amount of suffering on the individual and collective levels (Modvig and Jaranson 2004). Health professionals all over the world are confronted with the individual consequences of these atrocities and are called in by survivors to treat them. Patients labeled with terms such as *traumatized asylum seekers*, *illegal* or *undocumented immigrants*, *refugees*, or *victims of war and torture* appear in the healthcare systems of Western countries and confront local health systems with challenging needs (Drožđek and Wilson 2004).

Case Report

The following case report aims to give the reader an illustration of the concepts presented later in this chapter. It is written in the therapist's first-person perspective, a form that may appear unusual in a scientific publication. However, the eminent influence of the therapist's authentic personality on the therapeutic process is conveyed more accurately that way. When treating traumatized immigrants, authenticity, personal commitment, and appreciation are crucial, so the author requests that this uncommon form be allowed by the reader.

Ceylan was a 32-year-old married woman from Syria and was referred to our outpatient clinic by her GP. She lived with her husband and two daughters (2 and 6 years old) in a rural Swiss village, where the family was accommodated by the immigration authorities. Ceylan had arrived in Switzerland 2 years earlier, and the family was still waiting for its case to be decided by the immigration authorities. Her husband Awar had escaped from the Kurdish areas of Syria some 2 years earlier, leaving his wife and two daughters with her parents in their remote home, a small village near the Turkish border. Awar later helped to organize the journey for his wife and daughters from

Syria to Switzerland, a dangerous and confusing experience for Ceylan in the hands of facilitators.

At the time of referral, Ceylan could speak only a few words in German, and in the referring letter, the GP erroneously stated that her mother tongue was Arabic. In fact, she had learned only a little Arabic in school, and her mother tongue was instead a Kurdish dialect. The first appointment with her was therefore somewhat disappointing because the Arabic interpreter we had retained was not much help. Direct communication with her was hardly possible, and only the husband, who had learned a little more German in the meantime, could give me some information about her problem. As the GP had already mentioned in his referring letter, Ceylan was perceived as constantly sad, exhausted, uncommunicative, absentminded, forgetful, and confused. With her agreement – which was, in spite of the nebulous situation, very clearly given – I arranged a second appointment with a female Kurdish interpreter. The presence of the husband at the second appointment was a matter of course to both of them (as it seemed to me).

In the second appointment – which was later followed by many more – I explored some parts of the family's story. Both Awar and Ceylan came from the same Kurdish village in Syria near the Turkish border. Their families had been – like many others – settled there for generations and spread across the border between the two countries. They lived a spare and rural life in the mountainous Kurdish area, cultivating their own land and raising some cattle and sheep. Awar and Ceylan were relatives and had known each other since they were children; however, the two of them had freely made the decision to marry, which they related with pride. Like most of the villagers, Awar was a supporter of the Kurdish party, which was antagonized by the Syrian police and army. Most probably, he was an active member of the party, which is intimately allied to the militant PKK at the Turkish side of the border and works mainly covertly. He was arrested several times by the police and experienced beatings and ill treatment by state officials. To escape from further imminent detentions and even more violent treatment, he decided to immigrate to Switzerland, where some distant relatives already lived. For certain reasons, he was advised by friends to conceal his real identity when entering Switzerland and to register under a false name. This decision was a momentous mistake, as he realized later, because authorities refused at first to reunite him with his wife and children when they made it into Switzerland 2 years later. Only after the disclosure of his real identity was the family allowed to live together in an apartment assigned to them. This initial name deception, however, made Awar particularly suspicious to the immigration authorities and prolonged the procedure for granting the right for asylum. It was eventually decided only 4 years after his arrival in Switzerland, and Awar was not recognized as a refugee in legal terms.

Awar reported his wife to have started being altered in her mood and behavior only several months after her immigration. At first, he said, she was glad: happy to see her husband and joyful with her daughters. Only as time passed did she become increasingly peculiar, neglecting her housework, being erratic with her children and irritable, ill humored, sad, and weepy. She could (or would) not explain the reasons for her behavior to her husband, but obviously she suffered from it and was looking for help. Ceylan was a somewhat obese, pale woman, neatly dressed in Western style, rather shy, but not completely incommunicative. Initially, she merely answered questions I felt it was appropriate to ask and did not talk much spontaneously. But then, she gradually opened up, and it seemed to me that she started to like the kind of conversation we continued to have. From the very start of this therapy, I had different ideas about what could have happened to her and what could have been her experiences. However, I did not at all urge her to talk about specific issues but left it completely up to her to choose the subjects of the sessions. I felt unsure about what was psychologically and culturally appropriate for her to talk about and also realized that the situation – a male Swiss doctor and a Kurdish peasant woman sitting together in a room and having a conversation for 50 min – must be completely unfamiliar to her. Fortunately, our female interpreter was present, too, and helped to ease the situation.

During the first year of therapy in which I had appointments with her every 2 weeks, Ceylan mostly spoke about her feelings of insufficiency as a mother. Especially with her elder, now 7-year-old daughter, she had a lot of difficulties, because the girl (who was severely traumatized, as I guessed immediately and could confirm only much later from the story Ceylan told me) did not obey her and had severe learning problems in school. Ceylan felt responsible for her daughter's problems and asked me for advice. Together with the GP and a local social worker, I organized for her daughter to receive support from a child psychologist and for both of her children to visit with a neighboring Swiss family for lunch 3 days a week. She accepted these arrangements because they unburdened her somewhat and she realized that her children cheered up subsequently. Nevertheless, Ceylan's condition fluctuated considerably during the first year of treatment. Sometimes she was very depressed and desperate, and sometimes she seemed more self-confident and vigorous. Her husband was deeply worried about his wife's condition and supported her therapy. After several months of treatment, he agreed to have only the female interpreter and the therapist in the session with Ceylan while he remained in the waiting room. Often, Ceylan proposed that he (and sometimes also the two daughters) join us for the last 5 or 10 min of the session. Only much later, Ceylan revealed to me that she was always a little distressed by this setting as her husband used to question her after the sessions about the things we discussed.

Some 6 months after the beginning of our therapy, the family's claim for asylum was initially rejected. Not surprisingly, this decision caused a major relapse in Ceylan's condition. It took one more year to await the appeal court's decision, which assigned the family a temporary visa because of Ceylan's impaired mental health. The court argued that, given her current impaired health condition, it would not be reasonable to send Ceylan back to her home country where no proper medical treatment was available. The court decision was mainly based on the description of Ceylan's health condition that I had communicated to the authorities in an expert report. So in Ceylan's view, I had saved the family by writing the "right" letter, but in fact, it was Ceylan who unintentionally saved her family from expulsion through her illness. Fortunately, she did not fully realize the paradoxical implication of the authority's decision, but I realized at once the imminent dead end of this situation: the very moment that I declared Ceylan to be cured, the immigration authority would send the whole family back to their home country.

The granting of a regular, although only temporary, visa to the family had a remarkable effect on them: Awar was now entitled to work legally and to have his driver's license, and Ceylan felt visibly relieved. After a short time, Awar found a job as a handyman in a nearby spa resort, and Ceylan now had to function much more on her own as a housewife. Even after 2 years of treatment, she still felt unable to travel alone the 50 km from her home to my office. She would have to take a bus, then to change to a train, and finally to walk five blocks. She felt uneasy traveling on her own for several reasons; however, I knew one particular reason for her reluctance: Ceylan was illiterate. Only when her daughters went to school in Switzerland did she pick up the Roman alphabet and slowly learn to read and write in German. Because her husband now had to work when she had appointments with me, she simply had to jump into the cold water, as it were, and come to my office on her own. Initially, this necessity troubled her a lot, but then she visibly took some pride in her new daring. She also had learned to ride a bicycle in the meantime (something she never had the chance to practice in her home country), joined the local women's gymnastic club, and even attended the (mixed!) swimming lessons we organized in our treatment center. Around that time, she came to the appointment one day and proposed to me to continue the sessions without the interpreter. Indeed, she had learned to speak German fairly well now and communication was possible in a sufficient manner. Not astonishingly, the conversation changed in many ways after that. The subjects became much more personal, and she addressed different topics we had never discussed before: Ceylan wanted to talk about life in Switzerland, asking me about local traditions, family values, and religious practices, and even wanted to learn about delicate issues like contraception, dating and sex in adolescence, and marriage customs. I felt that by talking about all of these issues, she was in fact exploring *me*, and I prepared for something more to come.

Finally, after more than 3 years of continuous therapy, she started to tell me about traumatic and haunting experiences she had had in her home country before she left. After her husband had escaped to Switzerland, Ceylan lived with her small children (then a newborn baby and a 4-year-old daughter) with her parents in their farmhouse. One day, when her parents were away for work in the fields, three unknown men – civil officials of the military police – arrived suddenly at her door. They immediately entered the house and rudely asked for her husband. She said that he was abroad and that she had not seen him for some time. The policemen laughed at her and started beating and groping her. While both of her children were in the room, they forced her to undress, and they raped her brutally. They left her humiliated and injured but not without threatening her and her family with further troubles in case the family did not comply with the police. Ceylan was deeply frightened and scared not only by the horror she had just experienced but also by the imminent danger she was in now. If her father or husband were to find out what had happened to her, she would probably be outlawed and expelled by her own family. Ceylan confided in her mother and told her everything. Together, they managed to conceal the crime from the rest of the family. Ceylan was sick for several weeks; she had suffered from gynecological injuries and had to be treated at home. Fortunately, she recovered passably and could endure the adventurous escape together with her two children to Switzerland.

When Ceylan started to talk about these traumatizing experiences, she seemed to be determined that she wanted to tell it all. I did not have to persuade or urge her to do so. I was the witness, and she was the actor. When she was recalling her trauma over the next three sessions, she experienced deep pain, shame, and disgust and suffered from flashbacks and intensified nightmares between the sessions. However, it was doable, and she regained self-control and felt relief by the end. We could subsequently address some related issues such as sexual problems she had with her husband and her general anxiety towards male officials. She still did not want to tell her husband about her trauma. In my opinion, he already knew everything but did not want to embarrass her, and so they both remained silent about her secret.

Based on an amendment to the immigration law, the family could apply for a permanent visa after they had lived in the country for 5 years and were independent from welfare for more than 1 year. Proudly, Ceylan presented me a folder full of testimonials and letters of support written by dozens of neighbors, supporters, and friends from her new home village. This was a remarkable achievement because the village where they used to live was known as a rather conservative and close-minded area. Awar had gained a good reputation as a hardworking man, and Ceylan was well known among the women in the village because she had joined the local gymnastic club. After almost 5 years of treatment, Ceylan's family was given a permanent resident status. Her mental health condition was almost completely normalized. I ended our therapy and continued to see her once or twice a year for a follow-up.

21.2 Clinical Challenges

In the case vignette above, different specific problems linked to the treatment of traumatized immigrants are presented. Therapists must identify and address these problems to effectively improve the victim's condition.

21.2.1 Severity of Trauma, Shattered Assumptions, Loss of Self-Sameness

The severity of traumatic experiences in victims of war and torture often surpasses the levels of trauma that clinicians are used to treating in civil resident patients. The duration of traumatizing conditions, the number of traumatic events, the cruelty of the experienced trauma, the unsettling character of interpersonal violence, and the magnitude of loss are often extraordinary. In consequence, these patients not only suffer from "regular, classical" posttraumatic stress symptoms but also from a deep and fundamental blow to what could be called self-sameness or identity as a person (Bettelheim 1943; Mollica et al. 2001; Silove 1999; Wilson 2004). Severe depression, identity confusion, loss of meaning, and deep feelings of shame are challenges for clinicians working with traumatized refugees. In the WHO's ICD-10, the diagnosis of *enduring personality change after catastrophic experience* as well as the proposed ICD-11 Complex PTSD covers some of this severe and often persistent psychopathology (Chap. 6). However, the DSM classification does not endorse this diagnosis, and indeed, it is questionable that these posttraumatic features are correctly classified as personality change (Beltran and Silove 1999). For clinicians, it is important to realize that severely traumatized patients:

- Do not suffer only from intrusive memories and associated symptoms (i.e., hyperarousal, avoidance, dissociation). Although these "classical" features of posttraumatic stress disorder are often amenable to specific – and definitely successful – trauma-focused treatment (Başoğlu 1998; Lustig et al. 2004; Neuner et al. 2008; Nicholl and Thompson 2004; Schauer et al. 2005; van Dijk et al. 2003; Varvin 1998); some patients nevertheless continue experiencing suffering and despair. Many severely traumatized immigrants remain deeply depressed about their losses and cannot find a way to cope with helpless anger or recover from paralyzing shame.
- Have experienced a fundamental shattering of their assumptions about the trustworthiness of the world (Janoff-Bulmann 1992). Ordinary human life in the community with other people has lost meaning, and basic social values such as trust, respect, and compassion are mere words to these patients. Many have abandoned their faith in fairness and ethical values, and in consequence, some even abstain from any kind of religious practice. This feature is particularly dramatic for people who formerly had a deeply fundamental religiosity. Matters of faith are rarely addressed in psychotherapy; however, in the treatment of traumatized immigrants, the dimensions of faith, religion, and spirituality need to be explored

(cf. US Department of Veterans Affairs' guidelines for PTSD, p. 25). In some cases, advice from religious leaders may be helpful for therapists.

- Are deeply isolated in the world because they cannot share their experiences with anybody. Even if they live together with family members, they feel fundamentally alienated. "Whoever has succumbed to torture can no longer feel at home in the world" (Améry 1980).

21.2.2 Physical Disabilities and Complaints

Together with their psychological traumatization, most of these patients experienced significant physical injuries, too. Usually, physical injuries are healed in time; however, chronic pain or other residual consequences of earlier injuries often haunt patients and are intimately linked with altered psychological conditions (Amris and Prip 2000a; Otis et al. 2003; Thomsen et al. 1997). Physical complaints and symptoms often function as triggers for intrusions, and sometimes they *are* bodily flashbacks of traumatizing experiences (Salomons et al. 2004). When treating victims of war and torture, support from an experienced physician is very helpful. In an ideal treatment setting, the psychotherapist and physician collaborate closely, and the patient knows that these two health experts are coordinating their efforts. Often, a physiotherapist also can contribute to a favorable outcome (Amris and Prip 2000b). However, physiotherapists must be informed about the exact trauma history of a patient because they work directly with the body of a patient and must understand specific vulnerabilities in tortured patients. Intrusions and flashbacks can be provoked by physical contact or even when taking certain positions or performing certain motor actions (De Winter and Drožđek 2004). However, working with the body can be a clue to recovery for torture survivors (Karcher 2004). Experienced physiotherapists or body therapists are therefore welcome in the efforts to rehabilitate victims of war and torture.

Although survivors of torture prove to be physically strong and tough having survived unthinkable maltreatment, they often feel particularly sensitive and damageable in the posttraumatic situation. Many patients have irrational fears about supposed physical illnesses, sometimes to the level of hypochondriasis. Survivors of torture are focused on the body in a highly ambivalent manner: the body was the gateway for the torturers to break their minds; it was the weak link, the source of pain and suffering. At the same time, the body was their means of survival, the inseparable companion carrying them through danger and despair. So victims of torture feel shame and disgust about their body simultaneously with feelings of pride and gratitude. Psychotherapy should aim at a reconciliation of these ambivalent feelings and contribute to an acceptance of one's own body (Karcher 2004).

21.2.3 Insecure Residency Permit Status

Unfortunately, in traumatized immigrants, legal problems about residence often interfere with therapeutic interventions. Many traumatized immigrants live in chronic insecurity as asylum seekers awaiting their cases to be decided or even as undocumented immigrants. Some hosting countries barrack asylum seekers in run-down buildings, others put them in confinement, and still others virtually relinquish them to a social no man's land (Silove et al. 2001). Undocumented immigrants, the poorest of the poor, are in fact the invisible legions of victims traveling incognito through our orderly societies. They are helplessly at the mercy of slave traders, panderers, indifferent officials, and other doubtful characters. Only a few of them will ever appear in our services, and only a few of them will ever tell us their stories. Also, asylum seekers – who have a regular legal status – frequently remain with only minimal social, legal, and medical support. In many countries, only accepted refugees have access to professional treatment, although the need for treatment would be much more exigent in the earlier stages of immigration. The general stress of life for asylum seekers or even more for undocumented residents already affects the mental health condition of these individuals to a degree that is comparable to other extremely stressful life events (Hauff and Vaglum 1994; Heeren et al. 2012; Laban et al. 2004; Steel et al. 2002, 2004). For therapists, it is important to realize that legal problems of residence are paramount for most asylum seekers. Even those who have successfully endured long periods of insecurity as applicants for asylum and end up as recognized refugees often remain obsessed with fears of sudden expulsion, withdrawal of documents, nightly detention, and similar official orders. The very basic precondition of any trauma-specific treatment – safety – is not provided to many traumatized migrants. Even refugees often do not feel secure enough to engage in psychotherapy. This hesitancy sets limits on the possibilities of psychological treatment, and health professionals must first of all support their patients in the regulation of their legal situation. There is an undeniable responsibility for authorities, officials, and political leaders who are defining the legal frameworks of immigration policies.

21.2.4 Cultural and Social Uprooting

Immigrants who suffer from posttraumatic stress symptoms are often culturally and socially uprooted. Many lack social support and are distant from their families, their cultural background, and their traditional means of coping. This isolation is particularly distressing for traumatized individuals because the process of coping with extremely stressful experiences is always embedded in a cultural perspective (Aroche and Coello 2004; Charuvastra and Cloitre 2008). Ethnocultural beliefs, religious practices, and social behaviors are intimately linked to the process of how individuals integrate traumatic experiences into their lives and how they recover to a higher level of functioning. When treating victims of war and torture, clinicians must try to enter into the cultural and historical reality of their patients and evaluate the collectivistic dimension of individual traumata (Eisenbruch et al. 2004). In recent research, the social ecology of posttraumatic symptoms has been increasingly highlighted. Not only do PTSD symptoms lead to relational difficulties in the family and society, but the reverse is also true: Lack of social support leads to more severe PTSD symptoms. Factors like family acceptance, stigma, education, economic perspective, prosecution of perpetrators, and political development are intimately related to the course of posttraumatic stress symptoms. Despite the importance of societal and collective factors, however, most evidence-based treatment modalities for trauma victims focus on the individual.

> From a cross-cultural perspective, the social and relational aspects of trauma also can be more distressing than individual symptoms of PTSD. There is often a connection between social distress and post-traumatic psychosomatic complaints that resolve through community processes rather than solely through individual treatment (Kohrt 2013).

Therapists treating traumatized immigrants should always carefully explore the patient's social environment. Also, some knowledge about the patient's cultural background is very helpful for evaluating the context of the therapy. Even if a patient is reluctant to involve family members or friends in treatment, the significance of others for the patient's recovery has to be clarified before initiating therapy. If a patient feels like an outcast from his community or disregarded by the family patriarch because of his posttraumatic stress symptoms, the patient will not even be able to enter into therapy. In some cases, the involvement of cultural brokers facilitating the dialogue between patient and health professionals can be useful.

In addition to that, the language barrier is often a particularly complex issue in the treatment of traumatized refugees. The use of professional interpreters is highly recommended in various medical settings in order to assure sufficient communication and to achieve good treatment adherence (Karliner et al. 2007). However, the presence of a third person – the interpreter – is an irritating factor for both therapist and patient, especially when it comes to the recounting of traumatic experiences. Not only that the interpreter could be a member of the patient's local community, but also age/gender discordance, cultural, religious, ethnical, tribal or character differences may significantly interfere with the development of a therapeutic alliance. Therefore it is important for clinicians to collaborate with trained interpreters only and to establish a professional relationship with the interpreter (Crosby 2013). There are professional and ethical standards for medical interpreters (e.g., International Medical Interpreters Association 2014) as well as particular recommendations for the use of interpreters in psychotherapies with traumatized refugees (e.g., Tribe and Raval 2002; Miller et al. 2005).

21.2.5 Survivor's Guilt, Perpetrator's Guilt, Moral Injury

Traumatized immigrants have to cope not only with feelings of fear, helplessness, and horror but also with shame, guilt, hatred, and anger. This mixture of different emotions is sometimes hard to disentangle and unsettles patients and therapists, as well. Survivors of war and torture often believe they survived only because they could hide behind others who died. To survive is indeed sometimes the result of mere chance, and sometimes it is the result of the survivor's alert action. To survive in situations where reliable rules and moral values are annulled inevitably carries ethical dilemmas. The individual is challenged with the how to remain fair and honest in situations where the will to survive becomes a mere biological drive. Especially in contexts of war and torture, some experiences inevitably transgress deeply held moral beliefs. Transgressions that lead to serious inner conflict because the experience is at odds with core ethical and moral beliefs is called *moral injury* (Litz et al. 2009; Nickerson et al. 2014). From the comfortable armchair of the doctor's office, it is easy to moralize and to argue about right or wrong. Nevertheless, survivors of war and torture often rigorously apply moral reasoning to their acts and omissions, aggrieving themselves with reproaches and accusations. Feelings of guilt and persistence in self-reproach or even self-harm are, of course, symptoms of major depression; however, they also can be understood as reenactment of torture. In fact, torturers purposefully entangle their victims in moral dilemmas and inflict on them feelings of guilt (Modvig and Jaranson 2004). For therapists, the treatment of victims of war and torture always holds the potential for confusion, anguish, and pain, as in countertransference, the patient's horrors are reexperienced. In fact, patients' experiences can also involve acts of cruelty or even crime. Some severely traumatized patients desperately seeking help are, in fact, perpetrators at the same time. It is rare, however, that patients expose themselves as perpetrators and want to focus their therapies on committed acts of violence. The example of child soldiers or war veterans show, though, that even committed violence is potentially traumatizing and has detrimental effects on perpetrators, too. The crucial problem in these therapies is often the handling of actual guilt and moral injury, which is obviously not a psychotherapeutic issue. The therapist must wrestle with what to advise to a patient who believes he is guilty, probably not only morally but also legally. From a therapeutic perspective, the involvement of societal, religious, or legal authorities can pave the way to eventual recovery. When working in this field, clinicians must be prepared to enter into the most complex realities of patients, where truth, certainty, and clarity are not easy to recognize. They must find a way to address issues of morality, guilt, responsibility, and compensation without falling into a moralizing or condemning attitude.

21.2.6 Summary and Recommendations

The treatment of traumatized refugees and immigrants poses major challenges to healthcare professionals. Given the high and increasing number of affected individuals, healthcare providers should step up their efforts in providing effective treatments to these patients. As several studies have demonstrated recently, also in refugees and immigrants, trauma-focused psychotherapies are applicable and effective (e.g., Adenauer et al. 2011; Hinton et al. 2005; Neuner et al. 2004, 2008; Paunovic and Ost 2001). Owing to legal and language barriers, however, many affected individuals have no access to adequate treatment and remain untreated. Treatment should be made accessible to all individuals in need regardless of their legal status, their ethnical and cultural background, and their financial potency. The use of professional interpreters in mental health service provision should become part of the standard procedure.

References

Adenauer, H., Catani, C., Gola, H., Keil, J., Ruf, M., Schauer, M., & Neuner, F. (2011). Narrative exposure therapy for PTSD increases top-down processing of aversive stimuli – Evidence from a randomized controlled treatment trial. *BMC Neuroscience, 12*, 127. doi:10.1186/1471-2202-12-127.

Améry, J. (1980). *At the mind's limits: Contemplations by a survivor of Auschwitz and its realities* (trans: S. Rosenfeld & S.P., Rosenfeld). Bloomington: Indiana University Press.

Amris, K., & Prip, K. (2000a). Physiotherapy for torture victims (I): Chronic pain in torture victims: possible mechanisms for the pain. *Torture, 10*(3), 73–76.

Amris, K., & Prip, K. (2000b). Physiotherapy for torture victims (II): Treatment of chronic pain. *Torture, 10*(4), 112–116.

Aroche, J., & Coello, M. J. (2004). Ethnocultural considerations in the treatment of refugees and asylum seekers. In J. P. Wilson & B. Drožđek (Eds.), *Broken spirits. The treatment of traumatized asylum seekers, refugees, war and torture victims*. New York/Hove: Brunner-Routledge.

Başoğlu, M. (1998). Behavioral and cognitive treatment of survivors of torture. In J. M. Jaranson & M. K. Popkin (Eds.), *Caring for victims of torture*. Washington, DC: American Psychiatric Press.

Beltran, R. O., & Silove, D. (1999). Expert opinions about the ICD-10 category of enduring personality change after catastrophic experience. *Comprehensive Psychiatry, 40*(5), 396–403.

Bettelheim, B. (1943). Individual and mass behavior in extreme situations. *Journal of Abnormal and Social Psychology, 38*, 417–452.

Charuvastra, A., & Cloitre, M. (2008). Social bonds and posttraumatic stress disorder. *Annual Review of Psychology, 59*, 301–328.

Crosby, S. S. (2013). Primary care management of non–English-speaking refugees who have experienced trauma. A clinical review. *JAMA, 310*(5), 519–528.

De Winter, B., & Drožđek, B. (2004). Psychomotor therapy: Healing by action. In J. P. Wilson & B. Drožđek (Eds.), *Broken spirits. The treatment of traumatized asylum seekers, refugees, war and torture victims*. New York/Hove: Brunner-Routledge.

Drožđek, B., & Wilson, J. P. (2004). Uncovering: Trauma-focused treatment techniques with asylum seekers. In J. P. Wilson & B. Drožđek (Eds.), *Broken spirits. The treatment of traumatized asylum seekers, refugees, war and torture victims*. New York/Hove: Brunner-Routledge.

Eisenbruch, M., de Jong, J. T., & van de Put, W. (2004). Bringing order out of chaos: A culturally competent approach to managing the problems of refugees and victims of organized violence. *Journal of Traumatic Stress, 17*(2), 123–131.

Hauff, E., & Vaglum, P. (1994). Chronic posttraumatic stress disorder in Vietnamese refugees. A prospective community study of prevalence, course, psychopathology, and stressors. *Journal of Nervous and Mental Disease, 182*(2), 85–90.

Heeren, M., Mueller, J., Ehlert, U., Schnyder, U., Copiery, N., & Maier, T. (2012). Mental health of asylum seekers in the first two years of asylum: A cross-sectional study of psychiatric disorders. *BMC Psychiatry, 12*, 114.

Hinton, D. E., Chhean, D., Pich, V., Safren, S. A., Hofmann, S. G., & Pollack, M. H. (2005). A randomized controlled trial of cognitive-behavior therapy for Cambodian refugees with treatment-resistant PTSD and panic attacks: A cross-over design. *Journal of Traumatic Stress, 18*(6), 617–629.

International Medical Interpreters Association. http://www.imiaweb.org/default.asp. Accessed 22 Mar 2014.

Janoff-Bulman, R. (1992). *Shattered assumptions: Towards a new psychology of trauma.* New York: Free Press.

Karcher, S. (2004). Body psychotherapy with survivors of torture. In J. P. Wilson & B. Drožđek (Eds.), *Broken spirits. The treatment of traumatized asylum seekers, refugees, war and torture victims.* New York/Hove: Brunner-Routledge.

Karliner, L. S., Jacobs, E. A., Chen, A. H., & Mutha, S. (2007). Do professional interpreters improve clinical care for patients with limited English proficiency? A systematic review of the literature. *Health Services Research, 42*(2), 727–754.

Kohrt, B. (2013). Social ecology interventions for post-traumatic stress disorder: What can we learn from child soldiers? *British Journal of Psychiatry, 203*, 165–167.

Laban, C. J., Gernaat, H. B., Komproe, I. H., Schreuders, B. A., & De Jong, J. T. (2004). Impact of long asylum procedure on the prevalence of psychiatric disorders in Iraqi asylum seekers in The Netherlands. *Journal of Nervous and Mental Disease, 192*(12), 843–851.

Litz, B. T., Stein, N., Delaney, E., Lebowitz, L., Nash, W. P., Silva, C., & Maguen, S. (2009). Moral injury and moral repair in war veterans: A preliminary model and intervention strategy. *Clinical Psychology Review, 29*(8), 695–706.

Lustig, S. L., Weine, S. M., Saxe, G. N., & Beardslee, W. R. (2004). Testimonial psychotherapy for adolescent refugees: A case series. *Transcultural Psychiatry, 41*(1), 31–45.

Miller, K. E., Martell, Z. L., Patzdirek, L., Caruth, M., & Lopez, D. (2005). The role of interpreters in psychotherapy with refugees. An exploratory study. *American Journal of Orthopsychiatry, 75*(1), 27–39.

Modvig, J., & Jaranson, J. M. (2004). A global perspective of torture, political violence and health. In J. P. Wilson & B. Drožđek (Eds.), *Broken spirits. The treatment of traumatized asylum seekers, refugees, war and torture victims.* New York/Hove: Brunner-Routledge.

Mollica, R. F., Sarajlic, N., Chernoff, C., Lavelle, J., Vukovic, I. S., & Massagli, M. P. (2001). Longitudinal study of psychiatric symptoms, disability, mortality and emigration among Bosnian refugees. *JAMA, 286*, 546–554.

Neuner, F., Schauer, M., Klaschik, C., et al. (2004). A comparison of narrative exposure therapy, supportive counseling, and psychoeducation for treating posttraumatic stress disorder in an African refugee settlement. *Journal of Consulting and Clinical Psychology, 72*, 579–587.

Neuner, F., Onyut, P. L., Ertl, V., Odenwald, M., Schauer, E., & Elbert, T. (2008). Treatment of posttraumatic stress disorder by trained lay counselors in an African refugee settlement: A randomized controlled trial. *Journal of Consulting and Clinical Psychology, 76*, 686–694.

Nicholl, C., & Thompson, A. R. (2004). The psychological treatment of PTSD in adult refugees: A review of the current state of psychological therapies. *Journal of Mental Health, 13*, 351–362.

Nickerson, A., Bryant, R. A., Rosebrock, L., & Litz, B. T. (2014). The mechanisms of psychosocial injury following human rights violations, mass trauma and torture. *Clinical Psychology: Science and Practice, 21*, 172–191.

Otis, J. D., Keane, T. M., & Kerns, R. D. (2003). An examination of the relationship between chronic pain and post-traumatic stress disorder. *Journal of Rehabilitation Research and Development, 40*(5), 397–405.

Paunovic, N., & Ost, L. G. (2001). Cognitive-behaviour therapy vs exposure therapy in the treatment of PTSD in refugees. *Behaviour Research and Therapy, 39*, 1183–1197.

Salomons, T. V., Osterman, J. E., Gagliese, L., & Katz, J. (2004). Pain flashbacks in posttraumatic stress disorder. *Clinical Journal of Pain, 20*(2), 83–87.

Schauer, M., Neuner, F., & Elbert, T. (2005). *Narrative exposure therapy. A short-term intervention for traumatic stress disorders after war, terror, or torture.* Göttingen: Hogrefe & Huber.

Silove, D. (1999). The psychological effects of torture, mass human rights violence, and refugee trauma: Towards an integrated conceptual framework. *Journal of Nervous and Mental Disease, 187*, 200–207.

Silove, D. (2004). The global challenge of asylum. In J. P. Wilson & B. Drožđek (Eds.), *Broken spirits. The treatment of traumatized asylum seekers, refugees, war and torture victims.* New York/Hove: Brunner-Routledge.

Silove, D., Steel, Z., & Mollica, R. F. (2001). Detention of asylum seekers: Assault on health, human rights and social development. *Lancet, 357,* 1436–1437.

Steel, Z., Silove, D., Phan, T., & Bauman, A. (2002). Long-term effect of psychological trauma on the mental health of Vietnamese refugees resettled in Australia: A population-based study. *Lancet, 360*(9339), 1056–1062.

Steel, Z., Frommer, N., & Silove, D. (2004). Part I – The mental health impacts of migration: The law and its effects failing to understand: Refugee determination and the traumatized applicant. *International Journal of Law and Psychiatry, 27*(6), 511–528.

Thomsen, A., Madsen, J., Smidt-Nielsen, K., & Eriksen, J. (1997). Chronic pain in torture survivors. *Torture, 7,* 118–120.

Tribe, R., & Raval, H. (2002). *Working with interpreters in mental health.* New York: Routledge.

United Nations, Department of Economic and Social Affairs, Population Division. (2011). *International Migration Report 2009: A Global Assessment* (United Nations, ST/ESA/SER.A/316), online: http://www.globalmigrationgroup.org/uploads/gmg-topics/mig-data/International_Migration_Report_2009.pdf. Accessed 29 Sept 2013.

US Department of Veterans Affairs, Department of Defense. (2010). Clinical practice guideline for the management of post-traumatic stress. Guideline summary, online: http://www.healthquality.va.gov/ptsd/CPGSummaryFINALMgmtofPTSDfinal021413.pdf. Accessed 5 Oct 2013.

van Dijk, J. A., Schoutrop, M. J. A., & Spinhoven, P. (2003). Testimony therapy: Treatment method for traumatized victims of organized violence. *American Journal of Psychotherapy, 57*(3), 361–373.

Varvin, S. (1998). Psychoanalytic psychotherapy with traumatized refugees: Integration, symbolization, and mourning. *American Journal of Psychotherapy, 52*(1), 64–71.

Volkan, V. D. (2004). From hope for a better life to broken spirits: An introduction. In J. P. Wilson & B. Drožđek (Eds.), *Broken spirits. The treatment of traumatized asylum seekers, refugees, war and torture victims.* New York/Hove: Brunner-Routledge.

Wilson, J. P. (2004). The broken spirit: Posttraumatic damage to the self. In J. P. Wilson & B. Drožđek (Eds.), *Broken spirits. The treatment of traumatized asylum seekers, refugees, war and torture victims.* New York/Hove: Brunner-Routledge.

Considerations in the Treatment of Veterans with Posttraumatic Stress Disorder

22

Shannon E. McCaslin, Jessica A. Turchik, and Jennifer J. Hatzfeld

22.1 Introduction

> The soldier is the Army. No army is better than its soldiers. The soldier is also a citizen. In fact, the highest obligation and privilege of citizenship is that of bearing arms for one's country. – George S. Patton Jr.

Military service requires a commitment of service to one's country, motivated by very different passions which can range from the most patriotic to the most pragmatic. However, regardless of the reason a service member decides to enter military service, this commitment also demands a willingness to place oneself in situations that can mean exposure to unique stressors and traumas. As such, service members, particularly those who serve in combat, are at higher risk to experience potentially traumatic events. Traumatic events experienced while serving in the military may include not only exposure to combat and other life-threatening situations but also incidents that

S.E. McCaslin, PhD (✉)
Dissemination and Training Division, National Center for PTSD,
VA Palo Alto Health Care System, 795 Willow Road, Menlo Park, CA 94025, USA
e-mail: Shannon.McCaslin@va.gov

J.A. Turchik, PhD
Center for Innovation and Implementation, VA Palo Alto Health Care System,
795 Willow Road, Menlo Park, CA 94025, USA

National Center for PTSD, VA Palo Alto Health Care System,
795 Willow Road, Menlo Park, CA 94025, USA
e-mail: Jessica.Turchik@va.gov

J.J. Hatzfeld, RN, PhD
Defense Medical Research and Development Program,
Combat Casualty Care Research (JPC-6), MCMR-RTC, 504 Scott St, Building 722,
Fort Detrick, MD 21702, USA
e-mail: jennifer.j.hatzfeld.mil@mail.mil

© Springer International Publishing Switzerland 2015
U. Schnyder, M. Cloitre (eds.), *Evidence Based Treatments for Trauma-Related Psychological Disorders: A Practical Guide for Clinicians*,
DOI 10.1007/978-3-319-07109-1_22

occur during rigorous training and interpersonal violence (e.g., military sexual harassment or assault). In turn, greater trauma exposure can place service members at increased risk for the subsequent development of stress-related mental health difficulties such as posttraumatic stress disorder (PTSD), depression, and alcohol misuse. The majority of studies examining the prevalence of PTSD among veterans have sampled those exposed to combat. Estimates of current PTSD prevalence in national samples have included 15.2 % of males and 8.1 % of females among veterans who served in the Vietnam War (Kulka et al. 1990), 10.1 % among those serving in the Gulf War (Kang et al. 2003), and 13.8 % among veterans of Operations Iraqi Freedom (OIF) and Enduring Freedom (OEF; Tanielian and Jaycox 2008). Veterans with PTSD have reported greater interpersonal disturbances (e.g., Koenen et al. 2008), lower occupational functioning (e.g., Zatzick et al. 1997), and reduced quality of life (e.g., Schnurr et al. 2006).

Delivering high-quality treatment to veterans with PTSD and other trauma-related conditions requires awareness not only of evidence-based treatment practices but also of military-related stressors and the underlying military cultural context in which they occur. In this chapter, we aim to provide the clinician with a greater understanding of military-related stressors and increased insight into the military cultural context. Important aspects of the military experience are introduced, and additional resources are provided so that the clinician can learn more about each topic. Please note that the majority of our review and recommendations are grounded largely in the experience of US military service and veteran care.

22.2   Military Culture and Context

It can be argued that the military is a distinct culture, made up of a unique set of values, beliefs, and cultural rules. For example, service to community and country, courage, integrity, and loyalty are among core values. There is also a shared sense of purpose, and a fostering of strong bonds among service members. Service members begin the process of learning about this culture in basic training and become acculturated to various degrees. The degree to which a veteran continues to identify with military culture following separation from the military can influence how mental health symptoms are experienced and reported to the clinician. Hoge (2011) recognized this meeting of cultures by stating that the clinician should meet veterans where they are, literally and figuratively, in terms of culture. Separation from the military and transition back into the civilian setting can be challenging, even apart from stressful or traumatic experiences that may have been experienced while serving.

Recognizing sources of transitional stress in veterans can be an important part of an initial assessment. For example, factors such as whether individuals worked in the civilian sector prior to or after the military, if they are separating, retiring, or remaining connected in a reserve status, whether the separation from the military was planned or involuntary, and how well the job that the veteran had in the military translates to civilian work can all influence the ease of transition from the military context to civilian context. Additionally, military service-related achievements, experience, and recognition—easily seen on a uniform in medals and ribbons—become "invisible" in the civilian context. Rank and organizational hierarchy, clearly identified and articulated in the military setting, are less evident to the military member and may be difficult to navigate without understanding the unique cues and social norms in a civilian context. Another potential source of transitional stress involves the loss of social support from other service members. Social bonds with other service members can be extremely deep, and the loss of camaraderie and proximity of these relationships can be understandably difficult.

Treatment engagement and rapport with veteran clients can be improved by taking the time to learn about military culture. Unlike many other countries, the USA currently has an all-volunteer military, and those who serve make up a small minority of the population. Thus, civilian providers may not have had exposure to the military and may not have a deep understanding of military culture or context. In countries that require most civilians to serve within some component of the military for a period of time, there may be a deeper sense of connection with the veteran's military experience. Further, veterans vary broadly in their perceptions of their military service. For example, some will perceive their military service positively, whereas others may report more negative experiences and little to no continued positive identification with military culture. Thus, it is important to thoughtfully engage the veteran in conversation about their unique military experience and perceptions of their service. Respect for each individual's experience can be conveyed through sensitively inquiring about the veteran's military experiences such as their role and job, and whether they served in combat or not. Time in session should be dedicated to understanding their overall experience. At the end of this chapter, we provide links to resources that can help the treating clinician become more familiar with key values and beliefs of military culture and logistical and organization aspects of the military.

22.3 Combat Service

We few, we happy few, we band of brothers. For he to-day that sheds his blood with me, Shall be my brother; be ne'er so vile, This day shall gentle his condition; And gentlemen in England now a-bed, Shall think themselves accurs'd they were not here, And hold their manhoods cheap whiles any speaks, That fought with us upon Saint Crispin's day. – William Shakespeare (Henry V, Act IV, III)

As mentioned previously, there are various types of stressors that a service member may experience, including intense training and deployment experiences. Deployments are not limited to the direct support of combat operations and may include supportive roles well outside of the combat zone as well as humanitarian missions and actions. However, we focus on combat exposure in the next section because of the intense and often profound psychological impact of combat service. Combat stressors may include life-threatening situations, physical injury, witnessing death and dying, experiencing injuries and losses of comrades, and participating in actions that result in the injury or death of another. Additional factors that can compound these combat stressors include periods of intense action and long work hours interspersed with inactivity and downtime, separation from usual coping mechanisms or support systems, and a loss of control over the situation or environment.

Combat exposure has been associated with higher rates of PTSD, depression, and alcohol misuse (Hoge et al. 2004; Kulka et al. 1990; Kang et al. 2003). Post-deployment PTSD rates were found to vary between 11 and 22 % among veterans of OEF and OIF (Hoge et al. 2004; Seal et al. 2009). Length of deployment and higher level of combat exposure have been found to increase risk for PTSD (Schell and Marshall 2008). Among the many stressors that can be experienced in the combat environment, the consequences of losing comrades and of facing situations which conflict with one's deeply held beliefs and values are profound but often less addressed in traditional treatments for combat-related PTSD.

22.3.1 Grief and Loss

Many veterans who served in combat have experienced the sudden loss of comrades and continue to experience powerful symptoms of grief years later. Studies of US Army soldiers and marines who had deployed to Iraq and Afghanistan found that between 63 and 80 % of those surveyed knew someone who had been seriously injured or killed and 20–25 % experienced having a buddy shot or hit nearby (Thomas et al. 2010; Hoge et al. 2004; Toblin et al. 2012).

Strong bonds formed during training and combat and a sense of responsibility for the well-being of one's comrades can result in losses that deeply impact veterans who have survived combat (Papa et al. 2008). Among one sample of soldiers who had experienced the loss of a comrade, approximately 20 % reported difficulty coping with symptoms of grief (Toblin et al. 2012). In another study of 114 veterans who had served in combat during the Vietnam War, those who reported losses of comrades while serving reported a high level of grief symptoms (Pivar and Field 2004). Strikingly, the authors observed that the level of grief symptoms reported by the veterans was comparable to that endorsed by individuals who had experienced the death of a spouse within the past 3–6 months. Moreover, it was clear that grief symptoms could be distinguished from PTSD and depression symptoms and were most predicted by the losses themselves. Difficulty coping with such losses has also been associated with poorer physical health, occupational functioning, sleep disturbance, fatigue, and pain—including musculoskeletal and back pain and headaches (Toblin et al. 2012). Grief for the loss itself can be complicated by feelings of guilt about surviving when comrades did not or feelings of self-blame related to the belief that the service member or veteran could have prevented the death (Currier and Holland 2012).

In summary, symptoms of grief can remain unresolved, endure for decades (Pivar and Field 2004), and uniquely impact functioning (Toblin et al. 2012). Losses of comrades should be assessed and attended to in the same manner as one would assess traumatic experiences involving the death of a family member or close friend of a nonveteran client. For more information on the assessment and treatment of traumatic or complex (prolonged) grief, please see Chap. 15.

22.3.2 Moral Injury

Moral injury is a construct that has been increasingly researched during the past decade. It refers to psychological injury resulting from participating in, witnessing, or learning about events during war that violate the service member or veteran's deeply held values or moral beliefs about themselves and humanity (Currier et al. 2013; Litz et al. 2009). The types of experiences that may result in moral injury are broad and include betrayal by leadership or peers, betrayal of one's own values, inability to prevent harm to others, injuring or killing enemy combatants or civilians, witnessing or experiencing atrocities (e.g., inhumane acts), and facing ethical dilemmas (Currier et al. 2013; Stein et al. 2012).

Recent surveys have attempted to quantify the numbers of service members that have been exposed to such situations while serving in Iraq and Afghanistan. Among US Army soldiers and marines who served in Iraq and Afghanistan, 23–32 % reported being responsible for the death of an enemy combatant, 48–60 % reported seeing ill or injured women or children whom they were unable to help, over 50 % reported shooting or directing fire at the enemy, and over 5–9.7 % endorsed being responsible for the death of a noncombatant (Thomas et al. 2010; Hoge et al. 2004). Perception of betrayals from military leaders and of their own personal values, overly harsh treatment of civilians, and guilt about surviving combat were found to be the most endorsed items on a moral injury self-report measure among a sample of veterans who had served in Iraq and/or Afghanistan (Currier et al. 2013).

Studies have found greater PTSD symptoms among veterans who have injured or killed others during their combat service, after accounting for other combat exposure and stressors (Currier et al. 2013; Maguen et al. 2010, 2013; Litz et al. 2009 for review). One study indicated that certain categories of events may be more associated with specific clusters of PTSD symptoms. In this study, morally injurious events committed by self were the best predictor of reexperiencing symptoms, whereas those related to acts of others (such as betrayal or enemy violence) predicted state anger (Stein et al. 2012). Other psychological consequences related to morally injurious experiences include emotional responses, such as guilt and shame, and spiritual or existential concerns (e.g., loss of meaning, struggles with one's religious beliefs; Currier et al. 2013).

Psychological reactions related to morally injurious events such as guilt appear to be more likely to arise following an event versus during it, and it has been suggested that having time to reflect on and process the event may precede the development of some emotional reactions (Stein et al. 2012). The way in which the event is cognitively processed is the core component of the framework for understanding the cause and development of moral injury put forth by Litz et al. (2009). Key to this framework is the thesis that the individual is unable to contextualize or justify their own actions or those of others and that these experiences are not able to be successfully accommodated into preexisting moral schemas. This conflict then results in emotional responses, such as guilt or shame. Interestingly, a recent study reported that moral injury acts committed by self were related to the guilt-related constructs of *hindsight-bias/responsibility* and *wrongdoing*, but were not related to *lack of justification* (Stein et al. 2012). These findings suggest that service members may be able to understand the underlying rationale and context for their actions and simultaneously experience feelings of guilt.

Although the importance of addressing the impact of these types of experiences has been stressed (Currier et al. 2013), events with moral and ethical implications may not be given sufficient attention during a course of mental health treatment due to both clinician and veteran factors (Litz et al. 2009). Clinicians may not feel prepared to address what can be complex existential and spiritual questions, or they may be focused on other areas of the veteran's experience (e.g., experiences related to life threat). Veterans may hesitate to discuss actions by self or others that are related to feelings of guilt or shame and may be concerned about the potential reaction by the clinician (e.g., rejection, being misunderstood; Litz et al. 2009). Furthermore, some veterans may have fears of legal ramifications for themselves or others. Currier et al. (2013) suggested that these fears may limit the information provided to the clinician in response to questions that are specifically directed at the violation of rules of engagement, participation in atrocities, or other similar types of experiences and thus recommend exploring these topics within the bounds of a broader assessment.

Routinely assessing for these experiences can increase the likelihood that they will come to light and enable them to be addressed during the course of treatment. Such assessment and discussion should be done sensitively and can be guided by recently developed assessment instruments such as the Moral Injury Events Scale (Nash et al. 2013) and the Moral Injury Questionnaire—Military Version (Currier et al. 2013). Whereas clinicians should always provide the space and encouragement for veterans to share traumatic experiences, veterans may wish to share only limited information initially. Clinicians should be sensitive to a veteran's discomfort and allow him or her to determine the pace of any disclosures. Litz et al. (2009) proposed an eight-step treatment to address moral injury. This treatment touches on central components for processing such experiences, including components focused on strengthening the working alliance, providing education, important concerns such as self-forgiveness and social connection, and setting future goals. When appropriate, veterans struggling with spiritual or existential issues related to such experiences may benefit from referral to other services such as those of a chaplain or spiritual leader.

22.3.3 Considerations for Treatment

- Civilian clinicians who have limited experience working with service members or veteran clients may question whether they will be able to connect with or be accepted by the veteran. On the contrary, when speaking with clinicians, they often report that they are not only able to build strong therapeutic connections but also find the opportunity to serve veterans through providing treatment to be extremely rewarding. There are steps that the clinician can take to strengthen rapport, trust, and engagement in treatment. Analogous to working with other individuals from a different culture, it is important to learn about the military and veteran population. Conveying an interest in and understanding of the aspects of military culture demonstrates respect, can strengthen the therapeutic relationship, and can improve treatment formulation. Whenever possible, treatment providers should seek out training and information to increase their knowledge of military culture.

- In addition to gaining familiarity with military culture, it is essential to set aside stereotypes and assumptions about what it means to be veteran or to serve in combat. As noted earlier in the chapter, there is much variation among the veteran population including differences in reasons for joining the military, how veterans perceive or feel about their service, and their military assignments and experiences.

- In preparing to work with service members and veterans, clinicians should consider conducting a personal assessment of their beliefs and potential limits. For example, will one be able to set aside one's beliefs and judgments about war and politics, and how might one respond to or what is the extent to which one can tolerate themes that may arise in treating combat veterans such as gallows humor or situations involving moral ambiguity (e.g., inadvertently harming civilians in the context of combat)?

- Due to the great variation in experiences among veterans, the importance of a sensitive and comprehensive assessment cannot be overstated. For veterans that have served in combat, factors such as combat operation and era of service as well as individual characteristics such as the veteran's branch of service, job, and rank while serving may all influence the experiences and presentation of the veteran seeking treatment. Providing ample time for the veteran to share his or her personal experience can be critical to inform the direction of treatment. Sensitive experiences, such as those involving grief for fallen comrades and moral ambiguity, can be more difficult to share, accentuating the need to allow adequate time to develop a solid and trusting therapeutic relationship.

- The need for multidisciplinary care should be recognized. Veterans should be screened not only for comorbid mental health conditions but also comorbid physical health conditions and referred appropriately. For example, the physical demands of military service (e.g., physical training, combat injuries) can lead to chronic pain. Among a sample of 1,800 veterans who served in Afghanistan and Iraq, 46.5 % reported some pain, with 59 % of those exceeding a clinical threshold of greater than or equal to 4 (0–10 scale; Gironda et al. 2006). Both PTSD and chronic pain tax the coping resources of veterans, which can exacerbate both conditions and can negatively impact functioning and quality of life (Clapp et al. 2010; Sharp and Harvey 2001). Other physical injuries, such as traumatic brain injury, can also profoundly impact recovery.

- As stated above, combat veterans may present with a complex set of conditions including PTSD, pain, and sleep problems, which may feel overwhelming for the clinician to address. Awareness of one's own limits of clinical expertise and knowledge of where one might seek additional resources and support (e.g., consultation, supervision, referral for additional services) can be important to both the clinician and the overall success of treatment.

Case Illustration: Luis, Male, Operation Enduring Freedom (OEF) Combat Veteran

Luis joined the military at 18 years of age after graduating from high school. He had looked forward to serving in the military as both his father and grandfather had enlisted in the military. He served two tours in Afghanistan during which he engaged in many firefights, both receiving fire and firing at enemy combatants. During his second tour in Afghanistan, he experienced a blast caused by an improvised explosive device (IED). This same blast resulted in the death of one of his comrades.

Upon separation from the military, Luis decided to use the educational benefits he had earned through serving in the military to go to college. He was unprepared for the feelings of anxiety that struck him when he stepped onto the campus. He found that certain class material and comments by teachers or other students about the war brought up vivid memories of his experiences in Afghanistan, and he would find himself unable to concentrate for the rest of the day. He felt unable to connect with civilian students, and he spent much of his time on campus in the Veterans Resource Center where he met and engaged with other veterans. Luis felt that he should have been able to deal with his feelings, "just suck it up," as he had been able to do with many difficult experiences while serving, but no matter what he did, he found that the thoughts and images kept returning.

Luis started to wonder why, after separating from the military, things seemed to be getting worse, not better as he expected. He had looked forward to being home and to returning to his civilian life. While at his primary care appointment, his doctor conducted a number of mental health screenings, and Luis screened positive for PTSD. His doctor spoke with him about the symptoms, gave him information on websites that provided educational material, and suggested a referral to a mental health provider. Luis said he would think about it and took the information. That night he went home and looked up PTSD online, where he read about the symptoms and treatments, and noticed that other veterans were sharing similar stories and experiences to his own. Although ambivalent, he decided to call the number that was provided to him and set up an appointment to see a psychologist with experience in treating PTSD.

As Luis drove up to the clinic, he became anxious and had a strong urge to turn the car around and go home. His mind was racing with thoughts like, "Is it worth digging up all this stuff?" "What will a civilian know about any of this anyway?" "Will he/she judge me?" "I should be able to deal with this myself." Only halfway through the school semester, he was not sure he would be able to keep up his grades and maintain his GI Bill eligibility while taking medications that might "mess with" his mind. Still, he did not want to "no show" to his appointment, so he parked and checked in at the front desk, determined to avoid any medications that this doctor might give him.

Dr. Keast greeted Luis warmly, inviting him into the office. Although she had never served in the military, Dr. Keast had sought out information about military culture and consulted with colleagues to increase her knowledge. She asked how Luis felt about coming in, acknowledging that it can be difficult to ask for help, introduced herself and her professional background and expertise, noting that while she had not served in the military herself that she greatly appreciated his service and looked forward to working with him. Dr. Keast then provided him with an agenda for the session. She outlined that she would ask some general questions about his background, current living situation, military experience, and current symptoms—and that he was welcome to decline to answer anything he was uncomfortable with answering or discussing. She inquired about when, where, and in what role Luis had served, and she allowed him time to share and ask questions. Dr. Keast normalized the difficulties of transitioning out of the military. She also noted how certain behaviors, such as the ability to function on limited or inconsistent sleep schedules and remaining aware and prepared (hypervigilance), can be adaptive while in combat but may be inconsistent with life in the civilian context. In the course of the assessment, she learned that Luis was struggling with the meaning behind his service because of some of the things that he had witnessed while at the same time continuing to feel deeply connected to and proud of his military service. Dr. Keast normalized these experiences, providing information about moral injury to Luis and encouraging him to continue to discuss these issues in treatment. Dr. Keast inquired about blast injuries and learned that he had suffered a concussion following his exposure to the IED blast. She received his permission to refer him to a cognitive rehabilitation specialist for an assessment.

Luis decided to engage in a time-limited course of prolonged exposure therapy (PE) which allowed him to discuss his experiences and process through them, as well as to approach situations that he had been avoiding. After treatment, he continued to report residual symptoms of sleep disturbance for which Dr. Keast referred him to a sleep specialist for a course of cognitive behavioral therapy for insomnia. Dr. Keast also connected Luis with on-campus disability services so that he could receive accommodations, such as extended test-taking time and access to a notetaker, in the classroom for difficulties with concentration and anxiety symptoms. Luis began to feel more confident in his academic work, to engage in social activities again, and to feel more hopeful for the future.

22.4   Military Sexual Harassment and Assault

While serving in the military comes with the obvious risks to life and limb associated with combat exposure, too often sexual harassment and sexual assault are also a part of service members' military experiences. Sexual harassment is generally defined as unwanted sexual experiences that occur in the workplace and may include an array of behaviors, including offensive sexual comments, display of pornographic materials, promises of punishment or rewards related to performance of sexual favors, and sexual assault. Sexual assault is generally defined as unwanted physical sexual contact that includes a range of behaviors from unwanted touching of a sexual nature to nonconsensual vaginal, anal, or oral penetration (rape). Within VA, military sexual trauma is specifically defined as, "psychological trauma, which in the judgment of a VA mental health professional, resulted from a physical assault of a sexual nature, battery of a sexual nature, or sexual harassment which occurred while the Veteran was serving on active duty or [on] active duty for training" (US Code 1720D of Title 38).

There are some unique factors that contribute to the complexity of sexual harassment and assault in the military (Turchik and Wilson 2010). A key factor is the strong masculine orientation associated with military culture that reinforces strength and control. With women a clear minority in the active duty service (approximately 20 % of the force), inappropriate conversations and activities can easily develop that ultimately lead to an environment that condones sexual harassment and even sexual assault. Additionally, victims (either male or female) can be reluctant to report abuse as they may be seen as weak by other service members in the organization— either for contributing to the incident or not being able to stop it. Another important factor is the significance of rank structure and unit cohesion in the military. While these are valuable characteristics to accomplish a specific mission, they can also increase the vulnerability of lower-ranking service members and make the decision to report the incident that much more difficult if it occurs within the same unit.

22.4.1 Prevalence

It is difficult to determine the actual prevalence and incidence of sexual harassment and sexual assault in the military due to a number of factors (i.e., inconsistency in definitions across studies, underreporting); however, research suggests that it is not uncommon. In the 2006 Department of Defense (DoD) Workplace and Gender Relations Survey of Active Duty Members (Lipari et al. 2008), the annual prevalence of sexual assault was 6.8 % for women and 1.8 % for men. Rates were 9.0 and 3.0 % for women and men, respectively, for sexual coercion and 31.0 and 7.0 %, respectively, for unwanted sexual attention. It is important to note that while a higher percentage of women than men experience sexual assault/harassment during their military service, the actual numbers of women and men who experience military sexual assault/harassment are similar given the higher percentage of men in the military.

22.4.2 Mental Health Consequences

Research has demonstrated that veterans who report sexual trauma during military service are at greater risk for a number of physical health problems (Frayne et al. 1999; Kimerling et al. 2007; Turchik et al. 2012), mental health problems (Kimerling et al. 2007, 2010), and other impairments in functioning (Skinner et al. 2000), even years after the stressful experience. Research has found increased rates of mental health problems, including posttraumatic stress disorder (PTSD), depression, anxiety, substance use disorders, and sexual dysfunctions, among those who experienced sexual trauma during military service (e.g., Kimerling et al. 2007; Turchik et al. 2012). The condition that appears to be most highly associated with military sexual trauma is PTSD (e.g., Kimerling et al. 2007). This is consistent with other research which has found that rape leads to a higher risk of PTSD than any other trauma, including combat, in both veteran and nonveteran samples (Kang et al. 2005; Kessler et al. 1995; Yaeger et al. 2006).

22.4.3 Considerations for Treatment

- Many of the empirically supported PTSD treatments, including cognitive processing therapy (CPT; Resick and Schnicke 1993) and prolonged exposure (PE; Foa et al. 2007), were initially developed for and tested with sexual assault survivors, and these treatments have been shown to be helpful for those with sexual trauma-related PTSD. However, it should be noted that these treatments have primarily been tested with female sexual assault survivors, and further research may be needed for male sexual assault survivors. Additional PTSD treatments (e.g., skills training in affective and interpersonal regulation narrative therapy, STAIR; Cloitre et al. 2006, acceptance and commitment therapy, ACT; Walser et al. 2013) are also available and are being used with veterans who have experienced sexual trauma.
- Given that the sexual violence occurred within the military, the context may present additional concerns for victims. Providers should be attuned to confidentiality issues, stigma, concerns about effects on their job, perpetration retaliation, unit cohesion, and other issues that may be qualitatively different than for someone who experienced sexual trauma as a civilian.
- Given the gendered nature of sexual trauma, it is also important to ensure that screening and treatment is delivered in a gender-sensitive manner. If seeking care within the military or at Veteran Medical Centers, both men and women in particular may face barriers related to being immersed in and receiving care in a male-dominated environment. The gender of the provider should also be taken into consideration. Two qualitative studies have examined whether veterans who have experienced military sexual trauma have a provider gender preference in regard to seeking care related to their military sexual trauma experience (Turchik et al. 2014, 2013). These results found that the majority of men and women did have a preference, with women with a preference preferring a female provider

and men being more mixed in their preferences. Such findings suggest that asking sexual assault survivors whether they have a preference and honoring this preference when possible may better facilitate ensuring that these veterans receive the treatment they are seeking.

- It is important for providers to recognize that while an experience of a sexual trauma increases the risk for mental health problems, it is not a diagnosis and not all men and women who experience sexual trauma will want or need to seek treatment. Further, while PTSD is one of the most common diagnoses associated with sexual trauma, providers should be mindful that there are a number of other mental and physical health issues associated with sexual victimization.

Case Illustration: Janine, Female, Military Sexual Assault Survivor

Janine is a 35-year-old woman who experienced a recent sexual assault by an officer in her unit during her first assignment following boot camp. After the attack, the officer continued to make lewd comments and gestures, grab her inappropriately, and threaten to enter her bunk at night. When Janine attempted to describe her experience to some of her peers, she was told to "get over it" and "not make a big deal." She hesitated to report his behavior for fear of jeopardizing her military career and losing her friends who were also close with the perpetrator. While on active duty, Janine made every attempt to not think about the experiences by distracting herself with her work and telling herself she was "overreacting." However, after leaving the military, Janine's symptoms, including insomnia and hypervigilance, worsened. She insisted on sleeping with a gun under her pillow, and she avoided going out with friends because she "didn't trust men anymore" and feared that her male friends would attempt to make unwanted sexual advances.

Due to an inability to sleep, Janine could not hold a job and feared she would never be able to work again. After building a tolerance to over-the-counter sleep medications, Janine sought out a primary care physician, who she hoped would prescribe a stronger sleeping pill. During her visit, Dr. DuBois completed a military sexual trauma screening. Janine confided in her doctor that she had experienced military sexual trauma and was having nightmares involving her perpetrator. Seeing her distress, Dr. DuBois informed Janine of the treatment options available and provided her with a number to contact to set up an appointment with a psychologist with PTSD treatment experience.

Janine was embarrassed that she had never sought treatment before, even though she knew it probably would have helped. With several different job assignments and her self-imposed busy schedule, she had never taken the time to look up the number to the mental health clinic. She also wished that she had the courage to report the incident when it happened, instead of keeping it quiet. If she knew then how this was going to impact her, she could have found the right person to tell; she was pretty sure that the same perpetrator had assaulted other people after her. She really did not want to get caught up in an investigation or to have to testify against that officer; thankfully she had not seen him since her first assignment. However, she was not sure if the psychologist would need to make a formal report to the military police if she told too many details. With all of those conflicting thoughts and swirling emotions, Janine made an appointment. Without a job, she figured she had the time to deal with this now.

After an initial assessment, it was decided by Janine and her psychologist that cognitive processing therapy would be a good treatment to try. It was clear that Janine had developed a lot of self-blame related to the harassment and that she felt that she must have "led [him] on" or done something to warrant the harassment. She described believing not only that she could no longer trust men but that she was now "dirty" and "worthless" and that she did not "deserve a good man anyway." Janine described her fears that she would never get back to normal and that she was permanently damaged. Her therapist focused on examining and challenging the beliefs and thoughts that were impacting Janine's recovery. This included completing assignments to explore Janine's perception of events and tendency to self-blame. She also addressed Janine's insomnia by psychoeducation on sleep hygiene and a referral to a sleep specialist. Writing an account of the trauma and processing through this account during the course of therapy helped Janine to make sense of the events she has been adamantly avoiding and allowed her to feel the emotions associated with her harassment. By the end of treatment, Janine showed significant improvement in sleep duration and sleep quality, reduction of nightmares, and willingness to engage in coed social activities. She also showed significant decreases in her PTSD symptoms and no longer felt the need to check her locks or look over her shoulder constantly. She also expressed increased self-efficacy and is currently in the process of seeking employment. Janine also finally began to feel open to the possibility of a romantic relationship in the future. Even after the end of treatment, she continues to read back over her therapy materials and complete therapy worksheets when she feels "stuck" about something.

22.5 Summary and General Treatment Considerations

It is not within the scope of this chapter to fully cover the many different clinical presentations and issues that may arise in the clinical setting. The veteran population is incredibly diverse, spanning generations, ethnicity, and gender. Many veterans have served during war, and many others have served during times of peace; still others have served on humanitarian missions around the globe. Thus, the importance of listening to the unique narrative with which each veteran presents is emphasized and recommendations are offered within this chapter to provide some general guidance when treating veterans with PTSD.

22.5.1 Barriers to Seeking Mental Health Care

A significant number of veterans who are in need of mental health care for PTSD do not seek out services (Shiner 2011). A 2003 survey of US soldiers and marines who served in combat found that despite up to 17.1 % endorsing the presence of a mental illness, only 23–40 % of those who screened positive sought mental health care (Hoge et al. 2004). In another national random sample of OEF and OIF veterans, 20 % screened positive for probable PTSD (Elbogen et al. 2013). Among those, greater than two-thirds had sought mental health treatment. Studies have documented a number of barriers to seeking mental health care, including concerns about and readiness for mental health treatment (Stecker et al. 2013), stigma surrounding the ramifications of seeking treatment on one's future military career and self-stigma such as perceiving mental health treatment as a sign of weakness (Hoge et al. 2004; Stecker et al. 2007, 2013), and logistical barriers such as scheduling, distance from health care, and balancing multiple roles (e.g., employee, student, and parent) (Hoge et al. 2004; Stecker et al. 2013). Interestingly, among a sample of service members that had served in Iraq and Afghanistan, the most endorsed barriers to care included concerns about treatment such as limited choices for treatment (i.e., medication would be prescribed; preferences for individual versus group treatment), concerns that one's situation would not be understood by a mental health clinician (e.g., only those who had been deployed to war would understand), and the perception that treatment was not needed or that one was not ready for treatment (Stecker et al. 2013). Believing one should solve one's own problems was more often endorsed among veterans with probable PTSD who did not seek mental health treatment (Elbogen et al. 2013). Given these various barriers to care, provision of mental health treatment may be improved through consideration of the following:

- Outreach to veterans in the community is warranted in order to raise awareness for veterans with PTSD who do not readily seek out treatment. Provision of education about PTSD and availability of services in places outside traditional arenas of care (e.g., college campuses, veteran's organizations) may increase the likelihood that some veterans will seek and receive care.
- Successful retention in treatment relies on the establishment of a solid and trusting therapeutic alliance between client and provider. A provider's understanding of military culture can bridge the civilian-military divide, increasing the veteran's sense of being understood and trust in the competence of the provider. For providers with limited contact with military or veteran populations, gaining education in military culture can increase sensitivity to the unique experience of each veteran, and it can enhance the clinician's ability to appropriately screen for military history while also guiding treatment formulation.
- Cultural factors can influence how mental illness and treatment for mental illness are perceived. For example, during military service, strength, endurance, and the ability to solve problems quickly are highly valued characteristics. Mental illness may be perceived as a weakness, and this can lead to ambivalence about seeking

mental health care. Providing clear and direct education to the veteran about PTSD, treatment options, and what to expect during the course of treatment as well as allowing adequate time to answer any questions that arise can demystify mental health treatment and build confidence regarding potential helpfulness.

22.5.2 Assessment and Treatment

A comprehensive assessment should be completed prior to beginning treatment. Such an assessment should include information about military background and experience, and it should also elicit information about PTSD-related conditions and functioning, such as those discussed earlier. Co-occurring psychological and physical conditions should also be included in the assessment. During the recent wars in Iraq and Afghanistan, the use of improvised explosive devices (IEDs) by the enemy and increased survival rates for veterans with severe injuries due to better protective gear and medical care have led to an increase in particular comorbidities. Co-occurring PTSD, pain, and traumatic brain injury, resulting from these types of events, have been deemed "signature wounds" of combat. Assessing for these physical and functional concerns and connecting the veteran with appropriate specialty care is extremely important. For example, offering a referral to a pain or cognitive rehabilitation specialist should be done in conjunction with providing psychotherapy for PTSD.

Recent studies support the use of trauma-focused therapies such as CPT (Resick and Schnicke 1993) and PE (Foa et al. 2007) for veterans (Department of Veterans Affairs and Department of Defense 2010). Acceptance and commitment therapy (ACT) has also been shown to reduce symptoms of depression and anxiety in veterans (e.g., Walser et al. 2013). For veterans with complex presentations (e.g., multiple traumas, emotional regulation deficits), stage-based treatments such as skills training in affective and interpersonal regulation narrative therapy (STAIR; Cloitre et al. 2006) and dialectical behavior therapy (DBT; Linehan 1993) may be considered (Landes et al. 2013).

In addition to individual psychotherapy, both family and peer support interventions can be important modes of treatment for those who are ambivalent about receiving mental health care. Family members can be deeply affected by their loved one's mental illness, and they often play a key role in recovery. Specific interpersonal disturbances reported by veterans with PTSD include worse family relationships (Koenen et al. 2008), difficulties in intimacy and communication, and higher rates of separation and divorce (Riggs et al. 1998; Cook et al. 2004). Among a sample of US Army National Guard soldiers, family counseling was an appealing option to the majority of those surveyed (Khaylis et al. 2011). Peer outreach and support has also shown promise in enhancing access to and engagement in treatment for individuals with PTSD (Jain et al. 2013). Given the often unique bond that exists between veterans, the integration of peers into the treatment plan should be considered.

22.5.3 Online Resources

In recent years, a number of resources for providers have been developed to facilitate a deeper understanding of military culture and to support mental health treatment. The Community Provider Toolkit (http://www.mentalhealth.va.gov/communitypro-viders/) provides information on understanding the military experience, mental health and wellness, and available resources. The Center for Deployment Psychology, funded in part by the US Department of Defense, provides additional information and trainings for clinicians working with military service members (http://deploy-mentpsych.org/). The National Center for PTSD website provides extensive education on the assessment and treatment of PTSD for veterans including a searchable database, PILOTS, that is regularly updated (http://www.ptsd.va.gov/).

References

Clapp, J. D., Masci, J., Bennett, S. A., & Beck, J. G. (2010). Physical and psychosocial functioning following motor vehicle trauma: Relationships with chronic pain, posttraumatic stress, and medication use. *European Journal of Pain, 14*, 418–425.

Cloitre, M., Cohen, L. R., & Koenen, K. C. (2006). *Treating survivors of childhood abuse: Psychotherapy for the interrupted life*. New York: The Guilford Press.

Cook, J. M., Riggs, D. S., Thompson, R., Coyne, J. C., & Sheikh, J. I. (2004). Posttraumatic stress disorder and current relationship functioning among World War II ex-prisoners of war. *Journal of Family Psychology, 18*, 36–45.

Currier, J. M., & Holland, J. M. (2012). Examining the role of combat loss among Vietnam War Veterans. *Journal of Traumatic Stress, 25*, 102–105.

Currier, J. M., Holland, J. M., Drescher, K., & Foy, D. (2013). Initial psychometric evaluation of the moral injury questionnaire-military version. *Clinical Psychology and Psychotherapy*, [Epub ahead of print].

Department of Veterans Affairs & Department of Defense (2010). *VA/DoD clinical practice guideline for management of post-traumatic stress*. Retrieved from: http://www.healthquality.va.gov/ptsd/cpg_PTSD-FULL-201011612.pdf

Elbogen, E. B., Wagner, H. R., Johnson, S. C., Kinneer, P., Kang, H., Vasterling, J. J., Timko, C., & Beckham, J. C. (2013). Are Iraq and Afghanistan veterans using mental health services? New data from a national random-sample survey. *Psychiatric Services, 64*, 134–141.

Foa, E., Hembree, E., & Rothbaum, B. (2007). *Prolonged exposure therapy for PTSD: Emotional processing of traumatic experiences*. Oxford: Oxford University Press.

Frayne, S. M., Skinner, K. M., Sullivan, L. M., Tripp, T. J., Hankin, C. S., Kressin, N., & Miller, D. (1999). Medical profile of women Veterans Administration outpatients who report a history of sexual assault occurring while in the military. *Journal of Women's Health & Gender-Based Medicine, 8*(6), 835–845.

Gironda, R. J., Clark, M. E., Massengale, J. P., & Walker, R. L. (2006). Pain among veterans of Operations Enduring Freedom and Iraqi Freedom. *Pain Medicine, 7*, 339–343.

Hoge, C. W. (2011). Interventions for war-related posttraumatic stress disorder: Meeting veterans where they are. *Journal of the American Medical Association, 306*, 549–551.

Hoge, C. W., Castro, C. A., Messer, S. C., McGurk, D., Cotting, D. I., & Koffman, R. L. (2004). Combat duty in Iraq and Afghanistan, mental health problems, and barriers to care. *New England Journal of Medicine, 351*, 13–22.

Jain, S., McLean, C., Adler, E. P., Lindley, S. E., Ruzek, J. I., & Rosen, C. S. (2013). Does the integration of peers into the treatment of adults with posttraumatic stress disorder improve access to mental health care? A literature review and conceptual model. *Journal of Traumatic Stress Disorders Treatment, 2*, 1–9.

Kang, H. K., Natelson, B. H., Mahan, C. M., Lee, K. Y., & Murphy, F. M. (2003). Posttraumatic stress disorder and chronic fatigue syndrome-like illness among Gulf War veterans: A population-based survey of 30,000 veterans. *American Journal of Epidemiology, 157*, 141–148.

Kang, H., Dalager, N., Mahan, C., & Ishii, E. (2005). The role of sexual assault on the risk of PTSD among Gulf War Veterans. *Annals of Epidemiology, 15*(3), 191–195.

Kessler, R. C., Sonnega, A., Bromet, E., Hughes, M., & Nelson, C. B. (1995). Posttraumatic stress disorder in the national comorbidity survey. *Archives of General Psychiatry, 52*(12), 1048–1060.

Khaylis, A., Polusny, M. A., Erbes, C. R., Gewirtz, A., & Rath, M. (2011). Posttraumatic stress, family adjustment, and treatment preferences among national guard soldiers deployed to OEF/OIF. *Military Medicine, 176*, 126–131.

Kimerling, R., Gima, K., Smith, M. W., Street, A., & Frayne, S. (2007). The Veterans Health Administration and military sexual trauma. *American Journal of Public Health, 97*, 2160–2166.

Kimerling, R., Street, A., Pavao, J., Smith, M., Cronkite, R., Holmes, T., & Frayne, S. (2010). Military-related sexual trauma among Veterans Health Administration patients returning from Afghanistan and Iraq. *American Journal of Public Health, 100*, 1409–1412.

Koenen, K. C., Stellman, S. D., Sommer, J. F., & Stellman, J. M. (2008). Persisting posttraumatic stress disorder symptoms and their relationship to functioning in Vietnam veterans: A 14-year follow-up. *Journal of Traumatic Stress, 21*, 49–57.

Kulka, R. A., Schlenger, W. E., Fairbank, J. A., Hough, R. L., Jordan, B. K., Marmar, C. R., et al. (1990). *Trauma and the Vietnam War generation: Report of findings from the National Vietnam Veterans Readjustment Study*. New York: Brunner/Mazel.

Landes, S. J., Garovoy, N. D., & Burkman, K. M. (2013). Treating complex trauma among Veterans: Three stage-based treatment models. *Journal of Clinical Psychology: In Session, 69*, 523–533.

Linehan, M. M. (1993). *Cognitive-behavioral treatment of borderline personality disorder*. New York: The Guilford Press.

Lipari, R. N., Cook, P. J., Rock, L. M., & Matos, K. (2008). *2006 gender relations survey of active duty members*. Arlington: Department of Defense Manpower Data Center.

Litz, B. T., Stein, N., Delaney, E., Lebowitz, L., Nash, W. P., Silva, C., & Maguen, S. (2009). Moral injury and moral repair in war veterans: A preliminary model and intervention strategy. *Clinical Psychology Review, 29*, 695–706.

Maguen, S., Lucenko, B. A., Reger, M. A., Gahm, G. A., Litz, B. T., Seal, K. H., & Marmar, C. R. (2010). The impact of reported direct and indirect killing on mental health symptoms in Iraq war veterans. *Journal of Traumatic Stress, 23*, 86–90.

Maguen, S., Madden, E., Bosch, J., Galatzer-Levy, I., Knight, S. J., Litz, B. T., & McCaslin, S. E. (2013). Killing and latent classes of PTSD symptoms in Iraq and Afghanistan veterans. *Journal of Affective Disorders, 145*, 344–348.

Nash, W. P., Marino Carper, T. L., Mills, M. A., Au, T., Goldsmith, A., & Litz, B. T. (2013). Psychometric evaluation of the moral injury events scale. *Military Medicine, 178*, 646–652.

Papa, A., Neria, Y., & Litz, B. (2008). Traumatic bereavement in war veterans. *Psychiatric Annals, 38*, 686–691.

Pivar, I. L., & Field, N. P. (2004). Unresolved grief in combat veterans with PTSD. *Journal of Anxiety Disorders, 18*, 745–755.

Resick, P. A., & Schnicke, M. K. (1993). *Cognitive processing therapy for rape victims: A treatment manual*. Newbury Park: Sage.

Riggs, D. S., Byrne, C. A., Weathers, F. W., & Litz, B. T. (1998). The quality of the intimate relationships of male Vietnam veterans: Problems associated with posttraumatic stress disorder. *Journal of Traumatic Stress, 11*, 87–101.

Schell, T. L., & Marshall, G. N. (2008). Survey of individuals previously deployed for OEF/OIF. In T. Tanielian & L. H. Jaycox (Eds.), *Invisible wounds of war: Psychological and cognitive injuries, their consequences, and services to assist recovery* (pp. 87–113). Santa Monica: RAND Corporation.

Schnurr, P. P., Hayes, A. F., Lunney, C. A., McFall, M., & Uddo, M. (2006). Longitudinal analysis of the relationship between symptoms and quality of life in veterans treated for posttraumatic stress disorder. *Journal of Consulting and Clinical Psychology, 74*, 707–713.

Seal, K., Metzler, T., Gima, K., Bertenthal, D., Maguen, S., & Marmar, C. (2009). Trends and risk factors for mental health diagnoses among Iraq and Afghanistan Veterans using Department of Veterans Affairs health care, 2002-2008. *American Journal of Public Health, 99*, 1651–1658.

Sharp, T. J., & Harvey, A. G. (2001). Chronic pain and posttraumatic stress disorder: Mutual maintenance? *Clinical Psychology Review, 21*, 857–877.

Shiner, B. (2011). Health services use in the Department of Veterans Affairs among returning Iraq war and Afghan war veterans with PTSD. *PTSD Research Quarterly, 22*, 1–10.

Skinner, K. M., Kressin, N., Frayne, S., Tripp, T. J., Hankin, C. S., Miller, D. R., & Sullivan, L. M. (2000). The prevalence of military sexual assault among female Veterans' Administration outpatients. *Journal of Interpersonal Violence, 15*(3), 291–310.

Stecker, T., Fortney, J. C., Hamilton, F., & Ajzen, I. (2007). An assessment of beliefs about mental health care among veterans who served in Iraq. *Psychiatric Services, 58*, 1358–1361.

Stecker, T., Shiner, B., Watts, B. V., Jones, M., & Conner, K. R. (2013). Treatment-seeking barriers for Veterans of the Iraq and Afghanistan conflicts who screen positive for PTSD. *Psychiatric Services, 64*, 280–283.

Stein, N. R., Mills, M. A., Arditte, K., Mendoza, C., Borah, A. M., Resick, P. A., & Litz, B. T. (2012). STRONG STAR Consortium. A scheme for categorizing traumatic military events. *Behavior Modification, 36*, 787–807.

Tanielian, T., & Jaycox, L. (Eds.). (2008). *Invisible wounds of war: Psychological and cognitive injuries, their consequences, and services to assist recovery.* Santa Monica: RAND Corporation.

Thomas, J. L., Wilk, J. E., Riviere, L. A., McGurk, D., Castro, C. A., & Hoge, C. W. (2010). Prevalence of mental health problems and functional impairment among active component and National Guard soldiers 3 and 12 months following combat in Iraq. *Archives of General Psychiatry, 67*, 614–623.

Toblin, R. L., Riviere, L. A., Thomas, J. L., Adler, A. B., Kok, B. C., & Hoge, C. W. (2012). Grief and physical health outcomes in U.S. soldiers returning from combat. *Journal of Affective Disorders, 136*, 469–475.

Turchik, J. A., & Wilson, S. M. (2010). Sexual assault in the U.S. military: A review of the literature and recommendations for the future. *Aggression and Violent Behavior, 15*, 267–277.

Turchik, J. A., Pavao, J., Nazarian, D., Iqbal, S., McLean, C., & Kimerling, R. (2012). Sexually transmitted infections and sexual dysfunctions among newly returned veterans with and without military sexual trauma. *International Journal of Sexual Health, 24*, 45–59.

Turchik, J. A., McLean, C., Rafie, S., Hoyt, T., Rosen, C. S., & Kimerling, R. (2013). Perceived barriers to care and provider gender preferences among veteran men who have experienced military sexual trauma: A qualitative analysis. *Psychological Services, 10*, 213–222.

Turchik, J. A., Bucossi, M. M., & Kimerling, R. (2014). Perceived barriers to care and gender preferences among veteran women who experienced military sexual trauma: A qualitative analysis. *Military Behavioral Health, 2*, 180–188.

Walser, R. D., Karlin, B. E., Trockel, M., Mazina, B., & Taylor, C. (2013). Training in and implementation of acceptance and commitment therapy for depression in the Veterans Health Administration: Therapist and patient outcomes. *Behaviour Research and Therapy, 51*, 555–563.

Yaeger, D., Himmelfarb, N., Cammack, A., & Mintz, J. (2006). DSM-IV diagnosed posttraumatic stress disorder in women veterans with and without military sexual trauma. *Journal of General Internal Medicine, 21*(Suppl 3), S65–S69.

Zatzick, D. F., Marmar, C. R., Weiss, D. S., Browner, W. S., Metzler, T. J., Golding, J. M., Stewart, A., Schlenger, W. E., & Wells, K. B. (1997). Posttraumatic stress disorder and functioning and quality of life outcomes in a nationally representative sample of male Vietnam veterans. *American Journal of Psychiatry, 154*(12), 1690–1695.

Part VI
Special Treatment Modalities

Scott D. Litwack, J. Gayle Beck, and Denise M. Sloan

The technique of organized group therapy began around 1905 with J. H. Pratt. Pratt led instructional groups with tuberculosis patients designed to provide information about their illness, when he realized the emotional support that patients were experiencing in the group format (Barlow et al. 2000). Other early pioneers included the social worker Jane Addams, who organized immigrant support groups in Chicago, as well as the psychoanalyst Trigant Burrow, who began experimenting with group psychoanalysis techniques in 1925 (Ward 2010). Group therapy for trauma-related difficulties appears to first be documented after World War II, when large numbers of veterans struggled with "battle fatigue" and the resources of support and treatment were deficient (Grotjahn 1947). Group treatment of trauma-related problems was further popularized with the introduction of "rap groups" for combat veterans in the 1960s (Foy et al. 2000). Since this era, substantial advances have been made in individual psychosocial treatment approaches for trauma-related disorders, including the development and testing of several empirically supported treatments

This work was supported in part by Grant I01 CX000467-01A1, Veteran's Administration MERIT program awarded to D.M. Sloan and W. S. Unger, as well as funds provided by the Lillian and Morrie Moss Chair of Excellence at the University of Memphis (J. G. Beck).

S.D. Litwack (✉)
VA Boston Healthcare System, Boston, MA, USA

Boston University School of Medicine, Boston, MA, USA

J.G. Beck
Department of Psychology, University of Memphis, Memphis, TN, USA

D.M. Sloan
VA Boston Healthcare System, Boston, MA, USA

Boston University School of Medicine, Boston, MA, USA

Behavioral Science Division, National Center for PTSD, Boston, MA, USA
e-mail: Scott. Litwack@va.gov

© Springer International Publishing Switzerland 2015
U. Schnyder, M. Cloitre (eds.), *Evidence Based Treatments for Trauma-Related Psychological Disorders: A Practical Guide for Clinicians*,
DOI 10.1007/978-3-319-07109-1_23

(see Beck and Sloan 2012). Unfortunately, group treatments for trauma-related disorders have lagged behind these efforts, owing to considerable methodological issues that are intrinsic to the study of group therapy (see Beck and Sloan 2014; Sloan et al. 2012). This gap in our knowledge of effective group treatments is problematic as the group approach is frequently used in clinical settings (e.g., Rosen et al. 2004).

In this chapter, we will briefly review what is known about group treatment for trauma-related psychological disorders and describe the advantages of group treatment relative to individual-format therapies. Also, clinical aspects of group treatment for trauma survivors will be discussed, including various facets of clinical lore about treating trauma-related symptoms in a group setting. Finally, we will summarize key directions for clinical applications of group treatments for trauma-related disorders, as well as needed research directions.

23.1 History of Studying Group Treatment for Trauma Survivors

Early studies of group treatments for trauma survivors were conducted in the late 1970s and 1980s and examined the efficacy of group treatments for female survivors of child sexual abuse and sexual assault (e.g., Carver et al. 1989; Cryer and Beutler 1980). These initial studies often consisted of a single group of women in a supportive group environment without a comparison or wait-list condition. For example, Cryer and Buetler (1980) found that after 10 weeks of supportive group therapy, nine female sexual assault victims reported decreased distress, obsessiveness, and anxiety and increased expression of control. Although these findings were encouraging, the lack of a comparison condition in combination with the small sample size limited the conclusions that could be drawn from these studies.

Beginning in the mid- to late 1980s, there was a rapid shift to investigating more active group treatments, and researchers began to incorporate comparison conditions (e.g., Alexander et al. 1989; Resick et al. 1988; Roth et al. 1988). However, these studies continued to only include women survivors of child sexual abuse and sexual assault. In the late 1990s and early 2000s, researchers began to broaden examinations of the efficacy of active group treatments to survivors of other types of traumas, such as combat traumas (e.g., Schnurr et al. 2003) and motor vehicle accidents (Beck et al. 2009). The literature on group treatments for trauma-related symptoms has been growing considerably over the two decades.

23.2 Efficacy of Group Treatment for Trauma-Based Psychological Symptoms

With the increasing number of studies investigating the efficacy of group treatment for trauma-related symptoms, several recent reviews of group treatment for PTSD symptoms have been conducted. These reviews have focused on randomized controlled trials (RCTs) that included individuals who were at least 18 years old and either were identified as trauma survivors or diagnosed with PTSD (Beck and Sloan 2014; Sloan et al. 2013, 2012). Cognitive behavioral interventions that focus on exposure predominate in this literature, although a number of other therapeutic approaches are included (e.g., spiritually integrated therapy, interpersonal therapy). Overall, between-group effect sizes for group treatment in these RCTs are small to moderate; a meta-analysis by Sloan et al. (2013) noted that the average effect size was $d=0.24$. Notably, these effects are smaller than those reported for evidence-based individual treatments for PTSD, which tend to obtain large effect sizes of at least $d=1.0$ (e.g., Cahill et al. 2009). Another important aspect of the studies conducted to date is that the majority have included a no treatment, wait-list comparison condition. Thus, the significant between-group effect size indicates that group treatment for posttraumatic stress symptoms is better than no treatment. There are a number of group treatment studies for trauma survivors that are underway and include a treatment comparison condition. The findings of these studies will be important to advancing our knowledge of the efficacy of cognitive behavioral group treatments for trauma survivors.

Another important aspect of the studies conducted to date is that almost all of the cognitive behavioral group treatment approaches include exposure-based techniques as a central component of the intervention. This is not surprising given the evidence that exposure-based techniques are an essential feature of effective treatments for PTSD (Institute of Medicine 2008). However, the content of these exposure-based group treatments can vary considerably.

23.2.1 Exposure-Based Group Treatment

Several variations of exposure-based group treatment for trauma survivors have been developed, with considerable variability in the format in which imaginal exposure is conducted (e.g., written versus oral), the format of exposures (imaginal, in vivo), and the proportion of total treatment time that is dedicated to trauma exposure. In addition, the exposure-based group treatments involve a variety of treatment components, which can include cognitive restructuring, relapse prevention, and adaptive coping skills. For example, in their study of 360 male Vietnam veterans, Schnurr and colleagues (2003) conducted 30, 90–120-min sessions with 5 additional booster sessions. Of the 30 group treatment sessions, two sessions focused on autobiographical writing that included the trauma event, and 14 sessions focused on participants' verbal recounts of trauma experiences within the group session. Beck and colleagues (2009) administered a total of 14, 120-min sessions to 44 motor vehicle accident survivors. Participants engaged in written trauma accounts conducted within the group treatment sessions. In vivo exposures were conducted outside of the treatment sessions and then reviewed during group sessions. Both group treatments examined by Schnurr et al. and Beck and colleagues also included components of cognitive restructuring and relapse prevention.

An important aspect of exposure-based treatment groups is that the majority of the studies included participants who had the same type of trauma exposure (e.g., motor vehicle accident, Beck et al. 2009; child sexual abuse, Classen et al. 2011; combat veterans, Schnurr et al. 2003), although a few studies have included participants with mixed-trauma events (e.g., Hollifield et al. 2007). It is also important to highlight that although some promising findings have been observed for these treatments, there does not yet appear to be any specific group treatment approach for trauma survivors that meets the criteria of a "well-established" or even "probably efficacious treatment" according to the standards described by Chambless and Hollon (1998). Furthermore, while exposure-based techniques all have the commonality of incorporating imaginal and/or in vivo exposures, the considerable methodological differences among these treatment approaches make direct comparisons difficult.

23.2.2 Non-exposure-Based Group Treatment Approaches

There is limited information on the efficacy of non-trauma-focused group treatment approaches for trauma survivors. As previously indicated, most RCTs of group treatment for trauma symptoms have focused on exposure-based approaches. However, there have been several RCTs of group treatment that feature non-trauma-focused approaches. For instance, Zlotnick and colleagues (1997) studied the efficacy of an affect management group treatment for women survivors of childhood sexual abuse relative to a wait-list control condition. Affect management group is a 2-h, 15-session treatment that emphasizes skills in effective methods to manage negative affect. Techniques include distraction, distress tolerance, relaxation, and self-soothing. Material from dialectical behavior therapy (Linehan 1993) is also incorporated. Difficulties in managing negative affect are a core problem among individuals with PTSD symptoms; thus, the approach to develop effective affect management skills has much appeal. Despite this appeal, findings from Zlotnick et al. indicated no significant group differences between participants randomized to the affect management treatment group relative to those randomized to the wait-list condition (between-group effect size $d = .04$). No additional studies of affect management group treatment for trauma survivors have been reported since the study by Zlotnick and colleagues.

Krupnick et al. (2008) investigated the efficacy of group interpersonal psychotherapy (IPT) for women diagnosed with chronic PTSD resulting from interpersonal trauma. Women were assigned to either the group IPT condition or a wait-list control condition. IPT consisted of 16, 2-h sessions. The treatment was adapted from Interpersonal Psychotherapy for Depression (Klerman et al. 1984) with the goal of improving interpersonal skills which, in turn, were hypothesized to improve interpersonal functioning. The adaptation of IPT for PTSD addresses how trauma histories negatively impact interpersonal relations. The goal of improving interpersonal skills is important given the substantial difficulties individuals diagnosed with PTSD have with interpersonal relationships (American Psychiatric Association

2013). Findings from Krupnick and colleagues indicated that individuals assigned to IPT showed significant reductions in PTSD symptoms relative to participants assigned to the wait-list condition (large between-group effect size $d = .91$).

More recently, Harris and colleagues (2011) examined whether a 2-h, eight-session spiritually integrated group treatment for military trauma survivors was efficacious in reducing PTSD symptoms relative to a wait-list comparison condition. This treatment uses preexisting faith resources to manage the impact of trauma. Reconciling spiritual beliefs that conflict with trauma experience is one aspect of the treatment, along with enhancing areas of spiritual functioning that contribute to positive functioning. This treatment approach has much appeal as trauma survivors can have difficulty reconciling the occurrence of traumatic events with their spiritual beliefs (Litz et al. 2009). Harris et al. found significant reductions in PTSD symptoms for the spiritually focused treatment relative to the control condition (between-group effect size $d = .58$).

Another type of non-trauma-focused group treatment is anger management. Difficulties in managing anger are a prominent problem for trauma survivors, especially veterans (e.g., Lloyd et al. 2014; Morland et al. 2012). Patients are generally motivated to receive treatment for anger problems, even when they are reluctant to receive trauma-focused treatment (Morland et al. 2012). Morland and colleagues (2010) compared anger management group treatment delivered in person to group anger management treatment delivered via videoconferencing. Participants were military veterans diagnosed with PTSD. As anticipated, findings indicated that veterans in both anger management group treatment formats had significant reductions in anger symptoms. Significant symptom reduction in PTSD was not observed, although this finding was not surprising given the treatment focus on anger management skills. This study is notable as it demonstrates that group treatment can be effectively delivered with the use of videoconference technology, which has implications for delivering treatment to trauma survivors in rural areas or areas in which there is a shortage of therapists with trauma treatment expertise.

One additional non-exposure-based group treatment approach that should be considered is present-centered therapy (PCT). PCT has been included in a number of PTSD treatment studies (e.g., Classen et al. 2011; Schnurr et al. 2003). Although PCT has been included as a comparison condition to control for nonspecific therapy effects (e.g., therapist contact, empathy), findings in a growing number of studies suggest that PCT is an efficacious group approach. For example, in a study of veterans with chronic PTSD, no significant between-group differences were found in PTSD symptom severity following treatment for veterans assigned to the group PCT relative to veterans assigned to an exposure-based group treatment (between-group effect size $d = .14$, Schnurr et al. 2003). Similar findings were obtained by Classen et al. (2011) who investigated the efficacy of trauma-focused cognitive behavioral group treatment relative to group PCT for women survivors of childhood sexual abuse (effect size $d = .14$). Importantly, Classen and colleagues also included a wait-list comparison condition and found that both group PCT and group CBT had significant reduction in PTSD symptom severity following treatment, relative to the wait-list control condition. These findings indicate that the significant reduction in

PTSD symptoms observed for PCT and CBT was the result of the treatment and not some nontreatment-related factor (e.g., time).

These studies provide information on non-trauma-focused group treatment approaches that clinicians might consider. These group treatment approaches may be particularly useful for patients who are not willing to engage in trauma-focused treatment. The decision as to which group treatment approach to use will depend on the needs of the clients as well as the expertise of the clinicians. It should be noted that although efficacy has been found for group IPT, spiritually integrated group treatment, and group PCT, the comparison condition in each of the studies was a wait list (i.e., no treatment). It will be important to demonstrate that each of these treatment approaches is efficacious relative to a condition that controls for nonspecific group treatment effects (i.e., supportive counseling group).

23.3 Methodological Considerations of Group Therapy Studies

Although the evidence for group approaches to trauma-focused problems is growing, it remains considerably less developed than individual approaches for trauma survivors. A number of methodological considerations for conducting RCTs of group treatments have impacted the growth of this research area. First, a factor that must be accounted for in group treatment studies is the effect of the fellow group members on treatment outcome. Because members of a group affect each other, the group cohort effect needs to be accounted for in the analytic approach (Baldwin et al. 2005). This means that the degree of freedom for group treatment studies is the group cohort, not the individual participants, as would be the case for individual treatment studies. Accounting for the group cohort requires a much larger sample size to detect between-group effects than what is needed for individual treatment studies, which in turn increases the cost, time, and complexity of performing group treatment studies.

Another methodological consideration is that participants are randomized to groups, which means that a relatively large number of participants (e.g., 12–16) need to be gathered before randomization to two or more groups can occur. This requirement also means that participants need to be recruited in a relatively short period of time in order to prevent lengthy wait times prior to the start of treatment. Because participants will require some delay between enrolling in the study and starting treatment, there is a need to provide clinical management prior to the beginning of group treatment.

Relatedly, because a large number of participants are randomized and start treatment at the same time, this also means that the same group of participants needs to have follow-up assessments conducted at the same time. Conducting a large number of assessments in a very short period of time requires sufficient staffing. Thus, staffing needs for group treatment studies tend to be more demanding and complicated than what is required for individual treatment studies.

Another methodological consideration specific to research on group treatments of trauma-related disorders is whether to recruit groups of individuals who have experienced different types of trauma or to restrict the treatment to specific types of trauma (e.g., child sexual abuse, motor vehicle accidents, combat). While an advantage to mixed-trauma groups is a potential increase in the degree of generalizability and real-world application, such mixed-trauma groups also have the potential to increase intragroup difficulties and decrease the degree to which group members feel that they can relate to each other.

In considering this literature, it is notable that the most commonly studied individual treatments (PROLONGED EXPOSURE THERAPY AND COGNITIVE PROCESSING THERAPY; see Chaps. 8 and 10) have not been studied using the RCT design when administered in a group format, although RCTs are underway. Instead, most of the group cognitive behavioral approaches that have been studied are "package" interventions, treatments that include a mixture of some form of exposure, cognitive therapy, relapse prevention, treatment elements targeting depression, and the like.

One reason evidence-based treatments for PTSD have not been examined in a group format is because these treatments are difficult to conduct in a group setting. For example, a core component of PROLONGED EXPOSURE THERAPY is imaginal exposure of the trauma memory that is conducted in session. It may be difficult to conduct imaginal exposure within a group as one group member's trauma account may trigger trauma memories from the other group members. It would be difficult to manage such trauma reactions of multiple group members while simultaneously conducting imaginal exposure with a specific group member. Moreover, group members may find the group experience to be aversive because of the triggering they experience. One alternative approach would be to have group members write their trauma accounts rather than providing a verbal account of the memory; the written trauma narrative approach has been successfully used by others in a PTSD treatment format (e.g., Beck et al. 2009). Alternatively, Chard (2005) modified COGNITIVE PROCESSING THERAPY so that the treatment sessions that focused on the patient reading the trauma accounts and trauma impact to the therapist occurred during individual treatment, whereas other sessions were conducted within a group setting. Combining individual and group sessions allowed for the benefits of the group setting to be obtained, such as the social component and normalizing of symptoms, while still delivering the components of the treatment that are best conducted in an individual format. Beidel and her colleagues (2011) used a similar treatment approach. Specifically, exposure-based treatment sessions were first delivered individually, and the remaining treatment sessions that focused on social skills were conducted in a group setting. Although conducting exposure-based components of PTSD treatment can be challenging in a group setting, Ready and his colleagues (2008) have reported success conducting imaginal exposure by verbally recounting trauma events within the group treatment setting. This treatment uses an intensive outpatient program to deliver PTSD treatment with a veteran population.

23.4   Considerations for Different Trauma Populations and Different Settings

The majority of group treatment studies for trauma-related symptoms that have been conducted have included only adult survivors of childhood sexual abuse and/ or interpersonal violence. In addition, most of these studies included only women. Sloan and colleagues (2013) found that gender moderated within-group treatment effects for PTSD symptom severity; studies that included men were noted to have a significantly smaller effect size than studies that included women or mixed gender samples. However, a moderator effect was also observed for type of trauma, with studies that included combat veterans having a smaller within-group treatment effect than other trauma types. It is likely that the observed gender moderator effect was the result of trauma type as the studies that included men were also studies of combat veterans. The moderator finding suggests that combat-related PTSD may be more difficult to treat in a group format relative to other types of trauma. However, it may also be the case that participants with combat-related trauma represent a very chronic sample, and the chronicity of the disorder reduces the treatment outcome effect. Overall, the findings of group treatment for trauma survivors have limited application for clinical settings where mixed gender- and/or mixed-trauma-type groups are desired. Additional studies that mirror the clinical practice of groups with diverse patient members would be welcome in this literature.

Although we have limited information on the efficacy of group approaches for survivors of different trauma events, there is currently no evidence that any group treatment approach is more efficacious for a particular trauma sample. Survivors of traumatic events share common posttraumatic stress symptoms; thus, group treatment designed to target these symptoms (e.g., avoidance behaviors, cognitive restructuring skills, distress tolerance skills) should work equally well regardless of the specific trauma experience. As previously mentioned, it may be important to consider the chronicity of PTSD symptoms as more chronic (and severe) trauma-related symptoms may require more extensive treatment than what is included in most group treatments described in the literature (e.g., 12–16 sessions). It is also worth noting that the majority of studies examining group treatment for trauma-related symptoms have not required that participants meet diagnostic criteria for PTSD but rather display PTSD symptoms. Therefore, the group treatment approaches studied to date would be appropriate for individuals with PTSD symptoms, regardless of whether or not PTSD diagnostic criteria are met.

The clinical setting in which group therapies are conducted can also be an important factor that can influence the nature and focus of the group. For example, as previously mentioned, Ready and colleagues (2008) developed a treatment for an intensive outpatient setting in which patients attend 3 h of group therapy twice per week for 16–18 weeks. This treatment includes 4–5 weeks of psychoeducation and stress management skills, followed by 60 h of exposure (3 h of recounting the trauma memory verbally per each patient, 27 h of hearing other patients' trauma accounts, and 30 h of listening to recording of one's own trauma account). Findings indicated that veteran participants reported significant reductions in PTSD symptoms at follow-up assessment compared to pretreatment assessment (within-group effect size Hedges $g = 1.22$). Notably, of 102 veterans, only three dropped out of treatment. The unusually low treatment dropout rate may be attributable to the strong social connections that are developed in an intensive outpatient group treatment. Given the available evidence, it appears feasible to conduct an evidence-based treatment approach for PTSD in a group setting, although some modifications to delivering the treatment may be needed and using a combination of individual and group sessions might also be considered.

In considering group treatments for PTSD, it is notable that several approaches have been developed that expressly target patients with comorbid PTSD and an additional psychiatric disorder (see also Part IV, Chaps. 16, 17, and 18, this volume). Seeking Safety (Najavits et al. 1998) is perhaps one of the better known treatments in this category. This intervention is designed for men and women who suffer from comorbid PTSD and substance use disorders (SUDs). At present, only two RCTs have examined Seeking Safety, with a notable lack of differences between this intervention and psychoeducation on PTSD and substance use outcomes (Hien et al. 2009; Zlotnick et al. 2009).

A recent study by van Dam, Ehring, Vedel, and Emmelkamp (2013) investigated the efficacy of a combined treatment approach for PTSD and comorbid substance use disorder. The efficacy of combining structured writing therapy (SWT; Lange et al. 2001) with group treatment for substance use disorders was examined. SWT is an individual treatment approach in which individuals conduct multiple writing sessions during which they write about their traumatic experience and the impact the experience has had on their lives. In the van Dam et al. study, participants were assigned to either the SWT plus group substance use disorder treatment or group substance use disorder treatment only. Reductions were observed in substance use and PTSD symptoms for both treatment conditions, although no significant between-group differences were found. However, at follow-up assessment, the SWT plus group treatment condition displayed significantly lower rates of PTSD diagnosis relative to group treatment-only condition. Caution should be exercised when interpreting these findings as the study had a small sample size ($N = 34$). Nonetheless, the findings from this study suggest that comorbid PTSD and substance use disorder may benefit from a combined treatment approach.

Although the available research has not identified an effective treatment approach for comorbid PTSD and substance use, it is important to acknowledge that there is a pressing need to develop and investigate treatments that target the comorbidity that appears to be intrinsic to PTSD, particularly SUDs (Henslee and Coffey 2010). In particular, because substance abuse services tend to be distinct from mental health treatment services, it would seem timely to consider how best to integrate PTSD treatment into usual care models for SUDs.

Comorbid personality disorders are also fairly prevalent among patients diagnosed with PTSD and may require additional treatment components to address the personality disorder symptoms in combination with PTSD symptoms. A recent study conducted by Dorrepaal and colleagues (2013) addressed this question with a sample of women with child abuse-related PTSD as well as comorbid personality disorder symptoms. The cognitive behavioral group treatment consisted of 20 weekly 2-h sessions that included psychoeducation, emotion regulation skills, and cognitive restructuring. A treatment-as-usual (TAU) condition was included as the comparison group. When examining treatment completers, both treatments were found to be associated with a significant decrease in PTSD symptoms, with the CBT group approach having a large effect size and TAU having a medium effect size. Furthermore, women with PTSD who also had high levels of personality disorder symptoms were found to be equally responsive to the group treatment when compared to women with PTSD who had few personality disorder symptoms. Importantly, when intent-to-treat analyses were conducted, neither of the treatments was found to be associated with significant improvement from pretreatment scores. Additional group clinical trials examining comorbid personality disorders and PTSD are indicated, with particular attention paid to retention along with responsiveness to treatment.

Medical comorbidities, such as chronic pain and traumatic brain injury (TBI), have the potential to further complicate group treatments for PTSD. While considerations of comorbid medical conditions when providing individual treatment for PTSD have recently received increased attention (see Chap. 5), there is a lack of investigations or guidelines for group treatments for individuals with PTSD and comorbid medical concerns. There is some evidence to indicate that individual treatments (e.g., Prolonged Exposure Therapy) that have worked well for individuals with PTSD may also work well for those with comorbid PTSD and chronic pain (e.g., Blanchard et al. 2003) or TBI (e.g., Sripada et al. 2013). VA/DOD PTSD treatment guidelines (2010) note that there is no evidence to support withholding PTSD treatments while addressing symptoms of TBI. However, with regard to group treatment, it is important to consider the extreme range of symptoms and symptom severity that individuals with chronic medical conditions may present with. Attention to the severity of medical problems during the recruitment phase of the group, as well as a high degree of flexibility with regard to group focus and content, may be necessary.

When treating individuals with TBI and/or chronic pain, collaborative care teams are often recommended (Walker et al. 2010). With this in mind, it may be that group treatments for PTSD and these comorbid conditions may be best delivered within a broader formalized program of care (e.g., poly-trauma teams) simplifying the coordination of care for both providers and patients.

Importantly, there are many reasons why group treatments for PTSD-TBI and PTSD-chronic pain comorbidities may be particularly beneficial to individuals. The normalization of symptoms as well as increased socialization may be particularly important for individuals suffering from such comorbidities, as each of these disorders often contributes to greater levels of isolation and social impairment. In addition, group treatments allow for individuals to benefit from the experiences of other individuals with similar psychiatric and medical concerns.

23.5   Benefits of Group Treatment

Although much less is known about effective group treatments for PTSD, group treatment offers several advantages over individual treatment approaches. Individuals with trauma-related psychological disorders are often socially isolated and have difficulty trusting others (Brewin et al. 2000). The context of the group provides an opportunity for patients to develop social relationships and the opportunity to trust others in a safe environment. Indeed, some argue that the social aspect of group treatment is a central mechanism through which change occurs (e.g., Yalom 1995). Another benefit of group treatment is the opportunity for the patient to learn that other trauma survivors experience similar symptoms. The normalizing of trauma symptoms can lead to the patient feeling less distressed about their symptoms and less alone in their suffering. Group members may also be able to challenge each other in ways the therapist cannot because of the shared status of being a trauma survivor. Another potential advantage of group treatment is that it may be more cost effective for settings that have limited staff resources; however, there is no available data on the cost effectiveness of group treatment relative to individual treatment of PTSD.

23.6 Considerations for Group Treatment

Although group treatment is a good option for many patients, there are some factors that are negative indicators for group treatment. For instance, patients that are currently psychotic are not good candidates for group treatment as their psychotic symptoms may cause disruption within the group and may interfere with developing trust and rapport with other group members. Current substance abuse may also negatively impact the group process if group members attend intoxicated. Some personality characteristics may also be problematic in a group setting, such as narcissism or psychopathy. Moreover, patients who experience severe emotion dysregulation may not be good candidates for group treatment. Cloitre and Koenen (2001) investigated whether patients with borderline personality disorder (BPD) affected an interpersonal group treatment among a group of women with PTSD related to childhood sexual assault. These investigators found that groups that did not include individuals with BPD had greater treatment gains relative to groups that included patients with BPD. Moreover, group members reported greater anger at posttreatment when the group included patients with BPD. Cloitre and Koenen speculated that including patients with BPD in these groups leads to an "anger contagion." The results of this study suggested that caution be taken in mixing individuals with and without BPD, at least in groups that include exploration of interpersonal reactions and processes.

There are several other important patient characteristics that should be considered with group treatment. First, there may be some reluctance to mix patients who have been suffering from chronic PTSD for years with patients who have PTSD or other trauma-related disorders as a result of more recent and/or single-incident trauma(s) within the same group. This concern is common among clinicians working with combat veterans from different conflict eras. However, it is our experience that not only can veterans of different war eras (e.g., Vietnam, Iraq, and Afghanistan) be included in the same group, but there may be some advantages to doing so. For instance, older veterans may be able to talk with younger veterans about the importance of getting treatment for PTSD soon after the combat trauma based on their own life experiences living with chronic PTSD. This information can have a powerful impact on younger veterans in a way that would not occur if the information came from a therapist. Additionally, at times we have found older veterans to exhibit greater motivation to decrease avoidance behaviors and engage productively in treatment as a result of an expressed desire to act as a model for younger group members. It has also been our experience that combat veterans from different war eras share more commonalities than differences and this may also be true for civilians with different degrees of trauma-related symptom chronicity.

Although there are advantages to mixing patients of varying ages and backgrounds into a group, caution should be taken when including men and women in the same group. Women survivors of sexual assault may feel uncomfortable being in a group that includes men if they were assaulted by a man. A similar situation arises for men who have trauma-related disorders related to sexual assault perpetrated by a man. This is also the case for men veterans who have experienced military sexual assault. As the majority of veterans presenting for mental health services in VA care settings are men (United States Government Accountability Office 2011), treatment groups may solely or mostly consist of men. Thus, attention should be given to the trauma background and sex of the patients being considered for the group.

Groups introduce the considerable challenge of navigating many relationships (e.g., 40 dyadic relationships if group consists of six patients and two therapists) in each treatment encounter. Although group therapy can be an ideal context in which to increase social connectivity, trust, and self-esteem, there is also a potential for individuals to experience other group members as critical or unsafe, which can reinforce avoidance. An additional challenge of providing group therapy is the degree of time and energy required to support 6–8 group members outside of the group time. Although RCTs often have project coordinators who are able to provide much of this extra support, in "real-world" clinical settings such support staff typically does not exist. Effectiveness studies examining the provision of group treatments for PTSD in such real-world settings are indicated.

23.7 Summary

Group treatment for PTSD is frequently used in clinical practice, and patients report high levels of satisfaction with this approach; however, to date there are no evidence-based group treatments for PTSD. The evidence that does exist suggests that group treatment is efficacious relative to no treatment but may not differ from supportive counseling group treatment (e.g., present-centered group treatment). Nonetheless, caution needs to be taken when interpreting the literature given the limited work that has been conducted.

There are a number of advantages to using group treatment including the social aspect of the group and the ability of group members to motivate each other toward treatment goals. There are also a number of important factors to consider when deciding whether or not a patient may benefit from group treatment. These factors include personality characteristics, comorbid conditions, ability to regulate affect, and the gender composition of the group. Based on our collective experience, group therapy for trauma-related disorders can be successfully conducted with group members that vary in terms of age and trauma index event. In terms of deciding what type of group treatment is best to use, there is limited research that can be used in making this decision. We look forward to the results of a number of randomized controlled trials that are currently underway that will provide important information comparing individual versus group treatment approaches as well as cognitive behavioral versus supportive counseling group treatment approaches.

References

Alexander, P. C., Neimeyer, R. A., Follette, V. M., Moore, M. K., & Harter, S. (1989). A comparison of group treatments of women sexually abused as children. *Journal of Consulting and Clinical Psychology, 57*, 479–483. doi:10.1037/0022-006X.57.4.479.

American Psychiatric Association. (2013). *Diagnostic and statistical manual of mental disorders* (5th ed.). Arlington: American Psychiatric Association.

Baldwin, S. A., Murray, D. M., & Shadish, W. R. (2005). Empirically supported treatments or type I errors? Problems with the analysis of data from group-administered treatments. *Journal of Consulting and Clinical Psychology, 73*, 924–935. doi:10.1037/0022-006X.73.5.924.

Barlow, S., Fuhriman, A., & Burlingame, G. (2000). The therapeutic application of groups: From Pratt's "thought control classes" to modern group psychotherapy. *Journal of Group Dynamics: Theory, Research, and Practice, 41*, 115–134.

Beck, J. G., & Sloan, D. M. (Eds.). (2012). *Handbook of traumatic stress disorders*. New York: Oxford University Press.

Beck, J. G., & Sloan, D. M. (2014). Group treatments for PTSD: What do we know, what do we need to know?. In M. J. Friedman, T. M. Keane, & P. A. Resick (Eds.), *Handbook of PTSD: Science and Practice*, 2nd ed. (pp 466–481). New York: Guilford Press.

Beck, J. G., Coffey, S. F., Foy, D. W., Keane, T. M., & Blanchard, E. B. (2009). Group cognitive behavior therapy for chronic posttraumatic stress disorder: An initial randomized pilot study. *Behavior Therapy, 40*, 82–92. doi:10.1016/j.beth.2008.01.003.

Beidel, D. C., Frueh, B. C., Uhde, T. W., Wong, N., & Mentrikoski, J. M. (2011). Multicomponent behavioral treatment for chronic combat-related posttraumatic stress disorder: A randomized controlled trial. *Journal of Anxiety Disorders, 25*, 224–231. doi:10.1016/j.janxdis.2010.09.006.

Blanchard, E. B., Hickling, E. J., Devineni, T., Veazey, C. H., Galovski, T. E., Mundy, E., Malta, L. S., & Buckley, T. C. (2003). A controlled evaluation of cognitive behavioral therapy for posttraumatic stress in motor vehicle accident survivors. *Behaviour Research and Therapy, 41*, 79–96. doi:10.1016/S0005-7967(01)00131-0.

Brewin, C. R., Andrews, B., & Valentine, J. D. (2000). Meta-analysis of risk factors for posttraumatic stress disorder in trauma-exposed adults. *Journal of Consulting and Clinical Psychology, 68*, 748–766. doi:10.1037/0022-006X.68.5.748.

Cahill, S. P., Rothbaum, B. O., Resick, P. A., & Folette, V. M. (2009). Cognitive-behavioral therapy for adults. In E. B. Foa, T. M. Keane, M. J. Friedman, & J. A. Cohen (Eds.), *Effective treatments for PTSD. Practice guidelines from the International Society for Traumatic Stress Studies* (pp. 139–222). New York: Guilford Press.

Carver, C. M., Stalker, C. A., Stewart, E., & Abraham, B. (1989). The impact of group therapy for adult survivors of childhood sexual abuse. *Canadian Journal of Psychiatry, 34*, 753–758.

Chambless, D. L., & Hollon, S. (1998). Defining empirically supported therapies. *Journal of Consulting and Clinical Psychology, 66*, 7–18. doi:10.1037/0022-006X.66.1.7.

Chard, K. M. (2005). An evaluation of cognitive processing therapy for the treatment of posttraumatic stress disorder related to childhood sexual abuse. *Journal of Consulting and Clinical Psychology, 73*, 965–971. doi:10.1037/0022-006X.73.5.965.

Classen, C. C., Palesh, O. G., Cavanaugh, C. E., Koopman, C. E., Kaupp, J. W., Kraemer, H. C., Aggarwal, R., & Spiegel, D. (2011). A comparison of trauma-focused and present-focused group therapy for survivors of childhood sexual abuse: A randomized controlled trial. *Psychological Trauma: Theory, Research, Practice, and Policy, 3*, 84–93. doi:10.1037/a0020096002/jts.20214.

Cloitre, M., & Koenen, K. C. (2001). The impact of borderline personality disorder on process group outcome among women with posttraumatic stress disorder related to childhood abuse. *International Journal of Group Psychotherapy, 51*, 379–398. doi:10.1521/ijgp.51.3.379.49886.

Cryer, L., & Beutler, L. E. (1980). Group therapy: An alternative treatment approach for rape victims. *Journal of Sex and Marital Therapy, 6*, 40–46.

Dorrepall, E., Thomaes, K., Smit, J. H., Veltman, D. J., Hoogendoorn, A. W., van Balkom, A. J. L. M., & Draijer, N. (2013). Treatment compliance and effectiveness in complex PTSD patients with co-morbid personality disorder undergoing stabilizing cognitive behavioral group treatment: A preliminary study. *European Journal of Psychotraumatology, 4*, 2171. doi:10.3402/ejpt.v4i0.21171.

Foy, D. W., Glynn, S. M., Schnurr, P. P., Jankowski, M. K., Wattenberg, M. S., Weiss, D. S., Gusman, F. D., et al. (2000). Group therapy. In E. B. Foa, T. M. Keane, & M. J. Friedman (Eds.), *Effective treatments for PTSD: Practice guidelines from the International Society for Traumatic Stress Studies* (pp. 155–175). New York: Guilford Press.

Grotjahn, M. (1947). Experience with group psychotherapy as a method of treatment for veterans. *American Journal of Psychiatry, 103*, 637–643.

Harris, J. I., Erbes, C. R., Engdahl, B. E., Thuras, P., Murray-Swank, N., Grace, D., Ogden, H., Olson, R. H., Winskowski, A. M., Bacon, R., Malec, C., Campion, K., & Le, T. (2011). The effectiveness of a trauma focused spiritually integrated intervention for veterans exposed to trauma. *Journal of Clinical Psychology, 67*, 425–438. doi:10.1002/jclp.20777.

Henslee, A. M., & Coffey, S. F. (2010). Exposure therapy for posttraumatic stress disorder in a residential substance use treatment facility. *Professional Psychology: Research and Practice, 41*, 34–40. doi:10.1037/a0018235.

Hien, D. A., Wells, E. A., Jiang, H., Suarez-Morales, L., Campbell, A. N., Cohen, L. R., Miele, G. M., Killeen, T., Brigham, G. S., Zhang, Y., Hansen, C., Hodgkins, C., Hatch-Maillette, M., Brown, C., Kulaga, A., Kristman-Valente, A., Chu, M., Sage, R., Robinson, J. A., Liu, D., & Nunes, E. V. (2009). Multisite randomized trial of behavioral interventions for women with co-occurring PTSD and substance use disorders. *Journal of Consulting and Clinical Psychology, 77*, 607–619. doi:10.1037/a0016227.

Hollifield, M., Sinclair-Lian, N., Warner, T., & Hammerschlag, R. (2007). Acupuncture for posttraumatic stress disorder: A randomized controlled pilot trial. *Journal of Nervous and Mental Disease, 195*, 504–513. doi:10.1097/NMD.0b013e31803044f8.

Institute of Medicine. (2008). *Treatment of posttraumatic stress disorder: An assessment of the evidence*. Washington, DC: National Academies Press.

Klerman, G., Weissman, M., Rounseville, B., & Chevron, E. (1984). *Interpersonal psychotherapy of depression*. New York: Basic Books.

Krupnick, J. L., Green, B. L., Stockton, P., Miranda, J., Krause, E., & Mete, M. (2008). Group interpersonal psychotherapy for low-income women with posttraumatic stress disorder. *Psychotherapy Research, 18*, 497–507. doi:10.1080/10503300802183678.

Lange, A., Van de Ven, J. P., Schrieken, B., & Emmelkamp, P. M. G. (2001). Interapy: Treatment of posttraumatic stress through the Internet: A controlled trial. *Journal of Behaviour Therapy and Experimental Psychiatry, 32*, 73–90.

Linehan, M. (1993). *Cognitive-behavioral treatment of borderline personality disorder*. New York: Guilford Press.

Litz, B. T., Stein, N., Delaney, E., Lebowitz, L., Nash, W. P., Silva, C., & Maguen, S. (2009). Moral injury and moral repair in war veterans: A preliminary model and intervention strategy. *Clinical Psychology Review, 29*, 695–706. doi:10.1016/j.cpr.2009.07.003.

Lloyd, D., Nixon, R. D. V., Varker, T., Elliott, P., Perry, D., Bryant, R. A., Creamer, M., & Forbes, D. (2014). Comorbidity in the prediction of cognitive processing therapy treatment outcomes for combat-related posttraumatic stress disorder. *Journal of Anxiety Disorders, 28*, 237–240. doi:10.1016/j.janxdis.2013.12.002.

Morland, L. A., Greene, C. J., Rosen, C. S., Foy, D., Reilly, P., Shore, J., He, Q., & Frueh, B. C. (2010). Telemedicine for anger management therapy in a rural population of combat veterans with posttraumatic stress disorder: A randomized noninferiority trial. *Journal of Clinical Psychiatry, 71*, 855–863. doi:10.4088/JCP.09m05604blu.

Morland, L. A., Love, A. R., Mackintosh, M.-A., Greene, C. J., & Rosen, C. S. (2012). Treating anger and aggression in military populations: Research updates and clinical implications. *Clinical Psychology: Science and Practice, 19*, 305–322. doi:10.1111/cpsp.12007.

Najavits, L. M., Weiss, R. D., Shaw, S. R., & Muenz, L. R. (1998). 'Seeking Safety': Outcome of a new cognitive-behavioral psychotherapy for women with posttraumatic stress disorder and substance dependence. *Journal of Traumatic Stress, 11*, 437–456. doi:10.1023/A:1024496427434.

Ready, D. J., Thomas, K. R., Worley, V., Backscheider, A. G., Harvey, L. A., Baltzell, D., & Rothbaum, B. O. (2008). A field test of group based exposure therapy with 102 veterans with war-related posttraumatic stress disorder. *Journal of Traumatic Stress, 21*, 150–157. doi:10.1002/jts.20326.

Resick, P. A., Jordan, C. G., Girelli, S. A., Hutter, C. K., & Marhoefer-Dvorak, S. (1988). A comparative outcome study of behavioral group therapy for sexual assault victims. *Behavior Therapy, 19*, 385–401. doi:10.1016/S0005-7894(88)80011-X.

Rosen, C. S., Chow, H. C., Finney, J. F., Greenbaum, M. A., Moos, R. H., Sheikh, J. I., & Yesavage, J. A. (2004). VA practice patterns and practice guidelines for treating posttraumatic stress disorder. *Journal of Traumatic Stress, 17*, 213–222. doi:10.1023/B:JOTS.0000029264.23878.53.

Roth, S. H., Dye, E., & Lebowitz, L. (1988). Group therapy for sexual assault victims. *Psychotherapy, 25*, 82–93. doi:10.1037/h0085326.

Schnurr, P. P., Friedman, M. J., Foy, D. W., Shea, M. T., Hsieh, F. Y., Lavori, P. W., Glynn, S. M., Wattenberg, M., & Bernardy, N. C. (2003). Randomized trial of trauma-focused group therapy for posttraumatic stress disorder: Results from a Department of Veterans Affairs cooperative study. *Archives of General Psychiatry, 60*, 481–489. doi:10.1001/archpsyc.60.5.481.

Sloan, D. M., Bovin, M. J., Schnurr, P. P., Sloan, D. M., Bovin, M. J., & Schnurr, P. P. (2012). Group treatment for PTSD. *Journal of Rehabilitation Research and Development, 49*, 689–702. http://dx.doi.org/10.1682/JRRD.2011.07.0123

Sloan, D. M., Feinstein, B. A., Gallagher, M. W., Beck, J. G., & Keane, T. M. (2013). Efficacy of group treatment for posttraumatic stress disorder symptoms: A meta-analysis. *Psychological Trauma: Theory, Research, Practice, and Policy, 5*, 176–183. doi:10.1037/a0026291.

Sripada, R. K., Rauch, S. A. M., Tuerk, P. W., Smith, E., Defever, A. M., Mayer, R. A., Messina, M., & Venners, M. (2013). Mild traumatic brain injury and treatment response in prolonged exposure for PTSD. *Journal of Traumatic Stress, 26*, 369–375. doi:10.1002/jts.21813.

U.S. Department of Veterans Affairs & Department of Defense (VA/DoD). (2010). *VA/DoD clinical practice guideline for the management of posttraumatic stress*. Washington, DC: U.S. Department of Veterans Affairs & Department of Defense (VA/DoD).

United States Government Accountability Office. (2011). *VA mental health: Number of veterans receiving care, barriers faced, and efforts to increase access*. Washington, DC: Government Accountability Office.

van Dam, D., Ehring, T., Vedel, E., & Emmelkamp, P. M. G. (2013). Trauma-focused treatment for posttraumatic stress disorder combined with CBT for severe substance use disorder: A randomized controlled trial. *BMC Psychiatry, 13*, 172. doi:10.1186/1471-244X-13-172.

Walker, R. L., Clark, M. E., & Sanders, S. H. (2010). The "Postdeployment Multi-Symptom Disorder": An emerging syndrome in need of a new treatment paradigm. *Psychological Services, 7*, 136–147. doi:10.1037/a0019684.

Ward, D. R. (2010). Definition of group counseling. In R. K. Conyne (Ed.), *The Oxford handbook of group counseling* (pp. 36–51). Oxford: Oxford University Press.

Yalom, I. D. (1995). *The theory and practice of group psychotherapy* (4th ed.). New York: Basic Books.

Zlotnick, C., Shea, T. M., Rosen, K., Simpson, E., Mulrenin, K., Begin, A., & Pearlstein, T. (1997). An affect-management group for women with posttraumatic stress disorder and histories of childhood sexual abuse. *Journal of Traumatic Stress, 10*, 425–436. doi:10.1002/jts.2490100308.

Zlotnick, C., Johnson, J., & Najavits, L. M. (2009). Randomized controlled pilot study of cognitive-behavioral therapy in a sample of incarcerated women with substance use disorder. *Behavior Therapy, 40*, 325–336. doi:10.1016/j.beth.2008.09.004.

Couple Treatment for Posttraumatic Stress Disorder

Candice M. Monson, Anne C. Wagner,
Alexandra Macdonald, and Amy Brown-Bowers

Posttraumatic stress disorder (PTSD) affects not only the people suffering from the disorder but also those surrounding them. PTSD is one of the mental health difficulties most strongly associated with relationship distress (Whisman et al. 2000); it has a strong association with a range of family problems, including mental health difficulties in partners and children (Monson et al. 2009; Renshaw et al. 2011; Taft et al. 2011). PTSD can elicit responses from friends and family that are well-meaning but may maintain the symptoms of PTSD, such as helping the individual with PTSD avoid reminders of the trauma, which may over time erode these relationships and place increased burden on family members, leading to negative mental health outcomes (Caska and Renshaw 2011). These accommodative behaviors may also reinforce avoidance associated with PTSD (Figley 1989). Consistent with research documenting that negative social interactions in the wake of trauma are among the most robust risk factors for PTSD (e.g., see Wagner et al. under review for a review), negative family interactions have been linked to poorer individual cognitive-behavioral therapy outcomes (Monson et al. 2005; Tarrier et al. 1999). Moreover, individual evidence-based treatments for PTSD do not consistently improve relational functioning (e.g., Galovski et al. 2005; Monson et al. 2012c; Lunney and Schnurr 2007). Consequently, there have been efforts to develop and test dyadic treatments that improve relational functioning and PTSD and, in some

C.M. Monson PhD (✉) • A.C. Wagner, PhD • A. Brown-Bowers, MA
Department of Psychology, Ryerson University,
350 Victoria Street, Toronto, ON M5B 2K3, Canada
e-mail: candice.monson@psych.ryerson.ca

A. Macdonald, PhD
Department of Veterans Affairs, Women's Health Sciences Division,
National Center for PTSD, Boston MA, USA

© Springer International Publishing Switzerland 2015
U. Schnyder, M. Cloitre (eds.), *Evidence Based Treatments for Trauma-Related Psychological Disorders: A Practical Guide for Clinicians*,
DOI 10.1007/978-3-319-07109-1_24

cases, also improve the health and well-being of partners. The current chapter describes different ways to conceptualize couple treatment in the case of PTSD and reviews the efficacy of these interventions.

24.1 Conceptualizing Partner Involvement in Treatment

When making the decision to involve loved ones in the treatment of PTSD, it is necessary to establish the treatment targets. More specifically, it is important to establish whether the desired outcomes of treatment are reduction in PTSD symptoms, improved relationship functioning and satisfaction, or both. A heuristic has been developed to describe and categorize the different types of couple treatments for PTSD based on their intended focus – improving PTSD and/or relationship functioning (Monson et al. 2012b). This heuristic builds upon work in both couple and family therapy by expanding the description of couples to include other loved ones (Baucom et al. 1998). This also builds upon work in the substance abuse literature by including interventions that are used to enhance treatment delivery (Miller et al. 1999).

Dyadic interventions for PTSD can be categorized into four general types of intervention:

1. Disorder-specific couple therapy
2. Partner-assisted interventions
3. Generic couple therapy
4. Education and family-facilitated engagement

First, disorder-specific couple therapies are interventions explicitly designed to target both PTSD symptoms and relationship functioning and satisfaction. Loved ones are integrated into these therapies to simultaneously improve both of these targets. Interventions are typically developed to target mechanisms of action that contribute to both treatment targets.

Second, partner-assisted interventions involve loved ones in therapy by having them act as a "coach" to the individual with PTSD, and the treatment target is reduction of PTSD symptoms. The loved one is used to enhance the treatment for the individual with PTSD, and treatment is often delivered in an individual format. Relationship functioning or satisfaction is not the target of these interventions. Rather, the interventions educate loved ones about how to assist the individual with PTSD successfully complete a trauma-focused intervention.

Third, generic couple therapy refers to interventions designed to target relationship functioning. These interventions do not explicitly target PTSD symptoms but may improve PTSD symptoms and the psychological health and well-being of the loved one by improving interpersonal interactions. These treatments do not specifically target the mechanisms maintaining PTSD symptoms, however.

Fourth, interventions may use loved ones to help engage the individual in PTSD treatment and/or to provide psychoeducation about PTSD and evidence-based treatments. The target of these interventions is not PTSD symptom reduction specifically but, rather, engagement in treatment and/or education.

24.2   Evidence Supporting Couple Treatments for PTSD

The following section reviews the evidence for each type of intervention for PTSD, organized according to the heuristic described above (see Table 24.1 for an overview). The review begins with those interventions with the strongest evidence and dual treatment targets.

Table 24.1 Intervention descriptions and key outcomes

Intervention	Description	Key outcomes
Disorder-specific couple therapy		
Cognitive-Behavioral Conjoint Therapy for PTSD (CBCT for PTSD)	15-session dyadic intervention targeting relationship satisfaction and PTSD symptoms. Composed of three phases: (1) psychoeducation and safety building; (2) dyadic skill-building, including communication and in vivo-graded exposures; and (3) trauma-focused cognitive interventions	Three uncontrolled studies and a wait-list controlled trial have demonstrated significant improvement in PTSD symptoms and increased relationship satisfaction (Monson et al. 2004, 2011, 2012a, c; Schumm et al. 2013)
Strategic Approach Therapy (SAT)	10-session couple therapy consisting of three phases: (1) motivational enhancement and psychoeducation, (2) relationship enhancement, and (3) partner-assisted exposures	A sample of six couples found improvement in avoidance and numbing symptoms of PTSD. Relationship adjustment outcomes not reported (Sautter et al. 2009)
Emotionally Focused Couple Therapy for PTSD (EFCT for PTSD)	12–20 session couple therapy focusing on identifying and understanding trauma-associated emotions. Composed of three phases: (1) identifying negative interactions, (2) dyadic skill-building including acceptance and communication, and (3) interactional and coping strategies	Two case studies and one case study replication with 10 couples have found improvements in relationship satisfaction and PTSD symptoms (Greenman and Johnson 2012; Johnson 2002; MacIntosh and Johnson 2008). Several cases of increased emotional abuse were noted, however, in couples where abuse was already present (MacIntosh and Johnson 2008)
Partner-assisted interventions		
Lifestyle Management Course	Five-day group residential program for Australian veterans and partners. Wide range of topics covered, including psychoeducation, self-care, problem-solving, and stress management	Gains in veterans' PTSD symptoms at post-intervention were not maintained at 6-month follow-up. Sustained reductions in depression, anxiety, and stress. No improvement in relationship satisfaction (Devilly 2002)

(continued)

Table 24.1 (continued)

Intervention	Description	Key outcomes
Generic couple therapy		
Behavioral Couple/ Family Therapy (BC/FT)	Behavioral interventions used to improve communication skills and problem-solving	In a randomized controlled trial with BFT following individual exposure therapy versus individual exposure therapy alone revealed greater improvement in problem-solving with BFT. No additional gains in PTSD symptoms with BFT (Glynn et al. 1999). Likewise, uncontrolled trials reveal some improvement in relationship functioning but not PTSD symptoms (Cahoon 1984; Sweany 1987)
K'oach program	Month-long intensive treatment program for Israeli veterans with PTSD. Some spousal involvement. Program includes psychoeducation, communication skills, and problem-solving	Reported improvements in relationship satisfaction. No change reported in PTSD symptoms (Rabin and Nardi 1991; Solomon et al. 1992)
Education and family facilitated engagement		
Support and Family Education program (SAFE)	14-session educational program for family members of veterans with mental health difficulties. Workshop sessions include topics such as psychoeducation, skills training, problem-solving, and stress reduction	Few outcomes reported. Program evaluation noted very high participant satisfaction, and participation led to better understanding of mental health difficulties, awareness of resources, and engagement in self-care (Sherman 2003)
Reaching Out to Educate and Assist Caring, Healthy Families program (REACH)	16-session psychoeducation program for veterans and family members. Three phases included goal-setting and rapport building, psychoeducation, and maintenance of gains	Few outcomes reported. Program evaluation noted high program retention and high participant satisfaction ratings (Sherman et al. 2011)
Coaching into Care program	A telephone intervention available to family members of US veterans providing guidance to encourage veterans to access mental health services	Reports indicate some increase in veteran health-care service use after family members have used the program (Sayers et al. 2011)

24.2.1 Disorder-Specific Couple Therapy

Three types of disorder-specific couple therapy for PTSD have been examined thus far in the literature.

24.2.1.1 Cognitive-Behavioral Conjoint Therapy for PTSD

Cognitive-Behavioral Conjoint Therapy for PTSD (CBCT for PTSD) is a 15-session conjoint therapy designed to reduce PTSD symptoms and enhance relationship satisfaction. The therapy consists of three phases: (1) psychoeducation about PTSD and safety building; (2) dyadic skill-building, specifically focusing on communication skills and graded in vivo approach assignments to reduce avoidance and increase mutually satisfying activities for the dyads; and (3) trauma-specific cognitive interventions to address problematic trauma appraisals and beliefs maintaining PTSD and relationship problems. CBCT for PTSD has been tested in three uncontrolled studies with Vietnam veterans, Iraq/Afghanistan veterans, and community members, as well as a wait-list controlled trial (Monson et al. 2004, 2011, 2012a; Schumm et al. 2013). All four studies have revealed significant improvements in PTSD symptoms as well as increased relationship satisfaction, even when couples do not begin treatment relationally distressed. In addition, intimate partners participating in CBCT for PTSD showed evidence of improvements in their psychological functioning (Monson et al. 2005; Shnaider et al. 2014).

24.2.1.2 Strategic Approach Therapy

Strategic Approach Therapy (SAT) is a 10-session behavioral couple therapy that specifically targets avoidance and numbing symptoms of PTSD. The treatment consists of three phases: (1) motivational enhancement and psychoeducation about PTSD (focusing on avoidance symptoms in particular), (2) relationship enhancement and increased emotional intimacy, and (3) partner-assisted graded exposures for anxiety reduction. One study presenting findings from six couples (all heterosexual couples with male military veteran partners with PTSD) noted significant improvements in overall PTSD symptoms by patient, partner, and clinician ratings, but no reductions in reexperiencing or hyperarousal symptoms, except for patient ratings of reexperiencing. Relationship adjustment outcomes have not been reported (Sautter et al. 2009).

24.2.1.3 Emotionally Focused Couple Therapy for Trauma

Emotionally Focused Couple Therapy for Trauma (EFCT for Trauma) is a 12–20 session experiential couple therapy that focuses on identifying and understanding trauma-associated emotions. The therapy aims to determine how these emotions affect relationships, attachment, and communication. The intervention has three components: (1) identification of negative relational interactions, (2) dyadic skill-building through acceptance and communication, and (3) development and consolidation of positive patterns of interaction and coping strategies. Single-case and case replication studies report outcomes from the therapy (Greenman and Johnson 2012; Johnson 2002; MacIntosh and Johnson 2008). In the case study replication of ten couples, half of the participants reported improvements in relationship satisfaction at posttreatment and all participants with PTSD demonstrated clinically significant reductions in PTSD symptoms. Three couples in the study demonstrated an increase in emotional abuse and decreased relationship satisfaction over the course of the treatment. The authors caution that EFCT for Trauma may not be indicated for couples with ongoing emotional abuse (MacIntosh and Johnson 2008).

24.2.2 Partner-Assisted Interventions

24.2.2.1 Lifestyle Management Course

A 5-day, residential Lifestyle Management Course was developed for Australian military veterans and their partners to address quality of life and psychological symptoms (Devilly 2002). The course was delivered in a group format, and various topics were discussed throughout the week, including diet and nutrition, relaxation, communication, PTSD psychoeducation, self-care, stress management, medications, alcohol use, anger management, self-esteem, problem-solving, and goal-setting. Although there were reductions in PTSD symptoms following the program, by 6-month follow-up the effects were minimal. Reductions in veterans' depression, anxiety, and stress were sustained at 6-month follow-up. The partners of the veterans noted larger improvements on all measures except for anger. No improvements in relationship satisfaction were found.

24.2.3 Generic Couple Therapy

24.2.3.1 Behavioral Couple/Family Therapy

Behavioral Couple/Family Therapy (BC/FT) generally involves improving interactions among family members or partners and enhancing communication. A randomized controlled trial tested BFT following individual exposure treatment for PTSD with veterans (Glynn et al. 1999). Individuals who received BFT subsequent to individual exposure therapy had greater improvements in interpersonal problem-solving compared with those who did not. No additional improvements were seen in PTSD symptoms following BFT. Several uncontrolled studies of group BCT with veterans with PTSD and their female partners have yielded improvements in relationship functioning but not PTSD symptoms (e.g., Cahoon 1984; Sweany 1987).

24.2.3.2 K'oach Program

The K'oach program is a month-long intensive treatment program for Israeli military veterans with PTSD (Rabin and Nardi 1991; Solomon et al. 1992). The program provides PTSD psychoeducation, communication, and problem-solving skills. The program incorporates spouses at several times over the course of treatment to learn cognitive, communication, and behavioral reinforcement skills. Minimal empirical research has been conducted on the efficacy of the K'oach program, although participants reported improved relationship satisfaction. No change was found in PTSD symptoms (Solomon et al. 1992).

24.2.4 Education and Family Facilitated Engagement

24.2.4.1 Support and Family Education Program

The Support and Family Education (SAFE) program is a 14-session educational program for the loved ones of veterans with mental illness (Sherman 2003). The program is delivered in a monthly workshop format. It is designed for a range of mental health difficulties (e.g., PTSD, schizophrenia, depression) and for any family member to attend. The program includes psychoeducation about mental health difficulties, as well as four sessions of skills training, problem-solving, and stress reduction. Although no assessment of the impact of the SAFE program on PTSD symptoms and/or relationship functioning for the individual with PTSD or their loved ones has been conducted, 3- and 5-year program evaluations report very high participant satisfaction (Sherman 2003, 2006). Findings suggest that program participation led to increased understanding of mental health difficulties, awareness of resources, and increased ability to engage in self-care activities. Fewer attended sessions were associated with higher distress in loved ones (Sherman 2003).

24.2.4.2 Reaching Out to Educate and Assist Caring, Healthy Families Program

The Reaching Out to Educate and Assist Caring, Healthy Families (REACH) program is a 16-session psychoeducation program for veterans with mental health difficulties and their family members (Sherman et al. 2009b). The program consists of three phases. The first phase is a 4-week session conducted with the veteran and his or her family. This phase focuses on goal-setting and rapport building. The second phase is a 6-week session of diagnosis-specific psychoeducation for a group of four to six veterans and their families. The third phase is 6-month group session to support ongoing education and maintain gains. A preprogram motivational interviewing strategy was also used to engage veterans with the REACH program (Sherman et al. 2009a). Participants with PTSD had a relatively high rate of retention across phases I and II of the program (of those who began phase I, 90 % completed that phase, and 97 % who began phase II completed that phase), although there was 25 % attrition between phases I and II (Sherman et al. 2011). Data was not reported for phase III. Participants reported high satisfaction with the program (Sherman et al. 2011). No data regarding PTSD symptom change or relationship satisfaction was reported.

24.2.4.3 Coaching into Care Program

A program has been developed whereby loved ones of veterans who are suspected to have PTSD and other trauma-related symptoms can call a telephone support service to receive guidance on how to facilitate engagement of their loved one in treatment. The program provides information about available treatment options, allowing loved ones to assist the veteran in accessing care in a non-coercive manner. Initial program evaluation has demonstrated some increase in veteran engagement in mental health services after use of the program (Sayers et al. 2011).

24.3 Discussion

The mental health field is beginning to recognize the permeating effects of trauma and PTSD on interpersonal relationships and the role of these relationships in improving the lives and well-being of those with PTSD. There are a variety of ways in which partners might be incorporated into treatment, including disorder-specific couple therapy, partner-assisted interventions, general couple therapy, and education and engagement interventions. The class of disorder-specific couple therapy for PTSD has the strongest empirical support in terms of achieving multiple outcomes (i.e., reductions in PTSD, improvements in relational functioning, improvements in partners' psychological functioning). Because PTSD has systemic-level implications for relationships with loved ones, targeting both the individual with PTSD and their partner in treatment seems to have greater effects across both symptom and relational domains. If the client and the partner are both willing to participate in a dyadic intervention for PTSD, disorder-specific couple therapy is recommended, regardless of level of relationship distress, because these interventions have been tested with couples across the spectrum of relationship satisfaction. Caution should be heeded, however, if the couple has ongoing emotional abuse for interventions focused explicitly on emotions.

Depending on the desired focus of treatment and client preference, however, other types of treatment described in the aforementioned heuristic may be most appropriate. For example, should the client be engaged in individual PTSD treatment and/or not want their partner to participate in trauma treatment with them but are experiencing relationship distress, also engaging in generic couple therapy may be helpful. Decreasing stress in social relationships may help the client participate more fully in individual treatment and can help improve treatment outcomes (e.g., Price et al. 2013).

Evidence-based individual, couple, and group interventions for PTSD only matter if individuals with PTSD engage in them. Thus, using partners and other loved ones to facilitate engagement in assessment and treatment represents an important innovation in the traumatic stress field. Moreover, partner-assisted interventions may be beneficial if additional assistance is needed to implement individual interventions that have been shown to ameliorate PTSD. However, we recommend that partner-assisted interventions be chosen and implemented with caution and may be contraindicated if the couple is experiencing significant distress based on prior research on partner-assisted interventions for clients with agoraphobia (Barlow et al. 1981).

Given the importance of social variables in the onset of PTSD and other traumatic stress-related disorders, we argue that early intervention strategies for preventing acute stress disorder and PTSD incorporate significant others. There have been some efforts to include significant others in these interventions (Billette et al. 2008; Guay et al. 2004), but no full protocol has been developed and no randomized controlled trial has been conducted to date. Several have offered suggestions about the types of interpersonal interventions that might be used to reduce mental health problems in the early period after traumatization (e.g., Guay et al. 2006, 2011; Litz et al. 2002; Wagner et al. under review).

In addition to considering the inclusion of significant others in the early intervention and treatment of PTSD, couple therapy for PTSD may be particularly important for cases of "complex PTSD (C-PTSD)," which has been put forth by a number of authors (e.g., Cloitre et al. 2012), and is considered for inclusion in the upcoming version of the International Classification of Disorders (Maercker et al. 2012). One of the symptoms of C-PTSD put forth is disturbances in interpersonal relationships. Thus, interventions that simultaneously target interpersonal relationship functioning should address these symptoms postulated to comprise C-PTSD and may potentiate treatment for C-PTSD. Likewise, couple therapy may be particularly well suited for "complicated/protracted/prolonged grief" (Boelen and Prigerson 2013), especially when the loss is shared by the couple.

Couple interventions for PTSD, with its range of possible modes of delivery, present compelling preliminary data in terms of treatment outcomes. This area of research is still in its infancy, however, and additional research is warranted to further establish the long-term effectiveness of the interventions and to extend findings into community samples, as the vast majority of the work thus far has been done within the veteran population. Couple-oriented interventions for PTSD address the systemic nature of PTSD and provide hope for not only improvements in the client's PTSD symptoms but also the partner's functioning and improved relationship satisfaction.

References

Barlow, D. H., Mavissakalian, M., & Hay, L. R. (1981). Couples treatment of agoraphobia: Changes in marital satisfaction. *Behaviour Research and Therapy, 19*, 245–255. doi:10.1016/0005-7967(81)90008-5.

Baucom, D. H., Shoham, V., Mueser, K. T., Daiuto, A. D., & Stickle, T. R. (1998). Empirically supported couple and family interventions for marital distress and adult mental health problems. *Journal of Consulting and Clinical Psychology, 66*, 53–88. doi:10.1037/0022-006X.66.1.53.

Billette, V., Guay, S., & Marchand, A. (2008). Posttraumatic stress disorder and social support in female victims of sexual assault: The impact of spousal involvement on the efficacy of cognitive-behavioral therapy. *Behavior Modification, 32*, 876–896. doi:10.1177/0145445508319280.

Boelen, P. A., & Prigerson, H. G. (2013). Prolonged grief disorder as a new diagnostic category in DSM-5. In M. Stroebe, H. Schut, & J. van den Bout (Eds.), *Complicated grief: Scientific foundations for health care professionals* (pp. 85–98). New York: Routledge/Taylor & Francis.

Cahoon, E. P. (1984). *An examination of relationships between posttraumatic stress disorder, marital distress, and response to therapy by Vietnam veterans* (Unpublished doctoral dissertation). University of Connecticut, Storrs.

Caska, C. M., & Renshaw, K. D. (2011). Perceived burden in spouses of National Guard/Reserve service members deployed during Operations Enduring and Iraqi Freedom. *Journal of Anxiety Disorders, 25*, 346–351. doi:10.1016/j.janxdis.2010.10.008.

Cloitre, M., Courtois, C. A., Ford, J. D., Green, B. L., Alexander, P., Briere, J., Herman, J. L., Lanius, R., Stolbach, B. C., Spinazzola, J., Van der Kolk, B. A., & Van der Hart, O. (2012). *The ISTSS expert consensus treatment guidelines for complex PTSD in adults*. Retrieved from http://www.istss.org//AM/Template.cfm? Section=Home&WebsiteKey=e 9d45456-aa9f-4ed8-811b-b6a6d6969dc4

Devilly, G. J. (2002). The psychological effects of a lifestyle management course on war veterans and their spouses. *Journal of Clinical Psychology, 58*, 1119–1134. doi:10.1002/jclp.10041.

Figley, C. R. (1989). *Helping traumatized families*. San Francisco: Jossey-Bass.

Galovski, T., Sobel, A. A., Phipps, K. A., & Resick, P. A. (2005). Trauma recovery: Beyond posttraumatic stress disorder and other axis I symptom severity. In T. A. Corales (Ed.), *Trends in posttraumatic stress disorder research* (pp. 207–227). Hauppague: Nova Science.

Glynn, S. M., Eth, S., Randolph, E. T., Foy, D. W., Urbaitis, M., Boxer, L., Paz, G. G., Leong, G. B., Firman, G., Salk, J. D., Katzman, J. W., & Crothers, J. (1999). A test of behavioral family therapy to augment exposure for combat-related posttraumatic stress disorder. *Journal of Consulting and Clinical Psychology, 67*, 243–251. doi:10.1037/0022-006X.67.2.243.

Greenman, P. S., & Johnson, S. M. (2012). United we stand: Emotionally focused therapy for couples in the treatment of posttraumatic stress disorder. *Journal of Clinical Psychology: In Session, 68*, 561–569. doi:10.1002/jclp.21853.

Guay, S., Billette, V., St-Jean Trudel, E., Marchand, A., & Mainguy, N. (2004). Thérapie de couple et trouble de stress post-traumatique. *Revue Francophone du Stress et du Trauma, 4*, 81–88.

Guay, S., Billette, V., & Marchand, A. (2006). Exploring the links between post-traumatic stress disorder and social support: Processes and potential research avenues. *Journal of Traumatic Stress, 19*, 327–338. doi:10.1002/jts.20124.

Guay, S., Beaulieu-Prévost, D., Beaudoin, C., St-Jean Trudel, E., Nachar, N., & Marchand, A. (2011). How do social interactions with a significant other affect PTSD symptoms? An empirical investigation with a clinical sample. *Journal of Aggression, Maltreatment & Trauma, 20*, 280–303. doi:10.1080/10926771.2011.562478.

Johnson, S. M. (2002). *Emotionally focused couple therapy with trauma survivors: Strengthening attachment bonds*. New York: Guilford.

Litz, B. T., Gray, M. J., Bryant, R. A., & Adler, A. B. (2002). Early intervention for trauma: Current status and future directions. *Clinical Psychology: Science and Practice, 9*, 112–134. doi:10.1093/clipsy/9.2.112.

Lunney, C. A., & Schnurr, P. P. (2007). Domains of quality of life and symptoms in male veterans treated for posttraumatic stress disorder. *Journal of Traumatic Stress, 20*, 955–964. doi:10.1002/jts.20269.

MacIntosh, H. B., & Johnson, S. M. (2008). Emotionally focused therapy for couples and childhood sexual abuse survivors. *Journal of Marital and Family Therapy, 34*, 298–315. doi:10.1111/j.1752-0606.2008.00074.x.

Maercker, A., Brewin, C. R., Bryant, R. A., Cloitre, M., van Ommeren, M., Jones, L. M., Humayan, A., Kagee, A., Llosa, A. E., Rousseau, C., Somasundaram, D. J., Souza, R., Suzuki, Y., Weissbecker, I., Wessely, S. C., First, M. B., & Reed, G. M. (2012). Diagnosis and classification of disorders specifically associated with stress: Proposals for ICD-11. *World Psychiatry, 12*, 198–205. doi:10.1002/wps.20057.

Miller, W. R., Meyers, R. J., & Tonigan, J. S. (1999). Engaging the unmotivated in treatment for alcohol problems: A comparison of three strategies for intervention through family members. *Journal of Consulting and Clinical Psychology, 67*, 688–697. doi:10.1037/0022-006X.67.5.688.

Monson, C. M., Schnurr, P. P., Stevens, S. P., & Guthrie, K. A. (2004). Cognitive-behavioral couple's treatment for posttraumatic stress disorder: Initial findings. *Journal of Traumatic Stress, 17*, 341–344. doi:10.1023/B:JOTS.0000038483.69570.5b.

Monson, C. M., Rodriguez, B. F., & Warner, R. A. (2005a). Cognitive-behavioral therapy for PTSD in the real world: Do interpersonal relationships make a real difference? *Journal of Clinical Psychology, 61*, 751–761. doi:10.1002/jclp.20096.

Monson, C. M., Stevens, S. P., & Schnurr, P. P. (2005b). Cognitive-behavioral couple's treatment for posttraumatic stress disorder. In T. A. Corales (Ed.), *Focus on posttraumatic stress disorder research* (pp. 245–274). Hauppague: Nova Science.

Monson, C. M., Taft, C. T., & Fredman, S. J. (2009). Military-related PTSD and intimate relationships: From description to theory-driven research and intervention development. *Clinical Psychology Review, 29*, 707–714. doi:10.1016/j.cpr.2009.09.002.

Monson, C. M., Fredman, S. J., Adair, K. C., Stevens, S. P., Resick, P. A., Schnurr, P. P., MacDonald, H. Z., & Macdonald, A. (2011). Cognitive-behavioral conjoint therapy for PTSD: Pilot results from a community sample. *Journal of Traumatic Stress, 24*, 97–101. doi:10.1002/jts.20604.

Monson, C. M., Fredman, S. J., Macdonald, A., Pukay-Martin, N. D., Resick, P. A., & Schnurr, P. P. (2012a). Effect of cognitive-behavioral couple therapy for PTSD: A randomized controlled trial. *Journal of the American Medical Association, 308*, 700–709. doi:10.1001/jama.2012.9307.

Monson, C. M., Macdonald, A., & Brown-Bowers, A. (2012b). Couple/family therapy for posttraumatic stress disorder: Review to facilitate interpretation of VA/DoD Clinical Practice Guideline. *Journal of Rehabilitation Research and Development, 49*, 717–728. doi:10.1682/JRRD.2011.09.0166.

Monson, C. M., Macdonald, A., Vorstenbosch, V., Shnaider, P., Goldstein, E. S. R., Ferrier-Auerbach, A. G., & Mocciola, K. E. (2012c). Changes in social adjustment with cognitive processing therapy: Effects of treatment and association with PTSD symptom change. *Journal of Traumatic Stress, 25*, 519–526. doi:10.1002/jts.21735.

Price, M., Gros, D. F., Strachan, M., Ruggiero, K. J., & Acierno, R. (2013). The role of social support in exposure therapy for Operation Iraqi Freedom/Operation Enduring Freedom veterans: A preliminary investigation. *Psychological Trauma: Theory, Research, Practice, and Policy, 5,* 93–100. doi:10.1037/a0026244.

Rabin, C., & Nardi, C. (1991). Treating post traumatic stress disorder couples: A psychoeducational program. *Community Mental Health Journal, 27,* 209–224. doi:10.1007/BF00752422.

Renshaw, K. D., Blais, R. K., & Caska, C. M. (2011). Distress in spouses of combat veterans with PTSD: The importance of interpersonally based cognitions and behaviors. In S. M. Wadsworth & D. Riggs (Eds.), *Risk and resilience in U.S. military families* (pp. 69–84). New York: Springer.

Sautter, F. J., Glynn, S. M., Thompson, K. E., Franklin, L., & Han, X. (2009). A couple-based approach to the reduction of PTSD avoidance symptoms: Preliminary findings. *Journal of Marital and Family Therapy, 35,* 343–349. doi:10.1111/j.1752-0606.2009.00125.x.

Sayers, S. L., Whitted, P., Straits-Troster, K., Hess, T., & Fairbank, J. (2011, November). *Families at ease: A national Veterans Health Administration service for family members of veterans to increase veteran engagement in care.* Paper presented at the Annual Meeting of the Association of Behavioral and Cognitive Therapies, Toronto.

Schumm, J. A., Fredman, S. J., Monson, C. M., & Chard, K. M. (2013). Cognitive-behavioral conjoint therapy for PTSD: Initial findings for Operations Enduring and Iraqi Freedom male combat veterans and their partners. *American Journal of Family Therapy, 41,* 277–287. doi:10.1080/01926187.2012.701592.

Sherman, M. D. (2003). Rehab rounds: The Support and Family Education (SAFE) program: Mental health facts for families. *Psychiatric Services, 54,* 35–37. doi:10.1176/appi. ps.54.1.35.

Sherman, M. D. (2006). Updates and five-year evaluation of the S.A.F.E. program: A family psychoeducational program for serious mental illness. *Community Mental Health Journal, 42,* 213–219. doi:10.1007/s10597-005-9018-3.

Sherman, M. D., Fischer, E., Bowling, U. B., Dixon, L., Ridener, L., & Harrison, D. (2009a). A new engagement strategy in a VA-based family psychoeducation program. *Psychiatric Services, 60,* 254–257. doi:10.1176/appi.ps.60.2.254.

Sherman, M. D., Fischer, E. P., Sorocco, K., & McFarlane, W. R. (2009b). Adapting the multifamily group model to the Veterans Affairs system: The REACH program. *Professional Psychology: Research and Practice, 40,* 593–600. doi:10.1037/a0016333.

Sherman, M. D., Fischer, E. P., Sorocco, K., & McFarlane, W. R. (2011). Adapting the multifamily group model to the Veterans Affairs system: The REACH program. *Couple and Family Psychology: Research and Practice, 1,* 74–84. doi:10.1037/2160-4096.1.S.74.

Shnaider, P., Pukay-Martin, N. D., Fredman, S. J., Macdonald, A., & Monson, C. M. (2014). Effects of cognitive-behavioral conjoint therapy for PTSD on partners' psychological functioning. *Journal of Traumatic Stress, 27,* 129–136.

Solomon, Z., Bleich, A., Shoham, S., Nardi, C., & Kotler, M. (1992). The "K'oach" project for treatment of combat-related PTSD: Rationale, aims, and methodology. *Journal of Traumatic Stress, 5,* 175–193.

Sweany, S. L. (1987). *Marital and life adjustment of Vietnam combat veterans: A treatment outcome study* (Unpublished doctoral dissertation). University of Washington, Seattle.

Taft, C. T., Watkins, L. E., Stafford, J., Street, A. E., & Monson, C. M. (2011). Posttraumatic stress disorder and intimate relationship problems: A meta-analysis. *Journal of Consulting and Clinical Psychology, 79,* 22–33. doi:10.1037/a0022196.

Tarrier, N., Sommerfield, C., & Pilgrim, H. (1999). Relatives' expressed emotion (EE) and PTSD treatment outcome. *Psychological Medicine, 29,* 801–811. doi:10.1017/S0033291799008569.

Wagner, A. C., Monson, C. M., & Hart, T. L. (manuscript under review). *Social interaction and posttraumatic stress disorder: Toward a new conceptualization.*

Whisman, M. A., Sheldon, C. T., & Goering, P. (2000). Psychiatric disorders and dissatisfaction with social relationships: Does type of relationship matter? *Journal of Abnormal Psychology, 109,* 803–808. doi:10.1037/0021-843X.109.4.803.

Telemental Health Approaches for Trauma Survivors

25

Eric Kuhn, Julia E. Hoffman, and Josef I. Ruzek

25.1 Introduction

The past couple of decades have witnessed a veritable explosion of technology development and services with nearly ubiquitous uptake of innovative electronic products. In fact, today about 40 % of the earth's population has access to the Internet, and there are almost as many mobile phone subscriptions as there are people on the planet (International Telecommunications Union [ITU] 2014). Virtually overnight, we have become reliant on these technologies for many of our everyday activities, such as finding information, shopping, banking, and staying connected to friends and family. Modes of communication have multiplied to include options such as no-cost web-based video calling, instant messaging at home or on the go, and asynchronous microblogging tools for connected self-reflection. The latest generation of mobile phones, called smartphones, offers capabilities and functions that only a few short years ago were unimaginable or only available on stationary computers. As these technologies continue to transform our everyday lives, their potential to address the tremendous unmet mental healthcare needs of trauma survivors is also beginning to be realized through innovative telemental health (TMH) approaches.

In this chapter, we define TMH and discuss its potential and challenges in mental healthcare for trauma survivors. Three emerging TMH approaches that have been applied to the treatment of individuals with trauma-related mental health issues are reviewed. These approaches include clinical video-teleconferencing (CVT), web-based interventions, and mobile phone interventions. We conclude this chapter with a discussion of future directions of TMH for helping those affected by trauma.

E. Kuhn, PhD (✉) • J.E. Hoffman, PsyD • J.I. Ruzek, PhD
Dissemination and Training Division,
National Center for PTSD,
Department of Veterans Affairs Palo Alto Healthcare System, Palo Alto, CA, USA
e-mail: Eric.Kuhn@va.gov; Julia.Hoffman@va.gov; Josef.Ruzek@va.gov

© Springer International Publishing Switzerland 2015
U. Schnyder, M. Cloitre (eds.), *Evidence Based Treatments for Trauma-Related Psychological Disorders: A Practical Guide for Clinicians*,
DOI 10.1007/978-3-319-07109-1_25

461

25.2 Telemental Health (TMH)

Telehealth or telemedicine has been broadly defined as using telecommunications technology for delivering medical information and services (Perednia and Allen 1995). TMH is subsumed under this rubric as it entails using this technology to deliver information and services for mental health specifically. Modes of TMH delivery include plain old telephone services (POTS), video-teleconferencing, and web-, mobile phone-, and, more recently, smartphone-based interventions.

TMH has vast potential to help address the unmet mental health needs of trauma survivors by expanding access to and increasing efficiency of care. For example, TMH approaches can extend the geographic reach of care to rural areas that have a shortage of mental health clinicians (e.g., Morland et al. 2010). Likewise, asynchronous TMH approaches (e.g., web-based interventions) are highly scalable, easily being able to accommodate increasing numbers of users, and can serve as a force multiplier increasing the capacity of existing providers (Marks et al. 2004). By utilizing TMH approaches, providers can increase efficiency by seeing more patients while spending less time per patient (e.g., with groups, shorter sessions, and brief coaching calls) without necessarily compromising the quality of services. TMH approaches that employ evidence-based treatments (EBTs) for PTSD (Foa et al. 2009) could allow less highly trained providers to deliver quality care (i.e., task and skill shifting), expanding access to services while reducing cost.

TMH approaches could also improve the effectiveness of traditional care. For example, outcomes could be improved by better generalization of skills taught in in-person psychotherapy sessions being practiced and used when needed in the patient's natural environments (e.g., facilitated with smartphone interventions). Psychotherapy typically involves placing a tremendous responsibility on patients to learn materials during the session and then remember to apply what was learned in suitable contexts (at certain times, places, and situations) outside of session. Mobile TMH approaches can reduce this burden by providing cueing to use appropriate skills along with supportive practice materials when needed. In addition, communication between sessions is typically very limited; TMH can increase opportunities to communicate and get support through email or text messaging, which may improve outcomes.

TMH could confer other benefits as well, such as allowing clinicians to expand the range of problems they treat. For example, clinicians could attend to secondary or co-occurring problems by using web- or mobile phone-based self-management programs. They could also be employed after care has concluded to enhance relapse prevention, possibly preventing or delaying return to treatment or potentially even enhancing effects after treatment is over. Lastly, TMH approaches could improve outcomes by increasing provider and patient fidelity to EBT protocols by affording easy access to standardized materials and facilitating protocol adherence through highly structured programs.

In addition to their potential to improve effectiveness of care, TMH approaches also could increase access to care. Providers and service organizations could use TMH approaches to engage individuals with limited motivation or capacity to participate in traditional care as an initial step toward more intensive care, if needed. If care requires little or no face-to-face contact with mental health professionals, this may reduce stigma-related obstacles to help-seeking and privacy concerns of seeking care (e.g., in-home CVT).

While it is clear that TMH has great potential, various issues must be considered before it is used. Foremost among these is ensuring patient safety when practicing remotely. Before using TMH with a patient, providers should ensure that local emergency resources are known and that a plan is in place should the need arise. This plan should also include involvement of a supportive significant other (e.g., spouse, parent), if available.

Other professional and ethical issues must also be attended to, including prevention of information security problems, which could range from fairly innocuous breaches of privacy to situations that can truly endanger patients (e.g., when working in politically unstable regions or less than open societies). Thus, data must be secure when transmitted (i.e., strongly encrypted) and protected when stored (e.g., behind a firewall). Costs of the required devices and data plans must be considered as the aim is to expand access to those with fewer resources.

Providers adopting and using TMH will require guidance on ethical and legal use of TMH, as well as training to develop and maintain competence, given the rapidity at which technology changes. The American Psychological Association (2013) has created guidelines that cover everything from security of patient data to informed consent and clinical boundaries for successful and legal implementation of TMH (e.g., providing services outside of one's professional license jurisdiction).

25.3 TMH and Trauma

TMH can help to fill gaps in trauma care services across a number of contexts. These include assisting in covering mental health needs in places where traumas have recently occurred or are ongoing and therefore may be unsafe for mental health providers to be practicing in person. These include active war zones, politically unstable countries or regions, areas acutely affected by natural and manmade disasters lacking basic necessities (potable water, shelter, food), and regions with uncontained contagious disease outbreaks (e.g., avian flu). Aside from areas that may be too risky for providers, there are many places and trauma-exposed populations that lack sufficient access to mental health services. Many stable but developing nations have inadequate mental health infrastructures. But even in the most developed countries, coverage can be insufficient in certain areas, for example, in rural areas or in underserved communities of ethnic minorities. Likewise infirm, elderly, or disabled trauma survivors may not be able to get to needed care readily. Specialty trauma services may not be available in jails and prisons where populations have high rates of PTSD and other mental health conditions (Goff et al. 2007).

TMH approaches could also be used to monitor disaster-stricken populations, allowing for identification and triage of those most affected in order to ensure that limited resources are used most efficiently. Moreover, they could help provide care in disaster-stricken regions that have compromised transportation infrastructure that is restricting or entirely prohibiting patient travel or during disasters and other mass-scale traumas in which the demand for mental healthcare services has exceeded the supply. TMH also has the potential to provide more convenient access to care for trauma survivors facing a host of post-trauma and other logistical challenges. For example, trauma may cause physical injuries that could restrict mobility.

TMH may be a more palatable or less risky modality of care delivery relative to in-person traditional care for some trauma survivors, including individuals who are concerned about the social stigma associated with having been traumatized (e.g., raped) or those fearing possible untoward repercussions of disclosing trauma (e.g., military service members or members of certain ethno-cultural groups). Likewise, many individuals perceive stigma about having and disclosing post-trauma mental health issues and seeking treatment for them (e.g., Vogt 2011). In certain ethnic groups (e.g., Asian Americans), individuals may fear that seeking services will cause them embarrassment and shame (Jimenez et al. 2013).

Some TMH approaches (e.g., web- and mobile phone-based interventions) may offer help when no other options are available or accessible. For example, individuals who are socioeconomically disadvantaged who have limited or no healthcare coverage or cannot afford traditional MH care services could benefit from TMH services. Likewise, individuals who do not have the capacity to engage in traditional care due to time constraints because of employment requirements or childcare responsibilities could benefit from TMH approaches.

When considering using TMH approaches for traumatized individuals, clinicians and other service providers should weigh potential drawbacks. For example, most EBTs for PTSD are trauma-focused requiring patients to forego maladaptive avoidant coping strategies and instead engage in exposure by actively discussing or repeatedly confronting painful trauma memories and situations that provoke trauma-related distress. For some trauma survivors, venturing out to connect in person with a mental health provider can be an initial therapeutic step in overcoming avoidance, while remaining at home exclusively using a TMH approach (e.g., a web-based program) could serve to further reinforce avoidance.

TMH approaches, such as web- and mobile phone-based programs, require little motivation to initially access them. However, a great deal of motivation may be required to fully engage and sustain meaningful use over time, especially without some amount of regular support (e.g., telephone-based coaching). Thus, there is a risk that aborted or other unsuccessful attempts to use and benefit from TMH for self-management will lead to discouragement and beliefs that treatment in general does not work or will not work for the user in particular.

25.4 Examples of TMH Approaches Applied to Trauma Populations

25.4.1 Clinical Video-Teleconferencing (CVT)

CVT involves using video equipment, including cameras and monitors (e.g., television, computer, or mobile devices such as tablets or smartphones) to deliver mental health services remotely through telecommunications infrastructures (e.g., broadband). CVT affords a close approximation of traditional face-to-face care by allowing both patient and provider to see and hear one another in real time. However, compared to traditional care, CVT's primary advantage is that it can increase convenience by reducing or entirely eliminating travel requirements (e.g., with in-home CVT applications). CVT typically involves providers located in one healthcare setting (e.g., main hospital) and patients located at a distant healthcare facility (e.g., a rural clinic). Recent advances in and broader availability of video-teleconferencing technology (e.g., low-cost and smartphone cameras, expanded broadband access) have made CVT to patients' homes feasible, entirely eliminating travel and further reducing inconveniences associated with receiving care. It also overcomes the stigma of having to go to a mental healthcare setting, which could engage more patients, reduce missed appointments, and prevent premature termination of treatment.

CVT is a mode of care delivery that can be used for a variety of trauma-related mental health services, including screening and diagnostic assessments (e.g., Nelson et al. 2004), medication and case management (e.g., Shore and Manson 2005), and psychotherapy, both in individual (e.g., Tuerk et al. 2010) and group (e.g., Morland et al. 2011b) formats. Despite this broad applicability, some providers may be reluctant to use CVT because of concerns that patients will not want to use it or it may compromise the therapeutic relationship or negatively impact care delivery in other important ways. In fact, CVT has been shown to be an acceptable form of treatment delivery for PTSD patients, with some patients preferring this modality over in-person care (Thorp et al. 2012). Likewise, research has shown that a strong therapeutic relationship can be developed and maintained (Germain et al. 2010), although when it is used with groups, the alliance might suffer somewhat (Greene et al. 2010). Furthermore, providers have been shown to be able to deliver the same level of care in terms of adherence to and competence with therapy protocols using CVT for PTSD patients (Frueh et al. 2007a; Morland et al. 2011a).

Considerable evidence has been amassed establishing the efficacy of CVT for a variety of mental health conditions, with outcomes generally comparable to those of in-person care (Backhaus et al. 2012). For trauma care specifically, a number of studies have been conducted, including both CVT from clinic to clinic (Morland et al. 2004, 2011a, b; Frueh et al. 2007a, b; Germain et al. 2009; Tuerk et al. 2010; Gros et al. 2011; Hassija and Gray 2011) and more recently from clinic to patient's home (Strachan et al. 2012). Consistent with the broader CVT literature, comparable outcomes have been shown between CVT and in-person delivery of psychotherapy for PTSD patients (Gros et al. 2013). However, several studies suggest that outcomes for exposure therapy delivered by CVT, while good (and comparable to those found in the extant in-person delivery literature), may not be as good as those from in-person delivery (Gros et al. 2013).

There are a number of issues that should be attended to when using CVT. Foremost among these are equipment and technical considerations. Early applications of CVT required costly monitor and camera systems, but now inexpensive, ready-to-use off-the-shelf equipment and software that have adequate encryption capabilities are widely available. Once the hardware is in place, clinicians should be prepared for technical issues that can arise, such as unreliable or slow connections leading to dropped connections and delays in communication that disrupt the flow of the session. Having backup plans in place, such as reverting to telephones, will lessen the impact of these inevitable disruptions. Setting issues will also need to be managed when using CVT to a remote clinic. For example, patients will need a private office with video-teleconferencing equipment, and remote clinic personnel will be required to prepare the space for the patient and be available if clinical or technical issues arise. Finally, clinicians must also overcome other logistical issues when using CVT. For example, EBTs for PTSD such as prolonged exposure (PE) and cognitive processing therapy (CPT) routinely use self-report symptom measures and homework forms. Providing these to patients and having them completed and transferred back so they can be used in a timely fashion will require additional technology (e.g., scanners, fax machines). Obviously, for in-home CVT, all of these issues require additional careful forethought and contingency planning.

Specific clinical issues can also arise when using CVT with trauma patients. While CVT affords the opportunity to assess nonverbal signs, it can lack the sensitivity needed to detect or distinguish subtle emotional signs (e.g., soft crying, fidgeting) that are a routine part of trauma-focused care. Likewise, detection of other clinically relevant issues that arise in trauma care, such as recent alcohol or marijuana use and poor personal hygiene (Thorp et al. 2012), may be compromised. Depending on what can be brought into the video frame, the clinician may not be able to see the entire patient. A stark case of this is described by Thorp et al. (2012), who note a situation where the clinician did not know the patient was in a wheelchair because it was out of frame.

25.4.2 Web-Based Interventions

Web-based interventions provide a platform for reaching a huge proportion of the population. Anyone with Internet access can use web-based interventions, and once they are constructed, they can be used by large numbers of individuals with no additional costs. This makes them especially well suited for use in the aftermath of large-scale traumatic events that affect hundreds or even thousands of individuals.

But in addition to advantages of reach, web-based interventions have characteristics that may enable them to be particularly effective. EBTs typically incorporate common therapeutic components that are likely to contribute to their effectiveness. These include information and education, skills training with demonstration/modeling, individualized assessment, goal setting, behavioral task assignment, self-monitoring, and personalized feedback. Web-based interventions lend themselves to incorporation of these features, and many existing web programs have successfully included these elements (Amstadter et al. 2009). In this sense, it can be argued that many EBTs for PTSD are well suited for translation to and delivery via the Internet. Automated interactive programs essentially seek to replicate many aspects of face-to-face interventions that have been found to be effective.

In addition to preventive and treatment interventions, web-based programs can offer screening and assessment of trauma-related mental health issues. Individuals can screen themselves for problems and be offered customized feedback, in the privacy of their own homes. They can track their own progress in efforts to improve their symptoms. Their assessment information can be used to tailor the intervention by directing them to particular information, skills, or materials. This capacity for assessment means that web-based interventions can collect data, both in terms of usage and self-entered information and automatically collected site use data. Potentially, the gathering of data before, during, and after the intervention is used can help clinicians increase their ability to monitor progress and outcomes of treatment and more generally move toward evidence-based decision-making. A fundamental obstacle to routine measurement of mental health outcomes is a reliance on the use of paper and pencil questionnaires to provide information that cannot easily be integrated into electronic health records or viewed across time and treatment sessions. Web-based programs can potentially permit ongoing data entry by clients that can then be summarized in visual "dashboards" that can be reviewed by provider and client to review treatment progress and inform decision-making.

It is also possible that, if well-designed, web-based interventions may be motivating for those who might benefit from their use. The unlimited access and 24/7 availability of programs enables users to self-pace their experience getting as little or as much from the intervention as is desired at virtually any time they can access the Internet, including from the privacy of their own home. Individuals can use web-based interventions anonymously, so that perceptions of stigma or embarrassment at help-seeking are likely to be less significant impediments to care. Cost is also reduced or eliminated as a barrier, since many interventions are available at no or low cost.

Web-based interventions can vary in terms of the degree to which they are intended to include human service provider involvement. At one end of the continuum, they can be designed as entirely stand-alone self-help interventions, delivering symptom assessment and monitoring, psychoeducation, and instruction in a range of intervention tools (e.g., self-regulation skills) to be self-administered by the user. At the other end of this continuum, web-based interventions can serve as treatment augmentation tools in which care is delivered by human service providers but supplemented by the web program. It is possible that integration of web-based interventions into traditional care might serve as a force multiplier by reducing the amount of time required to treat each patient allowing more patients to be seen by a provider (Marks et al. 2004).

Between these two extremes is assisted self-help, in which individuals self-manage their problems or symptoms but are offered human support that is less intensive than that likely to occur during face-to-face mental health treatment. For example, support could include brief phone calls to provide caring support and coaching to reinforce program use, encourage persistence, and problem-solve difficulties with implementing intervention components. This contact would also increase accountability to help ensure consistent, meaningful engagement with the intervention. Support personnel could be mental health professionals, but a range of other helpers could also provide support (e.g., peer specialists, clergy).

Provider concerns about patient nonacceptance of this form of TMH and its effect on treatment may affect adoption. As with CVT, substantial research to date indicates that patients using web-based programs often find them to be acceptable and satisfying (Marks et al. 2007) and that incorporating web-based activities into therapy is not incompatible with establishing a good relationship with the therapist (Klein et al. 2009; Knaevelsrud and Maercker 2007). Evidence on effectiveness from several studies of web-based interventions for trauma survivors is promising (Lange et al. 2000, 2001; Hirai and Clum 2005; Knaevelsrud and Maercker 2007; Litz et al. 2007; Klein et al. 2009, 2010; Steinmetz et al. 2012; Wang et al. 2013). Most of the web-based programs evaluated in this literature have relied on significant provider involvement, and unfortunately, many of the programs studied have not been made widely available to the public. Fortunately, there are a number of very good, publicly available, free web-based programs that are available, which are informed by evidence-based intervention components commonly found on research sites. These include the VA National Center for PTSD's PTSD Coach online (www.ptsd.va.gov/apps/PTSDCoachOnline) designed for the general population and DoD's AfterDeployment.org (Ruzek et al. 2011; Bush et al. 2013) that was designed for military service members and veterans.

For clinicians considering using web-based interventions with PTSD patients, there are several issues that require attention. The most obvious is that the patient must have access to the web in a private or semiprivate setting. It is also important to select an appropriate web-based program that will match the patient's preferences, characteristics (e.g., motivation, self-efficacy), limitations (e.g., time), and severity of problems. Clinicians must also consider the optimal level of support and assistance that will be required for and desired by the patient. For example, highly motivated, self-reliant patients with good social support may need less support than patients lacking these characteristics. If asynchronous communication (e.g., email) will be included, clear expectations should be negotiated upfront about the type of information that should and should not be communicated through these channels and the expected time for responses.

25.4.3 mHealth

Mobile health or mHealth is a form of TH that uses electronic mobile devices, such as smartphones, to deliver health assessments and interventions. This subset of TH is defined by the devices from which materials are accessed (e.g., mobile phones, e-readers, tablet computers, personal organizers, and media devices) rather than the format of the materials themselves, which can include mobile-optimized websites, mobile applications, short message service (text messaging, "SMS"), or widgets. These applications and services can be used to support self-management or to enhance face-to-face treatment during and between sessions, much like web-based offerings. They are also most often free or very inexpensive, with the exception of the equipment and data plans needed (which are not specific to use of these functions but amortized over the entirety of the user's connected behavior). Generally, the benefits of web-based TMH are applicable to mHealth products as well; however, while similarities exist, mobile platforms have some major differences from typical web-based tools that should be noted.

First, mobile devices are more ubiquitous and personal than computers; according to the International Telecommunications Union (ITU) (2014), the penetration of mobile cellular subscriptions per 100 inhabitants is 128 in developed nations and 89 in developing nations. Smartphone ownership is also rapidly increasing and is estimated at 16.7 % penetration globally (ITU 2014) and is even more prevalent in developed nations, like the USA, where 55–65 % of adults own a smartphone (Duggan 2013; Nielsen 2013). This penetration, and the use of these devices for non-phone call activities such as texting (81 %), accessing the Internet (60 %), or downloading apps (50 %) is relatively consistent across various demographic groups (Duggan 2013). Unlike personal computers, mobile devices are not frequently shared between individuals, which enables opportunities to share private data and to maintain highly personalized tools.

Second, mobile devices – especially phones – are almost always within arms' reach and turned on, which allows for nearly constant opportunities to engage users or to support them in practicing treatment-consistent behaviors (e.g., coping effectively with acute distress, accomplishing assigned homework tasks) on a just-in-time basis. Notifications can be used to alert users to recommended tasks and are likely to be noticed immediately (as opposed to reminders sent by email), and assessments can be deployed in order to catch users at the moment of distress or at various points in their day to accurately identify micro-trends and gain insight into difficulties.

Third, mHealth options can support the parts of EBTs that specifically require mobility to accomplish – for example, participating in and recording in vivo exposure exercises in PE in various community settings. Fourth, mobile devices often include a distilled set of personal data and media that can be leveraged for intervention in ways that are unavailable on the web (e.g., contact lists to identify social supports, preferred music, or photos to inspire changes in perspective). Fifth, mobile devices have significantly less visual display space to use than typical computer monitors and tend to be used for shorter periods, which requires editing mobile materials for both length and complexity and results in fewer opportunities for in-depth intervention or instruction.

Mobile approaches offer some advantages that are ideally suited for trauma-related distress, whether or not users are engaged in EBTs for PTSD. First, PTSD and related disorders are defined, at least in part, by the acute exacerbations experienced by individuals when prompted by internal or external trauma cues. This makes the immediacy of mobile intervention especially valuable, as users can be provided with coping strategies to be used in moments of distress. For those in face-to-face care, mHealth options can provide the intersession support needed, while patients navigate the themes and emotional processing targeted in session. It is well known that for some patients, effective treatments for PTSD can cause a temporary increase in distress and mHealth may alleviate some of this difficulty, which could result in decreased suffering and possibly decreased attrition. One such app, developed by the VA National Center for PTSD and the Department of Defense National Center for Telehealth and Technology, is the PTSD Coach (Hoffman et al. 2011), which provides psychoeducation, self-assessment with a validated measure (PTSD Checklist; Weathers et al. 1993), and just-in-time self-management tools.

A second hallmark of PTSD is avoidance, which can manifest in various ways, some of which can be decreased by the use of mHealth tools. Individuals may avoid care entirely for reasons of stigma or fear of directly addressing traumatic material, and mobile options can be provided to engage users at the level at which they are comfortable. When an intervention resides on the user's smartphone or other mobile device – devices which are capable of almost every type of interpersonal digital communication – avoidance of others may be decreased as more opportunities to engage social connections are provided. Increased social support is a well-known positive prognostic indicator (Ozer et al. 2003). Avoidance of tasks related to treatment (e.g., homework assignments) may be decreased because timely reminders to engage with materials can be issued, prepopulated messages can help users overcome moderate concerns rooted in avoidance (e.g., "You've done this before, you can do this again"), and patients are unlikely to lose their mobile devices or to be without them either at times when tasks should be accomplished (between sessions) or reviewed (in session). It should be noted that some counter-therapeutic effects of mHealth options, with regard to avoidance, may be encountered, including unwarranted distraction from treatment targets (e.g., in vivo exposure) (Clough and Casey 2011). More speculatively, phone apps might be used by some clients as cues for safety that could impair exposure to avoided stimuli, in the same way that individuals with anxiety disorders might only be willing to approach feared situations if carrying a supply of medications.

Many interventions for PTSD bring with them a substantial burden of in-session tasks and between-session work, some of which can be eased by the use of mobile technology. For example, PE requires recording sessions and listening back to these recordings between sessions. Historically, this has required the purchase and maintenance of a specialty recording device and media storage. Considering the ubiquity of smartphones and other mobile devices with native recording features, this requirement can be satisfied with decreased burden to the patient with apps such as the PE Coach (Reger et al. 2013). Reminders for visits, assignments, and prescribed coping tools can all enhance typical care by ensuring full participation by patients. For those mHealth tools that pass data back to clinicians, these novel feedback mechanisms can guide care. Literature exists that has identified indicators of likely success or failure in EBT (Lambert 2011), and reports on treatment engagement via mobile tools can both identify cases of likely failure before they occur and contribute to a better understanding of the variables tied to clinical outcomes through aggregating data.

Evidence for the efficacy of mHealth interventions for individuals with trauma-related problems is very limited at this time. The field is young and it takes time to develop and refine the technologies before evaluating them, but there is some indication from related domains that mHealth holds much promise for trauma survivors (e.g., Rizvi et al. 2011). SMS initiatives have proven effective for the management of other behavioral problems from smoking (Free et al. 2011) to diabetes (Holtz and Laucker 2012) and depression (Agyapong et al. 2012).

Consistent with what has been mentioned previously for the other TMH technologies, providers correctly recognize that the realities – and challenges – of bringing novel devices into clinical care are yet to be fully realized. First at issue is to determine whether patients and providers are willing and interested in these technologies for the enhancement of traditional care delivery methods. Evidence is emerging that individuals will accept mobile technologies as healthcare support tools and find them helpful. For example, veterans with PTSD reported high satisfaction with PTSD Coach and perceived it as being moderately to very helpful in managing acute distress, PTSD symptoms, and helping with sleep (Kuhn et al. 2014). They also found that it helped them to learn about PTSD and explain it to their family and friends. There is also evidence that providers see the potential of using apps in care and would be willing to use them to support EBTs (Kuhn et al. 2014). For example, a survey of trained PE providers indicated that they believed that the PE Coach app could significantly improve their care, would not be too complex to integrate, would not change the therapeutic relationship, and three-quarters reported that they would use the app (Kuhn et al. 2014).

As with the other forms of TMH, access to the technology is a fundamental requirement. While smartphones and other smart mobile devices are now being carried by a substantial and ever-growing minority of individuals worldwide (ITU 2014), and in developed nations they are carried by a majority of individuals (Duggan 2013; Nielsen 2013), there are still many who do not yet have access to them. Furthermore, unlike web-based interventions that can be accessed and used across different types of computers, mobile apps are often built for a particular platform (e.g., Apple or Android) which can limit availability. Additionally, using apps independently can be limited by the level of insight of individuals in correctly identifying the types of tools needed and selecting appropriate and scientifically sound options from the crowded and difficult-to-navigate public marketplaces. Much like web-generated data, mHealth data can be sensitive and requires a level of sophistication to ensure its safe transmission and/or storage.

When combining mHealth apps with in-person care, additional challenges can emerge. Relatively little training exists for clinicians in how to use these tools generally, or any given app in particular. While patients may be comfortable identifying and procuring mobile tools and highly motivated to digitally enhance clinical care, clinicians may find that they are less fluent in one or more platforms and may find the task of integration difficult. Even for willing clinicians, trialability can be a challenge; it can be difficult to get clear documentation on the content of apps in order to ensure that they are appropriate for clinical use. Apps that are currently available are generally unconnected – they do not pass data to or from any existing structures that clinicians can access – which can create problems for clinicians trying to thoughtfully integrate these tools into care. Finally, assessments deployed on mobile platforms have hardly been validated (even if the same assessment has been validated in paper and pencil versions), and it is unclear if using these tools for assessment purposes will yield an apples-to-apples comparison.

25.5 Conclusion and Future Directions

Many of our patients – just like ourselves – have come to expect and rely upon the various comforts and efficiencies that technologies play in our lives. Industries have been transformed (e.g., banking, shopping) and we can expect no less for mental healthcare. As the ubiquity of technology continues to grow, the promise of leveraging these novel products for the care of trauma-impacted populations grows in parallel. This chapter has elucidated the currently available platforms that can be used by trauma survivors with or without clinicians, including the potential advantages and drawbacks of each. Much like technology itself, the potential of TMH seems virtually infinite. The obligations of scientists and clinicians alike are to act as thoughtful consumers of these new options, simultaneously ensuring that we are offering our patients the best options available and taking a critical eye to ensure that technologies are effective and usable and do not undermine the foundational elements of psychotherapeutic care.

Selection of the appropriate technology platform and interventions – ones that are best suited to the needs of both the patient and provider – is a critical first step to integrating technology into a trauma-focused practice. Special care should be taken to ensure that patient expectations and boundaries are not compromised by integration of novel technologies into PTSD care. Less than a generation ago, electronic communications with patients may have seemed completely unacceptable; now that many have integrated this into practice, it has become important to ensure that communications are secure and safe and do not increase the liability or burden of the clinician or healthcare system unnecessarily.

Technology will continue to evolve and create opportunities – and liabilities – for patients and providers. It is likely that background sensing – from the frequency and duration of phone calls made on the phone to the geodiameter traversed within the course of a day – will become available for integration into TMH applications shortly. Already GPS has been used to trigger location-based coping tools (Gustavson et al. 2011), and placeable and wearable sensors provide actigraphy data to better understand momentary biological signals (Morris and Aguilera 2012). The science and practice of mental health will likely benefit greatly from the additional capacities enabled by mobile and other technologies. Just as physical health assesses the multiple bodily systems, mental health needs to take a similar approach by assessing multiple systems including psychological, environmental, behavioral, and social systems. The richness of available information is incredible to consider, but conscientious clinicians will rightly work to ensure that any potential violations of privacy or consideration of the large number of variables that can be monitored via TMH are transparent to patients to avoid real or imagined breaches in therapeutic alliance.

It is likely that TMH can significantly improve care delivery processes. As noted above, the capacity for routine gathering of outcomes and use data means that this information can be used as a basis for clinician decision-making. Currently, decisions about treatment are seldom informed by data derived from validated assessment instruments, and TMH therefore holds promise to advance the potential for data-driven care. TMH also holds potential for advancing the development of stepped-care delivery systems in which frequency and intensity of intervention is matched to client need, problem severity, and preference (including pacing).

Having these capacities could result in providers being able to efficiently manage larger panels of patients without compromising quality.

Although not directly related to the primary focus of this chapter on providing TMH services to traumatized populations, TMH has applications for increasing provider access to and improving training in EBTs for PTSD. Availability of online training in EBTS is rapidly increasing, and several comprehensive web-based courses in EBTs for PTSD now exist, including CPT Web (https://cpt.musc.edu/), PE Web (http://pe.musc.edu/), and a web training for Skills Training in Affective and Interpersonal Regulation (STAIR; http://www.ptsd.va.gov/professional/continuing_ed/index.asphttp).

Finally, it is important to emphasize that much of the international burden of trauma falls on individuals living in geographical regions in which mental health-care infrastructures are not available. In such regions, trained mental health professionals are rare, and traditional delivery of mental health services is doomed to fail (Kazdin and Blase 2011). In time, as more of the world's population gains access to innovative technologies, TMH services hold untold promise of providing significant assistance to millions of affected trauma survivors.

References

Agyapong, V. I., Ahern, S., McLoughlin, D. M., & Farren, C. K. (2012). Supportive text messaging for depression and comorbid alcohol use disorder: Single-blind randomised trial. *Journal of Affective Disorders, 141*, 168–176. doi:10.1016/j.jad.2012.02.040.

American Psychological Association. (2013). *Guidelines for the practice of telepsychology*. Washington, DC: American Psychological Association.

Amstadter, A. B., Broman-Fulks, J. J., Zinzow, H., Ruggiero, K. J., & Cercone, J. (2009). Internet-based interventions for traumatic stress-related mental health problems: A review and suggestion for future research. *Clinical Psychology Review, 29*, 410–420.

Backhaus, A., Agha, Z., Maglione, M. L., Repp, A., Ross, B., Zuest, D., Rice-Thorp, N. M., Lohr, J., & Thorp, S. (2012). Videoconference psychotherapy: A systematic review. *Psychological Services, 9*, 111–131. doi:10.1037/a0027924.

Bush, N. E., Prins, A., Laraway, S., O'Brien, K., Ruzek, J., & Ciulla, R. (2013). A pilot evaluation of the Afterdeployment.org online posttraumatic stress workshop for military service members and veterans. *Psychological Trauma: Theory, Research, Practice, and Policy*. doi:10.1037/a0032179. Advance online publication.

Clough, B. A., & Casey, L. M. (2011). Technological adjuncts to increase adherence to therapy: A review. *Clinical Psychology Review, 31*, 697–710. doi:10.1016/j.cpr.2011.03.006.

Duggan, M. (2013, September 19). *Cell phone activities 2013*. Retrieved from Pew Research Center's Internet & American Life Project website: http://pewinternet.org/Reports/2013/Cell-Activities.aspx

Foa, E. B., Keane, T. M., Friedman, M. J., & Cohen, J. A. (2009). *Effective treatments for PTSD: Practice guidelines from the International Society for Traumatic Stress Studies* (2nd ed.). New York: Guilford.

Free, C., Knight, R., Robertson, S., Whittaker, R., Edwards, P., Zhou, W., Rodgers, A., Cairns, J., Kenward, M. G., & Roberts, I. (2011). Smoking cessation support delivered via mobile phone text messaging (txt2stop): A single-blind, randomised trial. *The Lancet, 378*, 49–55. ISSN 0140–6736, http://dx.doi.org/10.1016/S0140-6736(11)60701-0

Frueh, B. C., Monnier, J., Grubaugh, A. L., Elhai, J. D., Yim, E., & Knapp, R. (2007a). Therapist adherence and competence with manualized cognitive-behavioral therapy for PTSD delivered via videoconferencing technology. *Behavior Modification, 31*, 856–866. doi:10.1177/0145445507302125.

Frueh, B. C., Monnier, J., Yim, E., Grubaugh, A. L., Hamner, M. B., & Knapp, R. G. (2007b). A randomized trial of telepsychiatry for post-traumatic stress disorder. *Journal of Telemedicine and Telecare, 13*, 142–147. doi:10.1258/135763307780677604.

Germain, V., Marchand, A., Bouchard, S., Drouin, M. S., & Guay, S. (2009). Effectiveness of cognitive behavioural therapy administered by videoconference for posttraumatic stress disorder. *Cognitive Behaviour Therapy, 38*, 42–53. doi:10.1080/16506070802473494.

Germain, V., Marchand, A., Bouchard, S., Guay, S., & Drouin, M. (2010). Assessment of the therapeutic alliance in face-to-face or videoconferencing treatment for posttraumatic stress disorder. *Cyberpsychology, Behavior and Social Networking, 13*, 29–35.

Goff, A., Rose, E., Rose, S., & Purves, D. (2007). Does PTSD occur in sentenced prison populations? A systematic literature review. *Criminal Behaviour and Mental Health, 17*(3), 152–162.

Greene, C. J., Morland, L. A., Macdonald, A., Frueh, B. C., Grubbs, K. M., & Rosen, C. S. (2010). How does tele-mental health affect group therapy process? Secondary analysis of a noninferiority trial. *Journal of Consulting and Clinical Psychology, 78*, 746–750.

Gros, D. F., Yoder, M., Tuerk, P. W., Lozano, B. E., & Acierno, R. (2011). Exposure therapy for PTSD delivered to veterans via telehealth: Predictors of treatment completion and outcome and comparison to treatment delivered in person. *Behavior Therapy, 42*, 276–283. doi:10.1016/j.beth.2010.07.005.

Gros, D. F., Morland, L. A., Greene, C. J., Acierno, R., Strachan, M., Egede, L. E., Tuerk, P. W., Myrick, H., & Frueh, B. C. (2013). Delivery of evidence-based psychotherapy via video telehealth. *Journal of Psychopathology and Behavioral Assessment, 35*, 506–521. doi:10.1007/s10862-013-9363-4.

Gustavson, D. H., Shaw, B. R., Isham, A., Baker, T., Boyle, M. G., & Levy, M. (2011). Explicating an evidence-based, theoretically informed, mobile technology-based system to improve outcomes for people in recovery for alcohol dependence. *Substance Use & Misuse, 46*(1), 96–111. doi:10.3109/10826084.2011.521413.

Hassija, C. M., & Gray, M. J. (2011). The effectiveness and feasibility of videoconferencing technology to provide evidence-based treatment to rural domestic violence and sexual assault populations. *Telemedicine Journal and e-Health, 17*, 309–315.

Hirai, M., & Clum, G. A. (2005). An Internet-based self-change program for traumatic event related fear, distress, and maladaptive coping. *Journal of Traumatic Stress, 18*, 631–636. doi:10.1002/jts.20071.

Hoffman, J. E., Wald, L. J., Kuhn, E., Greene, C., Ruzek, J. I., & Weingardt, K. (2011). PTSD Coach (Version 1.0). [Mobile application software]. Retrieved from http://itunes.apple.com

Holtz, B., & Laucker, C. (2012). Diabetes management via mobile phones: A systematic review. *Telemedicine Journal and e-Health, 18*, 175–184.

International Telecommunications Union. (2014). Key 2005–2013 ICT indicators for developed and developing countries and the world (totals and penetration rates) [Data file]. Retrieved from http://www.itu.int/en/ITU-D/Statistics/Pages/stat/default.aspx

Jimenez, D. E., Bartels, S. J., Cardenas, V., & Alegría, M. (2013). Stigmatizing attitudes toward mental illness among racial/ethnic older adults in primary care. *International Journal of Geriatric Psychiatry, 28*, 1061–1068. doi:10.1002/gps.3928.

Kazdin, A. E., & Blase, S. L. (2011). Rebooting psychotherapy research and practice to reduce the burden of mental illness. *Perspectives on Psychological Science, 6*, 21–37. doi:10.1177/1745691610393527.

Klein, B., Mitchell, J., Gilson, K., Shandley, K., Austin, D., Kiropoulos, L., Abbott, J., & Cannard, G. (2009). A therapist-assisted internet-based CBT intervention for posttraumatic stress disorder: Preliminary results. *Cognitive Behaviour Therapy, 38*, 121–131.

Klein, B., Mitchell, J., Abbott, J., Shandley, K., Austin, D., Gilson, K., Kiropoulos, L., Cannard, G., & Redman, T. (2010). A therapist-assisted cognitive behavior therapy internet intervention for posttraumatic stress disorder: Pre-, post-and 3-month follow-up results from an open trial. *Journal of Anxiety Disorders, 24*, 635–644.

Knaevelsrud, C., & Maercker, A. (2007). Internet-based treatment for PTSD reduces distress and facilitates the development of a strong therapeutic alliance: A randomized controlled clinical trial. *BMC Psychiatry, 7*(1), 13.

Kuhn, E., Eftekhari, A., Hoffman, J. E., Crowley, J. J., Ramsey, K. M., Reger, G. M., & Ruzek, J. I. (2014a). Clinician perceptions of using a smartphone app with prolonged exposure therapy. *Administration and Policy in Mental Health and Mental Health Service Research*. doi:10.1007/s10488-013-0532-2. Advance online publication.

Kuhn, E., Greene, C., Hoffman, J., Nguyen, T., Wald, L., Schmidt, J., Ramsey, K. M., & Ruzek, J. (2014b). A preliminary evaluation of PTSD Coach, a smartphone app for posttraumatic stress symptoms. *Military Medicine, 179*, 12–18.

Lambert, M. J. (2011). What have we learned about treatment failure in empirically supported treatments? Some suggestions for practice. *Cognitive and Behavioral Practice, 18*, 413–420.

Lange, A., Schrieken, B., Van de Ven, J., Bredeweg, B., Emmelkamp, P. M., van der Kolk, J., Lydsdottir, L., Massaro, M., & Reuvers, A. (2000). "Interapy": The effects of short protocolled treatment of posttraumatic stress and pathological grief through the Internet. *Behavioural and Cognitive Psychotherapy, 28*, 175–192.

Lange, A., van de Ven, J. P., Schrieken, B., & Emmelkamp, P. M. (2001). Interapy. Treatment of posttraumatic stress through the Internet: A controlled trial. *Journal of Behavior Therapy and Experimental Psychiatry, 32*, 73–90.

Litz, B., Engel, C., Bryant, R., & Papa, A. (2007). A randomized, controlled proof-of-concept trial of an Internet-based, therapist-assisted self-management treatment for posttraumatic stress disorder. *American Journal of Psychiatry, 164*, 1676–1684.

Marks, I. M., Kenwright, M., McDonough, M., Whittaker, M., & Mataix-Cols, D. (2004). Saving clinicians' time by delegating routine aspects of therapy to a *computer: A randomized controlled trial in phobia/panic disorder. Psychological Medicine, 34*, 9–18.

Marks, I. M., Cavanagh, K., & Gega, L. (2007). *Hands-on help: Computer-aided psychotherapy*. Florence: Taylor & Francis.

Morland, L. A., Pierce, K., & Wong, M. (2004). Telemedicine and coping skills groups for Pacific Island veterans with post-traumatic stress disorder: A pilot study. *Journal of Telemedicine and Telecare, 10*, 286–289. doi:10.1258/1357633042026387.

Morland, L. A., Greene, C. J., Rosen, C. S., Foy, D., Reilly, P., Shore, J., He, Q., & Frueh, B. C. (2010). Telemedicine for anger management therapy in a rural population of combat veterans with posttraumatic stress disorder: A randomized noninferiority trial. *Journal of Clinical Psychiatry, 71*, 855–863. doi:10.1002/jts.20661.

Morland, L. A., Greene, C. J., Grubbs, K. M., Kloezeman, K., Mackintosh, M., Rosen, C., & Frueh, B. C. (2011a). Therapist adherence to manualized cognitive-behavioral therapy for anger management delivered to veterans with PTSD via videoteleconferencing. *Journal of Clinical Psychology, 67*, 629–638. doi:10.1002/jclp.20779.

Morland, L. A., Hynes, A. K., Mackintosh, M., Resick, P. A., & Chard, K. (2011b). Group cognitive processing therapy for PTSD delivered to rural combat veterans via telemental health: Lessons learned from a pilot cohort. *Journal of Traumatic Stress, 24*, 465–469. doi:10.1002/jts.20661.

Morris, M. E., & Aguilera, A. (2012). Mobile, social, and wearable computing and the evolution of psychological practice. *Professional Psychology: Research and Practice, 43*, 622.

Nelson, E., Zaylor, C., & Cook, D. (2004). A comparison of psychiatrist evaluation and patient symptom report in a jail telepsychiatry clinic. *Telemedicine Journal and e-Health, 10*(Supplement 2), 54–59.

Nielsen. (2013, December 16). *Consumer electronics ownership blasts off in 2013*. [Press release]. Retrieved from http://www.nielsen.com/us/en/newswire/2013/consumer-electronics-ownership-blasts-off-in-2013.html

Ozer, E. J., Best, S. R., Lipsey, T. L., & Weiss, D. S. (2003). Predictors of posttraumatic stress disorder and symptoms in adults: A meta-analysis. *Psychological Bulletin, 129*, 52–73.

Perednia, D. A., & Allen, A. (1995). Telemedicine technology and clinical applications. *Journal of the American Medical Association, 273*, 483–488.

Reger, G. M., Hoffman, J., Riggs, D., Rothbaum, B. O., Ruzek, J., Holloway, K. M., & Kuhn, E. R. (2013). The "PE coach" smartphone application: An innovative approach to improving implementation, fidelity, and homework adherence during prolonged exposure. *Psychological Services, 10*, 342–349.

Rizvi, S. L., Dimeff, L. A., Skutch, J., Carroll, D., & Linehan, M. M. (2011). A pilot study of the DBT coach: An interactive mobile phone application for individuals with borderline personality disorder and substance use disorder. *Behavior Therapy, 42*, 589–600.

Ruzek, J. I., Hoffman, J., Cuilla, R., Prins, A., Kuhn, E., & Gahm, G. (2011). Bringing Internet-based education and intervention into mental health practice: Afterdeployment.org. *European Journal of Psychotraumatology, 2*, 1–9.

Shore, J. H., & Manson, S. M. (2005). A developmental model for rural telepsychiatry. *Psychiatric Services, 56*, 976–980. doi:10.1176/appi.ps.56.8.976.

Steinmetz, S. E., Benight, C. C., Bishop, S. L., & James, L. E. (2012). My Disaster Recovery: A pilot randomized controlled trial of an Internet intervention. *Anxiety, Stress, and Coping, 25*, 593–600. doi:10.1080/10615806.2011.604869.

Strachan, M., Gros, D. F., Ruggiero, K. J., Lejuez, C. W., & Acierno, R. (2012). An integrated approach to delivering exposure-based treatment for symptoms of PTSD and depression in OIF/OEF veterans: Preliminary findings. *Behavior Therapy, 43*, 560–569. doi:10.1016/j.beth.2011.03.003.

Thorp, S. R., Fidler, J., Moreno, L., Floto, E., & Agha, Z. (2012). Lessons learned from studies of psychotherapy for posttraumatic stress disorder via video teleconferencing. *Psychological Services, 9*, 197–199. doi:10.1037/a0027057.

Tuerk, P. W., Yoder, M., Ruggiero, K. J., Gros, D. F., & Acierno, R. (2010). A pilot study of Prolonged Exposure therapy for posttraumatic stress disorder delivered via telehealth technology. *Journal of Traumatic Stress, 23*, 116–123. doi:10.1002/jts.20494.

Vogt, D. (2011). Mental health-related beliefs as a barrier to service use for military personnel and veterans: A review. *Psychiatric Services, 62*, 135–142. doi:10.1176/appi.ps.62.2.135.

Wang, Z., Wang, J., & Maercker, A. (2013). Chinese My Trauma Recovery, a web-based intervention for traumatized persons in two parallel samples: Randomized controlled trial. *Journal of Medical Internet Research, 15*, e213. doi:10.2196/jmir.2690. Published online 2013 September 30.

Weathers, F., Litz, B., Herman, D., Huska, J., & Keane, T. (1993, October). *The PTSD Checklist (PCL): Reliability, validity, and diagnostic utility*. Presentation at the annual meeting of the International Society for Traumatic Stress Studies, San Antonio.

Part VII

Pharmacotherapy

Pharmacologic Treatment for Trauma-Related Psychological Disorders

26

Lori L. Davis, Laura J. Van Deventer, and Cherry W. Jackson

26.1 Introduction

The goal of treatment of post-traumatic stress disorder (PTSD) is to manage core symptomatology, including intrusive reexperiencing, emotional numbing, cognitive distortions, avoidance, and hyperarousal, and improve the individual's social and occupational functioning. Pharmacologic treatments also aid in stabilizing psychiatric conditions, including mood, anxiety, psychotic, and substance use disorders, which frequently accompany PTSD or occur independently after a traumatic event. Based on clinical trials, approximately half of all PTSD patients will experience 30–60 % symptom improvement within 8–12 weeks of initiating an adequately dosed psychopharmacologic treatment. While the long-term goal is complete remission, a substantial

L.L. Davis, MD (✉)
Veterans Affairs Medical Center, Research Service,
3701 Loop Road East, Tuscaloosa, AL 35404, USA
e-mail: lori.davis@va.gov

Department of Psychiatry and Behavioral Neurobiology,
University of Alabama, School of Medicine,
Birmingham, AL, USA

L.J. Van Deventer, PharmD, BCPS
BayCare Health System,
Morton Plant North Bay Hospital,
6600 Madison Street, Port Richey, FL 34652, USA

C.W. Jackson, PharmD, BCPP, FASHP
Department of Pharmacy Practice,
Auburn University,
Auburn, AL, USA

Department of Psychiatry and Behavioral Neurobiology,
University of Alabama,
Birmingham, AL, USA

© Springer International Publishing Switzerland 2015
U. Schnyder, M. Cloitre (eds.), *Evidence Based Treatments for Trauma-Related Psychological Disorders: A Practical Guide for Clinicians*,
DOI 10.1007/978-3-319-07109-1_26

number of patients have treatment-refractory PTSD. In cases where full symptomatic relief cannot be achieved, improvements in psychiatric comorbidities, resiliency, functioning, and quality of life are achievable through a combination of psychological and pharmacological treatments. This chapter discusses the pharmacological treatments for PTSD; however, many of these principles apply to the treatment of depression, anxiety, and sleep problems associated with the broader trauma-related disorders.

How does a medication become part of a treatment guideline? Treatment guidelines require a recommended medication to have published evidence that the drug works better than a placebo or known active comparator. As with any medical or psychiatric disorder, the costly large-scale, randomized controlled trials (RCTs) necessary to achieve this level of evidence, as well as a US Food and Drug Administration (FDA)-approved indication, are typically supported by pharmaceutical companies. Therefore, the interests of the industry influence which drugs get developed and gain FDA approval, which, in turn, shapes treatment guidelines. For example, drug development for PTSD held great enthusiasm for several pharmaceutical companies in the 1980s, resulting in many large-scale RCTs of selective serotonin (SSRI) and serotonin-norepinephrine (SNRI) reuptake inhibitors and the subsequent FDA approval of sertraline and paroxetine. Since that time, industry has been reluctant to pursue PTSD as an indication, and no further FDA approvals for PTSD treatments have emerged. Obviously, a generic medication, such as prazosin, would not inspire a drug company to invest in its development. Over the past decade, the US Department of Veterans Affairs (VA) and US Department of Defense have invested more robustly in the research of pharmacologic treatments for PTSD, which has provided more evidence for other medications, such as prazosin, which are now being considered in treatment guidelines. These medications are approved by the FDA for other medical or psychiatric indications; however, they are considered "off-label" in their use for the treatment of PTSD.

The definition of response and remission in pharmacologic studies deserves mention, since it provides the clinician with a better understanding of the potential therapeutic impact of a medication. Although definitions vary, "response" is generally defined as a decrease in the PTSD rating scale by 30 % or more from the point in which the individual begins the medication. However, depending on baseline severity, some patients may simultaneously meet the definition of response and still remain quite symptomatic at the end of an 8- or 12-week trial. "Remission" or "recovery" is rarely mentioned as an outcome in published studies; however, when disclosed, it is typically defined as loss of the diagnosis of PTSD based on a scoring threshold for the outcome measure. For most antidepressants, less than 30 % of patients achieve full remission and response rates rarely exceed 60 %.

26.2   Antidepressants Are First-Line Medications for the Treatment of PTSD

In addition to their efficacy for the core symptoms of PTSD, antidepressants are effective for comorbid depressive and anxiety disorders. Serotonin reuptake inhibitors are considered by most treatment guidelines to be first-line medications for the treatment of PTSD. However, other classes of antidepressants, as discussed below, can also be effective. Paroxetine and sertraline are the only two medications FDA approved for the treatment of PTSD. Both are approved for acute PTSD treatment; however, sertraline is also approved for the long-term treatment of PTSD. Overall, paroxetine appears to be effective for all three of the core symptom clusters for PTSD, while sertraline shows consistent improvement in avoidance-emotional numbing and hyperarousal clusters and mixed improvement in reexperiencing symptoms. Antidepressant medications should be initiated at a low dose and increased as tolerated to a therapeutic dose. In general, PTSD symptoms show slow response to pharmacologic treatment. Once on a full dose of the agent, the patient should remain on that dose for 6–12 weeks in order to gauge response. In clinical follow-up, patients should be asked about target PTSD symptoms, as well as other symptoms including insomnia, irritability, psychosis, and suicidal ideation.

26.2.1 Serotonergic Reuptake Inhibitors

The efficacy of paroxetine was demonstrated in two pivotal studies (Marshall et al. 2001; Tucker et al. 2001). Paroxetine was beneficial in improving all three symptom clusters of PTSD for both genders, and results did not vary based on civilian or combat-related trauma. Both the 20 and 40 mg/day doses of paroxetine were effective and well tolerated. Compared to placebo, a significantly greater portion of those taking paroxetine achieved response and remission.

Similarly, two pivotal studies demonstrated that sertraline was significantly more effective than placebo in reducing PTSD symptoms with a little over half of the participants responding to treatment; however, these studies were in a sample of predominantly female civilians (Brady et al. 2000; Davidson et al. 2001b). Both studies showed significant improvement in avoidance/numbing and hyperarousal symptoms but yielded mixed results for the intrusive reexperiencing symptom cluster. Meanwhile, two large studies of similar design showed no advantage of sertraline over placebo [one unpublished study in a large group of mostly women with PTSD from physical and sexual assault (Pfizer Pharmaceuticals, written communication) and one trial in predominantly male US military veterans with combat-related PTSD (Friedman et al. 2007)]. A smaller study provided evidence that sertraline had positive effects in treating PTSD study in military veterans (Panahi et al. 2011). Other SSRI antidepressants, such as fluoxetine (van der Kolk et al. 1994; Connor et al. 1999; Martenyi et al. 2007) and citalopram (Tucker et al. 2003), have demonstrated some effectiveness in the treatment of PTSD, although results are very mixed.

These and other studies (Zohar et al. 2002) highlight the fact that the SSRIs do not always result in a clinically meaningful response for patients with PTSD. In an analysis of the evidence, the Institute of Medicine (IOM 2008) concluded that the clinical trials' evidence was inadequate to determine the efficacy of SSRI in the treatment of PTSD, although one member of the committee held a minority opinion stating that the effects of SSRI in general nonmilitary populations were suggestive, although not sufficient, to support their efficacy and that SSRIs were not effective in populations consisting of predominantly male veterans with chronic PTSD. Despite the debate, SSRI antidepressants continue to be recommended as evidence-based in several published treatment guidelines for PTSD (VA/DoD 2004; APA 2004; NICE 2005; Forbes et al. 2010). In addition, SSRIs are widely prescribed for individuals with PTSD, are well tolerated, and may improve concurrent conditions, such as major depressive, anxiety, and panic disorders, frequently seen in patients with PTSD.

26.2.1.1 Maintenance Treatment with SSRIs

Representative of the few long-term treatment studies, sertraline and fluoxetine have been shown to be better than placebo in maintaining PTSD symptom response. The majority of participants in the sertraline trial were women with PTSD from physical or sexual assault. Those treated with sertraline had significantly fewer PTSD relapses, fewer discontinuations due to relapse or insufficient response, and fewer exacerbation of PTSD (Davidson et al. 2001a). Compared to those treated with placebo, combat veterans with PTSD treated with fluoxetine had significantly fewer relapses and greater improvements in PTSD symptoms (Martenyi and Soldatenkova 2006; Martenyi et al. 2002). In conclusion, long-term treatment with SSRIs prevents PTSD worsening or relapses and also may bring about an improvement in PTSD symptoms over a longer period of treatment. Patients who respond to maintenance treatment should continue treatment for at least 1 year after they have achieved response. If the patient continues to have PTSD symptoms after 1 year, maintenance treatment should continue (International Psychopharmacology Algorithm Project: Post-Traumatic Stress Disorder 2005. Any consideration of discontinuing therapy should be based on current patient stressors, level of response to medication treatment, and side effects of the treatment. Discontinuation of medication therapy should occur slowly over at least a month to decrease the risk of relapse.

26.2.1.2 SSRI in Combination or Comparison to Behavioral Therapies

Patients with PTSD are most commonly treated with a combination of an SSRI and a type of behavioral therapy; however, very few studies have been conducted. For the studies that are available, evidence is very mixed and weak due to the very small sample sizes (Simon et al. 2008; van der Kolk 2007). The possibility of longer-lasting gains from behavioral therapy may be an advantage of treatment compared to medication alone. In a rare study focused on individuals with comorbid PTSD and alcohol dependence, sertraline was numerically, but not significantly, better than placebo in reducing PTSD scores (Brady et al. 2005). All participants received weekly cognitive behavioral therapy focused on their alcohol dependence. Patients with mild alcohol dependence did decrease their alcohol consumption during the study, while those with severe alcohol dependence had higher levels of alcohol consumption. While combination treatment is intuitively and clinically compelling, more research is needed to provide a better understanding of the comparative outcomes and to know the most efficacious combination that should be recommended.

26.2.2 Serotonin-Norepinephrine Reuptake Inhibitors (SNRI)

The SNRI venlafaxine is effective in the treatment of PTSD, particularly in regard to reducing the reexperiencing and avoidance symptom clusters and bringing about remission of PTSD (Davidson et al. 2006a, b). It also improves mood symptoms associated with PTSD. Venlafaxine has an early effect at week 2 on the symptoms for physiologic reactivity to cues, psychological distress to cues, irritability/anger, and intrusive recollections. Later in the course of treatment, at weeks 6–8, venlafaxine has significant effects on diminished interests, detachment, restricted range of affect, sense of foreshortened future, difficulty concentrating, hypervigilance, exaggerated startle response, and avoidance of thoughts, feelings, or conversations associated with the traumatic event. Treatment effects are essentially absent for distressing dreams; avoidance of activities, places, or people; inability to recall important aspects of trauma; and insomnia (Stein et al. 2009). These results are clinically informative in that the patient may show early improvements in physiological reactivity and psychological distress in response to cues, as well as irritability and anger, whereas symptoms of numbing and hyperarousal may take longer to improve. Nearly half of individuals achieve remission after 6 months of treatment with venlafaxine. The dose of venlafaxine should be initiated at 37.5 mg daily and titrated up to 225 mg/day or maximum dose of 300 mg/day, as tolerated. The results of another analysis suggested that higher pretreatment resilience is generally associated with a positive treatment response and remission to venlafaxine (Davidson et al. 2012). Venlafaxine improved resilience to varying degrees on a four-factor scale that included domains of hardiness, persistence/tenacity, social support, and faith in a benevolent or meaningful world (Davidson et al. 2008). These analyses did not find a significant gender effect on the efficacy of venlafaxine, but trauma type may have affected treatment outcome (Rothbaum et al. 2008a). Open-label studies of another SNRI, duloxetine, were positive (Walderhaug et al. 2010; Villarreal et al. 2010); however, placebo-controlled trials have not been published.

26.2.3 Other Antidepressants

Mirtazapine is primarily a α_2-adrenergic receptor and serotonin-2 receptor antagonist, which results in noradrenergic and serotonergic enhanced activity. Positive open-label trials of mirtazapine were subsequently confirmed by two small placebo-controlled trials (Davidson et al. 2003; Bahk et al. 2002). At lower doses, mirtazapine's sedation can be of use in treating insomnia associated with PTSD. However, at higher doses, the noradrenergic and serotonergic effects are more activating. Sexual side effects are lower than seen with SSRIs; however, there is more appetite stimulation which can lead to weight gain as compared to SSRI or SNRI medications.

Nefazodone is a α_1-adrenergic receptor and serotonin-2 receptor antagonist that also modestly inhibits serotonin and norepinephrine reuptake. Had it not been for the FDA black box warning of rare cases of liver failure (1:300,000 cases), practitioners may have taken more interest in nefazodone as a treatment for PTSD when positive results emerged in the literature (Hidalgo et al. 1999; Davis et al. 2004) However, two unpublished, industry-sponsored, placebo-controlled trials of nefazodone did not support these earlier findings. Two randomized double-blind studies comparing nefazodone and sertraline did not show group differences, but sample sizes were too small to support an active comparator trial (Saygin et al. 2002; McRae et al. 2004). Similar in its mechanism of action, the antidepressant trazodone has been shown to improve sleep and PTSD symptoms in open-label trials in veterans of the Vietnam War (Hertzberg et al. 1996). Both nefazodone and trazodone have sedating effects, which are a benefit for treating the insomnia associated with PTSD.

Bupropion is a unique antidepressant that has noradrenergic and dopaminergic enhancing properties. Small studies have shown that bupropion is helpful with treating severe depressive symptoms, but it is unreliable in treating the PTSD symptoms, especially in comparison to placebo (Canive et al. 1998; Becker et al. 2007; Davis et al. 1999; Herzberg et al. 2001).

Tricyclic antidepressants are fraught with side effects and hold the risk of being lethal in overdose. However, while not clinically appealing for these reasons, a practitioner may decide to choose a tricyclic in a patient who poses no risk of overdose and can medically tolerate these medications. Placebo-controlled studies provide some support for amitriptyline (Davidson et al. 1990) and imipramine (Frank et al. 1988; Kosten et al. 1991) and less with desipramine (Reist et al. 1989) in the treatment of PTSD. A small placebo-controlled trial of clomipramine showed a reduction in intrusive symptoms and obsessions in patients with PTSD and obsessive-compulsive disorder (Chen 1999).

Monoamine oxidase inhibitors (MAOI) in clinical trials for the treatment of PTSD have yielded mixed results. Studies of brofaromine did not differentiate drug from placebo for PTSD outcomes (Baker et al. 1995; Katz et al. 1994); however, phenelzine separated from placebo in two studies. Moclobemide was effective in reducing PTSD symptoms and inducing remission in approximately half of the 20 participants with PTSD (Neal et al. 1997). The disadvantage of MAOIs is the need for the patient to adhere to a low tyramine diet to prevent significant symptoms of serotonin syndrome, specifically causing elevated blood pressure.

26.2.4 Benzodiazepines

The reputation of benzodiazepines is mixed and professionals are fiercely divided on whether or not a patient with PTSD should be treated with benzodiazepines. Although benzodiazepines are frequently prescribed in patients with PTSD, evidence is lacking to support the use of this class of medication for the treatment of PTSD. To date, only one randomized double-blind, crossover trial with alprazolam compared against placebo has been conducted (Braum et al. 1990). This trial had high attrition, very small sample size, and other methodological limitations. Although there was no difference between treatment groups on PTSD measures, there was a significant effect of alprazolam on the anxiety scale. Due to lower central nervous system benzodiazepine receptors and neurotransmitter GABA levels, benzodiazepines may theoretically be somewhat pharmacologically inert in patients with PTSD. Eszopiclone, a non-benzodiazepine, GABA-A receptor agonist, demonstrated improvements on total PTSD symptom rating scale compared to placebo in a large clinical trial (Pollack et al. 2011). A replication study is warranted.

What are the consequences of using benzodiazepines immediately following a traumatic event, which may be medically appropriate as a form of sedation or anesthesia? Some animal studies suggest that benzodiazepine may interfere with post-trauma extinction and may actually potentiate the acquisition of fear responses. This phenomenon is limited to early stage of recovery during the acute post-trauma period when natural extinction processes are ongoing. Conversely, benzodiazepines may actually impede the ability to consolidate memories which could interfere with forming feared associations after a traumatic event (Makkar et al. 2010). For example, midazolam, a short-acting benzodiazepine impaired the reconsolidation of fear memories in animal models (Bustos et al. 2006). In a study investigating the prevalence of PTSD in burned soldiers who received perioperative midazolam compared to those who did not, investigators found that intraoperative midazolam was not associated with increased PTSD development or with increased intensity of memory of the traumatic event (McGhee et al. 2009).

Do benzodiazepines reduce the effectiveness of prolonged exposure therapy for PTSD? Some, but not all, animal research suggests that benzodiazepines interfere with extinction training (i.e., exposure therapy for rats). Thus, the field has been concerned with the possibility of a benzodiazepine interfering with the effects of prolonged exposure therapy. Although prospective studies are lacking, benzodiazepines have been shown to be associated with poorer outcomes after prolonged exposure therapy (Van Minnen et al. 2002). However, in a recently published study that reanalyzed results from a behavioral therapy trial to assess whether benzodiazepine use was associated with reduced response to exposure therapy, Rosen and colleagues (2013) found that patients prescribed benzodiazepines did not have weaker responses to prolonged exposure. In conclusion, while one would want to avoid initiating a new prescription of a benzodiazepine, patients who are taking benzodiazepines can benefit from prolonged exposure therapy.

Benzodiazepines have their advantages and disadvantages, especially when treating someone with PTSD. Benzodiazepines are contraindicated for patients with disinhibition and addictions, which are problems that many with PTSD face. Clearly, a person with alcohol or drug addiction is at risk of benzodiazepine addiction and misuse. This is why some practice guidelines list potential harm by the benzodiazepine drug class. While most clinical practice guidelines advise the clinician to avoid new prescriptions of a benzodiazepine in all patients with PTSD, the newly published 2014 treatment guidelines from the British Association for Psychopharmacology remind us that this class of medication has proven efficacy in the treatment of panic disorder, generalized anxiety disorder, and social anxiety disorder (i.e., common comorbid conditions in patients with PTSD) and that this class of medication is usually reserved for the treatment of patients who have not responded to previous treatments, arguing that "concerns about potential problems in long-term use should not prevent their use in patients with persistent, severe, distressing and impairing anxiety symptoms, when other treatment have proved ineffective" (Baldwin et al. 2014, p. 412). Cautious use and medical follow-up is advisable if a person with PTSD is prescribed a benzodiazepine.

26.2.5 Other Medications

26.2.5.1 Anti-adrenergic Agents

Perhaps one of the most exciting recent findings is that of prazosin in its ability to not only treat PTSD-related sleep disturbances (Raskind et al. 2003, 2008; Taylor et al. 2007) but also the full spectrum of combat-related PTSD symptoms (Raskind et al. 2013). Prazosin is used in the medical management of hypertension or benign prostatic hypertrophy and has been used as a treatment for PTSD, typically in combination with an SSRI. The average prazosin dosing is 2–4 mg in the morning and 7–16 mg at bedtime, with lower doses needed for the women. Prazosin is well tolerated, and blood pressure changes are not remarkable. Prazosin is not associated with many of the uncomfortable side effects like sedation, sexual dysfunction, dyslipidemia, hyperglycemia, or weight gain that accompany other psychotropic medications. Although uncommon, side effects include drowsiness, lightheadedness, and syncope due to orthostatic hypotension. Results from a larger multisite study in veterans will soon become available.

26.2.5.2 Atypical Antipsychotics

Most studies of atypical antipsychotics have been designed as adjunctive treatment to an antidepressant medication, which is in keeping with clinical practice. Although some evidence was initially compelling (Padala et al. 2006; Bartzokis et al. 2005; Monnelly et al. 2003; Reich et al. 2004), the overall evidence suggests little clinical benefit for risperidone or olanzapine (Stein et al. 2002; Butterfield et al. 2001) in reducing the core PTSD symptoms. Two small single-site studies did find an advantage of risperidone compared to placebo in ameliorating symptoms of insomnia and paranoia associated with PTSD (Rothbaum et al. 2008b; Hamner et al. 2003). Ultimately, the largest placebo-controlled study of an adjunctive risperidone in US veterans with chronic military-related PTSD who had ongoing symptoms despite at least two adequate SSRI treatments found no difference between groups in reducing PTSD symptoms, depression, anxiety, or quality of life after 6 months of treatment (Krystal et al. 2011). The rate of remission with risperidone (5 %) did not differ from placebo (4 %), nor did any differences emerge in terms of categorically definitions of response. Risperidone was associated with a statistically significant reduction in the reexperiencing and hyperarousal PTSD symptom clusters, but not the avoidance/numbing symptom cluster. However, these differences were not considered clinically meaningful. Compared to placebo, adverse events were more common in the risperidone group and included weight gain, fatigue, somnolence, and hypersalivation. Research in more diverse groups may be warranted, since other classes of medication appear to also fall short in a treatment-resistant, predominantly male population with military-related PTSD. Other types of antipsychotics, such as quetiapine, have more positive results of placebo-controlled study pending final analysis and publication.

Atypical antipsychotics can also be used to treat psychotic symptoms associated with PTSD (Hamner et al. 2003) or mood symptoms of depression or bipolar disorder in PTSD patients which is not adequately treated by SSRIs or mood stabilizers. Patients with PTSD may be more sensitive to the adverse effects of antipsychotic medications, so it is important to start at a low dose and titrate upwards as tolerated by the patient. Due to the risks of metabolic disorders, such as diabetes, patients should have their weight and waist circumference measured regularly, and their metabolic profile should be monitored at least annually.

26.2.5.3 Anticonvulsants

Clinical trials of anticonvulsants took a different route than antipsychotics, in that the drugs were used as monotherapy instead of adjunctive treatment in most studies. Placebo-controlled trials did not prove divalproex (Davis et al. 2008) or tiagabine (Davidson et al. 2007) to be beneficial in the treatment of PTSD. One very small placebo-controlled study of lamotrigine showed that this drug was better than placebo (Hertzberg et al. 1999), but replication in larger study is needed to confirm these preliminary findings. Although recent meta-analyses (Jonas et al. 2013; Watts et al. 2013) suggest that topiramate may have some effectiveness in the treatment of PTSD, larger placebo-controlled studies are warranted prior to reaching conclusive recommendations. Since there is no evidence for using anticonvulsants as monotherapy for the symptoms of PTSD, the only role that these medications have is for PTSD patients who have comorbid bipolar disorder.

26.2.5.4 Treatments Under Investigation

Clinical trials of investigational agents targeting neurotransmitter systems purported to be involved in the pathophysiology of PTSD, including glucocorticoids, corticotropin-releasing factor, yohimbine, beta-blockers, glutamate, neurosteroids, neurokinin receptor antagonists, oxytocin, opiates, endocannabinoids, methylene blue, methylenedioxymethylamphetamine, mifepristone, and rapamycin are under clinical study. Case reports and case series have reported benefits of adjunctive buspirone, cyproheptadine, and clonidine. None of these agents have reached the level of scientific evidence needed to be considered a recommended treatment.

26.3 Review of PTSD Treatment Guidelines

There are at least six published PTSD treatment guidelines, including those from the VA/Department of Defense, American Psychiatric Association (APA), National Institute for Clinical Excellence (NICE), International Society for Traumatic Stress Studies (ISTSS), International Psychopharmacology Algorithm Project: Post-Traumatic Stress disorder (IPAP), and the Harvard South Shore Program. Each set of guidelines has a different way of rating treatment recommendations based on the available evidence that support or refute specific therapies.

Five out of six PTSD treatment guidelines recommend SSRI antidepressants as first-line treatment with high ratings on strength of evidence. The use of prazosin is recommended as either monotherapy or augmentation for trauma-related nightmares by a majority of the guidelines. However, a recent placebo-controlled study demonstrated the efficacy of prazosin for PTSD, which should add to its strength of evidence. Antipsychotics are generally only recommended when there is an element of psychosis or bipolarity involved. There is a general consensus that benzodiazepines are not effective for PTSD. Most guidelines recommend against their use, although one set recommends them on an individual basis as adjunctive therapy for sleep and anxiety. Hypnotics are only addressed by the NICE guidelines which recommend temporary use and not as monotherapy. In slight contrast to the majority, the Harvard South Shore Program recommends addressing poor sleep first and using prazosin and trazodone before implementing an SSRI. If significant PTSD symptoms persist, an SSRI should then be considered. If inadequate response is seen with one SSRI, a different SSRI can be considered as well as switching to an SNRI or mirtazapine. If symptoms persist still, they should be treated according to specific symptom cluster.

26.4   Clinical Applications

The initial treatment of PTSD should start with pharmacotherapy, behavioral therapy, or a combination, depending on the patient's preference, availability of skilled therapists, and the urgency of the current clinical and psychosocial situation. However, evaluation for medications can be strongly considered when patients are diagnosed with comorbid disorders such as panic, psychotic, or bipolar disorders, with the goal of stabilizing the more serious mental conditions early in the course of treatment of the PTSD.

A psychotherapist or behavioral therapist should always have several providers in their professional network to refer their treatment-resistant patients for medication evaluation or intervention. These providers can be a psychiatrist, primary care physician, clinical pharmacist, or nurse practitioner with mental health experience. If the patient is not showing signs of stabilization with a few weeks of behavioral therapy or psychotherapy treatment, the therapist should suggest that the patient obtain an appointment with the medical professional for medication evaluation, especially since it may take some weeks or more before an appointment is available. Collaboration with a medical provider should include early stage communications of the core symptoms that may need medication, and follow-up communication may occur every few months as treatment response progresses.

First-line medication treatment usually includes an SSRI, such as sertraline or paroxetine, or an SNRI, such as venlafaxine, with an additional sleep aid, such as trazodone or prazosin, if needed. The use of benzodiazepines should be avoided because these medications are difficult to discontinue once a patient has become reliant on this class of medication. However, acute and severe panic attacks may require short-term use of a benzodiazepine until the SSRI and/or behavioral or psychotherapy can take effect.

Typically, antidepressant medications are initiated at a low dose and titrated to the maximum therapeutic dose, as tolerated by the individual patient. Explain to the patient that some symptoms that improve early in treatment are not necessarily the core PTSD symptoms (i.e., intrusive memories, flashbacks, and nightmares), but rather may be symptoms, such as irritability, hyperarousal, and emotional reactivity, which are not readily recognized by laypersons as symptoms of PTSD. Many patients with PTSD complain of having a "short fuse" and appreciate the concept of the medication having the ability to promote a longer fuse in the first 2–4 weeks of treatment. The longer fuse provides a space in which the patient can evaluate the situation and make the right choice rather than impulsively reacting without thinking. However, it is still up to the patient to make the right choice, which is where the therapist can come into the picture by reinforcing behavioral adaptations to promote recovery.

Typically, individuals with PTSD are resistant to taking medication due to fears of the potential side effects, such as sedation or sexual side effects, and the stigma of taking psychotropics. A therapist can help destigmatize medication and provide reassurance about the benefits of treatment compared to the side effects. Many patients consume high quantities of caffeine during the day in order to cope with the day-after effects of a sleepless night. Good sleep hygiene is important. Patients lead sedentary lives due to the avoidant behaviors that have developed. In addition, many patients may eat a diet high in sugar and fat – all of which contribute to insomnia, depression, and anxiety. In summary, therapists should encourage the basics, such as stressing the importance of adherence to the prescribed medication, good sleep hygiene, regular exercise or activity, and a healthy diet. Of course, mental health providers should remind women of childbearing potential to use adequate contraception when taking medication in order to avoid risks of birth defects.

Despite first-line treatment, more often than not, the PTSD symptoms persist beyond 12 weeks and the clinician is asked for next-step treatment recommendations. Prior to tampering the medications, it is important to ask about adherence and side effects, since poor adherence may be the reason medications are not working. Patients may have misunderstood the need to take these medications daily rather than as needed for symptoms. Also make inquiry into comorbid conditions or stressors, such as substance abuse; ongoing trauma, such as continued domestic violence or exposure to life-threatening events in the line of one's occupation; litigation issues, such as disability claims or law suits; and suicide risk, psychosocial stressors, or unemployment issues that might change clinical management and require additional support systems.

There are no research studies that provide guidance on second-level treatment for PTSD that has not remitted to first-line SSRI or behavioral therapy. In other words, head-to-head studies comparing a "switch" or "augmentation" approach have not been conducted. If PTSD symptoms require additional treatment, a switch from an SSRI to an SNRI, such as venlafaxine, is warranted. Alternatively, if the patient has not had a trial of prazosin augmentation, this approach would also be a strong candidate for next-step treatment. Mirtazapine or trazodone can be considered for PTSD with the added sedative benefit to help with sleep. Finally, if the patient has not participated in an evidence-based behavioral therapy (Part III), one should strongly seek out such treatment options.

Once medications are deemed ineffective, it is crucial that the provider taper and discontinue the medication, so that the number of medications is kept to a minimum whenever possible. Also realize that some side effects of medications can mimic symptoms of anxiety or PTSD, such as decreased concentration, irritability, agitation, and fatigue. Thus, a reduction or discontinuation of medication can sometimes alleviate unwanted psychosomatic symptoms.

26.5   In Summary

In conclusion, SSRI and SNRI antidepressant medications remain central to the pharmacologic treatment of PTSD. However, the clinician should not be surprised to find that most patients' PTSD symptoms do not remit. Next-step treatment is a common dilemma. Prazosin seems like a promising and low-risk alternative to consider as adjunct to the antidepressant and perhaps even as monotherapy in those who develop unwanted side effects to the SSRI or SNRI medication. The use of antipsychotic and anticonvulsive medications in the treatment of PTSD remains in doubt, especially given their unattractive side effect profiles. However, comorbid psychotic disorder, severe impulsivity, and frequent mood lability may compel the clinician to use these classes of medications. Benzodiazepines should be used sparingly, if at all, particularly in those with past histories of substance use disorders.

PTSD can manifest with a vast array of symptoms, making it an extremely heterogeneous and complex disorder, which adds to the challenge of selecting treatments. Advances in genetics research may provide more precision in matching the appropriate patient with the best treatment. Clearly, more research is needed to evaluate novel medications against placebo, to compare active medications against one another, to evaluate the combination of medications with behavioral therapies, and to find better, more personalized treatments for PTSD. Once effective treatments are supported by the evidence, an entirely separate problem is that of adherence to effective treatments. Fostering a strong therapeutic relationship to enhance treatment adherence is key to recovery. Keeping treatment patient centered and involving family support systems also improve the overall outcomes for persons with PTSD.

References

American Psychiatric Association. (2004). *Practice guideline for the treatment of patients with acute stress disorder and posttraumatic stress disorder.* Arlington: American Psychiatry Association. Available online at http://www.psychiatryonline.com/pracGuide/pracGuideTopic. Accessed 15 Dec 2013.

Bahk, W. M., Pae, C. U., Tsoh, J., Chae, J. H., Jun, T. Y., Lee, C., & Kim, K. S. (2002). Effects of mirtazapine in patients with post-traumatic stress disorder in Korea: A pilot study. *Human Psychopharmacology: Clinical and Experimental, 17,* 341–344.

Bajor, D. O., Ticlea, A. N., & Osser, D. N. (2011). The psychopharmacology algorithm project at the Harvard south shore program: An update on post-traumatic stress disorder. *Harvard Review of Psychiatry, 19*(5), 240–258.

Baker, D. G., Diamond, B. I., Gillette, G., et al. (1995). A double-blind, randomized, placebo-controlled, multicenter study of brofaromine in the treatment of posttraumatic stress disorder. *Psychopharmacology, 122*, 386–389.

Baldwin, D. S., Anderson, I. M., Nutt, D. J., Allgulander, C., Bandelow, B., den Boer, J. A., Christmas, D. M., Davies, S., Fineberg, N., Lidbetter, N., Malizia, A., McCrone, P., Nabarro, D., O'Neill, C., Scott, J., van der Wee, N., & Wittchen, H. U. (2014). Evidence-based pharmacological treatment of anxiety disorders, post-traumatic stress disorder and obsessive-compulsive disorder: A revision of the 2005 guidelines from the British Association for Psychopharmacology. *Journal of Psychopharmacology, 28*(5), 403–439.

Bartzokis, G., Lu, P. H., Turner, J., Mintz, J., & Saunders, C. S. (2005). Adjunctive risperidone in the treatment of chronic combat-related posttraumatic stress disorder. *Biological Psychiatry, 57*, 474–479.

Becker, M. E., Hertzberg, M. A., Moore, S. D., Dennis, M. F., Bukenya, D. S., & Beckham, J. C. (2007). A placebo-controlled trial of bupropion SR in the treatment of chronic posttraumatic stress disorder. *Journal of Clinical Psychopharmacology, 27*, 193–197.

Brady, K., Pearlstein, T., Asnis, G. M., et al. (2000). Efficacy and safety of sertraline treatment of posttraumatic stress disorder: A randomized controlled trial. *JAMA, 283*(14), 1837–1844.

Brady, K. T., Sonne, S., & Anton, R. F. (2005). Sertraline in the treatment of co-occurring alcohol dependence and posttraumatic stress disorder. *Alcoholism, Clinical and Experimental Research, 29*, 395–401.

Braum, P., Greenberg, D., Dasberg, H., et al. (1990). Core symptoms of posttraumatic stress disorder unimproved by alprazolam treatment. *Journal of Clinical Psychiatry, 51*(6), 236–238.

Bustos, S. G., Maldonado, H., & Molina, B. A. (2006). Midazolam disrupts fear memory reconsolidation. *Neuroscience, 139*, 831–842.

Butterfield, M. I., Becker, M. E., Connor, K. M., et al. (2001). Olanzapine in the treatment of posttraumatic stress disorder: A pilot study. *International Clinical Psychopharmacology, 164*(4), 197–203.

Canive, J. M., Clark, R. D., Calais, L. A., Qualls, C., & Tuason, V. B. (1998). Bupropion treatment in veterans with posttraumatic stress disorder: An open study. *Journal of Clinical Psychopharmacology, 18*(5), 379–383.

Chen, C. J. (1999). The obsessive quality and clomipramine treatment in PTSD. *The American Journal of Psychiatry, 148*, 1087–1088.

Cloitre, M., Courtois, C. A., Ford, J. D., Green, B. L., Alexander, P., Briere, J., Herman, J. L., Lanius, R., Stolbach, B. C., Spinazzola, J., van der Kolk, B. A., & van der Hart, O.. *The International Society for Traumatic Stress Studies (ISTSS) expert consensus treatment guidelines for complex PTSD in adults.* http://www.istss.org. Accessed 17 Dec 2013.

Connor, K. M., Sutherland, S. M., Tupler, L. A., et al. (1999). Fluoxetine in post-traumatic stress disorder. Randomized double-blind study. *British Journal of Psychiatry, 175*, 17–22.

Davidson, J., Kudler, H., Smith, R., et al. (1990). Treatment of posttraumatic stress disorder with amitriptyline and placebo. *Archives of General Psychiatry, 47*, 259–266.

Davidson, J. R. T., Pearlstein, T., Londborg, P., et al. (2001a). Efficacy of sertraline in preventing relapse of posttraumatic stress disorder: Results of a 28 week double-blind, placebo-controlled study. *The American Journal of Psychiatry, 158*, 1974–1981.

Davidson, J. R. T., Rothbaum, B. O., van der Kolk, B. A., et al. (2001b). Multicenter, double-blind comparison of sertraline and placebo in the treatment of posttraumatic stress disorder. *Archives of General Psychiatry, 58*(5), 485–492.

Davidson, R. T., Weisler, R. H., Butterfield, M. I., Casat, C. D., Connor, K. M., Barnett, S., & van Meter, S. (2003). Mirtazapine vs. placebo in posttraumatic stress disorder: A pilot trial. *Biological Psychiatry, 53*, 188–191.

Davidson, J., Baldwin, D., Stein, D. J., Kuper, E., Benattia, I., Ahmed, S., Pedersen, R., & Musgnung, J. (2006a). Treatment of posttraumatic stress disorder with venlafaxine extended release: A 6-month randomized controlled trial. *Archives of General Psychiatry, 63,* 1158–1165.

Davidson, J., Rothbaum, B. O., Tucker, P., Asnis, G., Benattia, I., & Musgnung, M. T. (2006b). Venlafaxine extended release in posttraumatic stress disorder. *Journal of Clinical Psychopharmacology, 26,* 259–267.

Davidson, J. R., Brady, K., Mellman, T. A., Stein, M. B., & Pollack, M. H. (2007). The efficacy and tolerability of tiagabine in adult patients with post-traumatic stress disorder. *Journal of Clinical Psychopharmacology , 27,* 85–88.

Davidson, J., Baldwin, D. S., Stein, D. J., Pedersen, R., Ahmed, S., Musgnung, J., Benattia, I., & Rothbaum, B. O. (2008). Effects of venlafaxine extended release on resilience in posttraumatic stress disorder: An item analysis of the Connor-Davidson resilience scale. *International Clinical Psychopharmacology , 23*(5), 299–303.

Davidson, J., Stein, D. J., Rothbaum, B. O., Pedersen, R., Szumski, A., & Baldwin, D. S. (2012). Resilience as a predictor of treatment response in patients with posttraumatic stress disorder treatment with venlafaxine extended release or placebo. *Journal of Psychopharmacology, 26*(6), 778–783.

Davis, L. L., Nevels, S. M., Farley, J., & Petty, F. (1999). *Bupropion sustained release for posttraumatic stress disorder-a placebo-controlled study.* International Society of Traumatic Stress Studies annual meeting, Miami.

Davis, L. L., Jewell, M. E., Ambrose, S., Farley, J., English, B., Bartolucci, A., & Petty, F. (2004). A placebo-controlled study of nefazodone for the treatment of chronic posttraumatic stress disorder: A preliminary study. *Journal of Clinical Psychopharmacology, 24*(3), 291–297.

Davis, L. L., Davidson, J. R., Ward, L. C., Bartolucci, A., Bowden, C. L., & Petty, F. (2008). Divalproex in the treatment of posttraumatic stress disorder in a veteran population. *Journal of Clinical Psychopharmacology, 28,* 84–88.

Forbes, D., Creamer, M., Bisson, J. I., Cohen, J. A., Crow, B. E., Foa, E. D., Friedman, M. J., Keane, T. M., Kudler, H. S., & Ursano, R. J. (2010). A guide to guidelines for the treatment of PTSD and related conditions. *Journal of Traumatic Stress, 23*(5), 537–552.

Frank, J. B., Kosten, T. R., Giller, E. L., et al. (1988). A randomized clinical trial of phenelzine and imipramine for posttraumatic stress disorder. *The American Journal of Psychiatry, 145,* 1289–1291.

Friedman, M. J., Marmar, C. R., Baker, D. G., Sikes, C. R., & Farfel, G. M. (2007). Randomized, double-blind comparison of sertraline and placebo for posttraumatic stress disorder in a Department of Veterans Affairs setting. *Journal of Clinical Psychiatry, 68*(5), 711–720. PMID:17503980.

Hamner, M. B., Faldowski, R. A., Ulmer, H. G., Frueh, B. C., Huber, M. G., & Arana, G. W. (2003). Adjunctive risperidone treatment in post-traumatic stress disorder: A preliminary controlled trial of effects on comorbid psychotic symptoms. *International Clinical Psychopharmacology, 18*(1), 1–8.

Hertzberg, M. A., Feldman, M. E., Beckham, J. C., & Davidson, R. T. (1996). Trial of trazodone for posttraumatic stress disorder using a multiple baseline group design. *Journal of Clinical Psychopharmacology, 16*(4), 294–298.

Hertzberg, M. A., Butterfield, M. I., Felman, M. E., Beckham, J. C., Sutherland, S. M., Connor, K. M., & Davidson, J. R. T. (1999). A preliminary study of lamotrigine for the treatment of posttraumatic stress disorder. *Biological Psychiatry, 45,* 1226–1229.

Hertzberg, M. A., Moore, S. D., Feldman, M. E., & Beckham, J. C. (2001). A preliminary study of bupropion sustained-release for smoking cessation in patients with chronic posttraumatic stress disorder. *Journal of Clinical Psychopharmacology, 21*(1), 94–98.

Hidalgo, R., Hertzberg, M. A., Mellman, T., et al. (1999). Nefazodone in posttraumatic stress disorder: Results from six open-label trials. *International Clinical Psychopharmacology, 14,* 61–68.

Institute of Medicine (IOM). (2008). *Treatment of posttraumatic stress disorder: An assessment of the evidence.* Washington, DC: The National Academies Press. Available online at http://books.nap.edu/openbook.php?record id=11955. Accessed 20 Dec 2013.

International Psychopharmacology Algorithm Project: Post-traumatic stress disorder. (2005). http://www.ipap.org

Jonas, D. E., Cusack, K., Forneris, C. A., Wilkins, T. M., Sonis, J., et al. (2013). *Psychological and pharmacological treatments for adults with posttraumatic stress disorder (PTSD).* Rockville: Agency for Healthcare Research and Quality (US).

Katz, R. J., Lott, M. H., Arbus, P., et al. (1994). Pharmacotherapy of posttraumatic stress disorder with a novel psychotropic. *Anxiety, 1,* 169–174.

Kosten, T. R., Frank, J. B., Dan, E., et al. (1991). Pharmacotherapy for posttraumatic stress disorder using phenelzine or imipramine. *Journal of Nervous and Mental Disease, 179,* 366–370.

Krystal, J. H., Rosenheck, R. A., Cramer, J. A., Vessicchio, J. C., Jones, K. M., Vertrees, J. E., Horney, R. A., Huang, G. D., Stock, C., & VA Cooperative Study No. 504 Group. (2011). Adjunctive risperidone treatment for antidepressant-resistant symptoms of chronic military service-related PTSD: A randomized trial. *JAMA, 306*(5), 493–502.

Makkar, S. R., Zhang, S. Q., & Cranney, J. (2010). Behavioral and neural analysis of GABA in the acquisition, consolidation, reconsolidation and extinction of new memory. *Neurpsychopharmacology, 35,* 1625–1652.

Marshall, R. D., Beebe, K. L., Oldham, M., & Zaninelli, R. (2001). Efficacy and safety of paroxetine treatment for chronic PTSD. A fixed dose, placebo-controlled study. *The American Journal of Psychiatry, 158,* 1982–1988.

Martenyi, F., & Soldatenkova, V. (2006). Fluoxetine in the acute treatment and relapse prevention of combat-related post-traumatic stress disorder: Analysis of the veteran group of a placebo-controlled, randomized clinical trial. *European Neuropsychopharmacology, 16*(5), 340–349.

Martenyi, F., Brown, E. B., Zhang, H., et al. (2002). Fluoxetine v. placebo in prevention of relapse in post-traumatic stress disorder. *British Journal of Psychiatry, 181,* 315–320.

Martenyi, F., Brown, E., & Caldwell, C. (2007). Failed efficacy of fluoxetine in the treatment of posttraumatic stress disorder: Results of a fixed-dose, placebo-controlled study. *Journal of Clinical Psychopharmacology , 27*(2), 166–170.

McGhee, L. L., Maani, C. V., Garza, T. H., DeSocio, P. A., Gaylord, K. M., & Black, I. H. (2009). The relationship of intravenous midazolam and posttraumatic stress disorder development in burned soldiers. *Journal of Trauma, 66*(4 Suppl), S186–S190.

McRae, A. L., Brady, K. T., Mellman, T. A., Sonne, S. C., Killeen, T. K., Timmerman, M. A., et al. (2004). Comparison of nefazodone and sertraline for the treatment of posttraumatic stress disorder. *Depression and Anxiety, 19*(3), 190–196.

Monnelly, E. P., Ciraulo, D. A., Knapp, C., & Keane, T. (2003). Low-dose risperidone as adjunctive therapy for irritable aggression in posttraumatic stress disorder. *Journal of Clinical Psychopharmacology, 23,* 193–196.

National Institute for Health and Care Excellence. (2005). *Post-traumatic stress disorder: The management of PTSD in adults and children in primary and secondary care* (Report No.: NICE clinical guidelines, No. 26), London, Available online at: http://guidance.nice.org.uk/CG26. Accessed 15 Dec 2013.

Neal, L. A., Shapland, W., & Fox, C. (1997). An open trial of moclobemide in the treatment of post-traumatic stress disorder. *International Clinical Psychopharmacology, 12,* 231–237.

Padala, P. R., Madison, J., Monnahan, M., Marcil, W., Price, P., Ramaswamy, S., et al. (2006). Risperidone monotherapy for post-traumatic stress disorder related to sexual assault and domestic abuse in women. *International Clinical Psychopharmacology, 21,* 275–280.

Panahi, Y., Moghaddam, B. R., Sahebkar, A., et al. (2011). A randomized, double-blind, placebo-controlled trial on the efficacy and tolerability of sertraline in Iranian veterans with post-traumatic stress disorder. *Psychological Medicine, 41*(10), 2159–2166.

Pollack, M. H., Hoge, E. A., Worthington, J. J., et al. (2011). Eszopiclone for the treatment of post-traumatic stress disorder and associated insomnia: A randomized double-blind placebo controlled trial. *Journal of Clinical Psychiatry, 72,* 892–897.

Raskind, M. A., Peskind, E. R., Kanter, E. D., et al. (2003). Reduction of nightmares and other PTSD symptoms in combat veterans by prazosin: A placebo controlled study. *The American Journal of Psychiatry, 160,* 371–373.

Raskind, M. A., Peskind, E. R., Hoff, D. J., et al. (2008). A parallel group placebo-controlled study of prazosin for trauma nightmares and sleep disturbance in combat veterans with post-traumatic stress disorder. *Biological Psychiatry, 41*, 8–18.

Raskind, M. A., Peterson, K., Williams, T., et al. (2013). A trial of prazosin for combat trauma PTSD with nightmares in active-duty soldiers returned from Iraq and Afghanistan 2013. *The American Journal of Psychiatry, 170*, 1003–1010.

Reich, D. B., Winternitz, S., Hennen, J., Watts, T., & Stanculescu, C. (2004). A preliminary study of risperidone in the treatment of posttraumatic stress disorder related to childhood abuse in women. *Journal of Clinical Psychiatry, 65*, 1601–1606.

Reist, C., Kauffmann, C. D., Haier, R. J., et al. (1989). A controlled trial of desipramine in 18 men with posttraumatic stress disorder. *The American Journal of Psychiatry, 146*, 513–516.

Rosen, C. S., Greenbaum, M. A., Schnurr, P. P., Holmes, T. H., Brennan, P. L., & Friedman, M. J. (2013). Do benzodiazepines reduce the effectiveness of exposure therapy for posttraumatic stress disorder? *Journal of Clinical Psychiatry, 74*(12), 1241–1248.

Rothbaum, B. O., Davidson, J. R., Stein, D. J., Pedersen, R., Musgnung, J., Tian, X. W., Ahmed, S., & Baldwin, D. S. (2008a). A pooled analysis of gender and trauma-type effects on responsiveness to treatment of PTSD with venlafaxine extended release or placebo. *Journal of Clinical Psychiatry, 69*(10), 1529–1539.

Rothbaum, B. O., Killeen, T. K., Davidson, J. R. T., Brady, K. T., Connor, K. M., & Heekin, M. H. (2008b). Placebo-controlled trial of risperidone augmentation for selective serotonin reuptake inhibitor-resistant civilian posttraumatic stress disorder. *Journal of Clinical Psychiatry, 69*, 520–525.

Saygin, M. Z., Sungur, M. Z., Sabol, E. U., & Cetinkaya, P. (2002). Nefazodone versus sertraline in treatment of post-traumatic stress disorder. *Bulletin of Clinical Psychopharmacology, 12*(1), 1–5.

Simon, N. M., Connor, K. M., Lang, A. J., et al. (2008). Paroxetine CR augmentation for posttraumatic stress disorder refractory to prolonged exposure therapy. *Journal of Clinical Psychiatry, 69*(3), 400–405.

Stein, M. B., Kline, N. A., & Matloff, J. L. (2002). Adjunctive olanzapine for SSRI-resistant combat-related PTSD: A double-blind, placebo-controlled study. *The American Journal of Psychiatry, 159*(10), 1777–1779.

Stein, D. J., Pedersen, R., Rothbaum, B. O., Baldwin, D. S., Ahmed, S., Musgnung, J., & Davidson, J. (2009). Onset of activity and time to response on individual CAPS-SX17 items in patients treated for post-traumatic stress disorder with venlafaxine ER: A pooled analysis. *International Journal of Neuropsychopharmacology , 12*(1), 23–31.

Stein, D. J., Rothbaum, B. O., Baldwin, D. S., Szumski, A., Pedersen, R., & Davidson, J. R. T. (2013). A factor analysis of posttraumatic stress disorder symptoms using data pooled from two venlafaxine extended-release clinical trials. *Brain and Behavior, 3*(6), 738–746.

Taylor, F. B., Martin, P., Thompson, C., et al. (2007). Prazosin effects on objective sleep measures and clinical symptoms in civilian trauma posttraumatic stress disorder: A placebo-controlled study. *Biological Psychiatry, 61*, 928–934.

Tucker, P., Zaninelli, R., Yehuda, R., et al. (2001). Paroxetine in the treatment of chronic posttraumatic stress disorder: Results of a placebo-controlled, flexible-dosage trial. *Journal of Clinical Psychiatry, 62*, 860–868.

Tucker, P., Potter-Kimball, R., Wyatt, D. B., Parker, D. E., et al. (2003). Can physiologic assessment and side effects tease out differences in PTSD trials? A double-blind comparison of citalopram, sertraline and placebo. *Psychopharmacology Bulletin, 37*(3), 135–149.

van der Kolk, B. A., Dreyfyss, D., Michaels, M., Shera, D., et al. (1994). Fluoxetine in posttraumatic stress disorder. *Journal of Clinical Psychiatry, 55*(12), 517–522.

van der Kolk, B. A., Spinazzola, J., Blaustein, M. R., et al. (2007). A randomized clinical trial of eye movement desensitization and reprocessing (EDMR), fluoxetine and pill placebo in the treatment of posttraumatic stress disorder: Treatment effects and long-term maintenance. *Journal of Clinical Psychiatry, 68*, 37–46.

Van Minnen, A., Arntz, A., & Keijsers, G. P. (2002). Prolonged exposure in patients with chronic PTSD: Predictors of treatment outcome and dropout. *Behaviour Research and Therapy, 40*(4), 439–457.

Veterans Health Administration, Department of Defense. (2004). *(VA/DoD) clinical practice guideline for the management of post-traumatic stress. Version 1.0.* Washington, DC: Veterans Health Administration, Department of Defense. Available online at http://www.healthquality. va.gov/ptsd/ptsd-full.pdf. Accessed 15 Dec 2013.

Villarreal, G., Canive, J. M., Calais, L. A., Toney, G., & Smith, A. K. (2010). Duloxetine in military posttraumatic stress disorder. *Psychopharmacology Bulletin, 43*(3), 26–34.

Walderhaug, E., Kasserman, S., Aikins, D., Vojvoda, D., Nishimura, C., & Neumeister, A. (2010). Effects of duloxetine in treatment-refractory men with posttraumatic stress disorder. *Pharmacopsychiatry, 43*, 45–49.

Watts, B. V., Schnurr, P. P., Mayo, L., Young-Xu, Y., Weeks, W. B., & Friedman, M. J. (2013). Meta-analysis of the efficacy of treatments for posttraumatic stress disorder. *Journal of Clinical Psychiatry, 74*(6), e541–e550.

Zohar, J., Amital, D., Miodownik, C., et al. (2002). Double-blind placebo-controlled pilot study of sertraline in military veterans with post-traumatic stress disorder. *Journal of Clinical Psychopharmacology, 22*(2), 190–195.

Part VIII
Conclusions

What Works for Whom?

27

Marylène Cloitre, Richard A. Bryant, and Ulrich Schnyder

27.1 Overview

We are very fortunate to have a volume with chapters that provide rich and detailed descriptions of various treatment programs across the spectrum of trauma-related disorders. This approach allows readers to select the chapter, which describes the type of patient or type of approach of interest, and obtain the desired information on a specific issue. It is also useful, however, for readers to consider the issues raised in chapters that may not seem to directly relate to their usual practice domain because the convergent lessons emerging from these chapters can inform and enhance our treatments for different types of patients. To this end, in this chapter we step back and summarize not only commonalities observed across treatments (see Chap. 1) but also consider differences across treatments and ask the larger question of how best to match treatments to patients. The phrase "what works for whom" asks the question what interventions are of demonstrated benefit to which specific patients groups. This question is of relevance to clinicians and patient consumers alike, as well as clinic administrators, insurers, and policy makers.

M. Cloitre (✉)
Division of Dissemination and Training, National Center for PTSD, Menlo Park, CA, USA

Department of Psychiatry and Child and Adolescent Psychiatry,
New York University Langone Medical Center, New York, NY, USA
e-mail: marylene.cloitre@nyumc.org

R.A. Bryant
School of Psychology, University of New South Wales, Sydney, NSW, Australia
e-mail: r.bryant@unsw.edu.au

U. Schnyder
Department of Psychiatry and Psychotherapy, University Hospital Zurich,
Zurich, Switzerland
e-mail: ulrich.schnyder@access.uzh.ch

© Springer International Publishing Switzerland 2015
U. Schnyder, M. Cloitre (eds.), *Evidence Based Treatments for Trauma-Related Psychological Disorders: A Practical Guide for Clinicians*,
DOI 10.1007/978-3-319-07109-1_27

The organization of the book reflects basic assumptions about matching treatments to different types of patients. Treatments are presented in a spectrum organized by acuity and complexity. Indeed, there are interventions for those who have severe stress reactions immediately post-event (ICD-10, acute stress reaction; DSM-5, acute stress disorder) and develop sustained reactions (PTSD) or more complex forms or variations of trauma reactions (complex PTSD, prolonged grief disorder). In doing so, it includes diagnoses described in both DSM-5 and ICD-10/ICD-11 but importantly extends beyond trauma-related diagnoses by including considerations of trauma-related disorders comorbid with borderline personality disorder and chronic pain.

The consideration of treatment matching to patient needs extends beyond symptom acuity and complexity. Age is recognized as an important consideration in intervention selection. Treatment interventions are described which have been designed with the cognitive, emotional, and social developmental needs of children in mind and are sensitive to the trajectory of rapid change and growth associated with the first decades of life. The slow decline in health, memory, and cognition of older adults is also addressed and includes recognition of age-specific life events such as the inevitable deaths of friends and family and the loneliness and loss of meaning and identity which may follow.

The volume also takes into consideration the social environment, identifying specific interventions that recognize the role of partners and family, as well as that of neurobiology via identification of state-of-the-science knowledge regarding the use of pharmacological agents and mapping of brain activity to behavior. Treatment matching to patients also requires consideration of access to care and logistical barriers. For this reason, we have included a chapter that discusses the way in which technology can be used to provide services to patients who cannot obtain or do not want face-to-face care. This is sometimes due to geographical barriers or work or family commitments or, alternatively, simply a preference to remain at a distance from provider sites. This may be the case with women veterans who have experienced sexual assaults by fellow military personnel during their service and state a preference for staying away from veteran healthcare facilities.

In this chapter, we first briefly discuss patient-treatment matching issues in regard to critical components of trauma treatment for which there seems to be broad agreement, specifically the therapeutic alliance, and the review and analysis of the traumatic experience. Yet, even here, unknowns remain regarding how to refine these elements to provide maximum benefit to each patient. We will discuss what has been traditionally considered the essential component to patient-treatment matching, namely, patient characteristics. It will be shown that, to date, research in the trauma field has provided little insight about how to optimize patient care. We provide some considerations about directions for future research. Lastly, we will discuss considerations regarding patient-treatment matching for which there seems to be less consensus. This includes the use of multicomponent therapies; the integration of different types of interventions into trauma-focused work such as coping skills training, emotion regulation, and stabilization strategies; and the debate about sequencing versus simultaneous implementation of interventions.

27.2 Common Factors

27.2.1 Therapeutic Alliance

Despite the fact that it is rarely explicitly discussed in any of the treatment chapters, a positive therapeutic alliance is uniformly revealed in the case examples and the interactions presented between the patient and therapist. It is expressed in the therapist's appreciation for and understanding of the patient's experience, the framing of the interventions in the context of the patient's experience, and a sense of warmth and kindness that emanates from the therapist. The therapeutic alliance is the most consistently identified predictor of psychotherapy outcome across types of treatments and patients (Horvath and Symonds 1991; Martin et al. 2000). It is typically defined as comprised of various dimensions including the patient's sense of being understood, sense of being liked by the therapist, agreement on treatment goals, and agreement on tasks or means toward reaching those goals.

27.2.2 Patient-Therapist Matching

Matching a patient to treatment can include a subset of considerations of matching patient and therapist on ethnic and cultural characteristics. Several studies have found that matches in culture, ethnicity, and gender can improve treatment engagement although effects on outcome are highly variable. Meta-analyses are uniform in finding a strong patient preference for and positive perception of therapists of the same ethnic background, particularly among minorities (Cabral and Smith 2011). However, the benefits of this match on treatment outcome are highly variable – so much so that a recent meta-analysis indicated that the effect size of patient-therapist match on outcome is nearly nil (ES = .09) (Cabral and Smith 2011).

Match on ethnicity and culture may be a proxy for factors potentially more directly aligned with the therapeutic outcome such as shared worldviews, values, and spiritual or religious beliefs. The benefits of the match may be eliminated without shared values and, indeed, potentially result in increased hostility and guardedness. Benefits may vary depending on severity of baseline symptoms and outcome of interest. For example, in a treatment study of PTSD/SUD patients, ethnic/cultural match produced better PTSD outcomes among those with more severe baseline PTSD, while it did very little to influence substance use outcomes (Ruglass et al. 2014). Additional factors may be the patient's interpersonal skill, determination, and overall resilience in managing the therapeutic relationship and working toward good outcome. For example, it has been found that Black Americans can be less impacted by therapist match than White Americans with the explanation that Black Americans are already quite acculturated to working outside their ethnic/cultural group than Whites (Ruglass et al. 2014).

In summary, ethnic/cultural matching has benefits in facilitating engagement into treatment and in the initial phases of the therapeutic alliance. However, the benefits of match on outcome are strongly influenced by contextual factors such as the presence or absence of shared values, the severity and nature of the problem, and the history behind the relationships of certain ethnic/cultural groups. Therapists need to develop multicultural competencies (e.g., understand different worldviews) while simultaneously avoiding the assumption that any one individual holds the beliefs of his or her ethnicity or culture. Therapists also need to be aware of their local cultural/ethnic context and the fact that racial and ethnic tensions and differences are dynamic and change over time and across regions.

27.2.3 Therapist Characteristics

It is also interesting to speculate whether certain dispositional characteristics in a therapist might be more or less appealing to a patient: the quiet therapist versus the more talkative person, the physically restless versus the more introverted and contained individual, and the directive versus open-ended therapist. For trauma work in particular, patients may be differentially sensitive to therapists' characteristic reactions and behaviors in response to trauma disclosure (e.g., sadness, outrage, disgust, embarrassment, concern, optimism about recovery) as well as the approach the therapist takes in introducing trauma-focused treatment elements. Some therapists quickly and explicitly introduce discussion of the trauma, while others wait for an inquiry from the patient. It might be valuable to ask patients what their preferred professional and personality characteristics might be as a means to increasing engagement and possibly improving outcome. Lastly, it is worth considering how the therapeutic relationship interacts with treatment activities and process. For example, an active therapist who provides repeated behavioral demonstration of interventions may facilitate better skills training outcomes, while a more contained, reactive (vs. proactive) therapist who focuses on attunement with the patient's emotional state may facilitate better outcomes during imaginal exposure. The therapist's capacity to flexibly shift in degree and kind of behavioral and emotional expression as the tasks of the treatment change may be an important therapeutic skill in treatment. To date, there is little research or information about the impact of therapist characteristics, attitudes, and behaviors on the patient and on treatment outcome.

Many therapists put significant emphasis on helping their patients regain control over their exaggerated emotional reactions (e.g., flashbacks) and encourage them to take charge of their lives. In psychoeducation at the beginning of treatment, they explain that one of the core elements of most traumatic events is the experience of an (in many but not all cases, sudden and unexpected) unwanted and extremely unpleasant loss of control. They also explain that the typical symptoms of PTSD, particularly the reexperiencing and hyperarousal cluster symptoms, can be seen as a repetition of that same loss of control. Therefore, they argue that regaining control is one of the main goals of trauma treatment. There is strong experimental evidence that believing one has control enhances capacity to manage distress (Bryant et al. 2014). Therapists also have good clinical reasons to facilitate control in their patients: once patients have regained control over their memories to the degree that they can decide at any given time whether or not they want to go back in their imagination to the time when the traumatic experience happened, much has been achieved! However, the emphasis on control may overwhelm other important goals of the treatment. Helping patients regain control always needs to be counterbalanced with the recognition that much of life is beyond our control. Many things in life, bad things as well as good, just simply befall us. We fall ill, we fall in love, and we can't and sometimes also don't want to do anything about it. Rather than pushing our patients to try to control everything in life, we might want to help them be better able to discriminate controllability. In a situation that is important to them and where they have some degree of control, they should learn to be assertive and courageous and try to exert their influence. However, in a situation beyond their control and power, they should learn to be wise enough to accept and adapt.

27.2.4 Review and Analysis of the Traumatic Experience

There is general agreement that direct attention to and explicit review of the traumatic events, when effectively done, produces superior reduction in PTSD and related symptoms compared to therapies that do not. In all of the interventions presented in this volume, the traumatic events are described in words and, occasionally, with additional representational media (drawings, letters, objects). Explicit attention to traumatic experiences and memories is carried out in different ways including through imaginal exposure, cognitive reappraisal, or narrative reconstruction. The goals of these activities are the same: to reduce or resolve feelings of fear, anger, shame, guilt, etc., to develop a coherent understanding of the events, and to create meaning from them.

Questions that clinicians often ask concern the timing of the trauma work and its intensity and duration. There is very little research to help guide the clinician in determining what is best and more particularly what is best for any one patient. Some therapies involve detailed and repeated review of the traumatic events, with an emphasis on sensory-perceptual detail (e.g., PE, NET). Others focus on the development of a narrative and emphasize attention to feelings that have been disregarded (e.g., BEPP) or to maladaptive beliefs (e.g., CPT) and do not emphasize repetition. Still others emphasize the development of an autobiography (NET) and focus on linking themes (e.g., self-identity) across narratives of different events (STAIR Narrative Therapy).

Randomized controlled trials comparing evidence-based trauma-focused therapies are few, and those available indicate that outcomes differ little between interventions (e.g., Nijdam et al. 2012; Resick et al. 2002; Rothbaum et al. 2005; Taylor et al. 2003). However, it is probable that patients are not equally interested in and motivated by all interventions. It is also probable that patients do not benefit equally from all interventions. Recent research in both pharmacological interventions and psychotherapies has found that patients do have treatment preferences and that providing patients with their preferred treatment provides superior results relative to assignment to a treatment by chance (i.e., randomization) (Swift and Callahan 2009). From a clinical perspective, these data would suggest that treatment decisions regarding type of trauma-focused treatment might best be made following the patient's preference, and options that occur during the course of treatment regarding timing, intensity, and duration of trauma-focused treatment include shared decision making. Research regarding the impact of patient preference on treatment selection and outcome is limited but of increasing interest.

27.3   Patient-Specific Characteristics

To date, there have been at least 20 studies assessing patient-specific characteristics as predictors of PTSD treatment outcome. A systematic review of all the studies indicates very little consistency in results (Cloitre 2011). For every study that has identified a particular patient characteristic which predicted outcome, there is at least one other study which obtained null results. Characteristics that have been evaluated include trauma history (e.g., childhood abuse), demographic characteristics such as age and education, severity of PTSD, and co-occurring symptoms including anger, anxiety, depression and dissociation, borderline personality features, and personality disorders as well as factors such as intelligence, self-esteem, and beliefs about self and the world.

Possible reasons for these inconsistencies include low sample size which limits power to detect real differences as well as great differences in study samples (e.g., inpatient versus outpatient) and interventions. More importantly, the statistical and conceptual approach to identifying predictors may be flawed. The traditional approach presented in reports has been to evaluate individual factors as predictors of outcome, in an effort to find the "silver bullet." However, as is well known, there are great symptom heterogeneity across PTSD patients and, by implication, a multitude of possible predictors, suggesting that the "silver bullet" approach will likely fall short of capturing clinical reality.

An alternative and potentially successful approach has emerged in general medicine which has been investigating disorders that, similar to PTSD, admit of significant complexity and heterogeneity (e.g., diabetes). Statistical analyses have revealed that there are typically multiple moderators of outcome, each of which is weakly predictive and where no single predictor is strong enough to provide information that is clinically meaningful. The alternative approach allows the statistical generation of a *combination* of factors (i.e., a profile) that provides the strongest predictor of outcome. For example, coronary heart disease is calculated on the severity of risk factors in combination with each other (e.g., age, blood pressure, cholesterol, diabetes, smoking). In this type of modeling, no one risk factor is critical, but rather each contributes a certain amount that leads to an overall "outcome" (occurrence of coronary heart disease). This approach has now been applied to treatment intervention outcomes in psychiatry (e.g., Wallace et al. 2013). For the treatment of PTSD, it may similarly be possible to identify a moderator "profile" that captures the key aspects of a patient that, as in the case of coronary heart disease, include a range of factors such as historical information (e.g., trauma history), symptoms (e.g., anger), current co-occurring disorders (e.g., dissociative disorder), and behaviors that can cumulatively predict outcome.

Although in its infancy, it is worth noting that there are preliminary studies indicating that treatment response is linked to certain neurobiological characteristics of PTSD patients. For example, there is recent work indicating that people differ in treatment response according to their genetic profile, in response to both psychotherapy (Bryant et al. 2010a; Felmingham et al. 2013) and pharmacotherapy (Mushtaq et al. 2012). Further, brain imaging studies indicate that brain structure impacts on how people respond to psychotherapy (Bryant et al. 2008a), as well as brain functioning prior to commencement of treatment (Bryant et al. 2008b; Falconer et al. 2013). Although this work is very new, it underscores the conclusion that at a fundamental level not all patients will respond to treatment equivalently.

Another critical aspect of matching that is receiving increasing attention in global mental health is the extent to which evidence-based interventions can be understood by poorly educated or poorly resourced people. Most of the world's trauma-affected populations come from low- and middle-income countries (LMIC), and accordingly it is not a simple task to transpose interventions that have been trialed in highly resourced (usually western) countries to these impoverished settings. There is a need to adapt evidence-based interventions to match the capacity of the patient to understand and engage in the intervention. For example, the motivation and capacity of a poverty-stricken person to allocate an hour to therapy may be compromised by the need to work in order to feed the family that day. Alternately, someone (who may be from a highly resourced country) may have marked difficulty in understanding cognitive strategies to identify and correct unhelpful thoughts if they are illiterate and had very little education. For this reason, low-intensity interventions are being developed to adapt evidence-based interventions so they are useful to people affected by trauma and adversity (Forbes et al. 2010).

Another "big picture" change that may improve prediction of treatment outcome is to consider patient strengths as well as symptoms. Clinicians often observe that two patients can present with equally severe PTSD and other co-occurring symptoms, but one will do well in treatment, while the other does not. The patient comes into treatment not only with symptoms that challenge him or her but also with strengths that they apply and that therapists can encourage during the course of treatment. While this observation may be self-evident, it is a reality that has not yet been translated into research or predictor modeling. Candidate strengths to include in outcome prediction might include social support, optimism, and "resilience." Ultimately, it may be that the best predictor of outcome is a ratio of negative (e.g., symptom severity) versus positive (e.g., social support) factors.

27.4 Multicomponent Therapies

There has been some debate about the benefits of multicomponent or multi-module treatments. Some researchers express concern that the introduction of elements to the therapy other than confronting the traumatic events is excessive and an unnecessary treatment and may even be an expression of therapist collusion with patients as avoidance of discussing traumatic events. It has been proposed that short trauma-focused therapies in fact do improve social adjustment and coping skills such as emotion regulation without directly incorporating training interventions. Moreover, researchers have sometimes pointed out that there is some, but at the present time limited, evidence that longer, more expansive treatments for more complex patients (complex PTSD, PTSD, and various comorbidities) produce better outcomes. In addition, it has been argued that randomized controlled trials of longer therapies with multiple components are expensive and take a great deal of time to complete and thus are challenging to fund and to conduct.

Nevertheless, it is unlikely that the "one-size-fits-all" approach to treatment will provide patient-centered care that delivers optimal outcome for each individual patient. It is also recognized that research systematically manipulating each component of multicomponent therapies creates financial and time burdens. Nevertheless, an important goal is to devise research strategies to determine how best to provide optimal care to each individual and to neither "undertreat" nor "overtreat" the patient.

Mental health research and services for children and adolescents have grappled with the problem of matching treatment to patient for the past decade. The treatment of children and adolescents is inherently complicated due to the complexities introduced by development. Treatments must be adapted to age-relevant problems (e.g., bed-wetting to substance abuse). Moreover, diagnoses are less clear as youth often show an admixture of problems that span across several disorders (e.g., phobias, mood problems, conduct disturbances). Lastly, engagement of parents and often teachers is necessary for effective treatment, and adults are typically integral partners in the treatment. These conditions have led to advances in research design which recognize the complexity of the patient and the involvement of the family and larger social environment. There are many research design and treatment strategies from this domain of mental health research that are applicable to the complex trauma patient who suffers from multiple symptoms or comorbidities and for whom the engagement of multiple social systems might be of benefit.

Multicomponent treatments have been found to be effective and superior to single-component treatments under a variety of conditions. For example, it has been found that outcomes for patients in the community are dramatically improved when a specific evidence-based protocol for a predominant class of problems or specific disorder (e.g., phobias) is implemented with additional components from other protocols as relevant to patients' problems (e.g., mood-boosting interventions for depression) as compared to single-protocol implementation (Daleiden et al. 2006). This does not necessarily mean that clinicians need to use multiple protocols to treat patients with multiple comorbidities, a tremendously inefficient enterprise as well as burdensome to patient and therapist. Interventions shared across protocols for specific types of problems have been identified. These intervention modules are relatively brief and specific (e.g., graded exposure hierarchy for fear-related problems, mood boosting for depression, differential attention for inappropriate conduct). The selection of the modules and the duration of their use are guided by weekly symptom measures and determined collaboratively by patient and therapist, which includes patient feedback about functioning during the week. This approach has been found superior to the use of full protocols either alone or in sequence and to treatment as usual in community settings (Weisz et al. 2012). This approach is akin to transdiagnostic approaches to treatment, which have garnered considerable support in recent years as a means of treating patients whose clinical presentations are not adequately described by distinct diagnostic categories (Barlow et al. 2011). This research highlights the role that flexibility plays in optimizing treatment outcomes and the potential value of integrating multiple interventions into a single treatment matched to identified problems.

Although there is not a similar body of research in the trauma field, the treatment development strategies described above are realized in many of the treatment programs presented in this volume. The psychological interventions for trauma-related disorders all contain a trauma-focused component (exposure or cognitive reappraisal) as a central or core intervention. The treatment programs for more complex patients introduce interventions that address additional, specific aspects to the patient's experience. For example, the death of a beloved spouse and the associated disorganization in identity that can occur (e.g., prolonged grief disorder) are addressed by including interventions that focus on the healthy revision of identity, roles, and responsibilities. Sustained and chronic trauma, particularly during childhood, is frequently associated with compromised socio-emotional capacities, and an intervention module can be introduced to provide skills training specific to these difficulties (STAIR, Chap. 14). The effects of torture and the consequent comorbid pain disorders that frequently develop can be treated with a therapeutic program which incorporates biofeedback and other interventions to reduce pain. Patients with significant self-injurious and chronic suicidal tendencies can be treated with a combination of interventions which address these "life-interfering behaviors" as well as traditional trauma-focused CBT (e.g., DBT+PE). Some newly reported trauma therapies have been careful not to unduly lengthen the therapies but provide and test the benefits of specific interventions for targeted and circumscribed problems, such as the cognitive restructuring and imagery modification (CRIM) for the feeling of being contaminated among adult female survivors of child sexual abuse (Jung and Steil 2013).

These are only a few examples of the ways in which interventions are built on to the central task of trauma-focused work (i.e., directly addressing the trauma) to treat a wide range of recognizable problems among trauma survivors and improve outcome. While this approach has not been tested, the history and experience of other mental health domains suggest that such approaches will be successful and superior to single protocols or sequencing of full alternative protocols.

27.5 Sequencing Treatment Components

The use and effectiveness of sequenced treatment components has been debated, and more particularly the use of treatment modules to function as "stabilizing" interventions preceding trauma-focused work. The goal of many multicomponent treatments is to strategically target and resolve specific problems which would otherwise remain a goal which is intended to improve functioning and quality of life for the patient. This is distinct from the "preparatory" nature implied in the stabilization function where goals include, for example, reducing the individual's suicidality and/or emotional reactivity (e.g., bipolar disorder symptoms, psychotic symptoms, or high baseline emotional reactivity), strengthening the relationship to the therapist, and ensuring an appropriate medication regime, which all have the purpose of eliminating clinical circumstances that might impede or interfere with the optimal use of exposure therapy. Recent studies suggest that the introduction of interventions which include the promotion of emotion regulation and other related skills preceding trauma-focused work is superior to the standard exposure therapies without skills training in both childhood abuse (Cloitre et al. 2010) and mixed trauma (motor vehicle, assault) populations (Bryant et al. 2010b) in regard to a range of outcomes such as PTSD symptom reduction, anxiety, and improved emotion regulation. There is also some evidence of the efficacy of this approach in hard-to-treat anxiety disorders (Keuthen et al. 2010).

There have been other studies which have reversed the order of the sequence, that is, where trauma-focused work preceded skills training. A recent RCT with Vietnam veterans found that multicomponent treatment in which social skills training and emotion management strategies were included after trauma-focused treatment was equivalent to the exposure therapy in reducing PTSD but superior in improving social functioning (Beidel et al. 2011). The rationale for the development and comparison of the sequenced treatment as compared to the exposure-alone therapy was to assess whether there was clinically significant benefit in adding social and emotional skills training to exposure, an outcome about which there has been doubt (see Cahill et al. 2004). Cloitre and colleagues (2010) completed a similarly designed study but differed in that the ordering of the sequence was reversed, that is, skills preceded exposure. A comparison of the effect sizes for the interpersonal and social outcomes targeted by the skills training in the Beidel et al. (2011) and the Cloitre et al. (2010) studies did not yield any differences, suggesting that the order of the sequenced components was not a significant factor influencing these outcomes. However, sequence order did impact PTSD reduction where skills training preceding the trauma-focused work (Cloitre et al. 2010) resulted in larger effect sizes than the reverse sequence (Beidel et al. 2011). While the caveat holds that results are being compared across two different studies, the data suggest that the order of sequencing may not always matter but may be relative to the outcome of interest and the patient population.

Still, the question remains – how best to select which in a series of interventions or modules goes first and how to order the sequence. Research on sequencing indicates that a flexible approach rather than implementation of a preset series produces better results in terms of greater reduction in all symptom measures and greater reduction in the total number of diagnoses (Weisz et al. 2012). Chorpita and colleagues (2014) describe a fairly straightforward strategy where the three top problem areas are identified with standardized measures and then rank ordered by patient priorities. The problem identified as most severe is treated first with an intervention or module that maps onto that problem domain; duration of the intervention or module is determined by weekly symptom assessment and patient feedback. This patient-treatment matching approach has been successful in producing large reductions in a range of outcomes (Weisz et al. 2012).

27.6 Choosing Among Similar Treatments

As the number of evidence-based interventions grows, the question confronting the clinician is how to choose a treatment when the treatments available appear relatively similar in interventions and outcomes. The efficacy of treatments and the identification of a "gold standard" treatment tend to be evaluated on a single criterion, namely, symptom reduction (typically PTSD symptom reduction). The reliance on a single indicator of outcome is a reasonable metric in initial efforts. It maximizes construct specificity (i.e., what exactly is this treatment good for?). However as multiple treatments emerge which perform in an equivalent fashion, the guideline of symptom reduction may not be sufficiently informative to support the discrimination task that the clinician faces (Schnyder 2005).

One approach is to consider how treatments fare with regard to multiple outcomes, particularly including functional improvement. Research to date indicates that most PTSD therapies still do not effectively resolve problems in functioning. While symptom severity and functional impairment may be positively associated, they are sufficiently distinct to warrant separate consideration. Indeed about one-third of PTSD patients who complete treatment end with significant impairment (Bradley et al. 2005). Moreover, from the patient's perspective, symptom severity may be of less interest than actual day-to-day functioning. Good functioning, like symptom severity, may be conceived of as on a continuum where the individual's capacity to adapt to the demands of and carry out daily roles differs or changes over time. The relationship to symptoms may vary depending on the individual (personal resilience, social supports) as well as on any number of symptoms which the person experiences. The association between functioning and symptoms is known to vary depending on the symptom. For example, anxiety symptoms tend to be associated with less functional impairment than depression (Siminoff et al. 1997). Thus, the level of functional impairment in trauma patients may not necessarily be best captured by assessment of or change in severity of PTSD symptoms. These observations suggest the relative autonomy of functional impairment from PTSD or other symptoms and the importance of the assessment of functional impairment in addition to symptoms.

Research in child mental health has experienced an explosion of treatment interventions and provides some "lessons learned" for the trauma field. An examination of 373 treatment trials found that while nearly two-thirds demonstrated efficacy regarding symptom reduction, only 19 % demonstrated evidence for reducing functional impairment (Becker et al. 2011). This was in large part because the majority of studies did not include measures of functioning. However, among those studies in which functioning was included, reduction in functional impairment was less frequently achieved than symptom reduction. In addition, some treatments resulted in improved functioning but little change in symptom status.

These data, in sum, highlight the lack of correspondence between symptom severity and functional impairment and have implications for assessment and treatment. Routine assessments should include evaluation of the severity and nature of functional impairments rather than just symptoms. While symptom reduction often enhances functioning, meta-analyses indicate that most interventions do not produce significant improvement functioning. Treatment programs that include skills interventions (e.g., social integration) may contribute to optimizing outcome when considering the overarching treatment goal of functional improvement.

Lastly, while we have focused on functional impairment as an important metric by which to select a treatment, other factors are likely to become important in decision making. These include patient engagement, treatment completion rates, and patient satisfaction. Data are rarely collected on how many patients refuse a proposed treatment and the reasons why. While data on treatment completion rates are routinely provided and, to some extent, patient satisfaction is reported, they do not figure importantly in the identification of preferred treatments. As therapies have become more successful in addressing symptom reduction, the opportunity to consider other factors has emerged. This is critical, not only for optimizing patient care but also for the dissemination and implementation of treatment in the community where such factors play a critical role.

27.7 Summary

This chapter has reviewed a wide range of factors that need to be considered in order to match patients to treatment for optimal outcome. Certainly, there is a need for the therapist to be educated about the values and culture of the patient and to respect and learn from the patient during the course of collaborative work. Traditional methods of identifying patient characteristics as predictors of outcome have largely failed and new approaches are necessary. This includes the identification of the cumulative burden of symptoms (rather than any one symptom) the patient experiences as well as the identification and utilization of the strengths the patient brings to treatment. In addition, recognition of patient preference is important. This includes identification and acknowledgment of the problems that bother the patient the most and aligning treatment consistent with these concerns and goals.

There is a need to investigate the benefits of combination treatments and to develop evidence-based strategies for selecting how to sequence interventions and when to move from one intervention to the next. Underpinning the issue of choosing between potential efficacious treatments is the recognition that many interventions have distinct labels and in a sense suggest they are distinct strategies. It is increasingly recognized that there are actually far more similarities between evidence-based treatments than differences. Conducting a thorough assessment, developing a problem formulation, providing the patient with a sense of control, activating trauma memories and facilitating emotional processing, and reframing unhelpful appraisals can be observed in nearly all psychological treatments for trauma-affected populations. Considering this overlap, it is useful for clinicians to keep in mind the importance of employing proven *strategies* rather than being overwhelmed by a choice between treatment *packages*. The reason for the commonalities across treatment packages is partly explained by the common components across different types of highly prevalent mental disorders (e.g., intrusive memories, avoidance, arousal), which has led to transdiagnostic approaches (e.g., Barlow et al. 2011).

References

Barlow, D. H., Farchione, T. J., Fairholme, C. P., Ellard, K. K., Boisseau, C. L., Allen, L. B., & Ehrenreich-May, J. C. (2011). *The unified protocol for transdiagnostic treatment of emotional disorders: Therapist guide*. New York: Oxford University Press.

Becker, K. D., Chorpita, B. F., & Daleiden, E. L. (2011). Improvement in symptoms versus functioning: How do our best treatments measure up? *Administration and Policy in Mental Health, 38*, 440–458.

Beidel, D. C., Frueh, B. C., Uhde, T. C., Wong, N., & Mentrikoski, J. M. (2011). Multicomponent behavioral treatment for chronic combat-related posttraumatic stress disorder: A randomized controlled trial. *Journal of Anxiety Disorders, 25*, 224–231.

Bradley, R., Greene, J., Russ, E., Dutra, L., & Westen, D. A. (2005). A multidimensional meta-analysis of psychotherapy for PTSD. *American Journal of Psychiatry, 162*, 214–227.

Bryant, R. A., Felmingham, K. L., Das, P., & Malhi, G. (2014). The effect of perceiving control on glutamatergic function and tolerating stress. *Molecular Psychiatry, 19*, 533–544.

Bryant, R. A., Felmingham, K. L., Falconer, E. M., Pe Benito, L., Dobson-Stone, C., Pierce, K. D., & Schofield, P. R. (2010a). Preliminary evidence of the short allele of the serotonin transporter gene predicting poor response to cognitive behavior therapy in posttraumatic stress disorder. *Biological Psychiatry, 67*, 1217–1219.

Bryant, R. A., Felmingham, K. L., Whitford, T., Kemp, A., Hughes, G., Peduto, A., & Williams, L. M. (2008a). Rostral anterior cingulate volume predicts treatment response to cognitive behaviour therapy for posttraumatic stress disorder. *Journal of Psychiatry and Neuroscience, 33*, 142–146.

Bryant, R. A., Felmingham, K. L., Kemp, A., Das, P., Hughes, G., Peduto, A., & Williams, L. M. (2008b). Amygdala and ventral anterior cingulate activation predicts treatment response to cognitive behaviour therapy for post-traumatic stress disorder. *Psychological Medicine, 38*, 555–561.

Bryant, R. A., Mastrodomenico, J., Hopwood, S., Kenny, L., Cahill, C., Kandris, E., & Taylor, K. (2010b). Augmenting cognitive behavior therapy for post-traumatic stress disorder with emotion tolerance training: A randomized controlled trial. *Psychological Medicine, 11*, 1–8.

Cabral, R. R., & Smith, T. B. (2011). Racial/ethnic matching of clients and therapists in mental health services: A meta-analytic review of preferences, perceptions and outcomes. *Journal of Counseling Psychology, 4*, 537–554.

Cahill, S. P., Feeny, N. C., Zoellner, L. A., & Riggs, D. S. (2004). Sequential treatment for child-abuse related posttraumatic stress disorder: Methodological comment on Cloitre, Koenen, Cohen and Han (2002). *Journal of Consulting and Clinical Psychology, 72*, 543–548.

Cloitre, M., Stovall-McClough, K. C., Nooner, K., Zorbas, P., Cherry, S., Jackson, C. L., Gan, W., & Petkova, E. (2010). Treatment for PTSD related to childhood abuse: A randomized controlled trial. *American Journal of Psychiatry, 167*, 915–924.

Cloitre, M. (2011). *Evidence for the efficacy of a phase-based approach to PTSD related to childhood abuse*. At the Expert Meeting on the Etiology and treatment of PTSD in Adult Survivors of Chronic Childhood Trauma (Chairs T. Ehring, P. Emmelkamp, & N. Morina), Netherlands Institute for Advanced Study in the Humanities and Social Sciences (NIAS). Wassenaar, The Netherlands.

Daleiden, E. F., Chorpita, B. F., Donkervoet, C., Arensdorf, A. M., & Brogran, M. (2006). Getting better at getting them better: Health outcomes and evidence-based practice within a system of care. *Journal of the American Academy of Child and Adolescent Psychiatry, 45*, 749–756.

Falconer, E., Allen, A., Felmingham, K. L., Williams, L. M., & Bryant, R. A. (2013). Inhibitory neural activity predicts response to cognitive behavior therapy for posttraumatic stress disorder. *Journal of Clinical Psychiatry, 74*, 895–901.

Felmingham, K. L., Dobson-Stone, C., Schofield, P. R., Quirk, G. J., & Bryant, R. A. (2013). The BDNF Val66Met polymorphism predicts response to exposure therapy in posttraumatic stress disorder. *Biological Psychiatry, 73*, 1059–1063.

Forbes, D., Fletcher, S., Wolfgang, B., et al. (2010). Practitioner perceptions of skills for psychological recovery: A training programme for health practitioners in the aftermath of the Victorian bushfires. *Australian and New Zealand Journal of Psychiatry, 44*, 1105–1111.

Jung, K., & Steil, R. (2013). A randomized controlled trial on cognitive restructuring and imagery modification to reduce the feeling of being contaminated in adult survivors of childhood sexual abuse suffering from posttraumatic stress disorder. *Psychotherapy and Psychosomatics, 82*, 213–220.

Keuthen, N. J., Rothbaum, B. O., Welch, S. S., Taylor, C., Falkenstein, M., Heekin, M., Jordan, C. A., Timpano, K., Meunier, S., Fama, J., & Jenike, M. (2010). Pilot trial of dialectical behavior therapy-enhanced habit reversal for trichotillomania. *Depression and Anxiety, 27*, 953–959.

Horvath, A. O., & Symonds, D. B. (1991). Relation between working alliance and outcome in psychotherapy: A meta-analysis. *Journal of Counseling Psychology, 38*, 139–149.

Martin, D. J., Garske, J. P., & Davis, M. K. (2000). Relation of the therapeutic alliance with outcome and other variables: A meta-analytic review. *Journal of Consulting and Clinical Psychology, 68*, 438–450.

Mushtaq, D., Ali, A., Margoob, M. A., Murtaza, I., & Andrade, C. (2012). Association between serotonin transporter gene promoter-region polymorphism and 4- and 12-week treatment response to sertraline in posttraumatic stress disorder. *Journal of Affective Disorders, 136*, 955–962.

Nijdam, M. J., Gersons, B. P. R., Reitsma, J. B., de Jongh, A., & Olff, M. (2012). Brief eclectic psychotherapy v. eye movement desensitisation and reprocessing therapy in the treatment of post-traumatic stress disorder: Randomised controlled trial. *British Journal of Psychiatry, 200*, 224–231.

Park, A. L., Chorpita, B. F., Regan, J., & Weisz, J. R. (2014). Integrity of evidence-based practice: Are providers modifying practice content or practicing sequencing? *Administration and Policy in Mental Health.* doi:10.1007/s104888-041-0559-z.

Ruglass, L. M., Hien, D. A., Hu, M.-C., Campbell, A. N. C., Caldeira, N. A., Miele, G. M., & Chang, D. F. (2014). Racial/ethnic match and treatment otucomes for women with PTSD and substance use disorders receiving community-based treatment. *Community Mental Health Journal, 50*, 811–822.

Resick, P. A., Nishith, P., Weaver, T. L., Astin, M. C., & Feuer, C. (2002). A comparison of cognitive-processing therapy with prolonged exposure and a waiting condition for the treatment of chronic posttraumatic stress disorder in female rape victims. *Journal of Consulting and Clinical Psychology, 70*, 867–879.

Rothbaum, B. O., Astin, M. C., & Marsteller, F. (2005). Prolonged exposure versus eye movement desensitization and reprocessing (EMDR) for PTSD rape victims. *Journal of Traumatic Stress, 18*, 607–616.

Schnyder, U. (2005). Why new psychotherapies for posttraumatic stress disorder? Editorial. *Psychotherapy and Psychosomatics, 74*, 199–201.

Simonoff, E., Pickles, A., Meyer, J. M., Silberg, J. L., Maes, H. H., Loeber, R., & Eaves, J. L. (1997). The Virginia twin study of adolescent behavioral development: Influences of age, gender and impairment on rates of disorder. *Archives of General Psychiatry, 54*, 801–808.

Swift, J. K., & Callahan, J. L. (2009). The impact of client treatment preference on outcome: A meta-analysis. *Journal of Clinical Psychology, 65*, 368–381.

Taylor, S., Thordarson, D., Maxfield, L., Fedoroff, I. C., Lovell, K., & Ogrodniczuk, J. (2003). Comparative efficacy, speed and adverse effects of three PTSD treatments: Exposure therapy, EMDR and relaxation training. *Journal of Consulting and Clinical Psychology, 71*, 330–338.

Wallace, M. L., Frank, E., & Kraemer, H. C. (2013). A novel approach for developing and interpreting treatment moderator profiles in randomized clinical trials. *JAMA Psychiatry, 70*, 1241–1247.

Weisz, J. R., Chorpita, B. F., Palinkas, L. A., Schoenwald, S. K., Miranda, J., Bearman, S. K., & Mayberg, S. (2012). Testing standard and modular designs for psychotherapy treating depression, anxiety, and conduct problems in youth: A randomized effectiveness trial. *Archives of General Psychiatry, 69*, 274–282.

Index

© Springer International Publishing Switzerland 2015
U. Schnyder, M. Cloitre (eds.), *Evidence Based Treatments for Trauma-Related
Psychological Disorders: A Practical Guide for Clinicians*,
DOI 10.1007/978-3-319-07109-1

CPSIA information can be obtained at www.ICGtesting.com
Printed in the USA
BVOW10*0819020215

385985BV00001B/1/P